# PHACOEMULSIFICATION: PRINCIPLES AND TECHNIQUES

# PHACOEMULSIFICATION: PRINCIPLES AND TECHNIQUES

*Edited
by Lucio Buratto*

SLACK Incorporated, 6900 Grove Road, Thorofare, NJ 08086

Publisher: John H. Bond
Editorial Director: Amy E. Drummond
Creative Director: Linda Baker
Editorial Assistant: Viktoria Kristiansson

Copyright © 1998 by SLACK Incorporated

Part of the content in Section I was translated from: Buratto L, Vitali D. Principi generali de facoemulsificazione. In: Camo, ed. *Chirurgia della Cataratta: Facoemulficazione Evoluzione e Stato Dell'arte*. Vol 2. Muggiò, Italy: Realizzazione Grafica e Stampa; 1996: 1-320.

All rights reserved. No part of this book may be reproduced, stored in a retrieval system or transmitted in any form or by any means, electronic, mechanical, photocopying, recording or otherwise, without written permission from the publisher, except for brief quotations embodied in critical articles and reviews.

Printed in the United States of America

Phacoemulsification: principles and techniques/[edited by] Lucio Buratto.
           p. cm.
     Includes bibliographical references and index.
     ISBN 1-55642-360-8
     1. Phacoemulsification.
I. Buratto, Lucio.
     [DNLM: 1. Phacoemulsification--methods. WW 260 P53195 1997]
RE451.P476 1997
617.7'42059--dc21
DNLM/DLC
for Library of Congress          97-34823

Published by:    SLACK Incorporated
                      6900 Grove Road
                      Thorofare, NJ 08086-9447 USA
                      Telephone: 609-848-1000
                      Fax: 609-853-5991
                      World Wide Web: http://www.slackinc.com

Contact SLACK Incorporated for more information about other books in this field or about the availability of our books from distributors outside the United States.

Authorization to photocopy items for internal or personal use, or the internal or personal use of specific clients, is granted by SLACK Incorporated, provided that the appropriate fee is paid directly to Copyright Clearance Center, 222 Rosewood Drive, Danvers, MA 01923 USA, 508-750-8400. Prior to photocopying items for educational classroom use, please contact the CCC at the address above. Please reference Account Number 9106324 for SLACK Incorporated's Professional Book Division.

For further information on CCC, check CCC Online at the following address: http://www.copyright.com.

Last digit is print number: 10 9 8 7 6 5 4 3 2 1

# DEDICATION

*Love to my wife, Marie,*
*who has always been at my side in my personal*
*and professional life.*

- Lucio Buratto, MD

# CONTENTS

DEDICATION .................................................................... v

ACKNOWLEDGMENTS ....................................................... xi

PREFACE ....................................................................... xiii

## SECTION I  PHACOEMULSIFICATION: STATE OF THE ART

**CHAPTER 1:** CATARACT SURGERY DEVELOPMENT AND TECHNIQUES ..................... 3
*Lucio Buratto, MD*

**CHAPTER 2:** THE PHYSICAL PRINCIPLES OF PHACOEMULSIFICATION ..................... 21
*Lucio Buratto, MD*

**CHAPTER 3:** THE INCISIONS .................................................... 33
*Lucio Buratto, MD*

**CHAPTER 4:** ANTERIOR CAPSULOTOMY ......................................... 49
*Lucio Buratto, MD*

**CHAPTER 5:** HYDRODISSECTION AND HYDRODELINEATION ..................... 65
*Lucio Buratto, MD*

**CHAPTER 6:** TECHNIQUES OF PHACOEMULSIFICATION .......................... 71
*Lucio Buratto, MD*

**CHAPTER 7:** IRRIGATION/ASPIRATION ........................................ 171
*Lucio Buratto, MD*

**CHAPTER 8:** POSTERIOR CAPSULE ............................................ 183
*Lucio Buratto, MD*

**CHAPTER 9:** INTRAOCULAR LENSES ........................................... 187
*Lucio Buratto, MD*

**CHAPTER 10:** SUTURES ........................................................ 205
*Lucio Buratto, MD*

**CHAPTER 11:** COMPLICATIONS ................................................ 211
*Lucio Buratto, MD*

**CHAPTER 12:** VISCOELASTIC SUBSTANCES AND CATARACT SURGERY ............ 263
*Lucio Buratto, MD*

## SECTION II PHACOEMULSIFICATION TECHNIQUES

**CHAPTER 13:** SURGICAL PHARMACOLOGY: INTRAOCULAR SOLUTIONS AND
DRUGS USED FOR CATARACT SURGERY ............................ 275
*Henry F. Edelhauser, PhD, David B. Glasser, MD*

**CHAPTER 14: TOPICAL ANESTHESIA** .................................................. **293**
*Matteo Piovella, MD, Ilvo Gratton, MD*

**CHAPTER 15: INCISIONS** ................................................................. **303**
*Antonello Rapisarda, MD*

**CHAPTER 16: THE LIMBAL INCISION** ................................................ **311**
*Paul H. Ernest, MD*

**CHAPTER 17: CAPSULORHEXIS: PRINCIPLES AND TECHNIQUES** ............. **321**
*Aldo Caporossi, MD, Stefano Baiocchi, MD, Paolo Frezzotti, MD*

**CHAPTER 18: PHACOEMULSIFICATION TECHNIQUE** ............................ **333**
*Stephen F. Brint, MD*

**CHAPTER 19: THE IN SITU (FOUR QUADRANT) PHACO FRACTURE TECHNIQUE** .... **341**
*John Shepherd, MD, FACS*

**CHAPTER 20: DIVIDE AND CONQUER NUCLEOFRACTIS TECHNIQUE** ........ **347**
*Howard V. Gimbel, MD, MPH, Michael T. Furlong, MD*

**CHAPTER 21: PERSONAL PHACOEMULSIFICATION TECHNIQUE** ............... **355**
*Kunihiro Nagahara, MD*

**CHAPTER 22: PHACOEMULSIFICATION: MODIFIED PHACO AND MINI CHOP** ..... **361**
*Ronald M. Stasiuk, MD*

**CHAPTER 23: CURRENT PHACOEMULSIFICATION TECHNIQUE** ............... **373**
*Richard Packard, MD, FRCS, FRCOphth*

**CHAPTER 24: PREFERRED PHACOEMULSIFICATION TECHNIQUE:
PHACO SLICE AND SEPARATE** ......................................................... **389**
*Steve Arshinoff, MD, FRCSC*

**CHAPTER 25: CHOP AND FLIP PHACOEMULSIFICATION TECHNIQUE** ....... **397**
*I. Howard Fine, MD*

**CHAPTER 26: PERSONAL PHACOEMULSIFICATION TECHNIQUE** ............... **407**
*James Davison, MD, FACS*

**CHAPTER 27: PERSONAL PHACOEMULSIFICATION TECHNIQUE** ............... **415**
*Harry B. Grabow, MD*

**CHAPTER 28: PERSONAL PHACOEMULSIFICATION TECHNIQUE** ............... **427**
*Tsutomu Hara, MD*

**CHAPTER 29: PERSONAL PHACOEMULSIFICATION TECHNIQUE** ............... **433**
*Paul S. Koch, MD*

**CHAPTER 30: PERSONAL PHACOEMULSIFICATION TECHNIQUE** ............... **443**
*Hiroko Bissen-Miyajima, MD*

**CHAPTER 31: PERSONAL PHACOEMULSIFICATION TECHNIQUE** ............... **447**
*Robert H. Osher, MD*

**CHAPTER 32: PERSONAL TECHNIQUE FOR CATARACT SURGERY** .................... 451
*Donald N. Serafano, MD*

**CHAPTER 33: CURRENT TECHNIQUE FOR PHACOEMULSIFICATION AND
IMPLANT OF INTRAOCULAR LENSES** .................................. 455
*Bo Philipson, MD*

**CHAPTER 34: PHACOEMULSIFICATION WITH LENS IMPLANTATION:
CURRENT TECHNIQUE** ................................................ 459
*Thomas Neuhann, MD*

**CHAPTER 35: THIRTY YEARS OF PHACOEMULSIFICATION: THE EVOLUTION OF MY TECHNIQUE
FROM 1967 TO 1997** ................................................ 465
*Charles D. Kelman, MD*

**CHAPTER 36: BIMANUAL IRRIGATION/ASPIRATION: BURATTO'S TECHNIQUE FOR REMOVAL OF
SUBINCISIONAL CORTEX IN PHACOEMULSIFICATION** .................... 469
*Lucio Buratto, MD*

**CHAPTER 37: FOLDABLE INTRAOCULAR LENSES AND DELIVERY SYSTEMS** ............ 481
*Lucio Buratto, MD*

**CHAPTER 38: FOLDING MANIPULATIONS AND OPTICAL QUALITY
OF A SOFT ACRYLIC INTRAOCULAR LENS** ............................. 487
*Tetsuro Oshika, MD, Yasuhiko Shiokawa, MD*

**CHAPTER 39: TECHNIQUES FOR INSERTING FOLDABLE LENSES** .................... 493
*Vittorio Picardo, MD*

**CHAPTER 40: POSTERIOR ASSISTED LEVITATION** ............................... 511
*Charles D. Kelman, MD*

**INDEX** ................................................................. 515

# ACKNOWLEDGMENTS

I would like to thank Steve Brint for his advice and for the time he spent revising the text. Steve contributed precious, important, and invaluable scientific support.

Thanks also to Richard Packard for his useful suggestions and for revising some of the text.

Last but not least, I would like to thank Maurizio Iori for his exceptional work with the text layout.

# PREFACE

It was the spring of 1978 when I performed my first cataract operation using phacoemulsification with the impalement of an intraocular lens in the posterior chamber. From that moment, I had no doubts that this was not only a winning combination, but that in the future, all cataract operations would be performed with this technique—and this technique alone.

The procedure has changed since then; it has evolved and improved. The technique has been perfected. The machine technology has progressed, knowledge is better, the quality of the IOLs has improved, but more importantly, surgeons throughout the world now trust and rely on the phacoemulsification technique.

However, the situation is still changing, the technique is still evolving, and there is no doubt that the procedure will change again the future. We can expect to see better machines, better lenses, and a perfected technique.

Future objectives include the development of the phaco laser, injectable lenses, prevention of capsular opacity, and means of accommodation. But this will be in the future; for the moment, we will concentrate on the present. As things stand, a number of procedures have been perfected. Some are fundamental and must be learned; others are necessary to understand the mechanics of the technique and must also be learned. Yet another group can be classified as variations of the basic techniques, but surgeons should nevertheless be aware of them as they may prove useful on occasion.

The main objective of this book on surgery is to give a detailed description, directly from the authors, of all of the more important phaco techniques. This will give the experienced surgeons, as well as those who aspire to be, an insight into the technique suitable for each surgeon, each ideal type of machine, and most importantly, the technique which best suits the particular clinical case. Only in this way can we guarantee optimal results for the patients affected by cataracts—by being able to tackle each individual situation with the most suitable technique.

*Lucio Buratto, MD*

# Section I

# PHACOEMULSIFICATION: STATE OF THE ART

# Chapter 1

# CATARACT SURGERY DEVELOPMENT AND TECHNIQUES

*Lucio Buratto, MD*

## INTRODUCTION

Phacoemulsification is a technique which was invented and developed by Dr. Charles D. Kelman during the 1960s. His objective was to perform the extracapsular cataract extraction (ECCE) through a small incision.

Some years passed from when the technique was invented to when it was actually put into practice. Because of the time needed to complete the experiments, tests, and improvements the irrigation/aspiration (I/A) system of phacoemulsification (Cavitron/Kelman), the mother of modern phacoemulsification equipment, was patented only in 1971.

The original machine, and to a certain extent modern day versions, consisted of an electromagnetic generator connected to a handle fitted with a titanium tip which vibrated longitudinally at ultrasonic frequencies.

The action of the tip breaks the lens into fragments which are then aspirated through the central aperture of the tip itself through the aspirating action of a vacuum pump fitted to the main piece of equipment.

The success of the procedure depends mainly on:
- The equilibrium between the fluid from a bottle (which flows along the irrigation line and enters the eye) and the material which is aspirated by the pump (in addition to the liquid which escapes from the main and side port incisions).
- The balance between inflowing and outflowing liquid guarantees maintenance of the spaces in the anterior segment.
- The ultrasound (U/S) tip can act on the lens material but avoids contact with the other eye structures which could cause irreparable damage.

This was not accepted immediately by Kelman's colleagues until the entire scenario of ocular surgery had developed sufficiently for this innovation.

There were many reasons for the low level of interest in the procedure. During the 1970s, the most popular technique for cataract removal was intracapsular cryoextraction and the optical correction of aphakia was basically achieved using spectacle lenses. Phacoemulsification changed all the rules. First of all, it introduced the concept of microsurgery (ie, under operating microscope). Moreover, the operation was performed through a minimal incision, another revolutionary concept. Then there was the return to extracapsular surgery considered obsolete by many surgeons. In addition, the numerous complications observed previously with this procedure had raised bitter criticism which seriously limited its acceptance.

However, phacoemulsification is one of the great techniques and slowly it was adopted by a wider group of surgeons and its popularity increased. It had numerous advantages over the more traditional techniques of the time (intracapsular) such as:
- The advantages of a small incision: a reduction in anatomical healing time, reduction in postoperative astigmatism, less postoperative flattening of the chamber, reduction of the hemorrhagic complications, and fewer sutures.
- Conservation of the posterior capsule separation of the anterior and posterior segments, less endophthalmodonesis, and posterior maintenance of the vitreous.
- Better and more complete aspiration of the cortex (aspiration in closed chamber, the chamber is deeper).
- Easier implantation and correct positioning of the intraocular lens (IOL) in the posterior chamber (the small incision favors the persistence of air in the chamber, an important factor considering that there were no viscoelastic substances (VES) available at that time).

One advantage of phacoemulsification, apart from the technique itself, is that it stimulated the development of planned extracapsular surgery.

According to Kelman, considered to be one of the true geniuses of modern eye surgery, manual ECCE was considered a *conversion* technique during phacoemulsification. It was used when the intraoperative conditions would not allow the surgeon to conclude the operation with emulsification. Thanks to the Kelman machine and other conditions (IOL implantation in the posterior chamber), planned ECCE has been established as a technique in its own right (ie, an elective technique). It has been adopted by those surgeons who, wishing to keep the posterior capsule in place for IOL insertion in the posterior chamber, also wished to sidestep the need to learn phacoemulsification or cope with the problems of using an instrument as complicated as the phacoemulsifier.

The increased interest during the 1980s for planned ECCE was also because surgeons became aware that the step from an intracapsular technique to a manual extracapsular did not require radical changes to the surgeon's instruments, but just a different mental approach to how the steps were performed.

Moreover, ECCE could be performed with relatively cheap instruments, did not require any specific training for the surgeon or his or her staff, could be learned within a short space of time, and resulted in a lower number of complications.

The advent of posterior chamber IOLs was a deciding factor for the rapid change in routine of many surgeons. At first, the orientation toward manual ECCE and then automated ECCE originated from the fact that this technique allowed intraoperative positioning and a safer postoperative recovery with the artificial lens when compared with the same operation with an intracapsular technique.

Nevertheless, phacoemulsification was not used extensively during the 1980s partly because many surgeons could not understand the sense in extracting the cataract through a small incision if they then had to extend the opening to insert the artificial lens. Only a handful of surgeons had realized the number of advantages of phacoemulsification.

It was only toward the mid-1980s that there was an increase in interest for the automated I/A systems for ECCE.

Surgeons have been drawn towards phacoemulsification for several reasons:
- An interest in foldable lenses allowed surgeons to use the same incision as in phacoemulsification without having to extend (or at least performing only minimal extensions), highlighting the advantages mentioned earlier.
- Capsulorhexis allows the extracapsular phacoemulsification to be performed so that the operation is safer, simpler, and programmable, and therefore easier to teach and learn.
- The introduction of instrumental variations and the surgical procedures allowed surgeons to highlight the advantages of phacoemulsification over manual ECCE (endocapsular phacoemulsification with the nuclear fracture technique).
- There are a greater number of theoretical-practical courses and therefore a better understanding of the principles of phacoemulsification.
- The possibility of performing the operation without sutures allows a good anatomical and functional result within a very short space of time with a reduction of postoperative astigmatism.

All of these factors have considerably improved the surgical and functional results, changing both the surgeon's and the patient's approaches to the operation.

Today patients request the operation more readily than they would have done some years ago, and the surgeon tackles it armed with a better possibility of providing the patient with an excellent result. Surgeons can use advanced techniques of phacoemulsification and the techniques are performed through a small self-sealing, noninducing astigmatism incision. These incisions allow rapid anatomical and functional recovery. Because they can be performed under a low level of anesthesia. The operation can be performed as an outpatient procedure with a significant reduction in the emotional, physical, and economic costs.

Phacoemulsification is one of the great procedures capable of giving enormously positive results. However, anyone wishing to embark on this experience must understand the technique, learn it, and practice it.

## THE BASIC PRINCIPLES OF PHACOEMULSIFICATION

In all surgical operations, every step influences the outcome of the following step. This is especially true for phacoemulsification. In this procedure, the precise sequence of events is of fundamental importance and even a minimal error during one of the various phases of the operation can alter the outcome of the steps that follow, increasing the difficulty for the surgeon, even to the point of jeopardizing the final outcome of the operation. Even the smallest details, those considered banal or taken for granted, play their part in the success of the planned operation and should be performed with special attention and precision.

In this description I will consider all the elements involved in phacoemulsification, giving a brief overview of the advantages and disadvantages of each component.

### Patient Selection

The current techniques and equipment for phacoemulsification have developed to such a degree that this technique can be used for the vast majority of patients. Naturally, the results change in proportion to the different clinical situations but also on the basis of the surgeon's experience. The most important factor is the selection of the correct surgical technique in relation to the professional capacity of the operator. The following are optimal conditions for the surgeon who is using phacoemulsification on cataracts for the first time. As

Table 1-1

# INTRAOPERATIVE AND POSTOPERATIVE ADVANTAGES OF PHACOEMULSIFICATION OVER ECCE

## Intraoperative

| | |
|---|---|
| Phacoemulsification allows excellent control of each phase of the operation for cataract removal | Capsulotomy. Removal of the nucleus. Aspiration of the cortex. Cleaning of the posterior capsule. IOL implant. |
| Capsulotomy | Phaco requires a continuous circular capsular opening which has considerable intra- and postoperative advantages. |
| Removal of the nucleus occurs | Through a continuous capsular incision (capsulorhexis). With the chamber closed and ample spaces. With positive pressure in the chamber for the entire operation. With a deep anterior chamber. With the tip far away from the endothelium, posterior capsule, and iris. |
| Aspiration of the cortex occurs | With a closed anterior chamber. With a deep chamber. With large mydriasis. With low risks of damaging the posterior capsule. More rapidly. With complete removal. |
| Cleaning of the posterior capsule occurs | With a closed chamber. With greater efficacy. With a minor risk of rupture. |
| IOL implant | The insertion of an IOL is safer and more rapid (particularly with capsulorhexis). Occurs through a smaller corneo-scleral incision. The planned implant is inserted in a high percentage of cases. |
| Sutures | Self-sealing incisions are easily obtained. Reduced need for sutures. |

## Postoperative

| | |
|---|---|
| Capsulorhexis | Gives better centering of the IOL. Greater isolation of the IOL in respect to the other structures. |
| The small incision of the phaco | More rapid anatomical healing. Earlier stabilization of the refraction. Absence of posterior synechiae. Absence of undesired leaking from the incision. |

discussed below, some important parameters must be taken into consideration.

### Hardness of the Nucleus

This is very important when planning the type of operation and for predicting the possibility of fragmenting the material within an acceptable space of time with a suitable method. Broadly speaking, particularly where the beginning surgeon is concerned, the rule is the harder the nucleus, the longer the phacoemulsification.

In the evolution of the cataract, the nucleus goes through various changes in color: from transparent to gray, then to a yellowish-gray, to amber, to amber-brown and black. Within certain limits, this color change corresponds to an increase in the hardness of the nucleus.

The age of the patient is important, as is the age when the cataract first appears. In two cataracts of the same color, the nucleus in a 60-year-old patient will be softer than in an 80-year-old patient.

Moreover, the cataract which takes longer to form will have a harder, larger nucleus.

The patient's history along with findings from slit lamp observation can give accurate indications regarding the consistency of the material. The following is a brief summary on how to classify the nuclei on the basis of their hardness.

*Soft nucleus (Grade 1)*—This nucleus is transparent or pale gray, and is generally associated with cortical or subcapsular opacities of recent onset, as in presenile metabolic cataracts.

These are cataracts that are easily pierced by the U/S tip and the accessory instruments (spatula or other), and require specific surgical methods. Normally not suitable for beginners.

*Slightly hard nucleus (Grade 2)*—This nuclear cataract is a pale gray or a gray-yellow color. It is present in presenile cataracts, mainly posterior subcapsular. These nuclei offer little resistance to the phacoemulsification tip and

| Table 1-2 | |
|---|---|
| **IDEAL CONDITIONS FOR PHACOEMULSIFICATION** | |
| Eyeball | Well-exposed |
| Cornea | Clear |
| Endothelium | Normal |
| Iris | Normotrophic |
| Mydriasis | Large |
| Anterior chamber | With physiological depth |
| Fundus reflex | Rosy, red |
| Anterior capsule | Visibly, normotensive |
| Nucleus | Moderately hard |
| Zonule | Intact |
| Lens | With normal shape |
| Ocular fundus | Normal |
| Patient's age | 60 years ± 10 |

| Table 1-3 |
|---|
| **ABSOLUTE AND RELATIVE CONTRAINDICATIONS TO PHACOEMULSIFICATION FOR BEGINNERS** |
| **Relative contraindications** |
| Dark ambroid cataract |
| Cataract in glaucoma treated with miotic medical therapy |
| Cataract in operated glaucoma, compensated or not |
| Cataract in eyes with a shallow chamber |
| Cataract in patients with endotheliopathy |
| Intumescent cataract |
| Uveitic cataract |
| Traumatic cataract |
| Cataract in severe myopia |
| Congenital cataract |
| Cataract in patients suffering from coagulation problems |
| Cataract in transplanted patients (eg, cornea, kidney, marrow, heart, liver, etc) |
| Cataract in vitrectomized patients |
| Cataract associated with one or more of the problems listed above |
| **Absolute contraindications** |
| Black cataract |
| Luxated cataract |
| More or less severely luxated cataract with vitreous in the anterior chamber |

other instruments that will tend to sink, so they are suitable for techniques that do not require maneuvers with the spatula.

*Moderately hard nucleus (Grade 3)*—This is the typical senile cataract. It is yellow when the cataract is predominantly nuclear and the nucleus also involves the peripheral portions of the lens. It may be gray in cataracts with a cortico-capsular component in patients more than 60 to 65 years old. It is the *perfect* cataract for beginning surgeons.

*Hard nucleus (Grade 4)*—This nucleus is yellow-amber in color and is found in advanced senile cataracts with large nuclear portions that took a long time to become opaque. The long time required for the fragmentation and the multiple manipulations required in surgery mean that this type of cataract is not suitable for the beginning surgeon. However, they can be easily tackled by expert surgeons particularly if using the techniques of nuclear fracture.

*Very hard nucleus (Grade 5)*—This nucleus tends towards a brown color with all the shades from amber to black. It is typical of the long-standing senile cataract. The consistency of the nucleus may involve the entire lens.

These cases are unsuitable for phacoemulsification by almost all surgeons—save a highly skilled operator equipped with all the necessary tools and who is well-informed on the most up-to-date techniques of nuclear-fracture.

### Red Reflex of the Fundus

The color indication given by the slit lamp examination can be integrated on the operating table by the observation of the red reflex of the fundus using a microscope with coaxial light.

The degree and the characteristics of the reflex, in addition to the possibility of focusing the planes of the lens, give good information regarding the density of the nucleus.

A soft nucleus will give a red reflex with marked luminosity diffused over the entire nuclear field.

A hard nucleus reduces the luminosity reflected to the point of giving a gray-brown color of the pupillary field.

The difference in luminosity of the reflex also allows the surgeon to evaluate the extension of the harder nucleus whose size is proportional to the length of time the cataract has been formed and how hard it is.

### Exposure of the Globe

The eye must be well-exposed to give optimal accessibility to the eye structures and a sufficiently large area for manipulation.

If the opposite is true, the U/S tip and the accessory tips must be held in a more vertical position, which is not only awkward for the surgeon, but can cause undesired traction pressure on the incision with a less stable hold and poorer visibility.

These conditions are essential for accurate control of all the operating steps and perfect visibility of the anatomical structures involved during phacoemulsification.

### Conditions of the Cornea

The cornea must be perfectly transparent with a normal endothelial cell count.

The surgeon must perform a specular microscopy (with a reflecting microscope or an Eisner contact lens) in order to give a qualitative and quantitative evaluation.

Table 1-4

## HARDNESS OF THE NUCLEUS

| Grade | U/S time | Color | Type of cataract | Red reflex |
|---|---|---|---|---|
| 1 | Minimal | Transparent or pale gray | Cortical or recent subcapsular | High |
| 2 | Reduced | Gray or gray-yellow | Subcapsular posterior | Marked |
| 3 | Moderate | Yellow or yellow-gray | Nuclear, cortico-nuclear | Good |
| 4 | Long | Yellow-amber or amber | Cortico-nuclear, dense | Poor |
| 5 | Very long | Dark brown or black | Totally dense | Absent |

In some cases a pachymetry of the central portion may be useful.

Normal corneal endothelium, particularly under a VES that is resistant to intraocular aspiration (eg, Viscoat), can allow for the almost inevitable small operating errors, reducing the risks of serious intraoperative and postoperative complications.

### Trophism of the Iris

The tissue of the iris must be normotrophic and allow wide, long-lasting mydriasis. A normotrophic iris will respond well to slight trauma, the pressure of the infusion liquids, and the VES allowing optimal conditions for the operation.

A dystrophic iris rarely dilates well and is extremely sensitive to hydrodynamic and instrumental stimuli. As a result, precocious miosis or pupillary irregularity tend to develop even as a result of small instrumental contact.

Preoperatively (but not during the 2 days prior to the operation), the surgeon should test the maximum possible dilatation.

This way the surgeon can prepare psychologically for any suspected operating difficulties, but more importantly, he or she can plan the correct operating procedure.

### Chamber Depth

The depth of the anterior chamber must be normal.

If the depth of the chamber is reduced, it may be difficult to insert the U/S tip and the surgeon may need to work with a reduced safety zone between the endothelium and the lens structures.

If the anterior chamber is too deep, the surgeon will need to keep the tip in an almost vertical position (ie, in an unnatural position), which will limit the depth of the microscope's field. The surgeon will have less control and all of the intraoperative maneuvers will be more difficult.

### Conditions of the Cataract

The lens must have a normal shape, both in the anterior and posterior capsules and in the zonular apparatus.

An irregular or membranous anterior capsule, such as those seen with exfoliation syndromes or in cortical cataracts with the phenomena of subcapsular rearrangement, can make the capsulotomy difficult, irrespective of which technique the surgeon has planned. A ruptured posterior capsule (traumatic cataract) can have serious consequences.

A weak zonule, particularly if the lens is large or hard, makes phacoemulsification dangerous with an increase in stress levels for the lens, the zonules, and the surgeon.

### Age of the Patient

The patient's age and the evolutionary characteristics of the cataract are of fundamental importance when choosing phacoemulsification patients.

The young patient often has a soft cataract that is not always easy to manipulate and which does not adapt well to the phacoemulsification techniques suitable for beginners.

In an elderly patient, the nucleus tends to be hard and large with a reduced cortical portion, often associated with slack zonules. In these cases, phacoemulsification may require a considerable amount of time for fragmentation, high U/S power, and prolonged manipulations that are possible sources of intraoperative and postoperative complications. The ideal patient for phacoemulsification is aged between 50 and 65 years.

### Associated Pathologies

It is better to avoid patients with severe ametropias or eyes that are affected by other associated pathologies, such as:

- Uveitis—Frequent presence of synechiae that exclude the previously described conditions.
- Glaucoma, with or without previous operations—It often happens that the surgeon will come across an iris that does not dilate well and a reduced anterior chamber. In addition, the intraoperative pressure is more difficult to control.
- Outcome of retinal detachment—This is often the case in hypotonic eyes with a very deep anterior chamber and weak zonules.
- Any sort of trauma—In these cases, the preoperative investigation does not highlight the clinical situation very precisely so very complex, dangerous intraoperative situations can be created.

## The Ideal Cataract

The ideal cataract is a moderately hard senile cataract with a nucleus which will allow easy manipulations, but which does not require high U/S power or phacoemulsification that is too long. In these cases the epinucleus and the peripheral cortex often have sufficient thickness to absorb the effects of the maneuvers on the nucleus and avoid excessive stimulation of the surrounding structures.

It is also very important that the pupil dilates well, that there is a good red reflex of the fundus, that the

Table 1-5
## ANESTHESIA

| Type | Advantages | Disadvantages |
|---|---|---|
| General | Excellent ocular calm.<br>Immobility of the eye.<br>Systemic hypotension.<br>Prolonged ocular hypotension. | Intra- and postoperative complications linked to the various associated pathologies of the patient. (diabetes, heart problems, bronchitis, elderly patients in general).<br>More stressful for the patient.<br>Requires an anesthetist.<br>More expensive. |
| Retrobulbar | Long experience.<br>Reduced amount of anesthetic injected.<br>Good akinesia. | Risk of retrobulbar hematoma.<br>Risk of perforation of the bulb or the optic nerve.<br>Sometimes insufficient anesthesia or akinesia.<br>Postoperative amaurosis.<br>Pain for the patient. |
| Parabulbar | Easy and safe to perform.<br>Excellent anesthesia and akinesia.<br>Excellent hypotony.<br>Long-lasting. | Abundant anesthetic use.<br>Quite painful.<br>Postoperative amaurosis. |
| Sub-Tenon | Free from important complications.<br>Very small quantity of anesthetic.<br>Immediate functional recovery. | Complete eyelid mobility.<br>Partial mobility of the bulb.<br>Subconjunctival hemorrhage possible. |
| Topical | Free from important complications.<br>Immediate functional recovery. | Complete eyelid and eye mobility.<br>Requires patient collaboration.<br>Painful during some steps.<br>Increased risk of intraoperative complications.<br>Complications are more difficult to resolve. |
| Intraocular | Simple to perform.<br>Smaller amounts of drugs.<br>No injection required.<br>Painless.<br>No intraocular sensitivity. | Intraocular injection of anesthetic.<br>Complete ocular and palpebral motility.<br>Patient's compliance is necessary.<br>Increased risk of intraoperative complications. |

endothelium is healthy, and that the patient receives adequate anesthesia.

The above selection criteria allows the surgeon to tackle phacoemulsification under ideal conditions with maximum predictability of the planned steps.

If the surgeon wishes to extend the operation outside the limits of these indications, the surgery must be supported by in-depth theoretical and practical knowledge of all the techniques of phacoemulsification and the instruments available for obtaining the desired results.

As the surgeon's experience increases, he or she can consider tackling a broader spectrum of clinical situations.

The expert phacoemulsification surgeon can undertake cases with a narrow pupil or with a particularly hard nucleus, even though the presence of both conditions should be considered a relative contraindication.

Once the surgeon has reached this level of operating safety, he or she can use phacoemulsification even in complex cases. With equal surgical capacity, the current phacoemulsification techniques are certainly more precise, controllable, and in the final analysis, less traumatic than any other extracapsular technique.

# ANESTHESIA

It is always better for the beginning surgeon to work with the patient under general anesthesia. This is also advisable for any difficult case or if the anesthetist believes it is necessary. The expert surgeon will be able to operate under local or topical anesthesia with excellent results.

## General Anesthesia

General anesthesia should be used when operating on children, patients with neurological pathologies, patients with severe psychic disorders, psychically or mentally unstable patients, or when the operation is particularly complex.

It should also be used when the operator is beginning to use the technique, as it allows him or her to work safely without worrying about being slow.

General anesthesia is the total responsibility of the anesthetist. It has the advantage of:
- Keeping the patient immobile and unconscious for the entire operation.
- Not changing the anatomy of the eye.
- Not imposing any restrictions on the duration of the operation.

- Controlling the eye pressure in an optimal manner both through the action of the drugs used and hyperventilation, but also through the variation of the degree of anesthesia.

However, just like all the other methods, it also has some important disadvantages; the patient may cough during or immediately after the tube is removed, resulting in an increase in ocular pressure.

I will not discuss the various techniques of anesthesia in this book as it is the responsibility of the anesthetist and not the ophthalmologist.

## Local Anesthesia

This method should never be used with children (for obvious reasons of their noncooperation) or in patients affected by neurological pathologies with severe psychological disorders.

If the above are excluded, one can safely assume that all the medium-length eye operations can be performed under local anesthesia, as there is no alteration of the cardio-circulatory or respiratory parameters, or liver and kidney function. This is one of the main reasons that local anesthesia is strongly advised for those patients affected by cardio-circulatory pathologies, severe bronchial pneumonia, severe liver or kidney failure, and in all those elderly patients where this form of disorder is common.

Until the surgeon feels confident about working under local anesthesia, the anesthetist must ensure good sedation of the patient. The surgeon must take a thorough case history and objectively evaluate the patient's general conditions, the preoperative test results (blood tests, electrocardiogram [ECG], and chest x-ray), and last but certainly not least, the psychological condition of the patient. The latter may actually be the most important condition and must be carefully evaluated prior to subjecting the patient to an operation under local anesthesia. Anyone facing a surgical operation, even the most elementary, will always be frightened to a certain degree. It is perfectly normal to be apprehensive about surgery.

The anesthetist and all staff who will come in contact with the patient during the operation must calm the patient, make him or her feel at home and more relaxed, and reassure the patient that he or she won't feel any pain and that the operation is certain to be a success. Even the way the preanesthetic drugs are administered is important. It is advisable to administer drugs orally as opposed to intramuscularly if that is what the patient wants, in order to avoid increasing his or her stress levels even further.

Benzodiazepins are preferable because of their low hypnotic effect and their considerable ansiolytic action. An antivagal drug is useful but not indispensable because of its action in reducing the bronchial secretions, which is especially important in the event that the surgeon has to convert to general anesthesia for any reason.

In patients with bronchial pneumonia, or those who have a tickly cough, administration of a cough sedative is necessary, given that sharp head movements could compromise the results of the operation.

Local anesthesia consists of premedication and local infiltration.

### Premedication

Preanesthesia or premedication is the responsibility of the anesthetist. The objective is to sedate the patient, reduce the bronchial and salivary secretions, and reduce the vagal stimulations. Drugs are dosed in proportion to the patient's age, weight, and emotional state. For a patient of around 70, about 30 to 40 minutes prior to the operation, the anesthetist should administer:

- Atropine intravenously (0.5 mg).
- Ten drops of an ansiolytic drug such as Valium (about 2 mg).

These dosages can be varied, at the anesthetist's discretion, depending on the patient's conditions. For example, an elderly patient in a precarious state of health should be administered lower doses of the drugs.

Once the patient has been settled on the operating bed, the various cardio-circulatory parameters should be monitored (ECG, AP) and a peripheral vein should be intubated for the administration of any emergency drugs.

### Local Infiltration

Local infiltration can be done by one of two fundamental methods:
1. Retrobulbar injection that requires separate akinesia of the orbicular.
2. Peribulbar infiltration that induces simultaneous peribulbar and palpebral akinesia.

### Akinesia of the Orbicularis Muscle and the Eyelid

Akinesia of the orbicularis muscle is performed to avoid contraction of the eyelid during the operation. Equal amounts of 0.50% Marcaine and 2% Carbocaine are used along with Hyaluronidase (0.5 cc for every 4 to 5 cc of anesthetic).

Carbocaine is used because it has an immediate effect; Marcaine is used to maintain the akinesic action for as long as possible; and Hyaluronidase is used to facilitate the diffusion of both products. This solution can be injected using the Van Lindt or the O'Brien techniques, or a mixture of both.

### The O'Brien Technique

This technique consists of blocking the conduction of the facial nerve at the mandibular condyle. In order to identify the exact point of administration, the patient is asked to open and close his or her mouth using a finger to locate the condyle. This is normally found about 1 cm in front of the ear tragus. In this area, a thin needle (No. 27) is used to inject 2 to 3 cc of liquid at a depth of about 1 cm aiming for the condylar process and noting that the needle is not inserted into the articulation.

The effect of this injection may be enough to anesthetize the entire area of the facial nerve. If the akinesia of the periocular area is not sufficient, a few minutes after this first injection the surgeon should proceed with the Van Lindt method.

### The Van Lindt Technique

This technique consists of blocking the distal fibers of the facial nerve near the lateral edge of the orbit. The

> Table 1-6
> **SUB-TENON ANESTHESIA**
>
> Preparation—Administration of 4% lidocaine in drops, one drop every 5 minutes during the 20 minutes prior to the start of the operation.
>
> Preparation of the eye (washing, application of the sterile drape, retractor).
>
> Cauterization of the conjunctiva in the inferior nasal sector 3 mm from the limbus.
>
> Incision of the conjunctiva with Westcott scissors to expose the scleral plane.
>
> Insertion of the sub-Tenon cannula by Alcon (Greenbaum cannula) or Asico.
>
> Injection of 1 cc of anesthetic (2% Carbocaine) toward the equator of the bulb.
>
> Diffusion of the sub-Tenon anesthetic around 360° with the sub-Tenon cannula.
>
> The operation can now begin.

surgeon starts 1 cm from the temporal canthus using a No. 25 insulin needle mounted on a 10 cc plastic syringe and injects 3 to 4 cc of the anesthetic cocktail. The needle is then partially retracted and reintroduced toward the lower edge of the orbit edge where an additional 2 cc are injected just under the central part of the lower eyelid. The needle is then retracted again and directed superiorly where an additional 2 to 3 cc are injected into the superior orbital edge in correspondence to the middle third.

With this technique, paralysis of the orbicular muscles is generally rapid and complete. Akinesia of the oculomotory muscles is obtained with a retrobulbar or peribulbar injection. These also induce general anesthesia of the eyeball.

### *Retrobulbar Injection*

A No. 23 or No. 25 needle, 3.5 to 4 cm long is used for this injection. The tip is blunted to avoid damaging the retrobulbar vessels or perforating the walls of the bulb.

For this akinesia 3 to 5 cc of a mixture consisting of 0.50% Marcaine, 2% Carbocaine and Hyaluronidase is used.

The patient is asked to look upward and medially (ie, to the left for the right eye, and to the right for the left eye). The needle is introduced into the skin at the junction point between the lateral third and the medial third of the eyelid, roughly at the notch of the orbit edge. The needle is aimed at the optic nerve (without reaching it). Injection of the drug begins when the needle starts to penetrate and continues until it is inserted for 1.5 to 2 cm or thereabouts. Once 3 to 4 cc have been injected, the needle is removed. A further injection is done in the area of the superior rectus. The upper eyelid is lifted with the thumb and the patient is asked to look downward. One to two cc are injected on the conjunctiva covering the superior rectus.

Immediately afterwards, an eye compress is applied and moderate pressure is applied for 30 to 40 seconds. In addition to lowering the ocular pressure on the eyebulb, it is also useful for blocking any peribulbar or retrobulbar hemorrhages provoked by the injection. The oculopressor is applied for 15 to 20 minutes.

Prior to beginning the operation, the patient is asked to move the anesthetized eye or, better still, to move both eyes in the four main directions (up, down, left, and right). If significant residual motility persists, an additional 2 to 3 cc retrobulbar injection of the anesthetic cocktail is administered. The behavior of the eyelids is evaluated in the same way and if they are still quite mobile, more anesthetic is injected.

In this way, complete akinesia is obtained, which is very important for a correct cataract operation. The ideal situation is total bulbar and peribulbar immobility.

## Peribulbar Anesthesia

A syringe containing 4.5 cc of 0.50% Marcaine and 4.5 cc of 2% Carbocaine is prepared. One cc of Hyaluronidase is added to these two products.

A 25 G blunt needle 3.5 to 4.0 cm long is used.

The patient is asked to stare at the doctor injecting the product and the needle is introduced into the skin of the lower eyelid above the orbit edge about 1.5 cm from the temporal canthus.

The needle is introduced to a depth of a couple of millimeters and the operator begins injecting. The needle progresses inward and more mixture is injected, which then progresses along the floor of the orbit toward the equator of the bulb to reach the bone plane (about 3.5 cm deep). At this point about 7 to 8 cc of the cocktail is injected after directing the needle upward and medially.

The needle is retracted and the eye and the contents of the orbit are compressed manually for 40 to 50 seconds in order to block any hemorrhages and to help diffusion of the injected products.

The oculopressor is applied for about 10 minutes; then the operator checks whether there is sufficient akinesia of the eye and the eyelid. If not, a second injection is performed superiorly and nasally about 1 cm from the nasal canthus. The oculopressor is applied once again for a minimum of 10 minutes.

The aim of the parabulbar infiltration is to reach the tissues around the muscular cone that are anesthetized by diffusion. The objective of the peribulbar injection is not to enter the cone but to stay as far away from the globe as possible. With this method, excellent oculomotory and palpebral akinesia is obtained. However, it is indispensable to have good active ocular pressure lowering (Super pinky, Honan's balloon/bubble). The passive method is of little use (sealed bag, mercury-filled bag, etc).

## Topical Anesthesia

This is a recent system that deserves special mention. Topical anesthesia is used in a procedure that uses anesthetics by instillation only (ie, anesthetic eyedrops). Topical anesthesia therefore excludes palpebral akinesia.

A lid speculum must be applied to guarantee adequate opening of the eyelids while leaving the patient acceptably comfortable and without interfering with the surgical maneuvers of the operation.

In order to obtain sufficient anesthesia of the structures involved in the operation, numerous anesthetics have been used to produce a long-lasting effect without any local or general toxic consequences.

At the time this was written, 4% nonpreserved lidocaine is the product that satisfies these requisites, thanks to the excellent corneal analgesia and partial conjunctival analgesia it produces.

There are very strict rules that apply to phacoemulsification under topical anesthesia. First of all, the surgeon must be an expert in phacoemulsification and the operation must be routine and free from any predictable complications.

During surgery, conjunctival and scleral manipulations must be avoided. However, small adjustments or incisions can be made without the patient's knowledge.

The stabilization of the globe (where required or necessary) must therefore be obtained using an accessory instrument (normally a spatula) inserted through the corneal side port incision (many operators are against the use of stabilizing instruments). Or, the globe can be left completely free with consequent increase in intraoperative difficulties.

During the operation, the patient is asked to perform specific eye movements to favor the surgeon's manipulations, so it is of the utmost importance that a relationship of maximum collaboration is created to produce optimal psychological harmony in every phase of the operation.

It is very important to talk to the patient with the right tone of voice so that he or she will willingly comply with the surgeon's needs without creating emotional tension or a state of psychological dependency. The surgeon must also practice what is called *vocal-local*.

## Methods of Topical Anesthesia

The patient is prepared as usual with premedication based on intravenous administration (Valium five to 10 drops depending on the age and emotional and psychic conditions of the patient). The patency of a peripheral vein and monitoring of the vital functions are guaranteed.

Neither akinesia nor oculopressure are performed. With topical anesthesia the bulb is just as soft as it is under local anesthesia because no liquid is infiltrated at an extrabulbar level and therefore no positive pressures are induced.

It is important to note that in local anesthesia by infiltration, particularly peribulbar, the aim of oculopressure is mainly to assist the periocular diffusion of the anesthetic, which can then determine a hypotony sufficient for the optimal surgery. Naturally, even the effect of the instrument has a certain amount of importance in reducing the pressure.

If 0.50% Tetracaine is used, two to three drops are instilled 15, 10, and 5 minutes prior to preparing the operating field and finally one to two drops prior to applying the lid speculum.

A further application is made once the blepharostat has been positioned, prior to beginning the operation.

Four percent nonpreserved lidocaine is used as follows:
- One drop every 10 minutes (three applications).
- One drop every 5 minutes (three applications).

The final instillation is performed when the patient is on the operating bed, prior to applying the lid speculum.

The product can be aspirated from a bottle with an insulin syringe (one dose and one syringe for each patient) or it can be instilled using the monodose preparations where available.

Recently, surgeons have started using an intraocular injection of 1% preservative-free lidocaine in association with the topical administration of anesthetic eyedrops.

This further reduces the irritating or painful sensations felt by the patient.

## OCULAR PRESSURE

Before the surgeon can begin an operation on a bulb that has been anesthetized by infiltration, it is important to reduce the ocular pressure and the volume of the orbit contents. This can be done through a variety of manual or instrumental methods, both simple and complicated. The simplest system is that of:

- Finger pressure—A gauze is placed on the patient's closed eyelids. The surgeon uses four fingers (excluding the thumb) to apply moderate pressure for approximately 1 minute. Then the surgeon releases the pressure for about 15 seconds to guarantee good blood flow to the optic nerve. The compression is repeated five to six times. This procedure should be used particularly in elderly patients, people affected by glaucoma, or in any patients with ischemic alterations of the optic nerve.
- Kelman's oculopressor—This consists of a sheath containing 300 g of mercury. The device is placed on the eye on top of a sterile gauze that prevents the sheath from coming in direct contact with the

---

**Table 1-7**
### TOPICAL ANESTHESIA

Administration of 4% lidocaine in drops, one drop every 5 minutes during the 20 minutes prior to the start of the operation.

Administration of one drop of 4% lidocaine in the counterlateral eye, once only to reduce blinking.

The operation can begin.

Additional drops of 4% lidocaine when necessary.

If painful and/or there is excessive movement, perform sub-Tenon anesthesia or inject 1% intraocular lidocaine preservative-free.

If there is excessive contraction of the eyelids and/or insufficient patient cooperation, perform akinesia according to O'Brien.

Table 1-8
**BASIC REQUIREMENTS FOR THE OPERATING ROOM**

| | |
|---|---|
| Minimum staff requirements | One surgeon |
| | One assistant surgeon |
| | One non-sterile nurse |
| | One anesthetist |
| Operating bed | Stable |
| | Adjustable height |
| | Comfortable |
| | Suitable for the temporal incision |
| Microscope | Coaxial |
| | Foot pedal controls |
| | Fitted with XY |
| | Fitted with zoom |
| | With eyepieces for the assistant |
| | Adjustable luminosity |
| | Suitable focal distance |
| | Ergonomic |
| Chair | Adjustable height |
| | With armrests |
| | Fitted with stop mechanism |
| | Comfortable |
| | With a back rest |
| | Ergonomic |
| Oculopressor | Active: Super pinky, Vorosmarthy's device |
| | Passive: Bag containing shot, bag containing mercury |

patient's skin and distributes the weight evenly (particularly for sunken or excessively protruding eyes). The oculopressor is left in position for about 10 minutes, a few minutes more in younger, stronger patients.

- Bags of lead shot—These are cheap, easy-to-use, and easily obtained. One bag contains a small-size lead shot, the same type used for hunting. The ideal situation is to have three different sizes available to suit the various characteristics of the eye and the specific clinical conditions (200, 300, and 400 g).
- A soft rubber ball with an elastic band (super pinky)—A soft rubber ball 8 cm in diameter is used. A small flap is made in the middle and an elastic band is passed through it. The ball is placed on the patient's eye and the elastic is passed around the patient's head and tightened to moderate tension.
- Honan's oculopressure—This consists of a strip of synthetic material. A rubber balloon is placed inside and then inflated using a pump. The pressure inside the ball is controlled and adjusted using a manometer calibrated to measure pressure variations of just a few mm Hg. With this method, a pressure of 30 mm Hg is used for about 10 to 20 minutes.
- Vorosmarty's balloon—This consists of an inflatable balloon which is held in place by an adjustable headband and fitted with an adhesive fastener. The balloon is connected to a manometer to keep the pressure under control.

All the oculopressors should be applied after having closed the eyelids with an adhesive strip because akinesia can favor spontaneous opening of the eyes that can cause the cornea to dry out.

Of the various devices mentioned, the Honan oculopressor is the simplest, most efficacious, and most popular because it allows the surgeon to obtain good hypotony and an excellent depletion of the orbital contents.

## THE OPERATING ROOM

Phacoemulsification requires a special set of instruments. The floor space and the cubature of the operating room must allow the staff to move easily around the patient and the various pieces of equipment. It must also be large enough to allow the surgeon to find the right position to perform the operation correctly.

The room must also be adequately ventilated and climate-controlled for the comfort of the surgeon, who must always be in a condition of maximum physical and psychological comfort, and for the patient, particularly if the operation is performed under local anesthesia.

The operating room must be quiet and isolated from other structures in order to guarantee the surgeon's indispensable peace and concentration.

The arrangement of the equipment must be studied in relation to the available space, the power points, the doors, and the light fixtures to allow safe, continual control of every single element.

Now I'll discuss the features every component should have to ensure the ideal conditions for phacoemulsification.

### Staff

The assistant and the nurse should be well-versed in the use of all the equipment and be able to recognize changes in both the function and appearance of situations that may cause problems during the operation. Both should be capable of remedying problem situations quickly.

The assistant must take care of the sterile instruments such as the tips, handles, and connecting tubes to guarantee the necessary operating tranquillity.

The *nonsterile* nurse has the job of preparing the microscope and the instruments, setting up the connections, and keeping a constant eye on the operating parameters of the phacoemulsifier, with the help of the *sterile* assistant.

Smooth operations between members of the surgical team can provide a high standard of safety and can contribute to abbreviating the operating times.

The high standard of assistance given to the surgeon is conducive to the calm he or she needs to concentrate on the operation without having to waste time looking after the technical and instrumental side of things—something that should not be underestimated.

### Operating Bed

The operating bed should be in a central position, equidistant from the various pieces of equipment. It should be stable and easily adjusted into the various positions to allow the surgeon to adjust quickly to the various situations that may arise during the surgical session.

It is indispensable that the bed, preferably motorized, has a broad range of positions. The bed's support structures must not interfere with the surgeon's freedom of movement, particularly of his or her legs, so it will also be suitable for movement around the patient's head.

The need for continuous control of the foot pedals and the microscope requires special attention, particularly in considering temporal incisions.

If the operation is being performed under local anesthesia, the bed must be comfortable and easy for the patient to climb on to.

It is always better to fit the room with units studied and produced exclusively for use by the eye surgeon.

## The Surgical Chair

During the operation with the microscope, the surgeon must be seated because this is the position that will give him or her the greatest stability and comfort during all the maneuvers. The surgeon will also tire less while sitting down.

Up until a few years ago the eye surgeon operated standing up and used spectacles or magnifying glasses. With the introduction of the operating microscope and extracapsular surgery, the seated position is required. If the surgeon is standing, he or she cannot use the foot pedal to bring the microscope into focus while simultaneously using the other foot to adjust the pedal of the machine to aspirate the fragments of the cortex. The surgeon's hands are also working so he or she needs good stability of the body and general control of movement that is obtained only in the sitting position.

The chair must satisfy some specific characteristics. First, it must be comfortable with an anatomical backrest to support the surgeon's spine. It must be easily adjustable in height with a control close to the surgeon's foot. It must be fitted with an armrest, which can also be adjusted in height, in order to give the surgeon's hands stability. The chair must be able to swivel in all directions and should be fitted with a blocking mechanism to allow the operator to fix it in a particular position. It should not be bulky so that it can fit easily beside the operating bed and not interfere with the position of the microscope's tripod and to give the surgeon easy access to the pedals of the equipment.

The height of the chair should be adjusted to suit the operating field. It should allow the surgeon to reach the eye piece of the microscope without straining and allow his or her hands to reach the patient's eyes. The surgeon's feet must reach the pedals easily.

The chairs that have a microscope incorporated are not practical because they do not adapt easily to the individual needs and various situations that may appear during the surgical operation. They are also bulky and difficult to maneuver.

## The Microscope

Before the operation, the surgeon must position the microscope so he or she can operate in a comfortable position. Uncomfortable positions can make the operation more difficult and increase surgical times on top of the useless fatigue of the surgeon that will be carried through to subsequent operations.

Once the staff has positioned the microscope correctly and the sterile plastic cover on the head of the instrument has been removed, the surgeon must proceed with the centering and final positioning of the head and the eyepieces.

Here the surgeon can wear a pair of fine, loose, sterile plastic gloves on top of the silicone operating gloves. These will allow the surgeon to move the head of the instrument as much as he or she wants while protecting the surgical gloves from any form of contamination.

The majority of instruments are fitted with metal or rubber handles that should be changed and sterilized after every operation. The operator can therefore complete all the preoperative or intraoperative adjustments without having to put on a second pair of gloves and without losing sterility.

During the operation, the surgeon may have to make further adjustments that he or she can do alone or have the assistant perform. The more modern instruments are fitted with an XY device that allows the operator to adjust the position of the head of the microscope using the controls on the instrument's foot switch.

The XY device must be positioned on zero before beginning in order to have suitable movement margins during the operation. The dioptric power of the eye pieces and the interpupillary distance must be regulated preoperatively according to the operator's needs.

Right from the start of the procedure the surgeon must adjust the luminosity of the instrument to a comfortable level. The light must be strong enough to allow the surgeon to see the operating area clearly but it should not be glaring, which would easily tire the operator's eyes. Moreover, strong light may damage the patient's retina. The correct intensity should take the operator's needs and the safety of the patient's eye into account.

When using the microscope, the type of light used plays an important role (eg, filament bulbs, halogen bulbs, etc) because of the effect the heat generated may have on the cornea. The evaporation of the epithelial film reduces the vision of the anterior chamber and necessitates frequent corneal washings. However, the more modern microscopes are fitted with good heat filters.

Low microscopic magnification is normally used at the beginning of the operation to cut the conjunctiva because the surgeon needs to be able to see the whole globe. The magnification is then increased for the capsulotomy, reduced slightly for the fragmentation and aspiration of the cortex, and then increased again for the emulsification and cleansing of the posterior capsule. The magnification is then reduced for the insertion of the IOL and the application of any sutures.

The inclination of the binocular tube and eyepieces must allow the operator to work with his or her head bent just slightly forward to avoid straining the back and neck muscles. The mask that covers the surgeon's mouth and nose must be mist-free so that the spectacles do not cloud over. To avoid interruptions during the operation

Table 1-9

## INSTRUMENTS NECESSARY FOR PHACO VIA SCLERA IN NARCOSIS

| | |
|---|---|
| Rectus muscles | Kratz or Barraquer specular (Asico AE1022). |
| | Large Castroviejo (Asico AE6230). |
| | Muscle forceps (Asico AE4430). |
| | Thread: 4-0 to 3-0 silk. |
| | 3 mosquito Hortman (Asico AE4815). |
| | Scissors to cut the thread and the plastic (Asico AE5703). |
| Conjunctiva | Colibri forceps (Troutman) (Asico AE4030). |
| | Westcott scissors (Asico AE5500). |
| | Coagulating forceps (Alcon 8065129601). |
| Phaco | Hoskin Forceps (Asico AE4039). |
| | Blade 30° (Alcon 5480). |
| | Crescent knife—straight (Alcon 1133). |
| | Crescent knife—bevel-up (Alcon 1134). |
| | 3.2 blade (Alcon 5485). |
| | 5.2 blade (Alcon 5661). |
| | Buratto's rhexis forceps (Asico AE4394S). |
| | Syringe with hydrodissection cannula (Alcon 4414), Asico. |
| | Viscoelastic: Provisc + Viscoat. |
| | Chop hook (Asico AE2517). |
| | Olive spatula to mobilize the nucleus (Asico AE2506). |
| | Two separate handles and cannulas for I/A (Asico). |
| | McPherson forceps (Asico AE4375). |
| | Universal forceps (Buratto) for IOL in PMMA (Janach J 2186). |
| | Buratto-Sinskey lens hook (Asico AE2208). |
| | Vannas scissors (Asico AE5490). |
| | Legacy phacoemulsificator (Alcon). |
| Suture | Buratto's needle holder (Asico AE6171). |
| | Corneal forceps (AE4081). |
| | 10-0 CU1 nylon (Alcon 1980). |
| | Bipolar forceps (Alcon 8065129601). |
| | Troutman Colibri (Asico AE4030) for conjunctiva closure. |

to clean the spectacles, the surgeon may apply an adhesive strip between his or her nose and the mask to prevent any escape of vapor.

Before starting the operation, the surgeon should ensure that:
- The focus control of the microscope is positioned halfway along the rail. Focus should be made on the iris first. This allows the operator to have a sufficient range of action during the subsequent phases of the operation.
- The eyepieces of the assistant are adjusted on the basis of the operator's focus to give correct vision during the operation.

The television camera should be fitted to the left of the optical divider so that the staff can observe all the operating phases. This allows the anesthetist to adjust the level of anesthesia and it allows the staff to have the necessary equipment ready at the right moment. The television camera must be focused on the basis of the operator's view so that the images transmitted are always in focus, clearly defined, and well-exposed.

Particularly interesting operations can be recorded and used as teaching material but also to safeguard the doctor from any complaints of malpractice at a later date.

The microscope must have coaxial illumination so there is good red reflex of the fundus. It also allows the surgeon to recognize the important structures (such as the posterior capsule and the cortical mass) involved in the operation and to do this safely, accurately, and quickly. Coaxial illumination permits easy identification of the anterior and posterior capsules, the masses, and the interdependent relationships between the various structures of the anterior segment.

The position of the patient's head and eye must complement that of the microscope to give a good red reflex of the fundus. This permits instant highlighting of the more important details of the operation. For example, the surgeon can witness the exact moment that the aspiration orifice captures the posterior capsule, etc.

Coaxial light also allows the surgeon to identify residual cortex on the posterior capsule and to evaluate the reflex that appears when the cleansing instrument is positioned. The contact of the scraper with the capsule causes the formation of a halo around the contact point, the size of which depends on the application power and the extension of the contact surface.

The microscope must also be fitted with a device that protects the macula from excessive exposure to light. In fact, during some phases of the operation, coaxial light is focused directly on the macula and can provoke serious and permanent damage. There are various methods used to reduce the amount of light exposure to the macula. The

surgeon can:
- Insert a filter to block light of a wavelength below 480 nm.
- Direct the light in an oblique fashion during the phases of the operation when coaxial light is not required.
- Place a disc of opaque material over the cornea.
- Insert an air bubble in the anterior chamber.

Among the microscopes currently available on the market, the following are ideal for phacoemulsification:
- OPM 1FR Zeiss—This is a very simple microscope, at a reasonable cost, and particularly suitable for the beginning surgeon. The only disadvantage is that it does not have a zoom lens.
- OPMI CS Zeiss—This is the latest addition to the range of microscopes from this company. It combines the excellent optical features and exceptional luminosity with a modern form. It is fitted with a two-grade illumination for a better red reflex. It is very expensive and is indicated for the surgeon with a heavy workload.

## The Phacoemulsifier

There are quite a few machines available on the market for phacoemulsification. One of the distinguishing features is the type of pump fitted on the machine. In my experience the best machines are those with a peristaltic pump. In this book, the surgical technique will be described using machines fitted with this type of device.

These instruments can function in two ways:
1. With preset or preselected vacuum values.
2. In linear suction (ie, with vacuum values that increase with the pedal pressure), the minimum and maximum values are selected by the surgeon when he or she is about to use the machine.

### *Preset Devices*

The minimum I/A is used with a value of 65 to 70 mm Hg, and maximum I/A, which is usually high (300 to 400 mm Hg). Each of these values can operate with a variable flow (minimum I/A slow, minimum I/A high; maximum I/A slow, maximum I/A high).

### *Devices in Linear Suction*

The operator selects the minimum and maximum vacuum. These values will persist until the surgeon changes them by changing the pressure on the foot pedal. This way, the surgeon can use the instrument very accurately to the needs of the individual case.

One very important characteristic of all the machines fitted with a peristaltic pump is that the vacuum increases in the aspiration line when the orifice is obstructed. In this case, the pump will continue to function. The advantages and disadvantages of this type of pump are described later in this book.

## Basic Instruments for Phacoemulsification

In addition to the basic equipment, the surgeon must have specific instruments available depending on the technique he or she plans to use.

For the *historical* phacoemulsification techniques no special instruments were needed compared with the manual extracapsular technique, with the exception of a calibrated blade (3.1 or 3.2 mm) and a spatula.

However, if the surgeon uses advanced endocapsular techniques, special instruments are required for every step of the operation. For the corneal or scleral tunnel incision, calibrated and angled diamond tools are available which have been studied and produced specifically for phacoemulsification. For the preparation of the tunnel and the extension of the incision, disposable blades are used.

Capsulorhexis can be performed using a normal bent insulin needle or special forceps.

Hydrodissection can be facilitated by the use of angled cannula, also available as disposables.

Mobilization and fragmentation of the nucleus are easier and more accurate with the use of a spatula and specific hooks.

In the traditional techniques and in some of the advanced techniques, the most popular accessory instrument is the cyclodialysis spatula or an angled spatula with a bulbous tip.

In cases of moderate-hard nuclei (Grade 1 to 2) the manipulation is facilitated by the use of an angled spatula with a forked tip.

In the advanced techniques of nuclear fracture, wider, flatter spatulas can be useful (eg, the Koch spatula) which assist the maneuvers in the grooves.

A special instrument is the *chopper* hook developed by Dr. Kunihiro Nagahara to cleave the nucleus, as described in the chapter on *Phaco Chop*.

The diffusion of foldable lenses for the small incision, available both in silicone and acrylic material, requires special systems and forceps which must be part of the instrument kit of any surgeon who intends to take full advantage of the excellent surgical possibilities offered by phacoemulsification.

Even the suture must respond to the same type of criteria and be ideal for the type of incision performed.

Modern cataract surgery requires instruments that can be used under the microscope and:
- They must be less than 100 mm long, so they are easy to handle.
- The end section must be short (less than 10 mm).
- The closing pressure must be low in order to prevent shaking hands and muscle fatigue.
- The material must be opaque or non-reflecting in order to avoid intraoperative glare which can irritate the surgeon.
- The instruments must be made from good quality material so that there is no rust formation or debris, and to avoid any loss of material.

The following must be available for a cataract operation:
- A disposable 25 G insulin needle which must be bent to become a cystotome.
- An I/A cannula with a 0.3 mm orifice.
- One scraper, an irrigating cannula with the end section sandblasted that is for the scraping of the posterior capsule (Storz E0508).

Table 1-10
## CONTENTS OF THE INSTRUMENT BOX FOR CATARACT SURGERY

| Name of the instrument | Model | Brand |
|---|---|---|
| Two retractors with elastic (Buratto) | AE1070 | Asico |
| Corneal forceps (eg, Bonn) | AE4081T | Asico |
| Hortman Mosquitos | AE4815 | Asico |
| Colibrì forceps with 1 × 2 0.25 teeth | AE4030 | Asico |
| Rectus muscle forceps | AE4430 | Asico |
| Rhexis forceps (Buratto) | AE43945 | Asico |
| Straight thread forceps | AE4360 | Asico |
| Straight Hoskin forceps 0.12 or 0.20 | AE4039 | Asico |
| Universal forceps for IOL in PMMA (Buratto) | AE4234 | Asico |
| Titanium corneal forceps 0.10 | AE4081T | Asico |
| McPherson forceps | AE4375S | Asico |
| Buratto's fine needle holder | AE6171 | Asico |
| Large Castrovjevio needle holder | AE6230 | Asico |
| Large, curved, blunt scissors | AE5703 | Asico |
| Scissors (Vannas), curved, 5 mm | AE5490 | Asico |
| Westcott scissors, curved, blunt | AE5505 | Asico |
| Back aus | AE4800 | Asico |
| Two I/A handles—bimanual I/A handpieces | | Asico |
| Iris hook (push-pull) | AE2172-AE2230 | Asico |
| Buratto or Sinskey lens hook | AE2208 | Asico |
| Olive spatula for the nucleus | AE2506 | Asico |
| Chop Hook | AE2517 | Asico |
| Loop for the nucleus for ECCE | AE2556 | Asico |
| Bipolar coaxial eraser | 8065806701 | Alcon |
| Bipolar forceps | 8065129601 | Alcon |
| Cannula for sub-Tenon anesthesia (Buratto) | AE7076 | Asico |
| Viscoat cannula | J 2641.31 | Janach |
| Healon cannula | J 2641.2 | Janach |
| Angled cannula for the anterior chamber | AS7001L | Asico |
| Hydrodissection cannula | AS57627 | Asico |
| Disposable 3 mL syringe | | |

- Two fine cannulas for air and saline solution. They should be fitted to two 5 cc syringes, either glass or plastic, to be used at any stage during the operation.
- One needle holder that must have thin, strong arms so that it takes a firm hold on the thin needles used in modern surgery. The arms must fit together perfectly to be able to catch even very thin suture threads such as 10-0 nylon. In that case, the needle-holder can also be used as a tying forceps. The arms must also be rounded to avoid snagging the thread.
- One pair of toothed forceps that can be straight but must be fitted with very fine teeth which will take a firm hold of the edges of the wound without causing damage or letting the tissue slip away. Another useful gadget is to have a short tying platform immediately behind the teeth which can complete the suture without having to replace the forceps with a smooth one. Alternately, a toothed angled forceps (Colibrì forceps) with long arms can be used. It has the advantage of having a small volume and remaining for the most part outside the operating field.
- Tying forceps that must be fitted with two terminal plates suitable for catching, tightening, and manipulating very thin threads without breaking them—threads as thin as 10-0 nylon.
- One pair of angled, smooth forceps, Kelman-McPherson type, with long, thin arms suitable for removing the anterior capsule and inserting the loops of the IOL.
- A pair of scissors, Vannas-type with thin blunt arms. These are used to perform the limbal peritomy, an iridectomy if required, and to cut any sutures.
- One lens-holding forceps. It must guarantee a good

hold of the IOL without damaging the optical zone.
- One pair of instruments to fold and insert soft IOLs.
- One lens hook (strong and thin).
- One thin iris retractor.
- One vial of VES (Viscoat), or two vials (Viscoat and Provisc).
- One 500 cc bottle of BSS (balanced salt solution) Plus (Alcon).
- One 10-0 nylon CU1 suture thread (Alcon 1980).
- One qualitative keratoscope.
- One thin, lightweight lid speculum.

## Position of the Instruments in the Operating Room

The position of the operator in relation to the patient and the instruments must respond to precise rules of comfort, safety, and space. The fulcrum point of the operating room is the patient's eye and the equipment and instruments must be placed strategically around the patient.

The following arrangement refers to a right-handed surgeon assisted by a right-handed scrub nurse, and an incision performed at the 12 o'clock position.

- The operator, in order to be comfortable, must place him- or herself at the 1 o'clock position when operating on the patient's right eye and at the 2 o'clock position for the left eye.
- The assistant must be positioned to the right of the operator. This way the assistant can pass the necessary instruments to the surgeon without having to cross the operating field. When the assistant is an expert and a good working relationship exists, the surgeon will receive the instrument he or she requires at any particular phase of the operation without having to remove his or her eyes from the microscope.
- The phacoemulsifier must be used under the visual and manual control of the assistant and should therefore be positioned between the operator and the assistant (ie, to the surgeon's right but slightly behind him or her). This will not interfere with the passage of the surgical instruments; moreover, the I/A tubes will not obstruct the movements.
- The tray of machine instruments (U/S handle, I/A handle, cystotome, cannulas, etc) must be positioned just in front of the machine.
- The table of surgical instruments necessary for the operation should be on the assistant's right. The microscope's tripod should be positioned to the left of the operator or suspended from the ceiling. The right binocular should be used by the assistant. A television camera or a camera is fitted to the left divider and the surgeon uses the central eyepieces.
- The pedals that control the microscope are positioned at the operator's left foot, and the pedals of the phacoemulsifier at his or her right foot. Both pedals must be easily reached so that all the movements made with them are simple and must not involve any movement or uncertainty on the surgeon's part.
- The position of the pedals must also allow the sur-

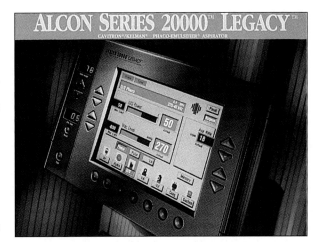

Figure 1-1. The top emulsifier: the Alcon Legacy.

geon to maintain good body balance during all the phases of the operation. They must therefore be placed so the surgeon remains comfortably seated and can rest his or her feet on the pedals with the same amount of pressure.
- The operating bed must be regulated to the right height in proportion to the height of the surgeon. Usually, a low bed is more comfortable than a high one. The body and the head of the patient must be on a plane parallel to the floor. This prevents pressure and vascular unbalance during anesthesia.
- The chin and the forehead of the patient must be on the same level. This places the eyeball in a comfortable position for the operation. Some surgeons prefer the chin slightly higher than the forehead. The latter must be fixed to the bed head with adhesive tape to keep the head still during the operation.
- The phacoemulsifier must be at the same height or slightly raised in relation to the patient's head (using the peristaltic pump as a reference point).
- Before the operation, the phacoemulsifier must be mounted and adjusted so it is ready to use when the surgeon sits down to begin surgery.
- The bottle of irrigating solution must be positioned about 60 to 65 cm above the patient's head. The infusion set must be free from bubbles and have a suitable flow rate. The correct function of the U/S tip and the I/A device must be controlled before the operation and must work properly. The irrigating flow and the vacuum levels of the I/A system must be regulated correctly.

## The Position of the Surgeon

Phacoemulsification is a physically stressful operation in that all four limbs must be used simultaneously in a controlled, coordinated fashion.

A personal ergonomic evaluation of the surgeon is recommended which should take some basic concepts into consideration.

The chair must give the surgeon an almost straight chest position and also limit the tilting of the head on the chest, which will also affect the position of the operating

> **Table 1-11**
>
> **INSTRUMENTS NECESSARY FOR PHACO VIA CORNEA UNDER TOPICAL ANESTHESIA**
>
> Corneal forceps (Bonn) in titanium (Asico AE4081T)
> Blade 30° (Alcon 5480)
> Disk knife (Alcon 6816)
> 3.2 blade (Alcon 5485)
> 4.1 blade for foldable IOL (Alcon 9940)
> Viscoelastic: Provisc and Viscoat
> Olive spatula (Asico AE2506)
> Buratto's rhexis forceps (Asico AE4394S)
> Syringe and cannula for hydrodissection (Asico AS7627)
> Phacoemulsificator Legacy (Alcon)
> Chop Hook (Asico AE2517)
> Two separate handles for I/A (Asico)
> McPherson forceps (Asico AE4375)
> Buratto's folding forceps for soft IOL (Asico)
> Buratto's insertion forceps for soft IOL (Asico)
> Syringe and cannula for the anterior chamber
> Cannula for sub-Tenon anesthesia (Asico AE7076)

microscope (tilting of the eyepieces).

The position of the footswitches and the height of the seat must allow the limbs to bend freely to avoid cramps or posture problems in the event of prolonged operations.

The surgeon should also have an arm and/or handrest to limit muscle fatigue when maintaining the correct hand position.

The operating microscope must be positioned at the beginning of the operation, calculating the various entrances for the chosen technique in order to avoid movements or interruptions during surgery.

## The Surgeon's Hands

In order to operate correctly and quickly, and for a prolonged period with minimal physical fatigue, the operator must assume a specific position in relation to the patient's eye and the microscope. The surgeon must be seated at a suitable height and have the operating bed at the right height. The surgeon must also keep his or her hands in a physiological position.

The hands must be prone, a position that prevents fatigue of the hand and forearm muscles. This also allows a better grip of the surgical instruments, and makes the surgical gestures easier, spontaneous, and natural.

The operating bed must be stable and immobile. The staff, the anesthetist, and the patient should also avoid moving the bed even slightly.

The surgeon's elbows and arms must have a solid support that will provide adequate stability for the hands. This can be obtained with two armrests fitted to the surgical chair or a device made from oval-shaped tubing to be placed around the patient's head.

The instruments (eg, forceps, needle-holders, spatulas, U/S handle, I/A handle, etc) must fit into the cavity on the palm between the thumb, forefinger, and middle fingers. They should be well-balanced and easily manipulated. The grip must be stable and suitable to guarantee safety, precision, and tremor-free surgical maneuvers.

The surgical instruments must suit the size of the surgeon's hand and their shape should be suitable for the micromanipulations and micromovements.

In addition, the surgeon should use appropriate surgical gloves.

## The Gloves

Rubber surgical gloves have three functions:
1. They protect the operating field, the instruments, and anything else used during the operation against contamination transmitted by the surgeon's hands.
2. They protect the surgeon against contamination that can be transmitted through contact with the patient's tears or blood which may pass through small scrapes or cuts on his or her hands. However, the gloves do not protect the surgeon against needle pricks, or nipping with the instruments, etc.
3. They improve the hold and the stability of the surgical instruments. Held by rubber, the instruments do not slide, all other conditions being equal. This reduces muscle fatigue in the hands and allows the surgeon to carry out a gentler, less traumatic operation on the ocular tissues. With phacoemulsification surgery, the gloves improve the surgeon's grip on the U/S and I/A handles.

However, gloves do have some drawbacks. For example, they release talcum powder, so before beginning the operation the surgeon should rub his or her hands with a damp gauze to eliminate the dust. Some surgeons feel that the gloves reduce the sensitivity of their hands but I feel that the extra-thin gloves available now maintain the natural sensitivity very well. Moreover, they are so thin and adherent that they almost become one with the hand and this can cause some of its own problems. The tightness and elasticity of the rubber causes poor blood circulation so that after a few hours of surgery using the gloves, the muscles may stiffen. The surgeon should remove the gloves between each operation and massage his or her fingers and hands to encourage good circulation.

## The Position of the Patient

The patient's head should be positioned so that the iridial plane is parallel to the floor and perpendicular to the coaxial light of the microscope.

The surgeon should check whether the patient's eyebrow is pronounced or whether the nose is unusually protrusive as he or she will have to take these features into account when preparing the operating field.

When planning surgery, it is very important to identify the location of the entrance sites to the anterior chamber so that the various structures are easily reached during the entire operation.

The current technique allows surgeons to adopt made-to-measure solutions for each patient. If, for example, the patient has a sunken eye or a protruding forehead, the surgeon can choose lateral access with a pure corneal tunnel. Vice versa, with a protruding eyebulb, a scleral tunnel can be used, giving the surgeon the possibility of tackling the nucleus with the tip in a more favorable position, preoperative astigmatism notwithstanding.

# PREPARATION OF THE OPERATING FIELD

## Preparation of the Eye

The periorbital skin, the eyelids, and the eyelashes must be washed with cotton steeped in Betadine or Ioprep and then dried with a sterile gauze. This should be done three to four times to remove the maximum amount of ciliary or cutaneous impurities (the eyelashes should not be cut).

The patient's face is covered with a sterile drape with a 10 cm diameter oval or round hole. A second drape is applied with a central self-adhesive part and a bag for fluid collection (Alcon 8065-102920).

The application of the drape may be done as follows. The surgeon removes the cellophane that protects the adhesive area and places the right index finger in the middle of the fold, holding the drape between the thumb and the index finger of the left hand. The assistant opens the eyelids as much as possible or the patient is requested to do so. The surgeon places the drape with the index finger placed along the palpebral rim so that the adhesive part is positioned on the cornea, the internal surface of the open eyelids, the eyelashes, and then on the periocular eyelid skin.

The drape extended completely to cover all the exposed skin. The surgeon then cuts in the middle of the eyelid opening starting from the external angle and proceeding toward the internal angle using straight scissors and a toothed forceps that allows the surgeon to lift the drape away from the underlying tissues to avoid corneal abrasions. After the first incision, which must correspond to the center of the eyelid aperture, four more perpendicular cuts are performed, two at the lateral canthus and two at the medial canthus. This produces two mobile edges of steridrape, one corresponding to the lower eyelid and the other to the upper eyelid.

The lid speculum is then applied so that the branches envelop the edges of the drape and the adhesive part sticks to the internal surface of the eyelid.

Two 4-0 silk sutures are applied as needed to the inferior and superior rectus above the eyelids. The threads are attached with thread-catchers and positioned at 12 and 6 o'clock in order to keep the eyelids divaricated. Then the lid speculum is removed. The sutures underneath the rectus muscles are not indispensable and in any case are applied only under general or local anesthesia, never under topical anesthesia.

These two sutures are applied using a low-magnification microscope. Apply the threads underneath the rectus muscles with a noninvasive procedure. This reduces the risk of annoying and unsightly hematoma of the rectus muscles which disturbs the operator during the operation.

The threads keep the eyelids open; the tension must avoid severe traction. The threads are also used to move the bulb up and down during some of the phases of the operation, and to give the eye a certain degree of stability particularly during penetration and the movement of the instruments in the anterior chamber.

The sterile drapes that define and isolate the operating field and collect the fluids must be fixed so they do not interfere with the movement of the tips and the instruments.

The adhesive drapes are applied for two reasons:
1. To completely isolate the eyelashes and the skin from the operating field and avoid any sort of contamination of the surgical instruments and other material used (ie, IOL, needles, threads) which come into contact with the operating tissues.
2. To prevent liquids from penetrating the operating area as they are collected and from falling to the ground and wetting the foot pedals, the floor, etc.

The operating liquids should not be allowed to fall to the ground. Apart from wetting the surgeon's and assistant's feet, they can also wet and corrode the electrical points of the pedals. A wet floor needs to be cleaned, thus increasing the staff's workload. It may become slippery and therefore dangerous for the staff.

The lack of BSS drainage from the conjunctival sac can create a *pool* around the globe which may cause irritating reflections and can even limit the visibility during the operation with very serious consequences. This problem should be prevented or resolved using a suitable drainer (Eye Drain, Merocel 400108).

The conjunctival sac is then washed repeatedly with a solution of Betadine (1 cc Betadine + 9 cc BSS) and then with a saline solution to remove any impurities. An antibiotic (Tobrex) can also be used.

As an alternative to the previous procedure, the operating field can be prepared as follows. Two sterile strips are applied (Steri-strip 3M R 1547) to divaricate the lower and upper eyelids. A self-adhesive drape is applied (Alcon 8065-103120) with a central hole and a lateral bag for fluid collection. Another drape with a central self-adhesive area is applied at the center of this hole. It is applied to the cornea, the conjunctiva, or the palpebral or periorbital skin.

With straight scissors, a central cut is made in the drape from the outer to the inner canthus and extending the two extremities with another two V-shaped openings. During this maneuver, special care must be taken to protect the cornea against scratching.

A lid speculum with closed arms is then inserted.

This preparation gives good exposition of the bulb with perfect isolation of the eyelids and the eyelashes.

The procedure just mentioned is used with general and/or local anesthesia through akinesia and is indicated for surgeons who are beginning phacoemulsification.

When the surgeon is experienced, he or she no longer needs to use the sutures that fix the rectus muscles. This means:
- Reduced postoperative ptosis.

- Reduced postoperative inflammation.
- Less trauma.
- Fewer hematomas.
- Less anesthesia.
- Reduced cost.

However, the lack of traction sutures causes:
- Greater mobility of the bulb particularly when the U/S or I/A tips are working inside the eye.
- Reduced possibility of obtaining the best red reflex and visibility for the fragmentation.
- Greater operating difficulties, in particular with sunken globes.

These considerations can be applied to topical anesthesia as well. In this procedure the surgeon requires the collaboration of the patient in order to have the globe in the right position during the various operating phases.

When applying the self-adhesive drape under topical anesthesia, the surgeon must ask the patient to open his or her eyes wide. The drape is then applied using the first method described previously in this chapter.

## Instrument Control

Once the preparation of the phacoemulsifier (see the instructions from the supplier) with all the relative connections has been completed, it is advisable to control the various operating parameters before beginning the operation.

The following controls are indispensable:
- The height of the bottle with the infusion liquid.
- The regularity of the irrigation flow and the absence of air bubbles along the line.
- The tightness of the irrigation control valve (or the correct insertion of the disposable cassette).
- The regularity and efficacy of the aspiration (avoid aspirating in air).
- The tuning of the U/S.
- The correct assembly and integrity of the tubes, points, and handles of the various tips.

In recently produced machinery, electronic management of the functions incorporates a computerized self-diagnosis of many of these parameters; therefore it is no longer the responsibility of the assistant.

## Holding the U/S Handle

The handle should be held like a pencil. This gives good stability to the handle and the U/S tip.

The fulcrum is the surgeon's wrist which can actually limit the movement of the tip and sometimes tends to raise the handle inadvertently.

This can be avoided by improving the support for the hand and the forearm.

Many operators hold the handle like a syringe. This position allows a wider range of movement for the tip but stability is reduced.

Some surgeons use two hands; one holds the handle while the other stabilizes it and controls the movements. This maneuver may be useful when the surgeon has still not gained enough confidence with the tip and when the surgeon's other hand is not needed for other maneuvers.

## Entrance of the U/S Tip

Prior to inserting the U/S tip, it is indispensable to extend the primary incision with a precalibrated blade (2.8, 3.0, or 3.2 mm depending on the tip and handle types used) and ensure that the anterior chamber is deep enough (if not, deepen the anterior chamber).

The U/S tip must be checked prior to insertion. The position of the silicone sleeve must allow the surgeon to view the entrance of the U/S tip and its edges.

The orifices of the sleeve itself must be positioned so that the flow is directed toward the two sides of the chamber angles. This way, the irrigation flow is directed from the peripheral iris toward the 6 o'clock position to then be aspirated by the tip in the central position of the anterior chamber.

In general, the tip is inserted with the orifice toward the surgeon (bevel-up), a position generally used for emulsification inside the eyeball.

In this position the surgeon can avoid rotating the tip once he or she is inside the anterior chamber with the possibility of creating folds in the silicone sleeve. In this case it is necessary to raise the anterior edge of the incision with forceps to facilitate the entrance of the U/S tip and avoid damaging Descemet's membrane.

If the anterior chamber is shallow naturally or with particular types of incisions, the entrance can be made with the orifice of the tip facing downward (bevel-down) to avoid lacerating or detaching the iris with the risk of hemorrhage and miosis which could jeopardize the outcome of the successive phases. With this maneuver, the surgeon enters without either irrigation or aspiration and the chamber is deepened previously using a VES.

# Chapter 2

# THE PHYSICAL PRINCIPLES OF PHACOEMULSIFICATION

*Lucio Buratto, MD*

## INTRODUCTION

In order to understand the phenomena that appear during phacoemulsification, it is of the utmost importance that the surgeon has a sound knowledge of two basic elements:
1. Fluid dynamics in a closed system such as the anterior chamber.
2. Function of the phacoemulsifier.

## Fluid Dynamics

Fluid dynamics and the physical phenomena that are observed in the anterior chamber during phacoemulsification can be exemplified by comparing the surgical environment with a closed hydrodynamic system, which lacks any physical contact with the external environment. The system consists of:
- A bottle with irrigation liquid.
- An irrigation tube.
- The eyeball.
- An aspiration tube.
- An aspiration pump.

The main objective of the operation is to perform all of the operative steps in a stable surgical environment under constant intraocular pressure (IOP). This is because the spaces of the anterior and posterior chambers should not vary to any great degree. Good equilibrium avoids the collapse of the eye structures.

Good equilibrium of the anterior chamber avoids damage to the structures of the eye because they will not come into contact with each other or with the instruments inside the eye.

In a system with no leakage that is connected to a bottle of liquid, the fluid flows spontaneously under the effect of gravity, (ie, in relation to the height of the bottle above the infusion system). The pressure inside the system depends on the height of the bottle. The flow stops when the pressure inside the system is equal to the gravitational pressure of the fluid.

In order to obtain a continual dynamic flow through the system, the liquid from the irrigation line must be aspirated using an aspiration pump. This way, the pressure inside the system will change in proportion to the height of the bottle and to the quantity of liquid aspirated by the pump in a time unit (or which escapes through one of the incisions, main or paracentesis).

In order to obtain constant pressure, the bottle is positioned at a certain height and the same amount of liquid should be aspirated by the pump at a steady rate. With an equal quantity of liquid aspirated in a unit of time, the internal pressure of the system can be changed by lowering or raising the infusion bottle.

In the same way, by keeping the bottle at a fixed height, the pressure inside the bottle (or anterior chamber) can be changed by varying the quantity of liquid aspirated in the unit of time.

In reality, the hydrodynamic behavior is dependent on the tightness of the incision, the size of the globe, and the rigidity of the sclera (the latter is more a static characteristic of the system as opposed to dynamic). Nevertheless, in the theoretical analysis of the system, these elements can be overlooked from a quantitative point of view.

The aspiration pump can be one of three types:
1. Peristaltic.
2. Venturi.
3. Membrane diaphragm.

At present, the more sophisticated instruments, such as Legacy by Alcon, use a peristaltic pump and the machine's computer has complete control of the pump's function.

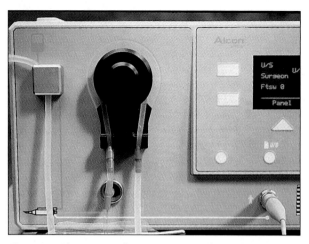

Figure 2-1. Alcon's peristaltic pump Universal II.

## Peristaltic Pump

This consists of a rotating drum fitted at regular intervals with cylinders that compress the aspiration tube wound around the rotating drum.

The rotation of the drum will produce the peristaltic wave that will draw the liquid in the direction of rotation.

With a low rotation rate, the quantity of liquid aspirated in the unit of time depends on the pump speed and the diameter of the orifice at the entrance of the aspiration line. With a high rotation rate, the diameter, the length, and the elasticity of the aspiration tubes come into play. These parameters modify the resistance along the aspiration line to increase the pressure difference between the anterior chamber and the pump and therefore the quantity of liquid aspirated per unit time.

The basic elements that condition the hydrodynamics of the system are:
- Flow rate.
- Vacuum and rising time.
- Occlusion.
- Venting.
- Reflux.

Occlusion, in reality, rather than being a fundamental element of the hydrodynamics, is an effect of it, and more precisely it is an effect of the vacuum and partly of the flow rate.

### Flow Rate

This indicates the quantity of liquid that is aspirated through the tubes over the time unit and therefore it measures the passage of liquid through the hydrodynamic system. It is measured in cc/min.

Clinically, this is translated into the possibility of controlling the rapidity with which the hydrodynamic phenomena are observed and consequently the events in the various steps of the operation. In practice the flow rate affects the speed with which the material is attracted to the ultrasound (U/S) or irrigation/aspiration (I/A) tip (followability).

Look at the case of an instrument that has a possible maximum flow rate of 40 cc/min (100% efficacy of the pump). If you set the pump on a flow rate of 20 cc/min the pump works at about 50% of its capacity. Under these conditions, a certain amount of liquid will travel in the system in twice the time compared with the maximum possibility of the instrument. For example, the aspiration is activated with the pump rotating at 25% of its potential and the aspiration line is free. The material that is found in the anterior chamber will be brought toward the aspiration orifice at a certain speed. This increases the pump action to 100%, the flow rate quadruples, and the material reaches the aspiration orifice with a speed almost four times greater than the previous case.

### Vacuum

In a system fitted with an aspiration pump it is the pressure difference that attracts the liquid and the materials it contains toward the aspiration orifice of the system.

The vacuum indicates the negative pressure that is created in the aspiration line of a system fitted with a peristaltic pump when the aspiration orifice is occluded by material which reduced the flow in the aspiration tube to the point of interrupting it.

In a machine fitted with a peristaltic pump, if the aspiration line is occluded by material, the negative pressure (or vacuum) which forms increases as long as the pump is functioning. In fact, if the entrance orifice of the aspiration line is occluded (eg, the orifice of the U/S tip), the pump continues to rotate and aspirates the liquid from the aspiration tube, creating a depression (vacuum) inside which gradually increases as the pump rotates, to reach the maximum preset values. At a certain point, the material which obstructs the aspiration orifice is aspirated.

The tip is freed in this way and the vacuum can be reduced or can drop to zero depending on whether the aspiration line is freed partially or totally.

In a system fitted with a peristaltic pump, when the aspiration orifice is occluded, the speed with which the maximum value is reached (rise time) depends on the value of the flow rate as well as the characteristics of the pump. For example, if the pump has a capacity of 40 cc/min and operates at 50% (ie, with a flow rate of 20 cc/min), the maximum level of vacuum set on the instrument (normally 400 mm Hg) is reached in 4 seconds. By bringing the flow rate to 40 cc/min (ie, with the pump at 100% capacity), the maximum vacuum level is reached in 2 seconds.

The way the vacuum in the aspiration tube is created and the speed with which the maximum values are reached therefore depend on the flow rate value set and by other factors such as the size of the aspiration orifice.

### Occlusion

This occurs with the obstruction of the U/S or I/A tip or the aspiration line (tube or other components). With the pump in action the occlusion activates the increase in vacuum along the aspiration line and therefore increases the capacity of the pump for aspirating material of size equal to or less than the size of the aspiration orifice, but also pieces that are larger.

The vacuum, which determines the occlusion through the effect of the flux that draws the material toward the orifice, is therefore the most important factor in the process of catching and fixing the lens material with the U/S or I/A tip.

Suppose that the aspiration orifice is 50% covered by material (which actually happens clinically at the start of cortex aspiration) and that the flow rate is at maximum, the vacuum value reached is 200 mm Hg in 2 seconds and 400 mm Hg in 4 seconds (rising time). On the other hand, if the orifice is completely occluded, with an equal flow rate, 200 mm Hg of vacuum is reached in 1 second and the maximum vacuum of 400 mm Hg is reached in 2 seconds.

By bringing the flow rate to 50%, the times exemplified in the two cases are roughly doubled.

### *Venting*

This is the phenomenon that cancels the vacuum in the aspiration tube thanks to a valve which restores the system to atmospheric pressure.

This way, suction of the material that occludes the aspiration orifice is interrupted.

This happens clinically when the wrong material is aspirated (eg, the iris and the capsule) and the surgeon completely releases the pedal that controls the functions of the phacoemulsifier.

Venting is also useful even if the vacuum reaches excessively high levels and the surgeon wishes to restore them to zero rapidly.

Therefore, venting is useful for releasing material or structures that have been involuntarily aspirated. However, this does not always happen and reflux may be necessary.

### *Reflux*

This is how positive pressure is created inside the aspirating tube to invert the direction of the flow and discharge the material that is already in the aspiration line. It is obtained by inverting the direction of pump rotation or by blocking the aspiration line and simultaneously opening a second line of infusion connected to it.

This function is important clinically in order to avoid tearing the tissue that has occluded the aspiration orifice in the event of iris or capsule capture. It is activated with a special device on the pedal of the phacoemulsifier.

If at all possible, reflux should be avoided because it causes a return to the eye of liquid and/or material that is found inside the aspirating line.

## The Venturi Pump

This consists of a compensation chamber connected on one side to the aspirating tube and on the other to a chamber containing compressed gas.

By modifying the volume of gas, a difference in pressure is created between the compensation chamber and the chamber containing the gas. This way, negative pressure that is transmitted to the aspiration line and this draws the liquid from the anterior chamber.

## Membrane or Diaphragm Pump

This pump consists of a chamber connected to an aspiration tube from a compensation chamber with a membrane moved by a rotating motor and by an expulsion chamber. The chambers are connected by two valves.

In the first phase, the membrane creates a difference in pressure between the first chamber and the compensation chamber, air passes into the compensation chamber, and the liquid is drawn into the first chamber. By continuing the movement of the pump air is pushed by the membrane into the second chamber, so the pressure in the compensation chamber returns to the initial value and the aspirating cycle is repeated.

## Function of the System (Venturi or Diaphragm Pump)

If the aspiration occurs with a Venturi or diaphragm pump, because of the intrinsic functional features of these systems, right at the initial phases of the operation a strong pressure difference is created in the aspiration tube which produces a negative pressure or vacuum even if the aspiration line is free from any material (the resistance is determined only by the structural features of the operating system). Moreover, the flow rate increases automatically in proportion to the vacuum.

With machines fitted with Venturi or membrane pumps, the hydrodynamic properties as a result of the vacuum are independent of the occlusion.

From an operative point of view, this characteristic supplies a series of advantages, but also has some disadvantages in comparison to the peristaltic pump.

Briefly, the peristaltic pump, thanks to the latency time needed to reach maximum vacuum levels, allows the surgeon to operate in all confidence even when close to the more delicate intraocular structures. This prerogative can be translated into greater versatility, so it is possible to tackle a very broad range of clinical situations with excellent control and a high level of safety.

However, the *vacuum effect* pumps offer greater speed of lens material removal even though the immediate aspiration action, which is independent of the occlusion of the U/S or I/A tip, requires particular skill in controlling the pedal action in order to avoid damaging or traumatizing the surrounding structures.

As the action of the pump is not affected by the hardness of the nucleus or by the shape of the material to be emulsified, when hard or soft nuclear segments are caught the procedure is more efficacious and less roundabout.

In reality, the modern Venturi systems, used by Storz, have sophisticated devices that simulate the behavior of the peristaltic pumps so the differences are not so important.

## Action of the Phacoemulsifier

Following the theoretical hydrodynamic system, I will discuss the components of a phacoemulsifier, analyzing the functional characteristics.

## THE PHACOEMULSIFIER

The phacoemulsifier is a machine with the following components:
- Machine body.
- Connection system.

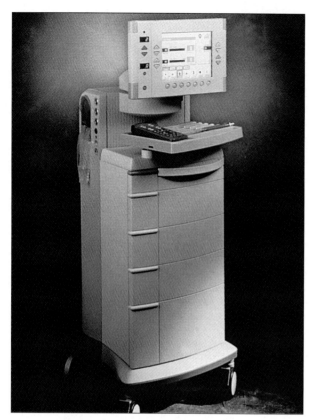

Figure 2-2. The Legacy phacoemulsifier by Alcon.

- Handles.
- Foot pedal.

## Machine Body (Console)

This is where the following functions are performed: production of the magnetic field, control of the irrigation, flow rate, and movement of the aspiration pump. It also usually incorporates a system for bipolar diathermy and for anterior vitrectomy.

## Connection System

This unites the various handles and cassettes of the machine, including the I/A tubes and the cables for transferring the electromagnetic energy to the U/S handle. This energy will be transformed into acoustic vibration and transmitted to the tip as mechanical energy.

## Handles

These are the surgical instruments used manually by the operator.

The U/S handpiece, in addition to the I/A system, contains the transducer which transforms electrical energy into ultrasonic vibration and thus into mechanical energy, producing an excursion of the U/S tip.

The irrigation handpiece sends the infusion liquid to the anterior chamber through cannulas or cystotomes.

The I/A handpiece carries the infusion liquid in the anterior chamber through the irrigation tube and aspirates liquid and cortical material through the aspiration tube.

In addition to these standard fittings, handles are available for diathermy, vitrectomy, ultrasonic hydrodissection (Hydrosonic), and ultrasonic or diathermic capsulotomy (Kloti-Oertli radio frequency instrument).

## The Foot Pedal

The pedal controls the action of the machine body and the handpiece used.

On the machines of the latest generation the pedal can also have a linear control of the functions so that the action can be regulated directly by the surgeon within the preset limits.

In general, the pedal has four positions.

Position 0 corresponds to the stand-by or resting position where the system is ready for operation but has been blocked. There is no irrigation flow, I/A, or U/S.

Position 1 is the first position of the pedal. It activates the irrigation flow by opening the pinch valve which compresses the corresponding tube. The flow in this case depends on the height of the bottle and the pressure that forms in the anterior chamber. This slows down with the increase in pressure. In order to increase or decrease the flow, the balanced salt solution (BSS) bottle must be raised or lowered.

Position 2 is the second position of the pedal. In addition to activating the infusion, it activates the aspiration pump.

In the more common machines fitted with a peristaltic aspiration pump, the flow rate is determined by the speed of the pump, ie, it increases with an increase in the pump speed and when it reaches the preset value it remains constant.

What follows is an example of what happens with an I/A tip.

If the aspiration orifice is free, the flow rate corresponds to the quantity of liquid that flows through the anterior chamber and then passes into the aspiration tube in the unit of time. The more aspiration, the more liquid is drawn in with equal bottle height, so the pressure is constant and the anterior chamber is stable.

In relation to the flow rate value, if the aspiration tip is partially or totally obstructed by material, negative pressure (vacuum) is created more or less rapidly in the aspiration tube. This causes the material to be removed by the tip with increased power (the induced vacuum depends on the values preset on the phacoemulsifier computer).

The maximum value of vacuum preset on the machine is reached gradually. With equal aspiration flow rate, it depends on the greater or lesser occlusion of the tip.

The set flow rate determines the speed at which these events are performed. The higher the flow rate, the higher the speed at which the liquid is aspirated and the material to aspirate occludes the tip (however, this also applies to the iris and the capsule).

If necessary, the vacuum can be eliminated even with the tip occluded by simply releasing the pedal completely. This way the aspiration line is restored to atmospheric pressure (venting) and the removal of the material that occludes the tip is interrupted.

On some machines there is a reflux control on the pedal which inverts the aspiration flow rate and the material aspirated is expelled into the anterior chamber by the tip.

Position 3 is last position on the pedal. It activates the U/S function of the U/S handle. With the pedal in this position, irrigation, aspiration, and U/S are always active.

The linear control pedal acts as an accelerator and the power of the U/S is controlled within preset limits, depending on how far the pedal is pushed (the surgeon controls the setting).

The various functions of the pedal can be independent to a greater or lesser degree. The period between the minimum and the maximum U/S can be short or long, just as the I/A function can be more or less separate from the previous irrigation action or the subsequent U/S action.

In the machines fitted with a peristaltic pump during the U/S phase with the pedal in Position 3, in the absence of occlusion, the flow rate is constant and there is no vacuum. Both the flow rate and vacuum parameters are preset on the machine prior to beginning the U/S phase.

On the other hand, in the event of occlusion, while the vacuum increases to the maximum preset values, the flow rate is reduced to complete stoppage. It is reactivated to different levels depending on the degree of disocclusion of the orifice (without exceeding the preset parameters).

In the more modern machines (Alcon Legacy) it is possible to determine different flow rates and vacuum values depending on whether the pedal is in Position 2 or 3 in order to adjust the parameters better to the different phases of the operation.

## U/S Handpiece

The U/S handpiece consists of a probe containing a transducer connected to a titanium tip. The transducer can be metal (magnetostrictive) or crystal (piezoelectric).

The magnetostrictive tip contains a series of connected metal sheets which vibrate in the presence of a magnetic field. This device heats easily and it is somewhat bulky and heavy. It is also difficult to sterilize (it cools down very slowly), but lasts longer.

The piezoelectric handpiece contains a crystal which vibrates at a specific frequency if excited by an electrical field. This device is light, easy to manage, easy to sterilize, and emits more homogeneous, regular U/S waves. However, it is more delicate and does not last as long.

The electrical energy supplied by the machine body creates a high frequency vibration in the transducer (from 28,000 to 60,000 Hz depending on the type of transducer). This is transmitted to the titanium tip as a longitudinal oscillation. The mechanical energy thus obtained contributes to the emulsification of the material that comes into contact with the U/S tip and which is subsequently aspirated.

It is very important to ensure tuning between the energy generator inside the machine and the U/S resonance system of the handpiece for maximum efficiency of the fragmentation action. The more modern machines are fitted with a computerized self-tuning system.

U/S is not heard by the human ear. However, when

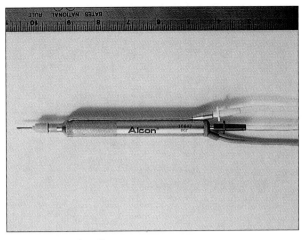

Figure 2-3. U/S handle.

the U/S tip is being used the operator will hear a buzzing noise. The intensity of this noise increases with the increase in power. The noise is produced by the harmonic overtones of the handpiece and the tip. An increase in the intensity is secondary to the increase in the width of the discharge caused by the increase in power.

The titanium tip is about 1 mm in diameter. It has high resistance and is suitable for the frequency of the U/S vibrations.

The aspiration orifice at the end of the tip is beveled at 15, 30, 45, or 0° nonbeveled.

The 15° tip has a greater occlusion capacity, the 45° tip has a greater cutting capacity, and the 30° tip is an excellent compromise between the two.

In addition to the traditional tips, the following are available:
- Tips with different angles (0° for the Phaco Chop).
- Anticavitation tips that reduce the presence of air bubbles as a result of turbulence during oscillation.
- Double-angled tips (15 to 60°) to increase the cutting capacity without losing any of the occlusion capacity (Kratz turbo tip).
- Fine tips (Shimizu) that easily obtain occlusion and take advantage of the vacuum to manipulate the nucleus.
- Tips with elliptical cross-section (Epsilon).
- Angled tips (Kelman) to increase the fragmentation capacity.

The contact surface of the tip is the most important factor to ensure the emulsification and aspiration of the nucleus, which does not occur if the material is not in contact with the tip.

The contact with the tip is also increased by the thickness of the edges of the tip, by a low U/S power, and high aspiration. Conversely, high U/S power with little aspiration causes the nucleus to move away and it will tend to bounce in front of the tip without being fragmented.

The capacity of the nuclear material to be attracted by the U/S tip for emulsification is called *followability* and is directly proportional to the flow rate and inversely proportional to the hardness of the nucleus. The material will be attracted to a greater degree when it is softer.

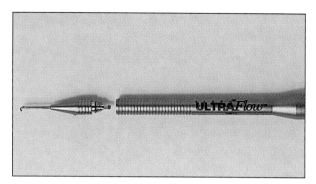

Figure 2-4. I/A handle with curved tip.

The U/S tip is covered by a silicone sleeve, which allows BSS to flow into the anterior chamber through both the distal opening and the lateral opening.

The irrigation liquid is also important for cooling the U/S tip, which heats considerably when functional.

## I/A Handpiece

The I/A handpiece includes a rounded tip with a lateral opening (diameter can be 0.2, 0.3, 0.4, or 0.5 mm) covered with a silicone or metal sleeve with two openings for infusion directly opposite each other (180°). The overall diameter is 2.0 mm (tip and sleeve).

Silicone sleeves guarantee greater flexibility and hold of the incision. In the final analysis, a silicone sleeve allows for a more homogeneous, regular anterior chamber during the various phases of the operation.

However, the metal sleeves allow a more regular flow rate, they are not affected by movements and the rotation of the tip, they are not compressed if the incision is small, and they do not break like silicone sleeves do. The metal sleeves separate the edges of the incision completely, allowing greater escape of BSS from the chamber and making the depth of the chamber more unstable.

The I/A tip is inserted into a metal unit which contains the I/A pathways which are connected to the tubes from the machine body.

The standard fitting consists of straight tips, but at present, angled (45 and 90°) and curved tips are available to aspirate the cortex below the incision.

In order to facilitate the aspiration in these areas, particularly with a capsulorhexis, I invented two separate handpieces, one for irrigation, the other for aspiration, to be inserted through two side port incisions positioned near the self-sealing, sclero-corneal tunnel incision.

## Irrigation Handpiece

This is a simple support connected to the irrigation tube. It is possible to fit a variety of cannulas for different usage and of different designs.

It is normally used in phacoemulsification to connect the cystotome and the rough cannula for cleaning the posterior capsule.

With modern phacoemulsification techniques the irrigation is not used a great deal. This may be because the capsulotomy is performed using forceps or a cystotome with the chamber shaped with VES or because cleaning

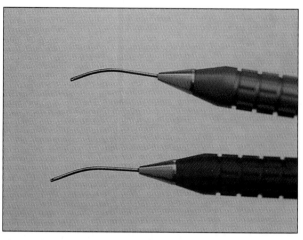

Figure 2-5. Buratto's separate handles for I/A.

the capsule is performed using the so-called vacuum cleaner technique using the I/A tip.

## Diathermy Handpiece

This is generally connected to the basic machine even though it is an independent element. It consists of forceps or a bipolar tip.

In the modern machines, the control of the diathermy value is linear, ie, it is controlled directly with the foot pedal (the more it is pushed, the greater the coagulation), but the value can be preset.

The coagulator can be used either to create a blood-free field in scleral incisions or to fix the conjunctiva at the end of the operation.

The sclera must be coagulated as little as possible, and the operation must be very delicate to avoid creating tissue retraction which may alter the hold of the incision and the astigmatism.

## Anterior Vitrectomy Handpiece

This consists of a sharp, guillotine tip mounted on a metal shaft connected to a specific socket on the phacoemulsifier.

The irrigation and the aspiration are connected to the respective tubes and the values of cut rate, flow rate, and vacuum can be set.

The anterior vitrectomy is normally performed dry, with irrigation blocked or by using a two-handed technique with a separate rather than coaxial infusion.

# OPERATING FEATURES OF THE PHACOEMULSIFIER

The main operating features of the phacoemulsifier are:
- Irrigation.
- Aspiration.
- Fragmentation with U/S.

During the operation, the main objective is to maintain the physiological distances between the structures in the anterior segment. Correct stability of the anterior segment will allow the operator to use the instruments in a predictable manner and reduce the overall surgical trauma with a deep anterior chamber.

Fluid exchange is necessary during phacoemulsification both for removing the fragmented material and to cool the U/S tip. The critical factors are irrigation and aspiration which are tightly linked to the characteristics of the machine and those of the incision.

## Irrigation

Irrigation is supplied by a bottle suspended on a pole which can be adjusted in height. It is connected to the instrument by a tube which passes through a pinch valve. This can compress the tube to interrupt the irrigation.

The liquid flows under the effect of gravity and the quantity of liquid that reaches the anterior chamber depends on the height of the bottle, the diameter of the tubes and the connectors, and the internal pressure of the anterior chamber.

As we have seen, this pressure sometimes depends on how much liquid is aspirated and any liquid loss from the incision(s).

The bottle should generally be placed 65 to 70 cm above the patient's eye considered the zero point. The eye must be on a level with the machine's aspiration pump.

The irrigation flow rate is controlled with the foot pedal.

With the pedal in Position 0, the valve compresses the tube and blocks the irrigation. By pushing the pedal into one of the three activation positions, the valve is opened and the irrigation liquid escapes from the handpiece in use.

## Aspiration

Aspiration in the phacoemulsifier occurs due to a pump which creates a pressure difference between the aspiration line and the anterior chamber. A precise quantity of liquid per unit time is removed from the anterior chamber (and simultaneously the material is emulsified or fragmented).

The most common type of pump is that with peristaltic action (see the following description). Some of the description has been deliberately repeated to ensure that the concepts are clear.

As previously mentioned, the two most important concepts of aspiration are the flow rate and the vacuum.

The flow rate measures the quantity of liquid aspirated from the anterior chamber per unit time. In the modern machines, the flow rate can be set according to the surgeon's needs and the characteristics of the instrument. The most common value is 20 cc/min.

The vacuum is the measurement of the negative pressure which is created in the aspiration line.

The flow rate is determined by the speed of the aspiration pump. The degree of vacuum is determined directly by the functional characteristics of the pump and is inversely proportional to the surface of the aspiration line.

So if the aspiration tip is free, the vacuum will depend solely on the action of the pump which determines the flow rate (with a low flow rate, the vacuum is zero; it will increase moderately with high flow and with an aspiration orifice of reduced diameter).

If the tip is occluded (and therefore the aspiration sur-

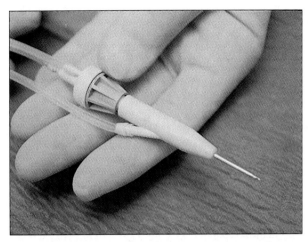

Figure 2-6. Anterior vitrectomy handle.

face is reduced) the vacuum will increase gradually (inside the handpiece, the tubes etc, ie, inside the aspiration system), causing the suction of the material that provokes the occlusion.

If the material can be aspirated, the pressure balance between the anterior chamber and the aspiration line will be redressed. However, if the material cannot be absorbed, the vacuum will continue to increase (until it reaches the preset value of the machine) so that the material will be *stuck* to the tip by suction.

For this reason, a maximum vacuum level is set on each machine. The value can be varied by the surgeon within the minimum and maximum values in relation to the surgical phase, the type of handpiece, etc. This way, the material is aspirated without provoking collapse of the anterior chamber.

The vacuum level during fragmentation using the U/S tip generally oscillates between 0 to 200 mm Hg depending on the type of machine and particularly on the needs of that particular surgical phase. During aspiration of the cortical masses (normally using a tip with a 0.3 mm orifice), the parameters are usually between 0 to 400 mm Hg.

The flow rate, in the machines fitted with a peristaltic pump, is not changed to any great degree with an increase in vacuum as a result of partial occlusion of the aspirating tip, whether U/S or I/A.

Nevertheless, the flow rate affects the speed at which the maximum values of vacuum are reached. The greater the flow rate, the less time required to reach the maximum preset vacuum level.

The speed at which the maximum preset vacuum level in the U/S mode is reached, occluding the tip, is directly proportional to the flow rate value.

In the I/A mode with linear pedal control, the level of vacuum with the tip occluded is controlled by the pressure exerted on the foot pedal. By pushing the pedal to its limit, the operator reaches the maximum preset value with a speed that is directly proportional to the flow rate.

## Fragmentation

During fragmentation, with the pedal in Position 3, there is simultaneous activation of irrigation, I/A, and U/S.

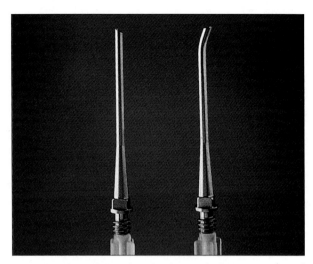

Figure 2-7. Two U/S tips. The curved one is the latest generation of Kelman's tip.

The strength of the U/S is the work (power x distance) done per unit time through the action of the U/S tip. This can be activated in four ways:
1. Mechanical impact of the U/S tip on the lens material at the end of each oscillation.
2. Acoustic soundwaves transmitted by the tip.
3. Impact of liquid and particles pushed forward by the tip with every oscillation.
4. Cavitation effect—At the end of the forward oscillation of the tip, liquid and particles in front of it are pushed forward. In the successive rapid backward movement, inertia prevents them from following the tip so a vacuum is created in front of it which draws the material to the sides of the tip with the effect of an additional mechanical wave.

The energy is transmitted in front of the tip with a cone-shaped conformation. It is therefore important to direct the tip correctly during phacoemulsification in order to avoid radiation of energy toward non-lens structures such as the edges of the rhexis, the iris, the endothelium, and the posterior capsule.

On every machine, the strength of the U/S is expressed as a percentage of the maximum value obtainable with the instrument.

The percentage of U/S that should be used in a specific phase of the operation depends on the characteristics of the instrument and should be selected in proportion to the hardness of the nucleus.

The intraoperative use of fragmentation with the U/S tip can be completed in three ways:
1. Cut or shaving—The tip is passed tangentially (shaving) with respect to the lens and the tip is occluded by the material not more than one-third of the width of the aspiration orifice.
2. Sculpting—The tip enters the lens tissue which occludes the tip for up to one-third of the aspiration orifice (sculpting).
3. Occlusion—The tip is positioned so that the orifice is totally covered by the lens material. With a short shot of U/S, the material is engaged by the tip and remains *stuck* thanks to the suction effect. With this maneuver the tip can shift the material or stabilize it and provide suitable resistance to another instrument.

## The U/S Mode

The action mode of the U/S can be continuous or pulsed. The continuous mode is standard in most cases.

The pulsed mode allows gentler, progressive fragmentation of the material by the aspiration tip. This characteristic may be useful in soft nuclei, in order to aspirate portions of the nucleus close to the posterior capsule and in the final phases of fragmentation when it is necessary to remove the residual fragments and the operator wishes to avoid oscillations in the depth of the anterior chamber.

## Thermal Effect

The transformation of energy from one form to another always involves some dispersion which generates heat. The transformation from electromagnetic energy to sound energy, and then to mechanical energy heats the components of the U/S handpiece which are then cooled with the infusion and aspiration liquids.

During fragmentation, if the flow rate drops excessively or if occlusion is performed frequently (also using the U/S) there may be a temperature increase of the tip which may cause serious burns to the incision. So if the U/S tip must be used for an extended period of time, a good flow rate must be ensured to keep the U/S tip cool.

## Adjustment of the Parameters

For the sake of the description, I will refer to machines fitted with a peristaltic pump which are the most common.

In the first phacoemulsifier by Dr. Charles D. Kelman and in the successive instruments up to the Cavitron/Kelman 8000 the parameters of the machine were fixed and set as follows:
1. With the pedal in Position 3:
   - U/S power—Pushing the pedal into Position 3, there was an *all or nothing* effect, so there was always the maximum of the preset value. Using a control with a range from 1 to 10, at the beginning of the operation the U/S power used was set on the basis of the particular case.
   - The flow rate value was set at 20 cc/min.
   - The vacuum was fixed permanently at 41 mm Hg in the U/S phase.
2. With the pedal in Position 2:
   - Aspiration—In the first series there was a selector for minimum and maximum I/A. In the second series there was also a selector for high and low speed for each of the two values (a total of four options).

Using a 0.3 mm I/A tip with the maximum I/A, a maximum value of vacuum of 370 mm Hg is obtained which is progressively reached by pushing the pedal and occluding the I/A tip to aspirate the cortex material.

With minimum I/A the limit of vacuum was 65 mm Hg, suitable for working near the posterior chamber.

In the latest generation of machines, the situation is

Table 2-1
## EXAMPLES OF VACUUM AND FLOW RATE BEHAVIOR

### With the tip open (without occlusion)

10% of total flow (20 revolutions / minute [ie, RPM]).

50% of total flow (100 RPM).

100% of total flow (200 RPM).

Vacuum stays at zero in all three cases. In actual fact, between 50 to 100% of the flow rate, the majority of the peristaltic pumps, will have a moderate increase of vacuum due to the resistance from the small orifice of the tip when maximum rate is active.

### With the tip obstructed (ie, with the orifice completely occluded)

The vacuum in a peristaltic pump increases with a rising time which is directly proportional to the flow. For example, with preset maximum vacuum of 400, the pedal pushed to the limit, and the preset flow rate at 50%:

After 0.1 sec, vacuum 0.

After 1.0 sec, vacuum 100.

After 2.0 sec, vacuum 200.

After 4.0 sec, vacuum 400.

### With the tip obstructed (ie, with the orifice completely occluded)

With the pedal pushed to the limit, the flow rate preset at 100%, and preset maximum vacuum at 400:
After 0.1 sec, vacuum 0.

After 1.0 sec, vacuum 200.

After 2.0 sec, vacuum 400.

After 4.0 sec, vacuum 400.

(Rising speed 100 mm Hg for every 0.5 sec).

### With the tip obstructed (ie, with the orifice completely occluded)

Flow rate 100% with occlusion; maximum preset vacuum at 400; pedal pushed only halfway:

After 0.1 sec, vacuum 0.

After 1.0 sec, vacuum 100.

After 2.0 sec, vacuum 200.

After 4.0 sec, vacuum 200.

The pedal halfway coincides with vacuum at half the preset value (rising speed 50 mm Hg for every 0.5 sec).

---

very different in that the parameters can be adjusted to the needs of the surgeon in the various phases of the operation, with the option of memorizing the values in more than one memory group. This is particularly true for very advanced machines such as the Master 10,000 and Legacy 20,000 by Alcon.

In the modern techniques of phacoemulsification what counts is that the instrumental values can all be changed in each phase of the operation so that it is the machine that satisfies the surgeon's needs and not the contrary.

The adjustment of the parameters is of basic importance and as they vary from technique to technique they will be treated in detail in the successive chapters. By way of an introduction, I have reported the most common parameters used with the current techniques of nuclear fracture.

In the initial phases of the operation:
- The vacuum is adjusted to 0 to 40 mm Hg.
- Flow rate from 10 to 20 cc/min.
- The U/S power from 40 to 100% (note: the parameters can vary considerably depending on the type of machine, the technique the surgeon intends to use, and the type of cataract).

These parameters are suitable for maximum fragmentation of the nuclear material when the lens is still a large mass offering considerable resistance to the effect of the U/S tip.

As the nucleus is reduced, it is usually better to change parameters.
- The vacuum is increased to 80 to 180 mm Hg. This way the holding power of the U/S tip on the nuclear material is increased with no risk of aspirating the posterior capsule. The adhesion of the material to the tip is increased thus reducing the speed (low flow rate).
- The flow rate is reduced to 10 to 15 cc/min.
- The U/S power is reduced to 40 to 50% (it is possible to control it directly with the linear pedal control).

If there are particularly hard nuclear remnants near the posterior capsule or for fragmentation of the free quadrants, it is advisable to reduce the flow rate further and increase the vacuum so that the occlusion determines a slow increase in vacuum until the nucleus is captured securely and fragmented in the pupillary field.

The I/A tip is used for the aspiration of cortical residues. With the 0.3 mm tip, the maximum vacuum is adjusted to 400 mm Hg. With a flow rate of 20 to 25 cc/min, the value of the vacuum can be controlled at any point in time with the linear control of the pedal. Nevertheless, the modern machines guarantee a large safety margin in the flow rate/vacuum ratio even with maximum values of the latter.

Naturally, it is advisable to read the instruction booklet of the machine used and follow the manufacturer's advice or the advice given by the technical staff.

Knowing the instrument means more safety, with the possibility of taking full advantage of the machine's characteristics. It also allows for rapidity in resolving problems and less time needed to fully appreciate the possibilities of each machine.

## General Rules

Before introducing the phacoemulsification tip, using a microscope, the surgeon must examine the condition of the edges of the U/S tip, the integrity of the silicone sleeve, the exposure of the tip, and the position of the irrigation orifices.

The pedal is then pushed into Position 1 to activate irrigation or reflux before the tip enters the anterior chamber. Position 2 must not be activated (I/A) before entering the anterior chamber as it introduces air into the aspiration line with consequent difficulties in aspiration once inside the anterior chamber.

If aspiration is insufficient, it may mean:
- Poor equilibrium of the anterior chamber.
- Overheating of the U/S tip due to reduction in the aspiration flow rate with a risk of burns, particularly around the incisions.
- Clouding of the irrigation liquid in the posterior chamber because of insufficient flow rate and aspiration of the material.

## Action of the Tip

Once the tip is inside the anterior chamber, phacoemulsification begins. With the current anti-turbulence and anti-cavitation tips, air bubbles rarely form during the U/S action. Nevertheless, should this happen, they should be removed quickly as they compromise visibility. In order to aspirate the bubbles, the tip must be directed toward the bubbles with the pedal in Position 2 (I/A only). Never push the pedal to Position 3 (U/S) during this maneuver because the tip is usually quite close to the endothelium and there is a possibility that other bubbles may be generated.

The U/S must only be activated when the tip is in contact with the nucleus or with nuclear or cortical material, when using the U/S in the progression phase of the tip itself. When the tip retreats toward the incision to continue fragmentation, return the pedal to Position 2.

In this way, the total power of the U/S is reduced, the aspiration line is freed from fragmented material, and overheating of the U/S tip is avoided.

One very important rule is that during the U/S action the tip must remain within the pupillary field. This is the safest area, equidistant from the non-nuclear structures which could be damaged by the mechanical action of the tip.

It is therefore of the utmost importance that the nucleus or parts of it are brought toward the U/S tip for the fragmentation and that the tip does not follow the fragments into potentially dangerous areas.

As the surgeon's skills increase, situations may occur where the rules will have to be bent, even though it is better to apply these rules as often as possible.

In the initial phases of phacoemulsification, the fragmentation must occur without ever totally occluding the tip. Complete occlusion must be deliberate and will be described later as a maneuver for mobilizing the nucleus. Inadvertent occlusion will fix the nucleus to the U/S tip under the effect of the vacuum increase and can cause traction, which when added to the U/S action, increases the risk of damage at various levels.

Now I will give a detailed description of all the steps of the various phacoemulsification procedures. They will be reported in chronological order as each one has been an important reference point in the evolution of this cataract removal procedure.

---

Table 2-2

### TWO COMPLICATIONS FROM THE PHACOEMULSIFIER

| | |
|---|---|
| Collapse | To avoid collapse: |
| | Disocclude gradually. When the tip has been occluded for a long time and the vacuum has reached the maximum preset value, disocclude gradually. |
| | Do not remain in occlusion for a long time, particularly with high vacuum and/or high flow rate. |
| | Use suitable parameters (ie, use vacuum suitable for every type of nucleus). |
| | Use a suitable phaco technique (does not involve prolonged occlusions in unsuitable sites). |
| | Use a machine with suitable technical characteristics. |
| | Make sure there is always BSS in the bottle. |
| | Avoid closure bends along irrigation line. |
| | Avoid squeezing or folding the aspiration tube. |
| Burning the wound | To avoid corneal burns: |
| | Have a suitable escape of BSS from the incision, so the incision should not be narrow. |
| | Use a suitable flow rate in aspiration (and consequently in irrigation). |
| | Keep the U/S power low. |
| | Reduce the times of continual U/S usage. |
| | Avoid nuclei that are too hard. |
| | Use cold BSS. |

It is important to analyze the individual original elements of each technique, as they are the maximum expression of a particular surgical sequence in a particular context. In addition to the historical and didactic value, there is the considerable practical use, as each technique can be updated with suitable variations in order to tackle the various clinical situations that the surgeon can encounter.

# Chapter 3

# THE INCISIONS
*Lucio Buratto, MD*

## INTRODUCTION

When we talk about small incision cataract surgery, we are usually referring to operations that involve a corneo-scleral opening of between 2.8 and 5.0 mm. In this event, the extraction of the cataract occurs almost necessarily through phacoemulsification. In these conditions the incision can be done classically and therefore requires the application of a number of sutures, or, according to the more recent techniques, it can be done so that it can be closed with a single suture or in the total absence of sutures. In these cases, the operation is usually done with a tunnel incision. This type of opening allows the surgeon to place the edges side-by-side so there is good spontaneous closure of even the wider apertures. The tunnel can be done in clear cornea, particularly when small openings are required (eg, for foldable intraocular lenses [IOLs]) or in the sclera (with a scleral tunnel). This technique is used particularly with lenses in polymethylmethacrylate (PMMA).

Self-sealing incisions all have in common the entrance to the chamber in the anterior cornea. They differ from the traditional incisions which sometimes have a limbal entrance.

These aspects have considerable practical importance for at least two reasons:

1. In the traditional incisions, at most two tissue planes are formed very close to each other, so in practice the cornea is cut more or less directly through the entire thickness. Therefore, the suture, in addition to being an important factor for the closure, transmits the changes to a large part of the cornea.

   In the tunnel incisions, there are three tissue planes and the primary incision is quite distant from the chamber entrance, so the forces induced by any suture act only on the first or second plane without extending through the entire cornea. Moreover, the two lateral extremes are not cut which confers stability and regularity inside the tunnel itself.

2. In the traditional incisions, the distance between the initial cut and the entrance to the anterior chamber is minimal and does not present problems when manipulating the instruments. In the tunnel incisions, the length of the cut and the more or less advanced position of the entrance condition the maneuverability of the instruments and determine the formation of corneal folds which limit visibility. These elements must be carefully evaluated when the incision is planned.

The incisions suitable for modern phacoemulsification can be classified as follows:
- Direct limbal incision.
- Limbal incision with a scleral plane.
- Sclero-corneal tunnel incision.
- Clear corneal tunnel incision.

## DIRECT LIMBAL INCISION

This is a classical incision used for many years for the manual extracapsular technique but it also has been used extensively in phacoemulsification. It involves a limbal preincision (of about half the depth) perpendicular to the plane, of sufficient width for the implant. It is followed by a direct incision toward the anterior chamber which is slightly angled. This allows the immediate entrance to the anterior chamber at an angle suitable for easy work procedures.

In this case the two planes of the incision coincide, so that the entire thickness of the cornea is cut. This may result in a poor overall stability, in addition to the fact that the traction on the tissue by the suture affects a large part of the cornea close to the incision.

Table 3-1

**ADVANTAGES OF THE SMALL INCISION IN PHACO COMPARED TO THE WIDE INCISION IN ECCE**

**Intraoperative**

| | |
|---|---|
| The small incision | Avoids air, aqueous, or VES loss from the anterior chamber. |
| | Makes it easier to maintain the depths of the anterior and posterior chambers. |
| | Allows easy separation between the various structures. |
| | Allows intraoperative control of the pressure and a reduction in the intraoperative and postoperative hemorrhage (including the choroid). |
| | Facilitates the positioning of the IOL and avoids any contacts during the procedure. |
| | Is a sutureless procedure or requires very few sutures. |
| | Reduces surgical times. |
| The incision for insertion of the IOL is a maximum of 6 mm; this | Reduces healing times. |
| | Reduces the amount of postoperative astigmatism. |
| | Causes minimal alterations to the anatomical structures of the bulb. |

**Postoperative**

| | |
|---|---|
| The small incision | Reduces the percentage of postoperative flattening of the anterior chamber. |
| | Allows rapid anatomical healing. |
| | Allows rapid stabilization of the refractive error. |
| | Reduces the time needed for the postoperative instrumental procedures. |

This incision is easy to perform and makes the maneuvers of entrance and instrumental manipulation easier. For these reasons it is the most suitable incision for the surgeon who is beginning to practice phacoemulsification.

However, it must satisfy certain characteristics of site, shape, and width in order to satisfy the needs of the operation.

Site—The most suitable position is median limbal because the U/S and I/A tip can penetrate easily.

Shape—A perpendicular-inclined incision is preferable because it allows optimal penetration of the tip/sleeve group. The silicone sleeve adapts well to the characteristics of the aperture. In addition the persistence of fluids in the anterior segment is facilitated through the shape of the opening and for the low amount of gaping by the edges caused by the tip.

Width—The incision must be wide enough to allow the tip to enter without any difficulty, so it must be proportional to the size of the tip.

## LIMBAL INCISION WITH SCLERAL PLANE

The scleral incision is performed parallel to the limbus and orthogonal to the scleral surface, about 1.5 mm posteriorly, with a width corresponding to the size of the lens to be implanted. With a blunt blade, the scleral plane is detached as far as the limbus and the surgeon enters the anterior chamber with the instruments or with a calibrated 2.8 to 3.2 mm keratome on a plane parallel to the sclera.

This type of incision guarantees a good hold of the anterior chamber and facilitates the entrance and the maneuvers of the instruments as well as the visibility during the operation. As the incision is performed on two planes, it cannot self-seal so interrupted or running sutures must be placed. The distance between the first incision plane and the entrance to the anterior chamber ensures good control of the astigmatism as it limits the effect of the suture on the superior portion of the cornea.

## SCLERAL TUNNEL

This consists of:
- A preliminary scleral incision, perpendicular to the plane, about 250 to 300 µm deep (external incision).
- A sclero-corneal pouch parallel to the scleral plane.
- An oblique (about 45°) entrance incision to the anterior chamber which creates a self-sealing valve effect (internal incision).

The first incision can have a variety of shapes. A curved incision is the most common, convex toward the limbus (frown incision) or alternately a straight incision tangential to the limbus. The width must be in function to the size of the optical disc of the lens to be inserted.

The distance from the limbus depends on the control of the astigmatism as a function of the width of the incision. Generally, for a 5 to 6 mm incision, a distance of 2 to 2.5 mm from the limbus (plus 1.0 to 1.5 mm in the cornea prior to entering the chamber) ensures almost neutral behavior. Whereas if the incision is shifted toward the limbus, there will be a tendency toward against-the-rule astigmatism (for an incision performed superiorly).

The surgeon tries to maintain this neutral behavior of the postoperative astigmatism by trying to cut a tunnel that has the same length and width so that the cleavage forms a square-shaped tunnel.

At this point the sclero-corneal cleavage is formed (ie, the true tunnel).

Using a blunt, angled blade, the surgeon continues parallel to the scleral plane, keeping the same initial depth, to reach the cornea 1.0 to 1.5 mm beyond the limits of the limbus.

Following the careful preparation of the desired width of tissue cleavage, the surgeon enters the sclero-corneal tunnel with a calibrated blade, better if angled, to reach the corneal limit of the tunnel.

It is better if the penetration of the chamber occurs with a certain degree of indentation directing the tip toward the anterior apex of the lens. This way the entrance to the chamber is simple and rapid, but above

Table 3-2

## DIFFERENCES BETWEEN CLASSIC AND TUNNEL INCISIONS

| Traditional incision | Tunnel incision |
| --- | --- |
| External and internal incisions are closed. | External incision is separated from the internal incision by the tunnel. |
| Straight internal incision. | Internal incision shaped like a flute mouthpiece. |
| The lateral extremities of the incision are cut radially. | Lateral extremities are not cut. |
| The chamber flattens between one surgical phase and the other. | The chamber remains deep. |
| Suturing is necessary and mandatory. | In most cases sutures are not needed. |
| The incision induces astigmatism. | The incision is astigmatically neutral or poorly astigmatic. |

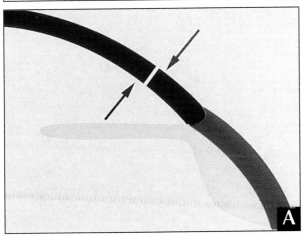

Figure 3-1A. In perpendicular single-plane incisions, the width of the wound margins in contact is narrow. Any force applied causes the division of the margins.

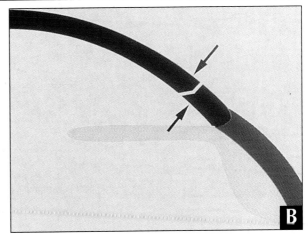

Figure 3-1B. In two-plane incisions, the wound margins have a wider surface of apposition. Forces applied tend to close the flaps.

all it forms an opening that is automatically self-sealing. The intracorneal cut must occur with the blade parallel to the iris plane so that a third incision plane is formed. In this phase it is better to have the cornea distended with tension similar to the physiological conditions, so if the globe is hypotonic it is better to increase the tone with injection of viscoelastic substance (VES) through a side port incision before entering the anterior chamber.

## Action Mechanism of the Sutureless Incision

How can an incision longer than 4.0 mm be self-sealing? What prevents it from reopening hours or days after the operation? Why does it not induce against-the-rule astigmatism? Look at how the classical incisions and the newer ones react.

- Standard limbal incision—In this aperture there is a marked separation of the tissues. They do not tend to stick together spontaneously because the external pressure on the sclera and the internal pressure of the anterior chamber react in such a way as to cause the edges to separate. If the wound is not closed carefully with numerous suture points, there will be a loss of aqueous, ocular hypotony, etc, in addition to induction of considerable against-the-rule astigmatism.

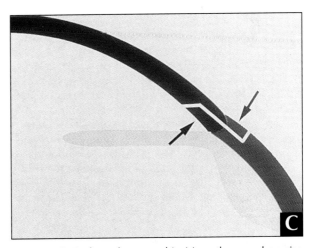

Figure 3-1C. In three-plane tunnel incisions, the wound margins have a wider surface area of contact. IOP and external forces tend to close the wound, pressing the flaps together and resulting in a valve mechanism.

- Posterior incision with scleral flap—An incision with the flap that begins posteriorly in the sclera at least a couple of millimeters from the limbus and which has a more anterior chamber entrance is more stable than the standard limbal incision. But it

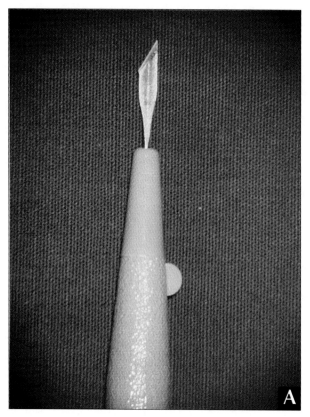

Figure 3-2A. Alcon 30° blade (5481).

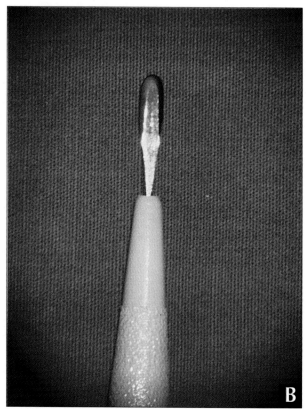

Figure 3-2B. Alcon straight bevel-up (1133).

is also subjected to gaping in response to the internal and external forces. This is because the external sides of the flap are cut radially to the entrance site in the anterior chamber and therefore the flap cannot adhere spontaneously to the underlying sclera. It is also because the ways for entering the chamber are such that the wound edges tend to separate spontaneously. This type of incision must therefore be supported by at least one or two interrupted sutures or a suitable horizontal suture.
- Posteriorized incision with a scleral tunnel—This incision is started posteriorly in the sclera and takes an intrascleral route which creates a large contact surface between the cut tissues. Moreover, as the lateral extremities are not cut radially, the tissues tend to stick together under the internal pressure. The penetration into the anterior chamber occurs further ahead in the cornea with the formation of a deep corneal flap which acts as a valve. Under the effects of the internal pressure, it can close the aperture and increase its adhesion to the more superficial flap favoring the self-sealing. So, it stands to reason that this type of aperture cannot require the use of sutures.

The intraocular pressure (IOP) is one of the elements that separates the edges of the wound when the aperture is corneal or limbal. In the event that a tunnel incision has been cut, the internal pressure acts positively to close the wound and the IOP brings the internal edge into contact with the external one thus avoiding the separation of the incision. This applies particularly if the length of the tunnel (the distance between the external and internal incision) is suitable.

## Surgical Limbus

The corneo-scleral limbus is not an anatomic structure as such but it is a transition area between the cornea and the sclera and the episclera and the conjunctiva. Under the operating microscope, the limbus is a gray, semi-transparent area which separates the transparent cornea from the opaque sclera. The limbus has a width of about 1.2 mm.

The transparent anterior surface of the cornea terminates with the insertion of the conjunctiva and the Tenon's capsule. The corneal insertion of the two membranes corresponds internally to a 0.5 mm zone in front of the Schwalbe's line. An incision perpendicular to the corneal surface, which begins from the conjunctival insertion, does not involve the trabeculum but remains just in front of it.

About 0.5 mm behind the insertion of the conjunctiva the transparent cornea gradually becomes opaque-white through a narrow bluish transition band of about 0.2 mm. This is called the *blue limbus* and is the most obvious reference point in the limbus. The Schwalbe line is found on the inside of the blue limbus and about halfway along it. The Schwalbe line is just in front of the Schlemm line and at the beginning of the trabecular line. When performing the corneo-scleral incision, if the surgeon remains anteriorly or on the posterior limits of the blue line, he or she

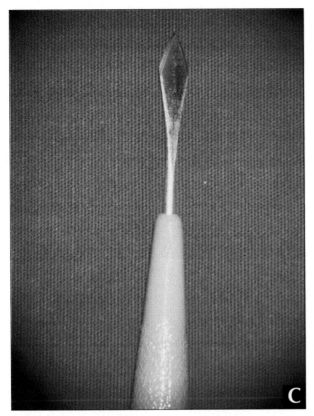

Figure 3-2C. Straight width 3.2 mm (Alcon 5485).

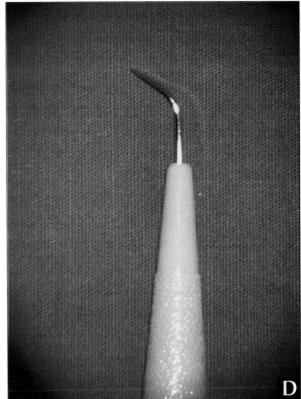

Figure 3-2D. Angled bevel-up (Alcon 1134).

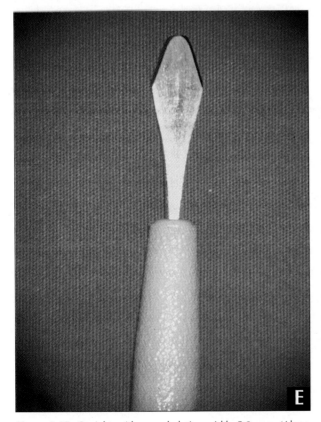

Figure 3-2E. Straight with rounded tip; width 5.2 mm (Alcon 6560).

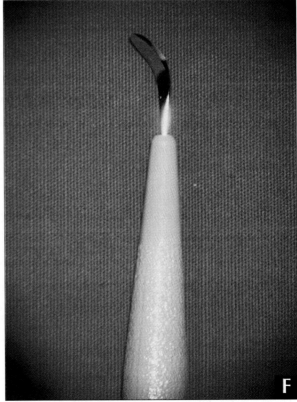

Figure 3-2F. Angled bevel-down (Alcon 8065-940003-1135).

Table 3-3

## SCLERAL TUNNEL: EQUIPMENT AND TECHNIQUE BY BURATTO

### Equipment

| | |
|---|---|
| External scleral microknife | Straight crescent incision (Alcon 1133). |
| Intrascleral dissection | Crescent microknife with angled bevel-up blade (Alcon 1134). |
| Entrance to the chamber | 3.2 angled blade (Alcon 5485). |
| Lateral incision | 30° angled blade (Alcon 5481). |
| Widening the tunnel for the IOL | Precalibrated 5.2 angled microknife, normal or stinted for implantation of PMMA IOL LX10 (Alcon). |

### Technique

| | |
|---|---|
| Conjunctival incision | With atraumatic forceps and Wescott's scissors. |
| Cauterizing of bleeding vessels | With bipolar tweezers. |
| Scleral preincision | Depth: About half the scleral thickness. The incision is preferably made with anterior convexity (frown incision). |
| Scleral dissection to form the pathway (channel of the tunnel) | Must be performed at the same depth. Separate the tissues to enter at least 1.0 to 1.5 mm the cornea. |
| Lateral incisions | With a 30° blade parallel to the iris plane. |
| Viscoelastic | Injection of Provisc. |
| Penetration in the chamber | With a 3.2 blade aiming at the center of the lens to make the internal mouthpiece incision. |
| Widening the tunnel for foldable IOL implantation | With a 4.1 mm angled blade for foldable AcrySof MA60 or with a 5.2 mm blade in a rigid lens LX90 by Alcon has been planned for implantation in the bag. |

will avoid the posterior portion of the limbus (which contains numerous blood vessels). Moreover, by not going in deep the surgeon will avoid the structures of the angle, the root of the iris, and the ciliary body.

The trabecular zone varies between 1.0 to 1.3 mm of width, so the surgeon must enter about 1.6 to 2.0 mm posterior to the insertion of the conjunctiva to the cornea to reach the extremity of the irido-corneal angle.

The easily visible external reference points are the insertion of the conjunctiva on the cornea and the line where the color change of the cornea begins (0.5 mm posteriorly—the blue limbus). The following average measurements for normal eyes may be useful reference points.

From the insertion of the conjunctiva:
- Color change of the cornea (blue limbus) at 0.5 mm.
- Schwalbe line at 0.6 mm.
- Trabecular meshwork between 1.6 to 1.8 mm.
- Root of the iris at about 1.8 mm.
- Pars plana between 3.2 to 7.5 mm.

These measurements must be reduced for hyperopic eyes and increased for myopic eyes in proportion to the length of the eyebulb.

## Characteristics of a Sutureless Scleral Tunnel Incision

Assuming that the incision is begun posteriorly in the sclera (1.5 to 3.0 mm), that a scleral dissection is necessary, that it continues to reach clear cornea, and that the right and left extremities are not cut radially, here are some suggestions for cutting a pouch which responds to the requisites of self-sealing.

- The wider the incision, the greater the distance between the limbus and the scleral incision (length). The wider the aperture, the greater the contact area between the superficial and deep edges to favor self-support and avoid the tissues sliding.
- The scleral incision can be straight or, better still, a frown line curve. However, the extremities of the aperture must be as far away from the limbus as they are from the central part of the incision. So the extremities of the incision contribute positively to supporting the tissues and to minimizing the variations induced in the eyeball and the cornea in particular.
- The scleral dissection should be done at half-thickness. A dissection that is too superficial will be fragile and therefore tend to tear during the operation. In addition, it will not adhere well at the end of surgery. A dissection which is too deep carries with it risks of deep penetration of the chamber, uveal prolapse, risks of damage to the underlying uvea, and greater intraoperative difficulties.
- The superficial scleral flap must be treated carefully as far as possible. The surgeon must minimize any manipulations of the dissected scleral tissue (ie, he or she must avoid trauma or snagging with the forceps or excessive pressure with the I/A tip etc). The surgeon must also ensure that the thickness is uniform and free from tears or holes.
- The penetration in the chamber must be in clear cornea. The entrance must be oblique to form a tissue flap which, inducing a certain amount of IOP, allows the deep portions to adhere firmly to the superficial portions (the mechanism of corneal valve closure). In relation to Descemet's membrane, the correct angle of penetration is 45°.
- The internal corneal flap must be cut obliquely with regular, continuous surfaces so that at the end of the operation the IOP allows the cut edges to adhere well.

Using these ideas as starting points, one can create some variations on the theme.

| Table 3-4 COMPARISON OF LONG AND SHORT TUNNEL INCISIONS ||
|---|---|
| **Retracted internal incision advantages** | **Advanced internal incision advantages** |
| Ease of instrument maneuvering | Very good self-sealing |
|  | Induced astigmatism reduced or absent |
| **Drawbacks** | **Drawbacks** |
| Greater iris trauma | Difficult instrument insertion |
| Possible iris prolapse during phacoemulsification | Formation of corneal folds |
| | Poor visibility |
| Possible formation of peripheral synechia | Poor maneuverability |
| | Poor access to subincisional cortex |
| Possible postoperative filtration | Difficult IOL insertion and positioning |
| Less self-sealing | |
| Induces more astigmatism | |
| Better postoperative refraction stability | |

| Table 3-5 CONTROL OF THE SUTURELESS INCISION |
|---|
| Aspirate the viscoelastic from the anterior chamber and the capsular bag. |
| Remove the I/A tip operating on irrigation so the anterior chamber remains formed. |
| Inject BSS with a thin cannula on both sides of the lateral incision(s) (edematization of the incisions) to increase tissue adhesion. |
| Inject BSS on both sides of the main incision (edematization of the main incision) with the same cannula. |
| Dry the cornea and/or the sclera surrounding the incisions with a surgical sponge. |
| Press with a dry triangular sponge 2 to 3 mm posteriorly to the main incision and check whether the chamber leaks. |
| With the same sponge (now damp) press on the cornea 1 to 2 mm centrally to the internal incision and check whether any fluid is leaking. |
| Repeat the procedure for the lateral incision(s). |
| If no leakage is present the operation is completed (when astigmatism permits). |
| If there is leakage, repeat the edematization of the incisions and repeat the test. |
| If the incision leaks apply one or more nylon 10-0 sutures. |

## Indications for the Sutureless Scleral Tunnel

It is better to choose globes that allow a good exposure of the sclera so the scleral tunnel can be performed easily.

In choosing the first cases for the sutureless technique, the surgeon should carefully check the preoperative astigmatism. At the beginning of training it is better to have eyes with 1 or 2 diopters (D) of with-the-rule astigmatism, because at least in first cases, there is a tendency to against-the-rule astigmatism due to tissue sliding, particularly where the larger incisions are involved.

The surgeon should avoid globes that may require an antiglaucoma fistulizing operation in the same area in the future.

The scleral tunnel is also not indicated in areas around antiglaucoma fistulas. It is better to avoid scleral tunnels in eyes that have already been subjected to conjunctival surgery for a number of reasons.

Scleral tunnels are preferred when the surgeon plans to implant a lens that requires an opening in excess of 5.0 mm (hard lenses). For the foldable lenses, the tendency is to perform the incisions in the clear cornea.

## Technique of Performing a Scleral Tunnel

What follows is a description of the procedure under peribulbar or general anesthesia. It also can be performed under sub-Tenon's anesthesia but not under topical anesthesia.

## Conjunctival Flap

A conjunctival flap is prepared with the base at the fornix (incision at the limbus) with a lateral extension of at least 7.0 mm and a posterior extension of at least 3.0 mm.

The control of the eyebulb can be obtained by two traction sutures under the superior and inferior rectus muscles; or the retraction of conjunctiva by just one superior suture internally to externally (ie, first through the Tenon's capsule and then through the conjunctiva [naturally after having cut and retracted the conjunctiva]). This allows sufficient exposure of the sclera to perform the posterior scleral incision necessary for the sutureless technique or for the technique with a single suture. This method, in relation to the superior rectus, also reduces postoperative ptosis.

## Scleral Cauterization

Cauterization of the episcleral vessels is performed with high frequency bipolar diathermy. This instrument is efficacious and does not burn the tissue. It reduces local congestion and postoperative inflammation of the interested tissues.

The cauterizing effect is created by the passage of current between the positive and negative arms of the device. For the best cauterizing effect, the operating field should be kept moist by a stream of saline drops falling on the treatment field. The two arms of the cauterizing field must be kept 1 to 2 mm apart (contact between the two arms will create sparks which will not cauterize).

## Creating the Tunnel

The posterior limit of the incision is marked with a caliper, then the lateral limits are marked. A dye should be used so that the reference points are easily seen. When phacoemulsification is performed and a foldable lens is inserted, the total width of the incision is about 4.0 mm. The tunnel (closest to the cornea) can be 2.0 mm from the insertion of the conjunctiva. When phacoemulsification is done and a PMMA lens is inserted (5 x 5, 5 x 6, or 6 x 6)

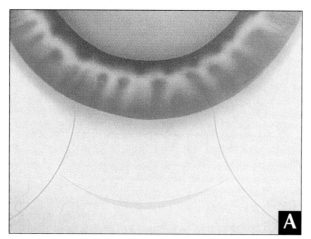

Figure 3-3A. Classical concave incision.

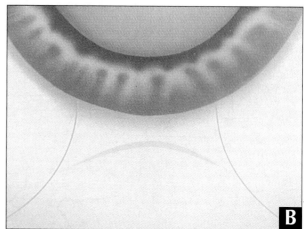

Figure 3-3B. Frown incision.

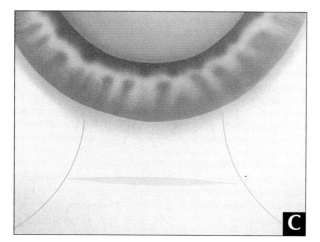

Figure 3-3C. Straight incision.

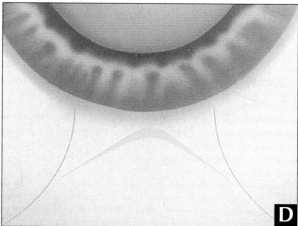

Figure 3-3D. Chevron incision.

the incision must be posteriorized by at least 2.5 mm. When an extracapsular extraction is done—an operation that may require an incision in the region of 6.0 to 8.0 mm—the tunnel must be made at least 3.0 mm from the limbal insertion of the conjunctiva.

Then the straight scleral incision is made to 40 to 50% of the scleral thickness (ie, to a depth of 250 to 300 μm for a length of about 5.0 mm [this aperture is ideal for the insertion of 5.5 to 6.0 mm lenses]).

The anterior edge is then caught with a Hoskin forceps with large teeth to reduce trauma to the edge. Special care must be taken to avoid damage to the anterior tissue of the tunnel. The surgeon then proceeds to dissect the sclera until a pouch has been formed (similar to a jacket pocket). An Alcon Crescent Knife, a Beaver 6900 blade, or a Grieshaber 681.22 blade can be used for this operation.

The scleral dissection must have the same width along the whole pouch. For example, if the primary scleral incision was 5.0 mm, the whole dissection must be 5.0 mm. The dissection must then be extended toward the cornea and into it for about 1.0 to 1.5 mm at half the corneal thickness.

At the end of this surgical phase, a scleral tunnel 5.0 mm wide and 2.5 mm long is obtained in the sclera, and a scleral tunnel about 1.0 mm is obtained in the cornea (corneal valve).

The penetration in the chamber must not occur too far forward or too close to the limbus. A flap of deep corneal tissue must be produced that will be able to stick to the anterior tissue at the end of the operation and close the eyebulb with a valve-like mechanism.

At this point, the surgeon penetrates the chamber with a 2.8 to 3.2 mm metal keratome.

The position of the entrance is of fundamental importance if the surgeon wishes to obtain a self-sealing incision. Penetration must occur inside the tunnel just in front of the Schwalbe line.

The tunnel must extend into the clear cornea for a number of reasons:
- To avoid the prolapse of the iris.
- To avoid even minor damage to the structures of the chamber angle.
- To avoid liquid loss at the end of the operation.
- Above all, to create a valve effect which will actually seal the wound at the end of surgery.

Penetration must occur at an angle of 45° with respect to the internal surface of the Descemet's membrane.

This way a thin, deep corneal flap is formed which

will allow contact first and then adhesion of the superficial portion of the cut cornea at the end of the operation when the ocular pressure increases.

The VES required in the successive stages of the operation is injected through the side port incision before entering the chamber through the main incision. Alternately, it can be injected directly into the tunnel after entrance to the chamber.

### *Some Suggestions to Simplify the Operation with a Tunnel Incision*

Some of the difficulties of the sutureless phacoemulsification operation derive from the fact that the tunnel begins 2 to 3 mm posterior to the limbus. This results in:
- Difficult access to the chamber.
- Limited movement of the instruments.
- Difficult access to the nucleus.
- Difficulty in aspirating the cortex, particularly the cortex immediately under the incision.
- Abnormal direction of the instruments and the IOL during penetration of the anterior chamber (in that they tend to move spontaneously, in relation to the shape of the incision, toward the cornea and not toward the capsular bag).

To make the procedure simpler, the surgeon should:
- Use the shortest tunnel possible, yet one that is compatible with the type of operation planned. This reduces to a minimum any difficulty regarding access or the maneuvers in the anterior chamber. It increases the need for one or more sutures.
- Slightly widen the posterior part of the tunnel that ends up wider than the anterior part. This way the instruments can move more easily.
- Use a VES to reduce the intraocular manipulations particularly during mobilization of the nucleus and during positioning of the IOL.
- Begin his or her approach to the sutureless technique with simple cases. The surgeon should start this technique gradually through a series of preliminary steps (that is, cutting short tunnels first and suturing at the end of the operation, etc).

## CLEAR CORNEAL TUNNEL

In this case the first incision is performed in clear cornea, in front of the limbal vessels, with a depth of 250 µm and a width dependent on the type of lens to be implanted.

This first incision is performed perpendicularly to the corneal plane, preferably with a calibrated diamond knife. Alternately, any other cutting instrument can be used although the precision and uniformity of the incision might be jeopardized.

The second plane, which creates a cleavage in the corneal stroma, can be performed in two ways. Using a diamond or ruby instrument that is calibrated and angled, a stromal groove is created for the desired length parallel to the corneal plane. Then the surgeon enters the anterior chamber directly along a plane parallel to the iris or better still engaging the blade and directing it toward the anterior apex of the lens.

Alternately, the surgeon can use a disk knife to cut a stromal tunnel of the desired length and then enter the anterior chamber with a calibrated lance.

The characteristics of stability depend almost exclusively on the construction of the internal corneal valve, and to a lesser degree on the total width of the incision and the length of the tunnel.

On the other hand, control of the astigmatism depends on the length of the tunnel. The neutral tunnel, as Paul Ernest has clearly demonstrated in numerous papers must be *squared* (ie, the length must be the same as the width).

For a 4 to 5 mm incision, a correct tunnel must have an overall length of 2.0 to 2.5 mm (even if it is not astigmatically neutral). In fact, a longer tunnel would create an entrance that was too far forward with negative consequences on the maneuverability and visibility during the operation.

If the incision is wide and the tunnel is short, it is advisable to place a suture to avoid the evolution of postoperative with-the-rule astigmatism (assuming that the incision is temporal).

Healing of the internal corneal valve allows early removal of the suture just 3 to 6 weeks postoperatively with no or only slight variations in the astigmatism.

The use of foldable lenses that can be inserted through a 3.2 to 4.0 mm incision allows the surgeon to perform a purely corneal sutureless tunnel of 1.5 to 2.0 mm with only minor variations in the preexisting astigmatism.

## Side Port Incision

The lateral side port incision is a paracentesis which should always be performed with the phacoemulsification technique for the following reasons:
1. It provides an access route for the introduction of VES.
2. It can be used to introduce the hydrodissection cannula.
3. It can be used to introduce the accessory instrument (spatula) during phacoemulsification, which can:
   - Stabilize the globe.
   - Cause the nucleus to move and control these movements.
   - Perform nucleofracture and facilitate the removal of the nuclear fragments.
   - Protect the posterior capsule during emulsification of the final fragments.
   - Keep the iris at a distance.
   - Facilitate the removal of the cortex.
   - Facilitate the insertion of the lens.

The side port incision is performed immediately in front of the limbal arches at approximately 70 to 90° to the left of the main incision.

Microknifers with a 30° blade (Alcon) are generally used for this procedure. The internal incision must be about 1 mm wide and the external incision about 1.5 mm. The route must be directed in order to produce an opening which is parallel to the iris plane so the hold at the end of the operation is guaranteed.

An incision that is too narrow will make it difficult to introduce large cannulas. An incision that is too wide will cause liquid to escape from around the instruments during the manipulations in the anterior chamber with a negative

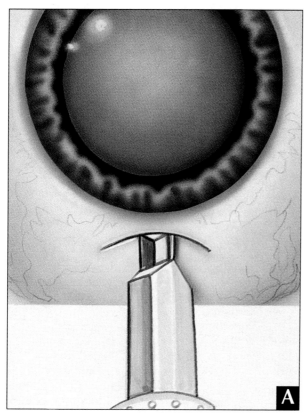

Figure 3-4A. Scleral tunnel. Following the incision and retraction of the conjunctiva, a frown incision is performed with a diamond blade to about half the scleral depth.

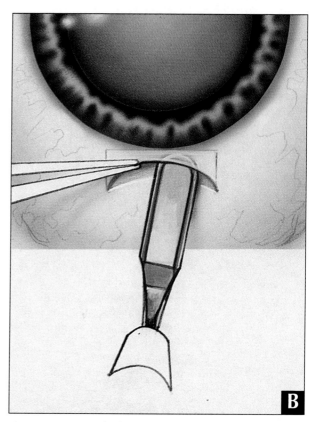

Figures 3-4B, 3-4C. The forceps with blunt tips lifts the superficial flap and places the tissue under tension to favor the dissecting action of the blade.

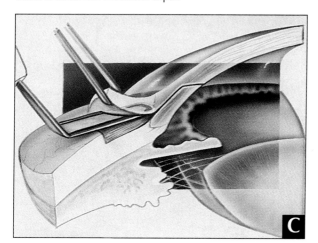

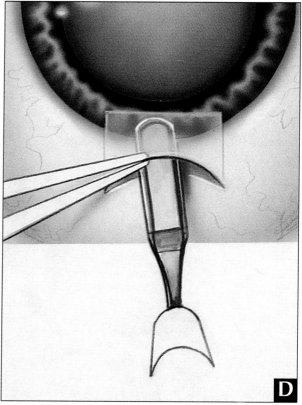

Figure 3-4D. The surgeon can clearly observe the action of the blade and control the width, length, and depth of the tunnel.

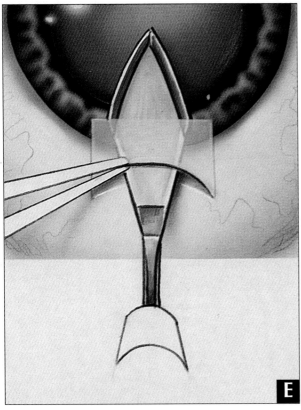 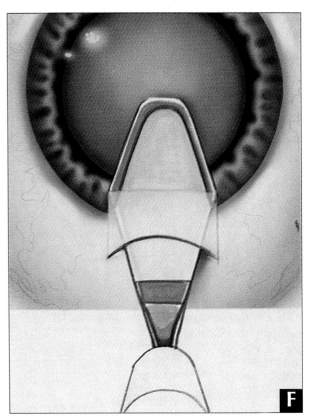

Figure 3-4E. The penetration in the chamber is done with a blade which provides the exact width of the opening ideal for the U/S tip. The penetration in the chamber occurs by directing the tip toward the anterior pole of the lens.

Figure 3-4F. Once I/A has been completed and VES has been injected, the incision is extended for IOL implantation

| Table 3-6 |  |
|---|---|
| **CORNEAL TUNNEL: EQUIPMENT AND TECHNIQUE BY BURATTO** | |
| **Instruments** | |
| Vertical preincision | Microknife with 30° blade (Alcon 5481). |
| Performance of intra-corneal delamination | Disk microknife (Alcon 6816). |
| Cutting lateral incisions | Microknife with 30° blade (Alcon 5481). |
| Entrance in the anterior chamber and incision for phaco (inside incision) | Angled 3.2 mm lancet microknife (Alcon 5485) or glazed (Alcon 93261). |
| Widening the incision to implant an AcrySof | Angled, glazed precalibrated 4.1 microknife (Alcon 64061). |
| **Technique** | |
| Vertical incision | Half thickness (250-350 μm) for 4.0-4.2 mm. Anteriorly to the vascular arcades. Temporal position (outer incision). |
| Formation of the tunnel | With the disc microknife the corneal tissue is cut—delaminated parallel to the epithelium in the depth of the preincision. |
| Lateral incision | One or two lateral openings parallel to the iris plane. Incision of about 1.2 mm inside and 1.7 mm outside. Lateral incisions are 70-80° separate from the main opening. One is on left and the other on the right of the main incision. |
| Viscoelastic | Injection of Provisc in anterior chamber. |
| Internal main incision | The 3.2 mm blade is introduced into the tunnel. The tip directed toward the lens anterior pole while the back is lifted (indentation). Penetration in the chamber is performed for the whole width of the blade. |

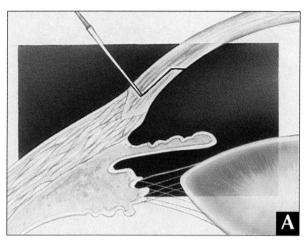

Figure 3-5A. Corneal tunnel incision with a metal blade. Drawing of the corneal tunnel incision.

consequence on the stability, hydrodynamics, and the possibility of maintaining suitable anatomical spaces.

When special techniques are used or when the I/A of the cortex is done with two separate handles, a second side port incision is performed on the opposite side to the first, both equidistant from the main incision.

## CONCLUSION

In the sutureless cataract operation, particularly if the aperture is wide, by the end of the operation the situation should be:
- Self-sealing (ie, there should be no aqueous loss or entrance of liquid or material from the outside). This can be controlled by exerting scleral pressure first posteriorly and then anteriorly from the incision with physiological ocular tone (a surgical sponge is used for this procedure).
- Absence of a postoperative opening aperture to the incision. In order to achieve this, the surfaces of the tunnel must be well-cut. Good rapid healing depends largely on a good matching of the edges.
- Absence of against-the-rule astigmatism. The position of the incision and the length and width of the tunnel are important in this case.

Generally speaking, when compared to other operations with wider apertures, small incision cataract surgery has a number of advantages. They are:
- Induction of less astigmatism.
- Quicker visual rehabilitation.
- Faster physical recovery for the patient.
- Fewer local disturbances.
- Faster local healing.
- Reduction of postoperative inflammation.

Take a look at these statements one by one.

### Induction of Less Astigmatism

Small incisions result in a reduction in the final astigmatism and less precocious astigmatism. Any astigmatism induced stabilizes more rapidly and is less likely to undergo late variations.

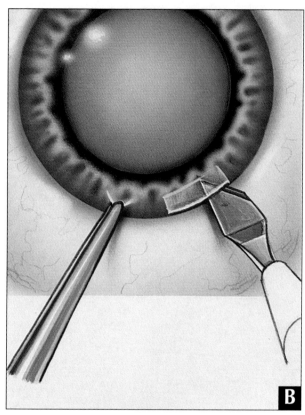

Figure 3-5B. Vertical incision with a 30° to half the corneal depth and for the extension planned for the IOL implantation.

In general, the amount of astigmatism induced by a cataract operation is dependent on a number of factors—the type, length, and site of the incision, the technique used, the suture material, etc. If all these factors are equal, the smaller the incision, the smaller the amount of induced postoperative astigmatism.

In addition, the smaller the incision, the greater the stability of the eye and the lower the shift toward against-the-rule astigmatism, all other conditions being equal (assuming that the incision is superior).

In the sutureless tunnel incisions, the induced astigmatism also tends to be greater when the incision is more advanced. In the event of posterior apertures (ie, scleral), the corneal variations induced are reduced and in this case depend on the width of the incision. If the surgeon increases the width of the incision, its position must be shifted proportionally posteriorly if he or she wishes to maintain the same variation of the corneal astigmatism.

### Quicker Visual Rehabilitation

Even though the visual result with the techniques that necessitate a wide incision are the same at the end of the healing processes and the stabilization of the suture, the time span between the operation and complete functional rehabilitation is important. The speed at which the patient visually recovers may be more important than previously thought. For example, in the elderly patients there is a significant correlation between visual disturbances and the

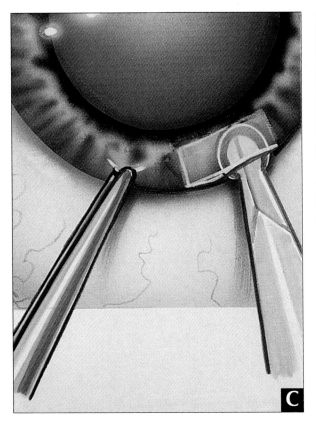

Figure 3-5C. Carving using a disk knife.

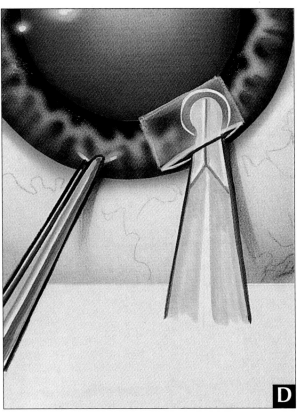

Figure 3-5D. Carving continues for the length of the tunnel.

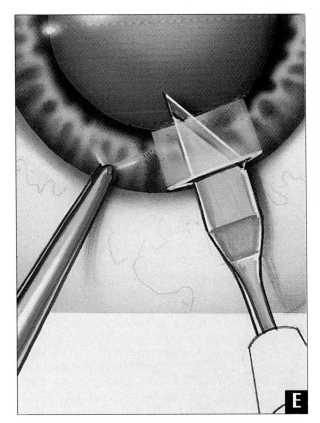

Figure 3-5E. Penetration in the chamber with a 30° blade (after the side port incision has been cut).

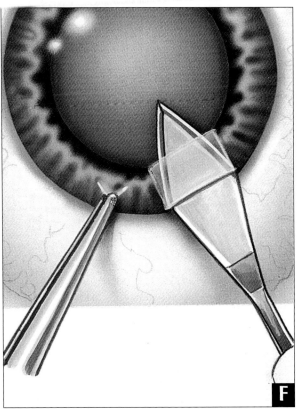

Figure 3-5F. Extension of the incision to a width suitable for phacoemulsification.

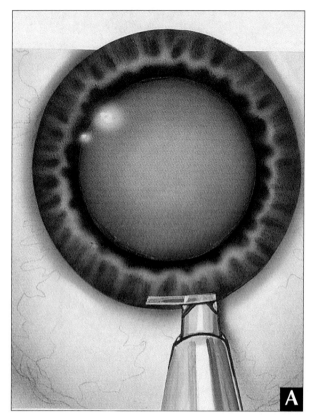

Figure 3-6A. Corneal tunnel with a diamond blade. Vertical 300 μm preincision with a preset diamond knife.

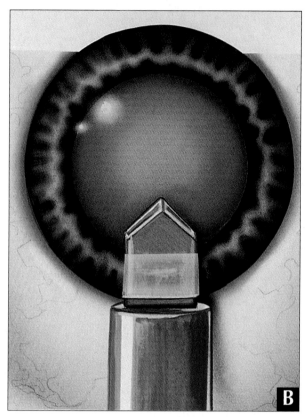

Figure 3-6B. The tunnel is cut with gradual and will-controlled progression of the blade. It proceeds parallel to the corneal surface for the entire length of the tunnel. Prior to entering the cornea, it is twisted to create the closure valve of the tunnel.

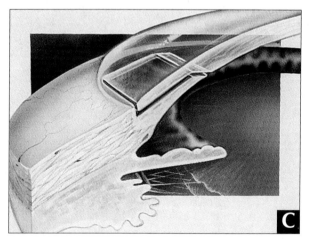

Figure 3-6C. The tunnel is cut with gradual and will-controlled progression of the blade. It proceeds parallel to the corneal surface for the entire length of the tunnel. Prior to entering the cornea, it is twisted to create the closure valve of the tunnel.

risk of fractures. The risk is particularly significant when there is poor vision in one eye and less so when the disorder is binocular and symmetrical. By the same measure, the risk is significant when there is poor stereoscopic vision.

Rapid functional recovery is naturally beneficial for the patients who have work commitments. For these patients, the fact that they can return to work just a few days after the operation with their usual workload is particularly advantageous both psychologically and economically. Also, patients who rely on a car for transportation find it extremely beneficial to drive again within a short space of time.

Generally speaking, the speed at which the patient recovers his or her visual function is tightly linked to the operation technique and particularly to the type and width of the incision and the type of suture applied. Because of the shape and the extension of the incision in sutureless cataract surgery, recovery is undoubtedly quicker than with all other previous techniques.

## Faster Physical Recovery for the Patient

The small incision, particularly if performed with a self-sealing tunnel, allows the patient greater freedom of physical activity as opposed to when there is a risk of rupture or the incision bursts. This is because the small size of the aperture minimizes the variations of the eyeball and restricts the areas of bulbar weakness. Moreover, the tunnel incision has greater resistance to the manipulations and the traumas compared to those with a sutured limbal or scleral incision.

## Fewer Local Disturbances

The application of one or more sutures is no problem for the surgeon, but it increases the local irritation for the

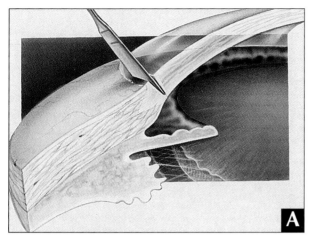

Figure 3-7A. Corneal tunnel with hinge. Vertical corneal incision to two-thirds of the depth.

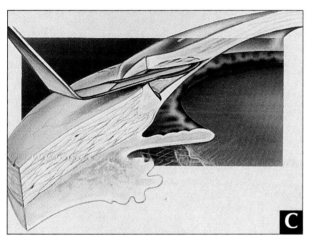

Figure 3-7C. Tunnel incision to one-half corneal depth for the entire length necessary.

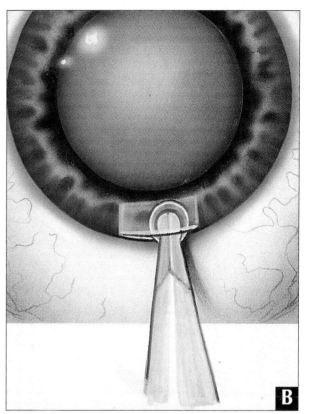

Figure 3-7B. Tunnel incision to one-half corneal depth for the entire length necessary.

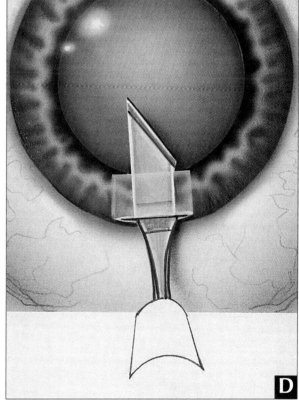

Figure 3-7D. Penetration in the chamber with the blade.

patient. It also involves the removal of the sutures in the postoperative period with consequent irritation for both the patient and possible refractive variations.

## Faster Local Healing

The tunnel incision heals faster and more permanently than a corneal or linear limbal incision because the contact surfaces are greater.

The healing surface of a linear incision is about 5.0 mm$^2$ (5.0 mm wide by 1.0 mm long). The healing surface in a scleral tunnel may be as much as 15.0 mm$^2$ (5.0 mm wide and 3.0 mm long).

This increase in healing surface confers mechanical properties to the cut area which makes the eyebulb very resistant even to postoperative trauma. This is very reassuring as it also supplies greater postoperative anatomical stability with minimal astigmatic variations and resulting rapid refractive stability.

## Reduced Postoperative Inflammation

According to recent studies, the width of the incision has a tight and direct correlation with the degree of post-

Table 3-7

## COMPARISON OF CORNEAL AND SCLERAL TUNNEL

|  | Corneal tunnel | Scleral tunnel |
|---|---|---|
| Anesthesia | Topical<br>Under Tenon's capsule | Under Tenon's capsule<br>Parabulbar<br>Retrobulbar<br>General |
| Conjunctiva | Intact | Open |
| Ability to work in the chamber | Very easy | More difficult |
| Visibility | Very good | Poor |
| Traction on the eyeball | Slight | Greater |
| Surgery time | Reduced | Longer |
| Endothelial damage | Greater | Lesser |
| Margin of error | Smaller | Greater |
| Type of nuclei | Not hard | Very hard |
| Difficulty in case of conversion | Relevant | Poor |
| Cost | Less expensive | More expensive |
| Ease of insertion for foldable IOL | Greater | Lesser |
| Ease of insertion for PMMA IOL | Lesser | Greater |
| Protection against infections | Lower | Higher |
| Foreign body sensation | Less intense | More intense |
| Cosmetic effect | Very good | Reddening |
| Induced astigmatism | More (with equal width) | Less |

Table 3-8

## LATERAL INCISION

| | |
|---|---|
| Site | 60-90° on the right or left of the main incision.<br>It can be single or double (one on each side with respect to the main incision).<br>Microknife with 22-5-30° angulation. |
| When | With the chamber still closed or with *suitable eyeball pressure*.<br>With the chamber open but with viscoelastic producing pressure. |
| Methods | Penetration in clear cornea, just in front of the limbal vessels.<br>Tangential incision of the iris. |
| Width | The external incision must be larger than the internal one to facilitate the introduction of the surgical tools (1.5-1.7 mm).<br>The width of the internal incision depends on what the surgeon requires, generally 1.0-1.2 mm is sufficient.<br>Learn to assess the width of the incision, particularly that of the outside cut, based on the width and length of the blade. |
| Objective | Insert the rhexis cystotome.<br>Insert the viscoelastic cannula.<br>Insert the cannula to inject BSS.<br>Insert the spatula for nucleus or IOL.<br>Insert the I/A cannula (in the two-handed technique). |
| Suturing | When performed correctly, the incision is self-healing.<br>If sutures must be applied use nylon 10-0. |
| Faults | Narrow—difficult to insert instruments.<br>Wide—fluid leakage, iris prolapse; suturing is required.<br>Too superficial—corneal folds.<br>Too deep—contact with the iris.<br>Poor positioning—uncomfortable working.<br>Too anterior—corneal folds.<br>Too posterior—iris trauma, iris prolapse. |

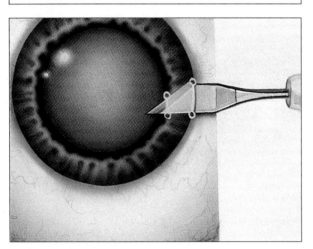

Figure 3-8. Side port incision—The 30° blade gives the right width of the external and internal incision. The incision must be parallel to the iris plane and must begin in transparent cornea at the end of the corneal vessels.

operative inflammation. This applies particularly in the first postoperative week. Being able to reduce the incision size has a significant positive result on the reduction of postoperative inflammation.

Concluding sutureless cataract surgery undoubtedly has some advantages, but in order for it to produce good results it must be done through a small incision. At present, good results can be obtained quite easily through phacoemulsification followed by the insertion of foldable or compressible IOLs which can be introduced through an incision suitable for phacoemulsification or a slightly larger incision. It can be done just as well with tunnel incisions of 5.2 to 5.7 mm (suitable for the insertion of hard lenses of 5.0 and 5.5 mm, respectively). The situation gets more complicated when the incision for the lens insertion reaches 6.2 or 6.7 mm (for lenses of 6.0 and 6.5 mm).

# Chapter 4

# ANTERIOR CAPSULOTOMY

*Lucio Buratto, MD*

## INTRODUCTION

The shape and size of a capsulotomy varies on the basis of the technique planned and the type of intraocular lens (IOL) to be inserted. Considering the type of operation, the capsulotomy should be planned and performed to adapt and blend well with all the successive operating phases.

The anterior capsulotomy, in the phases prior to implantation, must allow safe phacoemulsification of the nucleus and the complete aspiration of the cortex.

Another objective of capsulotomy is to leave enough lens capsule to allow safe IOL implantation in the capsular bag.

There are five common variations of capsulotomy:
- Can opener.
- Postage stamp.
- Christmas tree.
- Envelope.
- Continuous circular capsulotomy (CCC).

Two of these techniques are used frequently, the can-opener technique and the CCC, which is preferred for a number of reasons. However, there are pros and cons for each of these two methods.

## Can Opener Technique

The can opener capsulotomy introduced by Pearce in Great Britain in 1976 involves a series of incisions 360° around a diameter of 5 to 7 mm and the removal of the cut capsule. The main advantage of this capsulotomy, which was the most popular for many years, is the ease of execution.

The disadvantages are:
- Formation of radial fissures which tend to progress toward the equator.
- The possibility of bag rupture during the ultrasound (U/S) fragmentation.
- Difficulty in performing I/A because of the possibility of snagging the peripheral residual edges of the anterior capsule with the aspiration orifice.
- Difficulty in accessing the anterior edge of the bag during the insertion of the IOL particularly if there is an intraoperative reduction of mydriasis. This will leave the surgeon uncertain about the position of the IOL during the surgery and immediately postoperatively.
- Insufficient equatorial support for the loops. Because of postoperative capsular retraction, one loop will tend to escape with consequent decentering of the optical disc.
- Possibility of posterior irido-capsular synechia formation.
- Postoperative formation of traction lines through the adhesion of triangular flaps to the posterior capsule.

With this technique the capsulotomy consists of a series of small capsular openings which are very close together and which provide a wide regular opening that is free from any residual attachment bridges.

A cystotome can be made from a suitably bent disposable 25 G insulin needle.

The operation can be performed using various methods to fill the chamber.

## Features of a Good Cystotome

The cystotome must be sharp, which enables it to easily perform the capsular microperforation necessary to create the flap which is then used to perform a correct capsulorhexis.

The cystotome must have a lumen. This gives the operator the opportunity to introduce a saline solution or viscoelastic substance in the event the chamber flattens.

The cystotome must be small and not take up too much room. This allows the surgeon to maneuver the

Table 4-1
## CHRISTMAS TREE CAPSULOTOMY

| | |
|---|---|
| Instruments | Kelman's cystotome. |
| | Another needle bent at the tip. It is preferable if the shaft is large (23-21 G) and the tip is slightly blunt. |
| Incision | Anterior limbal. |
| | Width of about 1.0 mm. |
| Chamber | Shaped with air or BSS in the original technique. |
| | Provisc or Healon to modernize the technique. |
| Initial site | Draw point between the inferior and central thirds distally compared with the entrance point with the cystotome. |
| Method | Position of the cystotome. |
| | Slight pressure on the capsule. |
| | Controlled tearing of the capsule (as opposed to an incision). |
| | Pulling of the flap toward the incision. |
| | Extraction of the capsular flap with a cystotome or a McPherson forceps. |
| | Cutting the flap with straight Vannas scissors. |
| Completion | Two more triangular tear incisions (at 4 and 8 o'clock) to widen the opening. |
| Advantages | Simple and low cost. |
| | Provides a wide opening. |
| Disadvantages | In the attempts to luxate large hard nuclei in the anterior chamber there is a tendency to escape toward the equator, particularly if the Christmas tree capsulotomy is small (in the original technique). Capsular tearing is easy in the techniques in the posterior chamber. |

instrument easily in the anterior chamber. It gives the operator good visibility in the anterior chamber. As a result, each detail of the operation is observed better.

In addition, a fine cystotome must have a small entrance orifice so that it exerts minimal traction on the sclera and the cornea.

The cystotome must have an adjustable shape so that the instrument can be made to suit the specific needs of the surgeon. In some cases the operator must use a tip with a very short, acute angle. In other cases he or she may wish to use one that is more obtuse and longer. Under other conditions the surgeon may have to change according to the shape of the orbit so that he or she can work comfortably while keeping the cystotome in a comfortable position even in the event of very sunken bulbs or in patients with very prominent orbits.

It must be disposable and therefore changed for every operation. This guarantees sterility, proper hygiene, and the quality of the instrument.

It should be relatively cheap, which will contribute to reducing the running costs of the operation, and this makes it feasible to replace the instrument after every operation.

The cystotome must require little or no maintenance, which is only possible with disposable cystotomes. The reusable devices, even though they have a stronger tip, must be returned periodically to the manufacturer for sharpening. All of this is a waste of time—packing, dispatching, receiving, etc. The surgeon must have spares in perfect working order to cover this period of absence.

Cystotomes must be easy to obtain so the surgeon can guarantee that he or she has the right instrument at the right time. If the tip of an instrument breaks off or becomes blocked, it can be easily replaced with another.

In view of these facts, the insulin needle best satisfies these requisites when compared to the instruments available today. It is easy to obtain, it is sharp, the angulation can be changed when necessary, it does not require any maintenance, and it is cheap to buy. It is available in a range of lengths and thicknesses. The 25 G version combines a certain degree of elasticity with rigidity. The width and volume are limited and the insulin needle allows the surgeon to exert enough pressure on the corneal incision to penetrate the anterior chamber without having to perform any previous perforation.

## Technique with the Anterior Chamber Filled with VES

Through a 3.2 mm opening the chamber is uniformly filled with Provisc. The cystotome is then applied to the viscoelastic syringe.

The cystotome is inserted into the anterior chamber keeping the tip turned laterally. The insertion of the cystotome occurs by lifting the corneal edge of the incision with a forceps so that as it enters it does not tear Descemet's membrane, damage the endothelium, or tear the iris.

When the instrument is in the anterior chamber, the surgeon begins the capsular incisions.

The operator begins the capsulotomy in the superior quadrant with three to four centrifugal incisions between 11 and 1 o'clock. At this stage the surgeon pushes the cystotome further inside the anterior chamber and cuts the remaining 360° in a clockwise direction.

The surgeon must perform a large number of microincisions (at least 40 to 50) which are all very close to each other. This allows the surgeon to give the aperture a precise, regular shape, to reduce the size of the residual capsular flaps that remain in position and to exercise low-grade traction on the zonule.

The tip of the instrument has to perform a microperforation followed by a microaperture, ie, it has to perforate the capsule without penetrating the cortex or the nucleus.

The capsular openings must be very close together and very small so that only small-size flaps remain in their original position. Large fragments of capsule will interfere with the removal of the cortical material because they are easily trapped in the aspiration orifice and leave the residual capsule at a risk of tearing toward the equator.

Normally the surgeon starts cutting the capsule 1.5 to 2.0 mm inside the lens equator when the pupillary mydriasis allows him or her to see this boundary. In the event mydriasis is only moderate, the surgeon can use

Table 4-2
## CAN OPENER CAPSULOTOMY

| | |
|---|---|
| Instruments | Disposable cystotome obtained by bending the tip of an insulin needle (25-27-30 G). The tip is bent at an angle of 70-90° for a length of about 1.0.<br>Prepacked disposable cystotome (Alcon 4257). |
| Incision | Site—limbal or sclero-corneal or pure corneal.<br>Width—if VES used, incision of 3.2 for phaco. If BSS is used, the corneal wall is perforated with the cystotome to keep the chamber shaped. |
| Chamber | BSS.<br>VES—Healon GV, Healon, Provisc, Viscoat. |
| Site for beginning | The surgeon begins at 2 o'clock with a series of capsular incisions. |
| Method | The cystotome is introduced just inside the attachment point of the zonular fibers or about 3.5 mm from the center of the anterior capsule.<br>The tip of the cystotome is pushed slightly toward the capsule, and simultaneously, it is pulled gently toward the center (centripetal opening) or outward (centrifugal opening) creating a triangular opening with a base and height of about 1 mm.<br>About 30-40 incisions are performed in this way. |
| Capsular incisions | Very close to one another.<br>Around the entire circumference, prezonular.<br>The capsule opened in this way is detached from the various capsular points and the surgeon moves to the center of the lens surface. |
| Advantages | Allows an ideal wide capsulotomy for phaco both in the anterior chamber and the posterior chamber.<br>The opening is simple and safe.<br>It can be performed equally well with a chamber shaped by BSS or VES.<br>Aspiration of the cortex material is relatively easy. |
| Disadvantages | There is a certain frequency of radial openings starting from the apices (tips of the triangular openings).<br>Not suitable for the endocapsular techniques.<br>Capsular flaps can block the aspiration orifice during the I/A procedure.<br>The positioning of the IOL in the bag is often critical. With the postoperative phenomena of capsular retraction, one or both loops will tend to escape. A sulcus IOL is required even when the surgeon needs an implant in the bag. |

the point corresponding to the free edge of the iris as the incision site. In the event of poor mydriasis, the cystotome can penetrate slightly under the iris and the incision site is determined on the basis of the distance of the cystotome compared with the central limit of the iris in relation to the dimensions of the eye and the lens.

It is nevertheless important to avoid a capsulotomy that extends too far peripherally because this may encourage the progression of the aperture toward the equator or zonular tears.

The incisions of the capsule may be performed either in centrifugal or centripetal directions.

With centripetal incisions, the surgeon chooses the point he or she wishes to cut, the capsule is perforated, and then pulled gently toward the center of the anterior capsule to form a tiny triangular capsular flap. This method is easy, it has a low complication rate, and it can be applied to the majority of cases even when the pupil is poorly dilated. However, it has the disadvantage of unavoidable traction on the zonule.

In the centrifugal incisions, the surgeon chooses the point he or she wishes to cut, the capsule is perforated, and then the cystotome is moved toward the lens equator in order to create the aperture and the capsular flap. This technique is more difficult but it induces a lower degree of zonular traction.

However, if the surgeon's hand is delicate and if the instrument is sharp, there is no marked difference in trauma between the two techniques.

## Technique with the Chamber Filled with Balanced Salt Solution

During the capsulotomy, the depth of the anterior chamber can be maintained with irrigation of balanced salt solution (BSS). In this technique, in order to ensure maximum maintenance of the anterior chamber, the cystotome should penetrate the sclera-cornea with no preliminary aperture. The surgeon must therefore fine down the limbal wall with a preincision which involves three quarters of the thickness, and he or she must perforate the remaining tissue with the tip of the cystotome and penetrate directly to the anterior chamber.

This allows the surgeon to have a hole the same size as the needle shaft. This reduces liquid escape during the capsulotomy and maintains the volume of the anterior chamber at a constant level, with suitable irrigation if necessary.

In this technique, it is useful to use the cystotome connected to the phacoemulsification irrigation handle. This will provide a continuous or as-needed supply of saline solution to replace the aqueous humor that has escaped. With every amount of liquid loss, the surgeon can inject

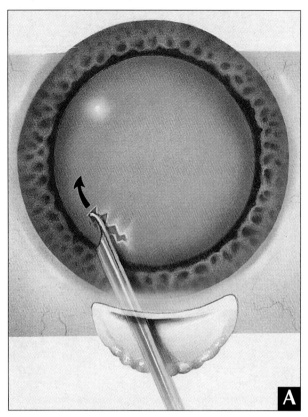

Figure 4-1A. Can opener capsulotomy. The irrigating cystotome, following the theoretical line just anterior to the insertion of the zonular fibers, rests on the capsule, perforates, and then tears it, creating a small triangular incision with an external point (if it is centripetal).

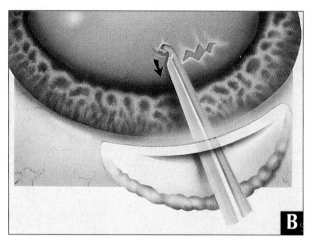

Figure 4-1B. If the action of the cystotome is centrifugal, the point will be internal (closeup).

saline into the anterior chamber without having to interrupt the operation or change the position of his or her hands. He or she simply moves the foot pedal into Position 1 and opens the valve to allow the flow of saline.

It is possible to regulate the irrigation flow within certain limits by changing the height of the bottle containing the saline solution. This may be very useful in view of the fact that some bulbs require just moderate irrigation to maintain the chamber at a constant depth whereas other bulbs need a more consistent degree of irrigation.

With the phacoemulsification irrigation handle, irrigation does not depend on the operator's hands. This allows the surgeon to use both hands in the movements of support and manipulation of the handle giving him or her a greater safety margin and freedom of movement.

The irrigation handle of the instruments is designed to provide a comfortable, easy grip. It is free from any protuberances that may interfere with the rotation which is often necessary during capsulotomy. It facilitates the surgeon's maneuvers. However, other supports for the cystotome—the syringe and the free outflow—are not so manageable.

The capsulotomy then continues with the technique we have just described.

## CAPSULORHEXIS

On the basis of what we just discussed, the can opener technique of capsulotomy sometimes cannot guarantee a safe implant of the IOL in the bag. The technique needed to be improved, ie, the surgeons had to find an opening that allowed them to position the IOL firmly inside the capsular bag. The only technique available at the moment that satisfies these requisites is capsulorhexis.

In 1984, this surgical technique was presented for the first time by Gimbel in North America with the name *continuous tear capsulotomy*, and had an almost simultaneous European development with Neuhann in Germany in 1985 who called it *circular capsulorhexis*. The Asian surgeon Shimizu called it *circular capsulotomy* in 1986.

The technique can be performed by a variety of methods which all give the same result. It involves a continuous, symmetrical linear opening of the anterior capsule. Capsulorhexis must satisfy some important requirements which condition the evolution of the entire operation and even the postoperative outcome, though to a lesser degree it must also have the following:

- Width—The aperture must be wide enough to allow easy emulsification of the nucleus. A large capsular aperture also makes it easy and quick to aspirate all the cortical material and completely clean the lens bag.

The capsulectomy must be sufficiently narrow to prevent the nucleus prolapsing in the anterior chamber during hydrodissection. This would mean that the surgeon would have to perform the phacoemulsification in the anterior chamber. A narrow capsulotomy will ensure that the loops of the IOL (and the lens itself) will stay inside the capsular bag. Between 5.0 and 5.5 mm is about the right size.

- Shape—As mother nature gave the principle structures of the eye a circular shape—and this includes the human lens and the pupil—and also because the optical part of the IOL is circular, the ideal situation is to have a round capsular opening.

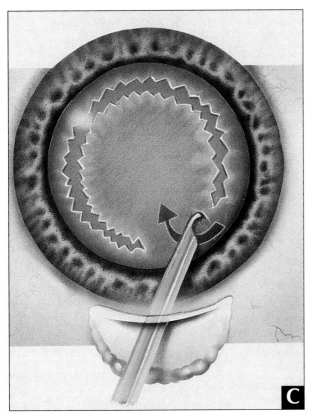 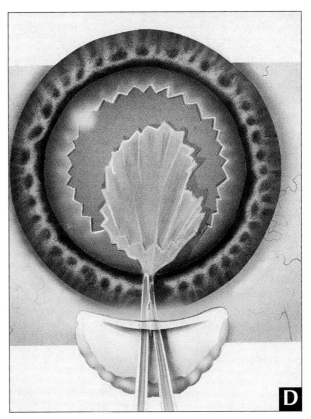

Figure 4-1C. The maneuver is done on the whole preequatorial anterior capsule with 30-40 incisions. The larger the number of capsular openings performed, the more uniform, accurate, and controlled the opening will be.

Figure 4-1D. Once the capsulotomy has been completed, the capsule is caught by a McPherson forceps and extracted. This maneuver will also allow the surgeon to check that all the capsular bridges have been removed. If any remain they could upset the successive phase of the operation.

- Continuous margin—an opening with continuous linear margins has a number of advantages:
1. The edges of the incision are strong and elastic and thus considerably reduce the risk of capsular rupture which extend toward the periphery. Every manipulation inside the capsular bag is therefore safer and easier so the techniques of endocapsular phacoemulsification can be performed.
2. The insertion of the artificial lens inside the bag is easier because the visualization of the capsule is better. In addition, the lens takes up a stable position inside the capsular bag and will not be subject to luxation.
3. The capsular bag will not tend to distort under the effect of postoperative capsular retractions.
    - Site—For optical and functional reasons, the capsulectomy must be centered on the pupil and the lens equator. This favors a homogenous distribution of the forces inside the sheath and therefore better centering of the IOL which can rest uniformly on the equator of the capsular bag.

Good centering of the rhexis will allow the surgeon to have a good view of the fundus and reduces the possibility of irido-capsular synechia formation. It also lays down the foundation for excellent functional recovery.

- Integrity of the zonules—The capsulectomy should leave the zonular fibers intact if possible, so it should be performed carefully in the equatorial and pre-equatorial zones to avoid damage to the peripheral or semiperipheral fibers. However, it should be remembered that following the central capsulectomy, the action of the zonular fibers changes.
- Suitability for IOL implantation—The capsulectomy must adapt to the IOL that will be inserted so it must have a shape suitable for the lens that the surgeon intends to implant. In view of the huge range of IOLs available today, the surgeon must first choose the lens and then perform the capsular opening to suit the planned insertion.

## Instruments for Capsulorhexis

The circular capsulotomy can be performed using different instruments—a cystotome or forceps for example. The majority of surgeons use just one instrument, but others may use two in succession. The anterior chamber can be formed using BSS or a VES, which is currently the more popular technique.

The cystotome can be:
- Reusable.
- Prepacked disposable.
- Modified disposable needles.

The advantages and disadvantages of each have been described in a previous chapter.

| Table 4-3 |
|---|
| **FOURTEEN RULES OF CAPSULORHEXIS** |
| 1. Always keep the anterior chamber well-filled to maintain its shape. |
| 2. Use high magnification during the operation. |
| 3. Look for the best red reflex. |
| 4. Use high molecular weight viscoelastic (Healon GV, Healon, Provisc). |
| 5. Operate slowly and carefully. |
| 6. Start in the middle with the formation of the flap and continue under the tunnel and then on the remaining 360°. |
| 7. Complete the rhexis from outside rather than inside the initial incision. |
| 8. Repeat capsular grasping several times (at least four times, but six or eight times would be better), which means opening by sectors. |
| 9. Keep the opening within the limit of the zonular fibers. |
| 10. A small rhexis is easier to perform than a large one. |
| 11. A small rhexis can be widened at the end of implantation, whereas a large one will tend to escape. |
| 12. An irregular rhexis is better than one with a tendency to escape. |
| 13. Should the smallest sign of escape appear, use viscoelastic with high molecular weight to reform the chamber. |
| 14. If problems appear, convert to a different technique to reduce complications. |

The forceps can be:
- Pointed or blunt with converging arms.
- Coaxial.

The viscoelastic substances can be high or low molecular weight, with high or low cohesion.

A number of rhexis techniques exist depending on which instrument is chosen and which substance is used to form the chamber.

## The Capsulorhexis Forceps

The forceps must have fine, strong arms. It must be in a non-reflecting material that avoids glare. The endings must allow a firm hold on the tissue without the arms coming into contact; this will avoid snagging the iris.

There are two capsulorhexis forceps available on the market at the moment:
- Forceps with opposed arms—Some are blunt and therefore not suitable for perforating the capsule (Buratto's forceps). The surgeon must use a cystotome to create a triangular capsular flap which is then caught by the forceps and the rhexis is completed.

Other forceps are pointed and can open the anterior capsule (Utrata, Gimbel, Shimizu, Corydon, Buratto).
- Coaxial forceps (Caporossi, Dossi)—These are fitted with blunted arms which require the additional use of the cystotome.

# Technique with the Cystotome and Viscoelastic

The viscoelastic substance makes the technique of capsulorhexis safer, easier to control, more precise, and simpler. It should therefore be used in routine surgery.

The surgeon should proceed as follows. A cannula is introduced through a side port incision or through the main incision and the aqueous is replaced with Provisc or Viscoat. The chamber is completely filled with the product leaving no residual bubbles of air or aqueous; the chamber depth must be slightly greater than the physiological depth to allow better control of the rhexis. The cystotome is attached to the viscoelastic syringe and the surgeon then proceeds with the capsulotomy. Generally, the procedure is simple because the guide flap is kept still and attached to the underlying capsule by the viscoelastic substance so manipulation with the instrument is relatively easy. The progression of the opening is well-controlled and therefore very safe.

The chamber depth is constant during the entire procedure so there is a lower tendency of uncontrolled escape of the rhexis.

## The Technique

The needle is placed on the anterior capsule at the center of the lens. The surgeon pulls slightly in the direction of the needled entrance point without perforating in order to create a small triangular capsular opening (guide flap). The flap is folded back on itself allowing the tip of the needle to rest on top of it and to guide the aperture with small, repeated tears.

The initial aperture is extended about 2 to 3 mm. Then the surgeon begins the clockwise rotation of the cut capsule toward the 6 o'clock position. The tip of the cystotome pushes the capsular flap gently toward the underlying anterior capsule and performs a circular pull and tear movement in a clockwise direction.

The position of the needle must be changed frequently and always applied to the flap that has already been torn and folded back over the area remaining to be torn. The pressure must be not be excessive, just enough to cause the tear. Excessive pressure will result in perforation or laceration of the underlying capsule and a loss of control of the aperture. Moreover, cortical material will be mobilized which can interfere with the surgeon's view and perception of the red reflex of the fundus. In the final analysis it may affect the end result of the entire operation.

The pressure from the needle must be directed at an angulation of 40 to 50° centrally to the desired direction of the aperture. If the needle is pushed in the direction of the aperture, it will extend toward the periphery with the risk of extending toward the equator. If it extends under the iris and the surgeon loses control of the aperture, he or she must interrupt the operation and convert the technique. The surgeon must inject more VES and continue the procedure with forceps.

In order to perform a continuous smooth capsulorhexis, it is necessary to:
- Limit the extension of the capsular incision within the attachment points of the zonular fibers.

Table 4-4
## CAPSULORHEXIS

| Tool | Cystotome | Forceps |
|---|---|---|
| Incision | Corneal or scleral tunnel. | Corneal or scleral tunnel. |
| Contents of the chamber | Viscoelastic, BSS, or air. | High molecular weight viscoelastic (Healon GV, Healon, Provisc). |
| Instrument | Cystotome. | Preventive opening of the capsule with the cystotome and then use of bevel forceps on both, using sharp-tip forceps. |
| Starting technique | Formation of capsular flap. | Formation of a flap ending in a point. |
| Continuing technique | The flap is laid on the underlying capsule. Quadrant after quadrant controlled tearing of the capsule is performed. | The flap is grasped by the forceps near the opening and torn, sector after sector, always keeping the opening within the planned diameter. |
| Indications | Simple cases. | All cases, and in particular: Miosis. Intumescent cataracts. Congenital cataracts. Tendency to escape. |
| Advantages | It can be performed without viscoelastic. | It provides better control of the opening. Difficult situations can be handled. |
| Drawbacks | Difficult control of the opening. | Viscoelastic required. |
| In case of escape or difficulty | Replace BSS or air with Provisc. Continue with the forceps. | Inject more viscoelastic. Continue with the forceps. |

- Always catch the mobile flap above and close to the point of join of the residual capsule.
- Proceed sector-by-sector, ie, tear less than one quadrant of the capsule, then reposition the needle point above the mobile flap.
- Avoid mobilizing the underlying cortex.

The cut capsule must be completely detached (360°) from the peripheral capsule. Ideally, closure of the capsulorhexis should occur from the outside to the inside (ie, with a greater radius compared with the remaining aperture).

The more circular the capsulorhexis and the more centered it is on the pupil, the better the result. However, an oval, slightly decentered opening can produce satisfactory results as long as the capsulorhexis is continuous and free from any escape points toward the equator.

The use of viscoelastic substance is advisable particularly for those surgeons who are approaching rhexis for the first time. However, it is indispensable when operating on very young patients, in patients with a shallow chamber, in poorly dilated or miotic pupils, or in cases where there is vitreous pressure.

It is also necessary if the surgeon wishes to operate under safe conditions because its use reduces the damage to the endothelium and the iris.

### Variations of the Technique

#### First
With the cystotome curved at an angle of about 90° about 1.0 mm from the tip, the surgeon performs a capsular incision at the 6 o'clock position in the middle third of the sheath. The instrument is moved laterally. The capsular opening proceeds in a counterclockwise direction toward the 3 o'clock position, leaving a stabilizing bridge between 2 and 3 o'clock. The cystotome is then positioned at the apex of the initial opening and the tear is directed in a clockwise direction toward 9 o'clock and then proceeds to reach the previous opening. At the end of the procedure the stabilizing bridge is detached.

#### Second
The capsular opening is done at the 2.30 position in the middle third. With the cystotome hook, the aperture is extended toward the 12 o'clock position. The tip of the cystotome is used to engage and guide the capsular flap that is being created without perforating, pushing it toward the 6 o'clock position in a counter clockwise direction. The opening is then directed to obtain an all-round tear (360°).

The stabilizing bridge at the 3 o'clock position is then torn.

#### Third
The surgeon performs the capsular incision at the 12 o'clock position about 2.5 to 3.0 mm from the center of the capsule. The initial incision is then pulled laterally with an arch-shaped movement. Normally the surgeon proceeds in a clockwise direction, repeatedly engaging the capsular flap.

The surgeon continues with the needle as close as possible to the limits of the aperture under the capsule using a combined action. He lifts the edge and pushes it forward in the direction desired. The surgeon then cuts the second flap, again starting from the first perforation, in a counterclockwise direction. The two flaps meet at 6 o'clock.

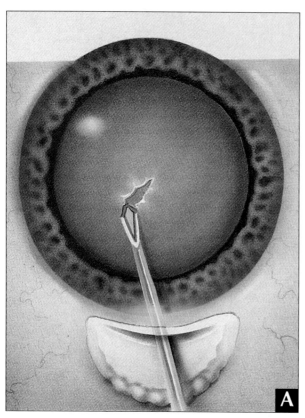

Figure 4-2A. Capsulorhexis with the cystotome. The cystotome with a very sharp cutting tip is brought to rest at the center of the capsule and performs a small radial opening. This must extend toward the outside to where the rhexis will be extended.

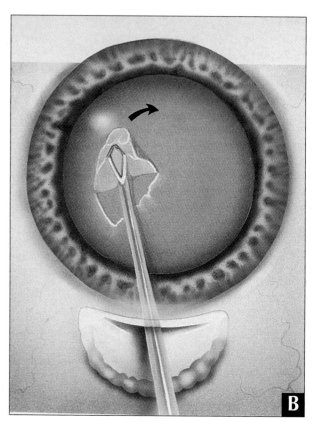

Figure 4-2B. The cystotome is inserted just below the capsule, and raising it performs a small capsular flap. The cystotome is then placed above the flap and directs the flap in relation to the desired diameter of the rhexis. It is always better to use the cystotome to draw a theoretical circumference of at least 1.0 mm less than the desired width of the rhexis.

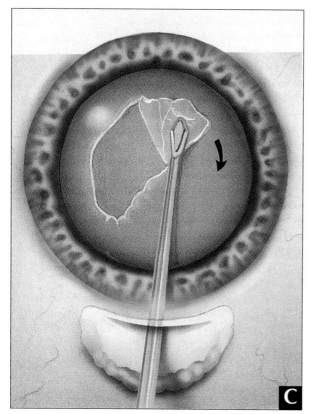

Figure 4-2C. The cystotome is repositioned at least five to six times (above the flap, near the end of the previous sector). In this way, the flap can be guided well and the surgeon can control the behavior of the opening. Positioning the cystotome above the flap, the surgeon must perform the action without perforating the flap itself (or the underlying anterior capsule).

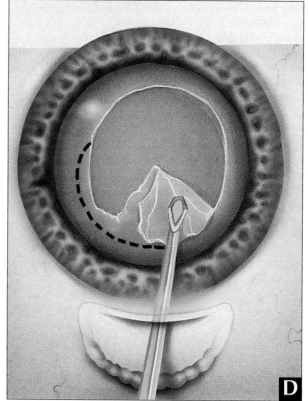

Figure 4-2D. The tear should ideally close outside the theoretical line (so it is better to keep the beginning of the tear narrow as it is only too easy to widen out in the final stages).

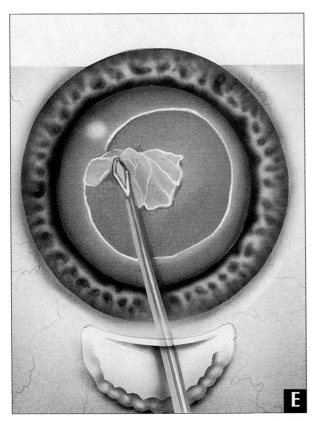 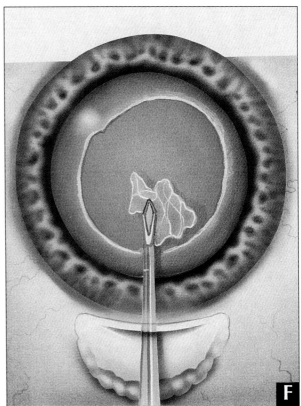

Figure 4-2E. Just before the rhexis is completed, it is possible that the opening will tend to widen (through reduction of the chamber, reduction of the control exerted when the cystotome is working close to the corneal incision).

Figure 4-2F. The capsule is gathered in the center. It is then extracted with a forceps or aspirated with the U/S tip.

### *Technique Using BSS*

The cystotome is applied to the irrigation handle of the instrument. Some drops of BSS are allowed to flow to remove any air from the circuit. In this case the eye has been prepared with a superior limbal preincision, and the chamber has not been opened.

The surgeon lifts the sclero-corneal flap with a Bonn forceps held in his or her left hand. The right hand is used to push the cystotome into the anterior chamber in the region of the 11 o'clock position. As the chamber is opened with the cystotome the entrance orifice is automatically obstructed by the needle shaft so its internal volume can be easily maintained with BSS irrigation alone.

The surgeon then continues with a continuous circular incision, similar to the one previously described.

Capsulorhexis with irrigation generally allows excellent visibility. However, the flow of the saline solution may create movement of the anterior capsular flap and therefore control may be difficult. A secondary miotizing effect may sometimes be produced.

## Capsulorhexis Under Air with the Cystotome

This technique involves inflating the anterior chamber with air once all the aqueous humor has been removed. The amount of air introduced must only slightly increase the physiological depth of the chamber. It should be introduced gradually to ensure the complete removal of the aqueous.

If air escapes during the operation, the surgeon must replace it to avoid abnormal contacts between the structures or an incorrect progression of the aperture.

The capsulotomy can be performed with the same cystotome and a similar technique to the ones described previously. Ideally the surgeon should begin at the anterior apex of the cataract and cut a triangular capsular flap. In a second phase, the capsular tear is completed for the 360°.

Air is used in capsulorhexis to provide the surgeon with a clear view of the zonular fibers and where they are attached to the capsule. However, it is also used to keep the capsule in position during the incision thus preventing it from rolling around freely in the anterior chamber making the entire procedure more difficult.

It gives the surgeon a clear view particularly in those cases where there is poor or no red reflex of the fundus in black or over-mature cataracts. In the latter, air also reduces the cloudiness in the anterior chamber which appears when the capsule is perforated and is due to escape of a milky liquid from the capsular sheath.

## Capsulorhexis with Forceps and VES

A high molecular weight VES is needed when forceps are used.

Low molecular weight VES will tend to escape during the maneuvers in the anterior chamber even though the arms of the forceps largely obstruct the aperture. The loss of VES causes a reduction in the depth of the anterior chamber, facilitates an upward movement of the lens, and puts the zonular fibers under tension making the correct completion of the operation much more complicated.

### *Technique with Buratto's Blunt Forceps with Opposed Arms*

The surgeon performs a 3.2 mm sclero-corneal opening and fills the anterior chamber with Provisc. A cystotome is used to create a triangular capsular opening with the formation of a mobile triangular flap. The flap must be large enough to be caught by the forceps. The capsulorhexis forceps then catch the base of the capsular flap and rotate it for one quadrant in a clockwise direction, keeping the progression of the aperture well under control.

The forceps then release their hold on the flap and catch it again at the base. The maneuver is repeated two to three times. The capsulorhexis is then completed with no points of capsular escape. The capsule is then extracted.

It may happen that during the progression of the aperture some substance will escape and the chamber will tend to flatten. If the aperture is well-controlled the surgeon can continue. If the opening tends to move toward the equator, the surgeon should inject some more Provisc through the side port incision without removing the forceps from the chamber.

### *Technique Using Buratto's Pointed Forceps with Opposed Arms*

The surgeon performs a 3.2 mm incision (with a calibrated blade, ideal for creating the right incision for phacoemulsification and the correct penetration of the forceps) and enters the chamber with the forceps arms closed. The chamber is shaped with high molecular weight viscoelastic substance. The tips rest perpendicularly on the center of the capsule. They are opened and then closed, catching the capsule which tears under the effect of the perforation and tearing movement. A flap is created which is then used in the rhexis, as described previously.

In the forceps technique, the progression of the capsulotomy under the incision is a particularly delicate phase. The width of the forceps arms and the variation in transparency of the tissues induced in the tunnel restricts visibility considerably. The surgeon must tilt the forceps laterally raising the flap and bringing it toward the center of the pupillary field to get a better view of the capsulotomy edge.

### *Forceps or Cystotome for the Capsulorhexis*

The choice of a technique with a cystotome or forceps is very much a question of individual dexterity. Nevertheless surgeons should learn both techniques as they each have specific applications in particular intraoperative conditions.

The technique using the cystotome is preferable when a viscoelastic substance is not available or when the available VES has a low molecular weight.

The forceps technique is preferable if the surgeon has a high molecular weight VES available. This technique should also be used in the more difficult cases (narrow pupil, intumescent cataract, etc). The technique using forceps is also more suitable for surgeons with a low work-load.

It is also the preferred technique of the experts because it is the simplest, the safest, and the fastest. It also allows surgeons to perform an excellent rhexis in the vast majority of cases.

## Principles of Capsulotomy

How the anterior capsule of the lens is removed has an important effect on the successive phacoemulsification. If it is removed correctly, it will have a positive effect on all the subsequent phases of the operation. If removal is inaccurate, the steps that follow will be consequently more difficult.

Before beginning the operation, the surgeon should remember that every mistake made during capsulotomy will be carried through to the subsequent phases. So it is of the utmost importance that the surgeon pays maximum attention to even the smallest details.

The operator must use high microscope magnification. This allows the operator to control every step of the procedure, to adjust the site and width of the incision where necessary, and to avoid unnecessary traction forces, etc.

The light beam must be angled to provide a good red reflex of the fundus (when the density or consistency of the cataract permits). This facilitates the detailed perception of the capsular incision.

The luminosity must be sufficient to provide a clear view of the capsule.

The pupil must be in maximum mydriasis. Wide mydriasis makes it easier for the surgeon to perform the capsulotomy. The surgeon can make it wider and shape it to suit his or her needs. So, contact between the cystotome and the iris (miotic stimuli) are avoided.

A wide pupil also facilitates the good red reflex of the fundus and therefore the surgeon has a better perception of the maneuvers necessary for completion of the capsulotomy.

The depth of the anterior chamber must be maintained during the entire capsulotomy. This simplifies penetration and the use of the cystotome or the forceps, and the movement for one sector to another, etc.

A deep chamber reduces the risk of abnormal contact with the endothelium and the iris. Above all, it prevents the upward movement of the lens toward the cornea and gives the surgeon better control of the capsulotomy procedure.

The high molecular weight viscoelastic substances are a valuable tool in maintaining the depth of the anterior chamber.

The capsular opening must respect the attachment of the zonular fibers. With a good red reflex of the fundus and a suitable microscopic magnification, the surgeon should be able to identify the insertion points of the fibers on the anterior capsule and begin the incision halfway between them. If this is not possible, the capsular aperture should not extend more than 3.0 mm peripherally from the center of the cataract's anterior pole.

The shape and size of the capsulotomy must take into account the phacoemulsification technique planned and the shape and size of the lens to be implanted, so prior to beginning the capsular aperture, the surgeon must have the surgical plan clear in his or her mind.

The entrance to the chamber must be studied carefully. It must not be excessively anterior or excessively posterior in the cornea. The entrance site must take into account the anatomical variations between individual globes (very deep chamber in severe myopia, greatly reduced spaces in elevated hyperopic, etc). It must be in an optimal working position with respect to the planes of the anterior capsule and the iris—this will have a positive effect on the outcome of the entire operation.

### *Correct Use of the Instrument*

During the corneal aperture, the surgeon's hands must be relaxed and must keep traction forces on the instrument entrance point to a minimum to restrict the formation of corneal folds. The forceps or the cystotome must be handled gently and carefully. They must be used on the surface with little pressure exerted on the crystalline mass.

The surgeon must also avoid any mechanical contact with the iris because each stimulus reduces the pupillary dilatation.

The surgeon must reduce manipulations and operating times. Good pupillary mydriasis will be maintained particularly if the surgeon works quickly.

The technique must be adapted to the type of capsule. The thickness and elasticity of the capsule changes with age and the type of cataract. In younger patients the capsule is thin and elastic and the capsulotomy tends to extend easily toward the equator. In the more elderly patients, the capsule is thicker, harder, and will often resist removal. The surgeon may have to use a different strength and a different removal method on the basis of the patient's age.

Even the state of greater (intumescent cataract) or lesser (shriveled cataract) tension of the capsule has a considerable influence on the capsular incision. When the lens is swollen the capsule is easier to open but it often happens that the shape and the extension of the capsulotomy slip out of the surgeon's control. In very advanced cataracts the capsule is thick and rigid making the incision difficult. So the surgeon often has to exert a considerable amount of traction on the capsule which can easily detach the zonular fibers (facilitated by the relaxed state of the fibers in these eyes). In these cases, it is often advisable to perform the capsular incision with scissors.

If any difficulties arise, the surgeon should stop what he or she is doing and fill the chamber with viscoelastic substance (or add additional material if it was previously injected). The VES will allow the surgeon to keep the spaces well-formed and contrast vitreous pressure or the formation of corneal folds. It also allows the operator a greater margin for maneuvers and errors.

### *Diameter of the Capsulorhexis*

The ideal diameter of capsulorhexis for phacoemulsification and the implantation in the sac of an IOL in polymethylmethacrylate (PMMA) is between 5.0 and 6.0 mm. If the rhexis is greater than 6.0 mm problems can arise as the operation can be difficult to control. Implantation of the IOL in the capsular bag can also be difficult, particularly if the pupil is narrow.

A small rhexis, though easier to perform, may cause difficulties in the successive phases of the operation, with undoubted problems with the endocapsular insertion of the IOL.

Moreover, it will be difficult to examine the fundus in the postoperative, the peripheral retina in particular. The anterior capsule that remains in its original position frequently becomes opaque blocking the vision.

Sometimes, in the postoperative period, the central edges of a small rhexis will close tightly like a sphincter because of fibrosis and capsular retraction. Sometimes, in the postoperative period, it is necessary to perform relaxing incisions with the YAG laser on the extremes of the central capsule to avoid excessive traction on the zonules.

After I/A if the surgeon realizes that the rhexis is too small for the implant, he or she must widen the opening as follows. The surgeon must inject abundant Provisc. Using curved microscissors, he or she should cut the capsular margin to create a new triangular tear or *dog ear* with a larger radius. Then with a capsulorhexis forceps, the surgeon should catch the flap and remove a portion of the anterior capsule between the primary rhexis and the attachment of the zonular fibers, if possible, a full 360°. If the opening is still not wide enough, the scissors are used to repeat the cut on the opposite side of the rhexis and the procedure is repeated.

## Advantages of Capsulorhexis

### *Intraoperative Advantages*

- The edges can be distorted during the operation. Thanks to its round shape and intrinsic structure, the capsule can be stretched considerably.
- A continual circular aperture limits the risk of tears or radial cracks which tend to extend toward the equator and toward the posterior capsule during the operation, particularly in younger patients. This usually happens during the phase of nuclear removal (phacoemulsification or nuclear expression), during I/A of the cortex material, and during insertion of the IOL.
- Hydrodissection is safe and allows the surgeon to perform the phacoemulsification with all the advantages this entails.
- It contributes to restricting the intraoperative turbulence inside the capsule.
- The intraoperative stress on the zonules is minimal and is distributed evenly over the equator.
- It allows easy aspiration of the cortex because it does not leave any gaping anterior capsular flaps that may occlude the aspiration orifice. In addition, the anterior capsule separates better from the posterior capsule. This makes it easier for the surgeon to enter the equatorial capsule to aspirate the more peripheral fragments. Finally, the edge of the rhexis is easily identified which makes the procedure safer and simpler.
- If the opening of the capsulorhexis is small, it can

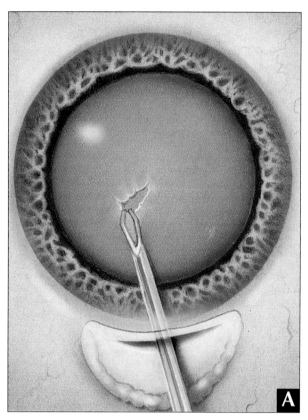

Figure 4-3A. Capsulorhexis with blunt-ended forceps. The capsule is opened at the center with the cystotome as described previously. A small flap is created in either a clockwise or counterclockwise direction.

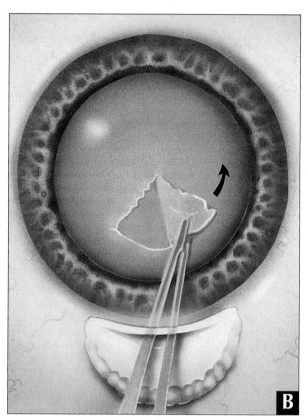

Figure 4-3B. The flap, which in this case has been created in a counterclockwise direction, is caught with forceps and pulled carefully to obtain a capsular tear along the desired circumference. The chamber must be shaped with VES of suitable molecular weight.

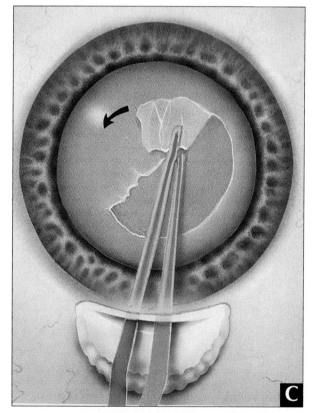

Figure 4-3C. As each sector is torn, the forceps are repositioned. One arm is placed on the internal face and the other on the external face of the anterior capsule. In order to have accurate and controlled action, the forceps must catch the flap as close to the opening point as possible (closer than shown in the drawing)

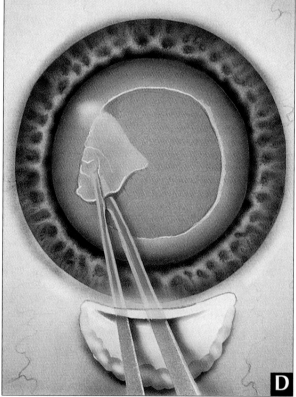

Figure 4-3D. Then the opening is controlled with a controlled tear which must not involve more than one-eighth to one-sixth of the planned width of the rhexis.

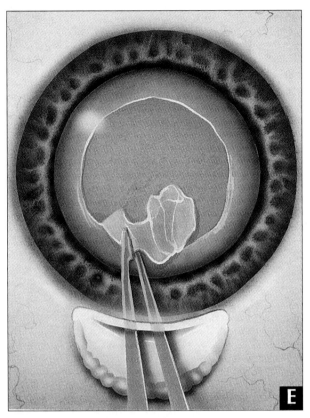

Figure 4-3E. The capsule has been released and is caught once again by the forceps to guide the final part of the capsulotomy.

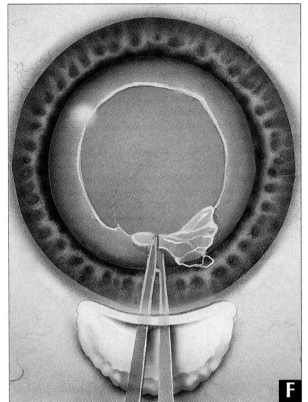

Figure 4-3F. The rhexis is loose and the capsule is extracted using forceps.

be extended to facilitate the insertion of the IOL and limit the amount of residual capsule which may become opaque and retract at a later stage.
- It permits the IOL to be positioned safely and symmetrically in the bag because the surgeon has an excellent view of the anterior capsular rim.

### *Postoperative Advantages*

The technique:
- Allows the uniform distribution of the forces within the capsular bag so that the IOL maintains its physiologic position and assumes a very stable position, protected from displacements and the effects of mechanical pressure.
- Produces an extensive contact area between the loop of the IOL and the anterior capsule which reduces the possibility of decentering.
- Ensures that there is no contact with the ciliary body. The possibility of iris contact, pigment dispersion, hyphema, and inflammation is reduced.

If the posterior capsule ruptures, the large anterior capsular flap supports the IOL and can be used to support the lens in the sulcus. In addition:
- There is no need for miotics.
- There is no need for an iridectomy.
- Pupillary capture is avoided.
- The risk of degradation of the loop material is reduced (if a three-piece lens is used).

- The implant is safer even when performed in children's eyes, and in eyes affected by anterior segment pathologies such as glaucoma, uveitis, etc (because of the excellent isolation of the IOL).

## Difficulties During Rhexis

### *Rhexis Escape*

In a certain number of cases, during capsulorhexis, the aperture opens excessively and progresses toward the equator. If this happens, the surgeon must ensure that the chamber is adequately deep. If not, he or she must inject a high molecular weight viscoelastic substance (or replace any that has escaped).

There are many techniques for recovering an escaping rhexis:
- If the escape occurs during a capsulotomy with BSS and a needle, the surgeon should inject Provisc and then continue with a forceps because this will guarantee a safer, firmer hold. In this case, the flap should be caught close to the split point in the capsule. The surgeon should then exert controlled pressure directed toward the center of the pupil.
- Another alternative is to fill the chamber with Provisc. Then using very curved microscissors cut the capsule right at the escape point to redirect the opening back to the initial route.
- Yet another solution involves starting a new rhexis

Table 4-5
## ADVANTAGES AND DRAWBACKS OF THE RHEXIS
### Advantages

| | |
|---|---|
| Deformable opening | Allows traction with U/S tip, spatulas, IOL, etc. |
| Resistant opening | Allows pressure to increase inside the bag with low risk of rupture (hydrodissection/hydrodelamination). |
| | Allows splitting of the nucleus in quadrants and/or maneuvers of nucleus fragmentation and/or Phaco Chop. |
| | Allow nucleus extraction in case of ECCE also when this slightly exceeds the rhexis diameter. |
| Suitable for IOL implantation | The CCC provides very good visibility during implantation. |
| | Allows self-centering of the IOL. |
| | Provides uniform distribution of IOL stretching forces. |
| | Allows IOL isolation from the other structures (iris, ciliary body, etc). |

### Drawbacks
Difficult to perform.
Opacification of part of capsule over the optic disc.
Difficult to examine retinal periphery.
Possible capsular block.
Possible shrinkage effect.

---

in another position working in a counterclockwise direction this time while attempting to join up with the first rhexis at the escape point.

- In the event that the aperture is blocked by one or more zonular fibers (either because these have a more central insertion or because the aperture is extended too close to the peripheral areas) and if these are visible, the surgeon can lacerate the two or three fibers involved using the cystotome and then continue as planned. This procedure must be done under very high magnification and the surgeon must limit the disinsertion of the fibers to a minimum; otherwise he or she risks weakening the zonular support of the bag in that area.
- The last alternative is to abandon the idea of a rhexis. In this case the surgeon can perform a can opener capsulotomy.

## Other Problems Related to the Rhexis

It can be difficult for the surgeon to:
- Obtain a capsular flap ideal for performing the procedure correctly.
- Guide the flap in a circular fashion. The greater the radius of the rhexis, the more difficult it will be to complete it correctly.
- Keep the limits of the capsular incision distant from the attachment point of the zonular fibers.
- Adapt the intraoperative behavior to the different consistency, elasticity, and thickness of the capsule.
- Remove the cortex in the sector adjacent to and beneath the incision when a coaxial I/A cannula is used.
- Completely clean the posterior capsule below the entrance point.

Sometimes the rhexis obtained will be too small. If that is the case, it may happen that the rhexis opens during emulsification, during the attempts of nucleofracture, or during the removal of the cortex. The surgeon will have to continue the procedure using special techniques (please refer to the specific chapter).

- If the rhexis is too large, it may facilitate luxation of the nucleus in the anterior chamber and make phacoemulsification and the insertion of the IOL in the capsular bag more difficult.
- If the capsulorhexis is grossly decentered, the IOL may become decentered in the postoperative because the capsular fibrosis shifts the lens toward the longest edge. If at all possible the surgeon should remove the excess capsule during the operation.

### Capsulorhexis in Special Cases
#### Newborn

In the newborn the capsulorhexis is performed in very small spaces. Moreover, the reduced scleral rigidity determines a certain tendency to positive vitreous pressure. This favors easy loss of control in the direction of the capsulotomy, with an increased risk of peripheral escape.

The high degree of elasticity of the capsule in infancy also contributes to this phenomenon.

For these reasons, the initial incision must be small. That way it is easier to control with forceps as opposed to the cystotome. Another important factor is the prompt availability of high molecular weight viscoelastic substance (Healon GV, Healon, Provisc).

## Pseudoexfoliation

In this case the capsule is relatively fragile so the capsulorhexis must be small and not reach the zonules or create traction forces.

If possible, it can be extended after the insertion of the IOL or some weeks after the operation with radial incisions using a YAG laser.

### *Over-Ripe or Intumescent Cataract*

In these cases, the lack of the red pupillary reflex makes the capsulorhexis extremely difficult because there is no perception of the capsular flap. In addition, the cataract is swollen, meaning that there is greater tension on the anterior capsule and a greater tendency to peripheral escape.

With the intumescent cataract, if the content is thought to be very liquid or milk-like, it is advisable to perform a central incision initially which will permit the escape of the semiliquid cortex. This can be removed with I/A, followed by further introduction of clean viscoelastic substance (Healon GV, Provisc, Healon).

However, if the intumescence is observed in an elderly patient where the nucleus is more likely to be hard and large and there is only a small amount of semiliquid material, it is wiser to proceed immediately using forceps. The preparation of the flap must be done under high magnification and with maximum illumination, taking care to keep the diameter of the capsulorhexis reasonably small.

The forceps allow good control of the aperture even in the absence of capsule visualization.

This precaution reduced the risk of capsulorhexis escape and does not jeopardize the possibility of widening the diameter of the capsulotomy at the end of the operation or in the postoperative period by YAG.

The surgeon may find it useful to turn off the light on the microscope and use a fiber optic to illuminate the capsule obliquely.

An alternative that should not be ignored is performing the capsulotomy under air, the presence of which prevents the escape of liquid material after the anterior capsule has been punctured by the cystotome. For the anterior chamber to remain well-formed by the air bubble, the capsulorhexis must be done using the cystotome. This increases the risk of escape of the edge toward the periphery, in that the maneuver is more difficult to control with forceps.

## Brunescent or Black Cataracts

Capsulorhexis can be difficult if there is no good red reflex of the fundus. The surgeon may find it useful to increase the magnification of the microscope and use a highly transparent viscoelastic substance. It is sometimes useful to illuminate the area with a fiber optic obliquely.

### *In Miotic Pupils*

The capsulorhexis can be performed blind, ie, without the surgeon being able to see what he or she is doing because the area is covered by the iris. Alternately, the pupil can be widened using one of the techniques described in another chapter.

## Posterior Capsulorhexis

This is a linear, continuous, circular capsulotomy that has all the intrinsic advantages of the anterior capsulorhexis, particularly where elasticity, stability, and long-term resistance are concerned.

This technique developed because there was a need to manage small-size posterior ruptures.

The technique consists of a small, continuous, circular opening (1.5 to 3.0 mm) performed using forceps after the capsular bag has been filled with viscoelastic substance.

The posterior rhexis can be decentered, in each of the quadrants of the posterior capsule, in line with the idea of keeping the zonular fibers intact.

The main indications for the posterior capsulorhexis are:
- Tears in the posterior capsule with or without vitreal prolapse.
- Central fibrotic opacity that requires surgical removal.
- Prevention of secondary capsular opacity.
- Removal of a portion of the posterior capsule for vitrectomy (particularly in children).

Tears in the posterior capsule are irregular and frequently tend to progress toward the equator with possible lysis of the zonules. This situation is suitable for correction with posterior capsulorhexis which optimizes the integrity of the residual capsule.

In the event of vitreous prolapse, a posterior rhexis is useful for a correct vitrectomy without having to widen the capsular opening. The vitreous is contained by a viscoelastic substance. The surgeon then performs the posterior rhexis followed by the vitrectomy.

This will allow safe implantation of an IOL in the bag without risking any progression of the posterior opening.

In cataract surgery in very young patients or in patients with congenital cataract, surgical removal of the posterior capsule can be used as prevention against fibrotic opacification, a frequent consequence of this operation. The frequency of central fibrotic opacity is extremely high in these cases and this technique can be used as an alternative to a secondary operation.

## CONCLUSION

The recently developed technique of CCC, an elective choice for many cataract surgeons, brings enormous advantages to cataract surgery. There is no question about the advantage of maintaining greater integrity of the capsule with a smooth, symmetrical, highly-resistant opening and these are the bases for the ideal situation for positioning an IOL in the capsular bag and its long-term stability.

These claims are supported by the positive results of many surgeons—despite the fact that many different techniques were used, the results were all astonishing.

Results of middle- and long-term follow-up have shown that the IOL implants in the posterior chamber have enjoyed a greater percentage of success with the technique of capsulorhexis combined with phacoemulsification. The higher percentage of optimal IOL centering proves that this technique offers a greater possibility of obtaining a stable implant in the capsular bag with the optical disc well-isolated and centered on the pupil.

# Chapter 5

# HYDRODISSECTION AND HYDRODELINEATION

*Lucio Buratto, MD*

## INTRODUCTION

Hydrodissection is an extremely important surgical step in the overall procedure of endocapsular phacoemulsification. It allows the surgeon to free the nucleus in the capsular bag. In addition to simplifying all the surgical maneuvers on the nucleus itself, it also prevents all the pressure exerted on the nucleus from being transferred to the capsule and zonular apparatus.

The possibility of facilitating the removal of the nucleus by injecting fluid between the lens planes was studied initially by surgeons who practiced the intercapsular techniques with a linear anterior capsulotomy (envelope). This maneuver used to be called hydrodelineation. It referred to the cleavage of the cortex and the nucleus, a maneuver useful to facilitate endocapsular mobilization and consequently the manual removal of the nucleus itself.

With the development of the techniques of capsulorhexis, the lenticular hydrodissection has become a fundamental step in all the techniques of endocapsular phacoemulsification.

There are numerous concepts of lenticular surgical anatomy that have significant practical importance, but they have also created an excess of terminology.

Even though we are still not in a position to adopt a universally accepted classification, we will try to present a general picture of what is referred to in the description of the phacoemulsification techniques.

## HYDRODELINEATION

According to Anis, this is the general term used to describe the cleavage of the lens structures through the injection of fluid, irrespective of the instrument used.

The term should be accompanied by indications as to

---

**Table 5-1**

### HYDRODISSECTION

**Hydrodissection is an important surgical step in endocapsular phacoemulsification**

Hydrodissection—Separation, by means of a fluid, of the nucleus from the external cortex adhering to the capsule.
Hydrodelamination—Separation of the central harder nucleus from the softer peripheral portion.

**Rules of hydrodissection to optimize the results**

The nucleus should be loosened as much as possible.
As much as possible of the capsule and external cortex should be detached from the inside contents.
The least amount of cortex should remain inside the bag.
The hydrodissection should be performed as quickly as possible.
A small amount of fluid should be used.
The number of fluid injections should be minimal.
The amount of time the cannula stays in the chamber should be as short as possible.

**Two techniques can be used**

A cannula mounted on a syringe (currently the most popular).
A specific instrument (Hydrosonic).

**Factors involved in hydrodissection**

1. Anterior chamber contents (BSS, Healon, Viscoat, etc.).
2. Type of syringe and cannula used.
3. Modality of BSS injection.
4. Fluid flow.
5. Site of fluid injection.
6. Diameter of the rhexis.
7. Type of nucleus.
8. Opening through which the cannula enters.

### Table 5-2
### HYDRODISSECTION AND CONTENTS OF THE ANTERIOR CHAMBER

The performance of hydrodissection varies depending on whether BSS or viscoelastic is used to fill the chamber. If the chamber is filled with viscoelastic, methods change depending on the properties of viscoelastic used. After injecting BSS, it is important to know whether or not it escapes, and if it does, from what leakage site (this is relevant, especially when BSS injection is made through the lateral incision).

| Saline solution | Viscoelastic material |
|---|---|
| BSS. | Healon GV. |
| | Healon. |
| | Provisc. |
| | Viscoat. |
| | Other materials. |

| Advantages of BSS | Advantages of viscoelastic |
|---|---|
| It leaves the chamber easily. | Eases introduction of the cannula in the chamber. |
| | Allows the cannula to find the right position for injection. |
| | Prevents the nucleus from luxating in the anterior chamber. |

| Drawbacks of BSS | Drawbacks of viscoelastic |
|---|---|
| The depth of the chamber tends to change easily. | If it remains in the chamber during injection there is risk of excessive deepening or stretching of the capsular bag. |
| The iris is stimulated to miosis. | If viscoelastic is very cohesive it will tend to exit in a lump. |
| The nucleus tends to luxate in the anterior chamber. | |

### Table 5-3
### SYRINGES AND CANNULAS FOR HYDRODISSECTION

| Syringe | Cannula |
|---|---|
| The right syringe: 3 mL size. The piston moves easily (best if made of glass). BSS filling 2-3 cc without air. Small, light and easy to handle. Luer-rock joint. | A large size (25 G) is preferable. Able to deliver large amount of BSS. With a flat end. With a flat hole. With a smooth tip. |
| The smaller the piston surface, the smaller the force required for pressing. The surgeon's sensitivity during injection is crucial. | The wider the diameter of the port, the greater the amount of fluid that can be injected. However, excessive injection should be avoided. |
| Fluid flow: The BSS flow depends on the pressure exerted on the piston as well as on the diameter and shape of the cannular lumen. | The cannula with small round hole: The fluid is injected in one spot only (localized flow). It tends to form a localized hydrodissection. Requires several injections in different sites. The cannula with wide flat hole: The fluid tends to produce a wide diffusion (laminar flow). |

### Table 5-4
### HYDRODISSECTION AND DIAMETER OF THE RHEXIS

| Small rhexis | Eases penetration and shifting of BSS into the bag. Eases separation of the nucleus from the external cortex. Keeps the nucleus inside the bag. |
|---|---|
| Large rhexis | Greater diffusion of BSS in the anterior chamber and poorer hydrodissection. Greater probability of nucleus luxation in the anterior chamber. Greater dispersion of cortex. |
| Open, escaped rhexis, or can opener capsulotomy | Avoid hydrodissection, or perform it very cautiously. There is risk of anterior luxation, as well as widening of the capsular opening. Risk of equatorial and posterior laceration of the capsule (risk of posterior nuclear luxation). |

### Table 5-5
### HYDRODISSECTION AND TYPE OF NUCLEUS

| Nuclei with 1-2-3a hardness with good red reflex | Easy hydrodissection. The diffusion wave is visible. Safe procedure. |
|---|---|
| Nuclei with 3b-4 hardness | The diffusion wave is not visible. Poor control by the surgeon. |

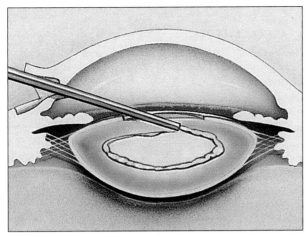

Figure 5-1. Hydrodelineation—The cannula is inserted into the cortex and then into the epinucleus. When the surgeon meets any difficulties in progressing, he or she injects BSS separating the hard core from the softer nucleus or epinucleus.

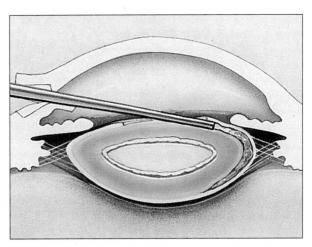

Figure 5-2. Hydrodissection—The cannula enters below the edge of the rhexis. It proceeds slightly and raises the anterior capsule slightly. The surgeon then injects BSS, separating the capsule with the cortex from the nucleus (soft nucleus and hard nucleus).

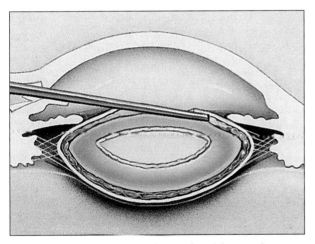

Figure 5-3. The injection of BSS has produced the complete separation of the nucleus from the capsule.

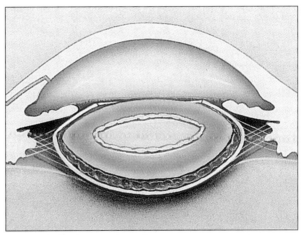

Figure 5-4. The injection of BSS is excessive and the escape of liquid from the capsular bag is not permitted. This risk situation should be avoided.

where the separation takes place (eg, hydrodelineation between the nucleus and the cortex).

In fact, the majority of authors use this term to indicate the separation of the internal nucleus (consisting of compact lamellas that cannot be separated through a simple fluid injection) and the external nucleus or epinucleus (consisting of less compact lamellas which can be separated by the fluid injection). I would agree with this definition; the term is therefore used as a synonym of hydrodelamination.

## HYDRODISSECTION

Technically this consists of injecting a variable amount of fluid immediately below the anterior capsule with a blunt cannula connected to a syringe.

Because of the fluid pressure and because of the effect of gravity on the fluid itself, it settles between the cortex and the epinucleus and not between the capsule and the cortex as one would imagine.

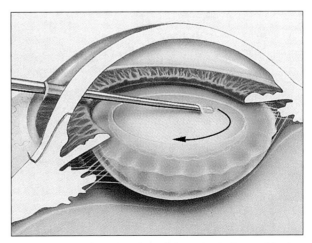

Figure 5-5. After having performed the BSS injection and having observed the wave of liquid following behind the nucleus, the surgeon must check whether the nucleus moves inside the bag.

### Table 5-6
### HYDRODISSECTION AND THE MODALITIES OF BSS INJECTION

| | |
|---|---|
| Site of BSS injection | The ideal site is between the capsule and the external cortex. Hydrodissection is quicker. Requires less injection of fluid. Less cortex is left in the site. |
| Rapid injection (with controlled pressure) | Effective diffusion of BSS, which results in effective dissection. |
| Slow injection | Dispersion of the fluid, which results in poor dissection. |
| Amount of fluid | Small amounts. Decompression of the capsular bag must be performed each time. |
| While injecting observe | The trend of the diffusion wave. The pressure exerted by the fluid, through the nucleus, on the rhexis. |
| With one BSS injection correctly performed | At least 70-80% hydrodissection is achieved. The remaining 30% is achieved with a second or third injection. |
| Injection just inside the rhexis | Achieves the best effect for various reasons: The fluid finds no resistance by the cortex. Posterior and equatorial capsule are natural chutes and suitable walls for its passage. |
| The injection must be performed close to the anterior capsule | When the capsule is slightly lifted with the cannula, the fluid detaches the outside cortex from the capsule (less residual cortex) more efficiently. |
| Hydrodissection must be followed by mechanical rotation of the nucleus | To check the hydrodissection. To break any remaining adherence. To check nuclear mobility inside the bag. |

### Table 5-7
### HYDRODISSECTION AND NUCLEUS HARDNESS

| | |
|---|---|
| Besides being surgical procedures, hydrodissection and hydrodelamination are very important diagnostic tests | They allow the surgeon to assess nuclear hardness. They allow the surgeon to determine the size of the hard inner nucleus. |
| The quality of hydrodissection is assessed based on the features of the diffusion wave | Shape. Range. Speed. |
| Good hydrodissection | Has a broad homogeneous wave that involves the whole capsular bag. Makes the posterior capsule stretch posteriorly toward the vitreous so the fluid present in the bag induces moderate shifting of the nucleus upward, toward the rhexis. |
| Cortical cleaving hydrodissection (I. Howard Fine) | Involves the separation of the equatorial and posterior capsule from the outer cortex (whereas in traditional hydrodissection, the separation concerns the inner and outer cortex). When correctly performed, no cortex material is left at the end of phaco. |

During the execution of these maneuvers, it is possible to see the wave of liquid that separates the cortex (more or less external) from the nucleus. This would indicate a successful hydrodissection, but does not mean that the objective has been reached—to free the nucleus from all the cortico-capsular adhesions.

The possibility of using hydrodissection to cordon-off the nucleus from the cortex depends on a variety of factors such as the patient's age, the hardness of the nucleus, how compact the lamellas are, the type of instrument used, etc.

Recently, I. Howard Fine stated that it was possible to create a cleavage between the capsule and the cortex (cortical cleaving hydrodissection) by performing a small capsulorhexis, introducing the cannula immediately below the capsular edge while keeping it slightly raised, prior to injecting with the cannula directed toward the anterior capsule. In this way, the amount of residual cortex to be removed by I/A is considerably reduced.

Practical experience has shown that this doesn't happen very often and it only happens with relatively soft nuclei (Grade 1 to 2, juvenile, or presenile) where the lamellas are not very compact thus permitting delineation of a large number of lenticular components or in

| Table 5-8 |
|---|
| **HYDRODISSECTION AND OPENING TO INTRODUCE THE CANNULA** |
| Regardless of which viscoelastic is used, the surgeon should use the main port for hydrodissection when: <br> • Pressure in the chamber or the bag increases beyond a certain limit, the contents of the chamber can easily leak out, either partially or completely. <br> • The risk of an excessive increase in internal pressure is reduced, and the inconvenience of posterior capsule rupture is avoided. <br> • It becomes easier to inject the fluid and thus achieve good flowing of BSS in the capsular bag. |

advanced cataracts (Grade 3 to 4) where the nucleus occupies almost the entire lens.

Good cleavage may sometimes not be possible because the compact part of the nucleus occupies almost the entire lens.

This is very important in practice because it will give the surgeon basic information regarding the real possibility of emulsifying the cataract with ultrasound and can indicate a more suitable technique for the specific case.

## HYDRODELAMINATION

This procedure is also called hydrodemarcation. It involves separating the superficial part of the nucleus (epinucleus of lower consistency) from the internal compact nucleus (inner nucleus or hard core) by fluid injection.

It is obtained using a thin cannula that is pushed into the nucleus just inside the edge of the capsulorhexis until it meets the resistance of the harder nucleus.

At this point the fluid injection is completed. It should create a cleavage between the nucleus and the epinucleus, identifiable by the formation of a luminous golden ring.

If this is not observed after repeated injections, it means that the nucleus is hard and compact. The phacoemulsification technique will be decided on the basis of this important indication.

As with hydrodissection, hydrodelamination must produce complete cleavage between the structures the surgeon is trying to separate, to obtain complete mobilization of the nucleus which will facilitate the entire operation.

Good separation of the nucleus from the epinucleus allows the surgeon to intervene using high power u/s in the central portion of the capsular bag with good protection of the softer material of the posterior epinucleus. This can then be captured and emulsified at the pupillary center once the harder part has been removed.

## HYDROFRACTURE

This involves cleaving the lamella of the internal nucleus with a combination of fluid injection and U/S and is possible with Alcon's Hydrosonic. According to preliminary reports by a number of authors, phacoemulsification is easier with this unit and the surgeon can also tackle particularly hard nuclei.

In order to keep the descriptions simple and for practical reasons, we will refer to the more popular methods of hydrocleavage: hydrodissection and hydrodelamination.

| Table 5-9 | |
|---|---|
| **DECOMPRESSION OF THE ANTERIOR CHAMBER AND/OR THE BAG** | |
| Decompression | Means reducing pressure by allowing fluid to leak out to reduce tension inside. |
| Decompression of the anterior chamber | Is performed by pressing on the deep lip of the incision and forcing out some drops of BSS and/or viscoelastic: <br> When the chamber becomes too deep (the pupil dilates). <br> When pressure in the chamber increases (this may induce zonular weakening). |
| Decompression of the capsular bag | Is performed by pressing gently with the back of the cannula on the central portion of the nucleus so that the BSS injected in the bag tends to leak out at the equator, which increases the splitting effect of the material: <br> When the nucleus is pushing on the rhexis. <br> When there is no evidence that the injected fluid is escaping. <br> When the bag has apparently become swollen (should the pressure in the bag increase there is risk of posterior capsule rupture). |
| Each fluid injection must be followed by decompression (ie, fluid leakage) | It allows an increase in the effect of dissection. <br> It decreases the pressure of the fluid present in the bag and on the posterior capsule. <br> It mobilizes the equatorial cortex. <br> It prevents luxation of the nucleus in the anterior chamber. <br> It allows reinjection of fluid. |

## FUNCTIONS AND OBJECTIVES OF HYDRODISSECTION

Hydrodissection has a number of objectives. It allows the surgeon to:
- Obtain complete mobilization of the nucleus so that it can rotate freely inside the capsular bag. This is a fundamental condition for correct completion of all the basic steps common to all techniques of endocapsular phacoemulsification.
- Accurately evaluate the degree of hardness of the nucleus and the degree of difficulty of the emulsification. This information can be obtained by observing the progression of the liquid between the lenticular layers and the formation of the wave of fluid along the posterior planes of the lens. This gives the surgeon a good idea how compact the lamellas of the nucleus are thus indicating the real consistency of the material.
- Free a large part of the capsulo-cortical and cortico-nuclear adhesions facilitating the removal of the residual material at the end of phacoemulsification.
- Create the space between the capsule and the nucleus for the insertion of the VES when the intraoperative conditions require the nucleus to be brought into the pupillary field or into the anterior chamber to complete the emulsification or to convert to a manual extracapsular technique.

## FUNCTIONS AND OBJECTIVES OF HYDRODELAMINATION

Hydrodelamination has the following objectives:
- It separates the internal compact nucleus, with its inseparable lamellas, from the epinucleus which is more attached to the peripheral cortex. This procedure is a fundamental step in the techniques of phacoemulsification which considers the emulsification of the central nucleus an independent step from the emulsification of the external nucleus.
- It allows the surgeon to evaluate the hardness of the nucleus. He or she does this by examining the penetration of the cannula between the cortical lamellas but also by how well the balanced salt solution (BSS) can separate the them.

In clinical practice, cleavage of the various planes (hydrodelamination) does not occur very often. As a result hydrodissection is used more often as it involves cortical cleavage alone—mainly between the superficial and the deep cortex and more infrequently between the capsule and the superficial cortex.

# Chapter 6

# TECHNIQUES OF PHACOEMULSIFICATION

*Lucio Buratto, MD*

## CLASSICAL PHACOEMULSIFICATION TECHNIQUES

### Introduction

Removal of the nucleus by U/S can be performed using a number of techniques that have evolved from Charles D. Kelman's original concept.

The technique has evolved because of non-stop development of both the machines and the application methods, the combination of which produces an extraordinary wealth of knowledge.

The constant development in this branch of ocular surgery is quite unique and can present a problem for surgeons who attempt to describe the state of the art at any one particular time.

On the other hand, the growing interest and the constant diffusion of phacoemulsification indicates a need for an overview of the procedure, with emphasis placed on a whole series of theoretical-practical elements. Some are almost obsolete, but they are important milestones in the history of the technique.

Cataract surgery was not equipped to take full advantage of the enormous potential of phaco upon its initial arrival. Nevertheless, as time went by, intraocular lenses (IOLs) became more perfect, even *bending* to the surgeon's needs; capsulotomies have become miniature works of art and precision. Viscoelastic substances (VES) have been transformed into surgical instruments in the true sense of the word; the incisions have become increasingly smaller and can be favorably compared to a project of structural engineering and architecture.

So finally, after many years, phacoemulsification is now the protagonist on the stage of cataract surgery.

### Rules and Basic Maneuvers

Some surgical maneuvers of phacoemulsification surgery have a *universal* value because they are repeated without substantial variation in all the techniques described. Some are simple and suitable for the beginner; others are more advanced and indicated for the more expert surgeons only.

The reference conditions between the various techniques will be normal shaped eyes and nucleus with Grade 3 hardness. Suitable variations of each technique will be suggested for very soft or very hard nuclei.

### Classification of the Phacoemulsification Techniques

The techniques will be split into two groups: those developed before the advent of capsulorhexis and those invented afterward.

Capsulorhexis is a procedure that has completely changed the face of phacoemulsification; it separates the past from the present, the historical techniques from the modern ones, the traditional techniques from the advanced ones.

The former used a Christmas tree or can opener capsulotomy; moreover, the nucleus is either luxated in the anterior chamber prior to U/S treatment, or it stays in the posterior chamber and is emulsified without being mobilized.

The latter are performed only after a continuous circular capsulotomy and once the nucleus has been mobilized inside the capsular bag.

### Phacoemulsification in the Anterior Chamber: Kelman's Technique (1970)

This is the original technique developed by Charles D. Kelman. However, by introducing a number of varia-

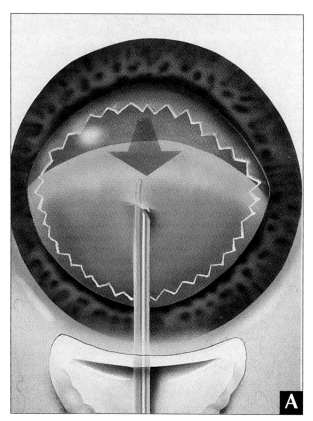
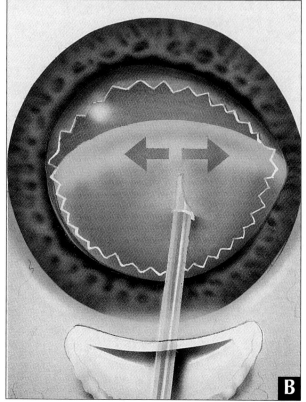

Figure 6-1A. Vertical seesaw maneuver. Sclero-corneal incision at 12 o'clock. The Kelman cystotome is pointed distally in the passage point between the third and fourth quarter. It is then pulled toward the incision, raising the inferior equator.

Figure 6-1B. With the vertical movement, the surgeon might find it useful to perform a slight rotation movement.

tions and modifications, it can still be used in modern cataract surgery.

It consists of the following steps:
- Preliminary steps.
- Mobilization of the nucleus.
- Fragmentation with U/S.
- Final steps.

### Preliminary Steps

The preparation of the operating field is done by fixing the eyelids and the superior and inferior rectus muscles. Methylene blue is instilled in the conjunctival sac; it is distributed uniformly over the sclera with a sponge to reduce irritating reflections during the operation.

The conjunctiva is cut at the limbus using scissors, and the dissection of the conjunctiva and Tenon's capsule is completed toward the fornix in order to expose the sclera.

For first operations, it is advisable to prepare a large scleral exposure so that the initial wound can be extended if the nucleus has to be removed manually.

A blood-free zone is created with a bipolar cautery. However, care must be taken not to involve the sclera within the coagulation.

A 3.1 mm incision is cut with a calibrated blade in correspondence to the posterior third of the surgical limbus. The anterior chamber is inflated with air, and the Kelman's irrigator cystotome is inserted with irrigation closed. The cystotome is inserted with the irrigation orifice toward the iris. The surgeon uses it to press lightly on the inferior edge of the incision, and, if necessary, he or she can carefully lift the superior flap with corneal forceps.

A *Christmas tree* anterior capsulotomy is performed with the main incision from 6 to 12 o' clock. Two more capsular incisions are cut at 4 and 8 o'clock to expose the nucleus.

Following the capsulotomy, the air is replaced with balanced salt solution (BSS) using the cystotome itself. The foot pedal is moved to Position 1, and the nucleus is mobilized and must be brought into the anterior chamber.

The capsulotomy must be as wide as possible to allow easy luxation of the nucleus in the anterior chamber.

The technique involves a wide Christmas tree capsulectomy; every other capsulotomy technique, and this applies to a wide can opener or capsulorhexis, will permit luxation of the nucleus in the anterior chamber. At this point, one might ask why the nucleus has to be fragmented in the anterior chamber. This is a valid question, as some conditions may reduce safety and control of phacoemulsification in the posterior chamber, though this is a rare occurrence. The conditions are:
- Rapid reduction of the mydriasis at the end of the capsulotomy.
- Reduction of the space in the posterior chamber.
- A restless patient under local or topical anesthesia.

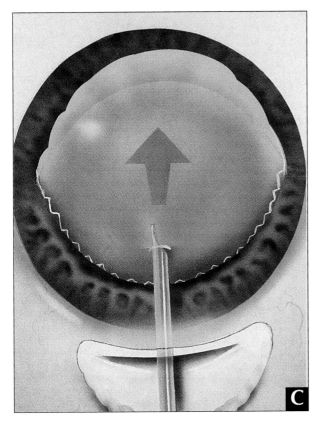

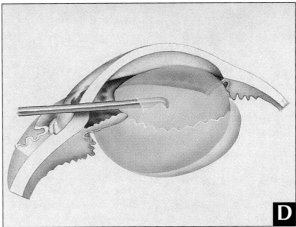

Figures 6-1C, 6-1D. The maneuver is repeated superiorly pointing the instrument between the first and second quadrant and pushing the nucleus downward, raising the superior equator. The maneuver must allow the surgeon to free the superior cortical adhesions. At the same time, it must exit the equator from the capsular bag superiorly. Then it must anteriorize the iris plane. One maneuver is probably not enough to obtain a satisfactory result so the maneuver should be repeated two, three, and sometimes four times.

In these cases, if the surgeon still wishes to perform phacoemulsification, the nucleus should be brought into the anterior chamber so that visual control is better.

High molecular weight, cohesive VES (Provisc, Healon) are irreplaceable during the phase of nuclear luxation because they provide excellent protection of the posterior chamber; dispersive VES which are resistant to aspiration, such as Viscoat, should be used during phacoemulsification to provide greater protection of the endothelium.

Mobilization begins with the classical seesaw movement, either vertical or horizontal; the equator of the nucleus is brought almost to the center of the anterior chamber and luxated above the iris.

Under special conditions (reduced depth of the anterior chamber, poorly dilated pupil), the surgeon can resort to alternative maneuvers of mobilization of the nucleus, such as the bed sheet or tire tool maneuver or impalement of the nucleus.

What follows is a description of the possible maneuvers of mobilization and luxation of the nucleus.

### Mobilization of the Nucleus

It is important to note that all of the maneuvers described are performed with no prior removal of the cortico-nuclear adhesions (ie, no hydrodissection, hydrodelamination, or other).

The nucleus is freed mechanically from the cortex, so it stands to reason that the surgeon must proceed gradually, gently but firmly. A wide capsulotomy is absolutely necessary to prevent the nucleus from moving in the anterior chamber, inducing tears (that may extend

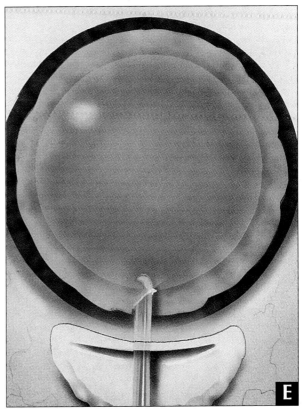

Figure 6-1E. The nucleus is raised above the iris and then into the anterior chamber. The vertical seesaw is indicated particularly for nuclei that are moderate-hard to hard.

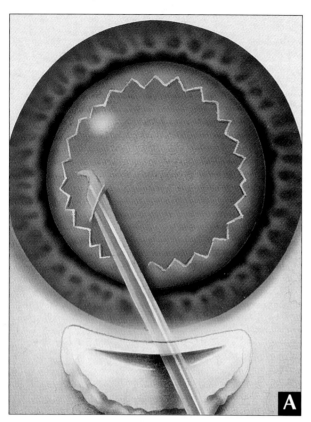

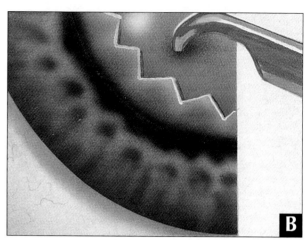

Figure 6-2B. Closeup of the operation.

Figure 6-2A. Lateral seesaw technique. Instead of being performed vertically, the maneuver can be lateral. In this case, the cystotome, given its shape, has a greater hold. This maneuver is more suitable for soft nuclei. The cystotome is positioned at the 3 or 6 o'clock position close to the capsulotomy.

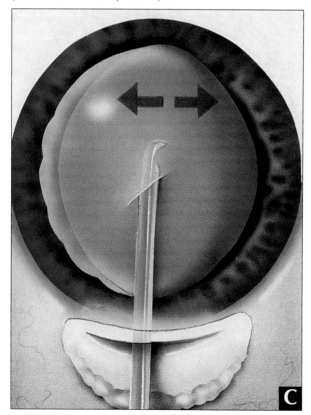

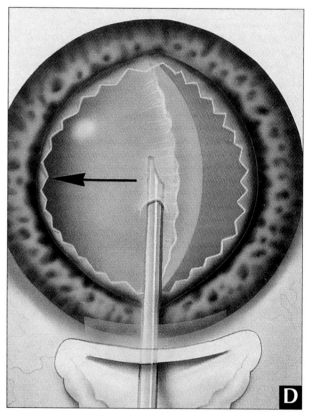

Figure 6-2C. The nucleus is moved toward the right-hand sector and raised slightly.

Figure 6-2D. The maneuver is repeated from the opposite side.

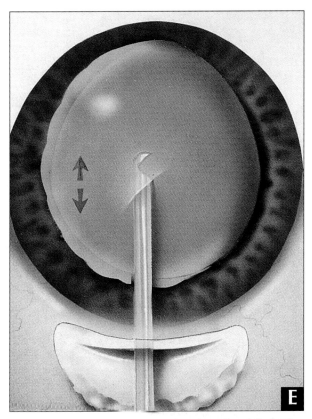

Figure 6-2E. In order to free the nucleus from the residual adhesions, the surgeon can use a slightly vertical movement or rotate slightly.

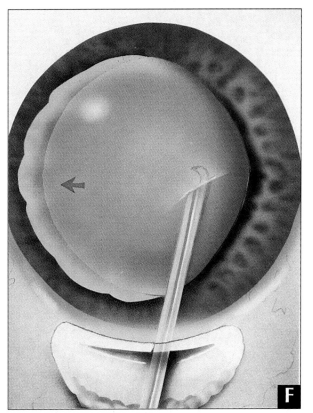

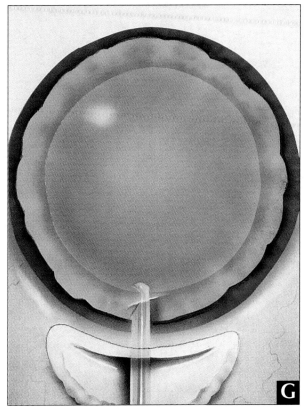

Figures 6-2F, 6-2G. In the end, the nucleus exits from the capsulotomy and enters the anterior chamber.

toward the equator) during the prolapse of the nucleus in the anterior chamber.

Another important factor is that the pressure in the anterior chamber should be relatively low; this will allow the surgeon to take full advantage of the vitreal thrust to prolapse the nucleus into the anterior chamber. A small incision will guarantee sufficient pressure to avoid oscillation of the anterior chamber.

The mobilization maneuvers are as follows:

*Seesaw maneuver*—This can be performed with a vertical or horizontal movement. In both cases, Kelman's cystotome (or similar type with a strong shaft and long tip) is inserted through an incision of around 1 mm, so that the anterior chamber is sufficiently shaped with irrigation alone.

In order to control the maneuver better and to protect the endothelium, a moderate quantity of low molecular weight VES can be injected. During this phase, the use of a high molecular weight VES could obstruct the luxation of the nucleus.

*Vertical seesaw*—The cystotome must be engaged in the nucleus at an intermediate point between the anterior pole and the equator of the lens in a position opposite to the incision (ie, at 6 o'clock) in order to avoid coming into contact with the zonular fibers.

The surgeon must slowly pull the nucleus toward the incision, progressively lifting the inferior equator, so that

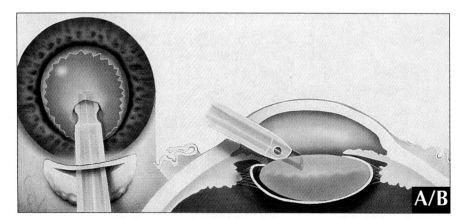

Figures 6-3A, 6-3B. Lollipop Maneuver. The U/S tip is directed toward the center of the nucleus. It enters the material under the effect of U/S. The surgeon must have obtained occlusion in order to have good implementation.

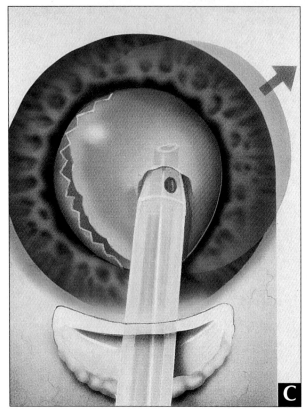

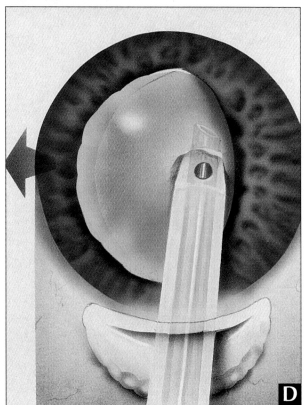

Figures 6-3C, 6-3D. With the pedal in Position 2 (ie, no U/S), the tip is used to move the nucleus first to one side and then to the other until all the adhesions in the capsular bag are freed. The nucleus is then brought into the anterior chamber.

he or she can see the detachment of the cortico-nuclear adhesions from the posterior capsule.

While the surgeon is performing this slow yet constant traction, the nucleus is moved backward and forward on a horizontal plane to free the residual adhesions and bring the inferior equator above the capsule and the iris.

The cystotome is then released from the nucleus and brought toward the incision to fix the nucleus in a superior position; the point of traction is symmetrical to the previous one. The maneuver is repeated pushing the nucleus downward, while lifting it above the iris close to the incision.

Mobilization of the nucleus is completed with gentle seesawing lateral movements to free the residual adhesions.

*Horizontal seesaw*—The principle is the same as previously; it differs in that the cystotome is applied at 3 and 9 o'clock. The surfaces of the Kelman's cystotome, which act on the nucleus, are larger than those used in the vertical seesaw maneuver (thanks to the particular design of this instrument), so better results are obtained if the pupil is only partially dilated (less than 8 mm), or the nucleus is relatively soft.

*Lollipop technique*—This is also a classical maneuver for the mobilization of the nucleus with the one-handed technique. The U/S tip is pushed into the nucleus with the foot pedal in Position 3 to obtain occlusion with a

Table 6-1

## MANEUVERS TO LUXATE THE NUCLEUS IN THE ANTERIOR CHAMBER ACCORDING TO KELMAN

**Phaco incision at 12**

| | |
|---|---|
| Preliminary statement | All maneuvers have been made without preliminary reduction of cortico-nuclear adhesions. |
| Aim | To mobilize the nucleus inside the bag. <br> To luxate it subsequently in the anterior chamber. |
| Vertical seesaw maneuver suitable for nuclei with hardness equal to 3-4 | Step 1: Apply the cystotome toward 6 (midway between the center of the nucleus and the distal end of capsulotomy). Act traction toward 12 and at the same time lift the nucleus distally. <br> Step 2: Cystotome at 12 and push toward 6 with elevation of the proximal equator. <br> Step 3: Both maneuvers are repeated until the nucleus is freed inside the bag and can be luxated in the anterior chamber. |
| Lateral seesaw maneuver suitable for nuclei with hardness equal to 2-3 | Step 1: Cystotome at 3 and shifting of the nucleus toward 9. <br> Step 2: Cystotome at 9 and pulling toward 3. <br> Step 3: In case, both maneuvers are repeated with nucleus elevation until complete luxation in the anterior chamber is accomplished. |
| Impalement or lollipop suitable for nuclei with hardness equal to 3-4, and particularly in case of small pupil diameter | With the U/S tip, the center of the nucleus is penetrated operating U/S; then aspiration is maintained. <br> The US/ tip is used to mobilize both on the right and the left and then upward, using the incision as a support. |
| Tire tool suitable when the other procedures fail | A bevel irrigation cannula is passed under the nucleus and progressively lifts the nucleus, thus *turning back* the iris underneath. |

short burst of U/S. This maneuver is easier with the modern instruments because greater vacuum can be used (100 to 200 mm Hg) and occlusion can be obtained more easily. Naturally, this is not part of Kelman's original technique.

Once the nucleus has been engaged, emulsification is interrupted but aspiration is maintained (foot pedal in Position 2) to engage the opening of the tip so that the vacuum fixes the nucleus to the U/S tip like a lollipop stick (thanks also to an increase in vacuum caused by the occlusion).

At this stage, the surgeon can mobilize the nucleus as he or she prefers. This maneuver is suitable for a poorly dilated pupil and is used in the one-handed techniques or for partial mobilization of the nucleus in the two-handed techniques.

It is a very important maneuver because many advanced techniques of phacoemulsification are based on the very same principle, including techniques such as the Phaco Chop, which will be described later.

The surgeon should only impale the nucleus once it has been freed from a large part of the cortical adhesions. Particularly in very elderly patients, impaling the nucleus can hold some unpleasant surprises such as capsular openings or zonular dialysis.

*Bed sheet or tire tool maneuver*—This two-handed technique brings the nucleus in front of the iris in the anterior chamber and is particularly useful if the pupil is narrow; a cyclodialysis irrigating spatula is passed underneath the nucleus after retracting the iris slightly and inserting the tip of the cannula under the equator of the nucleus. Then slowly, with irrigation open, the spatula passes underneath the nucleus, first temporally, then underneath the center, and then nasally, bringing it above the iris with progressive rotation.

The maneuver can be facilitated and made safer by injecting a VES under the nucleus to create a barrier from the posterior capsule, which helps lift the nucleus.

### Fragmentation with U/S

After having luxated the nucleus in the anterior chamber with one of the described methods, the U/S tip is inserted.

The angle of the tip orifice must be chosen prior to surgery in relation to the technique planned or the surgeon's personal preferences; Kelman used a 15° tip but the 30° tip is better for most cases.

Once the nucleus is in the anterior chamber, it can be emulsified in a variety of ways. However, there is a common factor—in all the emulsification methods, the nucleus must be in direct contact with the tip.

With phacoemulsification in the anterior chamber, the entire nuclear mass must be emulsificated by the U/S tip; the nucleus is first attacked at the equator to reach the central portion.

In the original technique, with the Cavitron/Kelman 8000, the parameters of vacuum and flow were factory set during the U/S phase, and only the U/S power was regulated in proportion to the hardness of the nucleus.

Once emulsification begins, the surgeon will become more aware whether the U/S levels chosen are suitable for the operation in hand. During the U/S action, the nucleus must be almost immobile, without any vibrations or very low vibrating, and the anterior chamber must be well-formed.

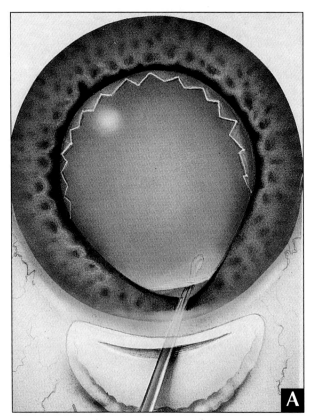

Figure 6-4A. Bed sheet maneuver. With a spatula, or better still, a blunt-ended cannula, irrigating to the side, the iris is gently retracted until the edge of the capsulotomy is visible. The capsule is also retracted slightly, and the tip of the instrument is introduced into the capsular bag under the nuclear equator.

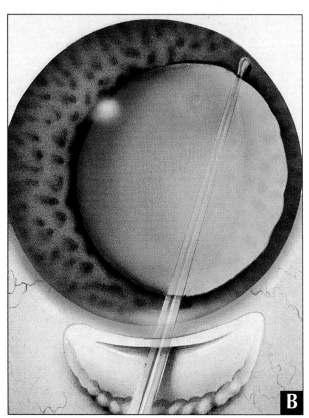

Figure 6-4B. The cannula is slowly introduced underneath the nucleus and is raised at the same time. Irrigation is opened to facilitate the maneuver.

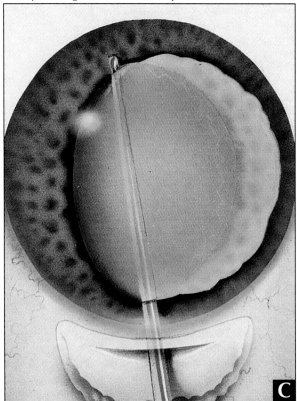

Figure 6-4C. The maneuver continues by directing the spatula toward 6 o'clock to move the nucleus above the iris in the sector involved in the procedure.

A frequent problem occurs when the nucleus vibrates through excessive U/S power.

The surgeon should not forget that the nucleus is free in the anterior chamber and that he or she is using a technique that was one-handed at the outset. Once he or she has acquired sufficient experience, he or she can begin to use an accessory instrument (such as a cyclodialysis spatula) with the other hand. Nevertheless, with the nucleus in the anterior chamber, the surgeon must proceed with extreme caution.

Modern machinery provides the option of selecting the operating parameters. The following can be used depending on the hardness of the nucleus:

- Soft—Vacuum 80; flow rate 15; U/S: 50%.
- Medium—Vacuum 100; flow rate 20; U/S 65%.
- Hard—Vacuum 120; flow rate 20; U/S 85%.

*Croissant technique*—This is a one-handed technique suitable for a medium-hard nucleus (Grade 2 to 3). The technique involves sculpting the nucleus to the point of giving it the *crescent/croissant* shape and is the technique that Kelman would still recommend to doctors learning phacoemulsification.

With irrigation active, the U/S tip is introduced into the anterior chamber. With a limbal incision, the tip directly engages the equator of the nucleus at 12 o'clock. The U/S can be activated by moving the foot pedal to Position 3.

Each U/S shot must be short, about 2 to 3 seconds, in order to avoid the U/S tip getting trapped in the nucleus, returning the foot pedal to Position 2 to maintain suitable flow rates. The nucleus is attacked throughout its

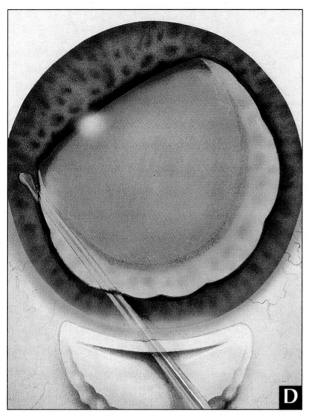 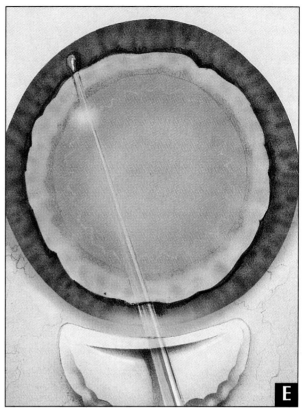

Figures 6-4D, 6-4E. At this point, the cannula is retracted and introduced from the opposite side to repeat a similar maneuver, which involves total luxation of the nucleus in the anterior chamber.

### Table 6-2
### TECHNIQUES FOR EMULSIFICATION IN THE ANTERIOR CHAMBER

| Croissant technique | Procedure |
|---|---|
| One-handed procedure suitable for nuclei with hardness equal to 2-3 | First fragment the nucleus in its whole thickness proximal to the incision and then turn it 180° to repeat the procedure until a croissant shape is obtained. Split the nucleus distally in two; then fragment each piece separately. |
| **Carousel technique** | **Procedure** |
| One-handed procedure suitable for nuclei with hardness equal to 2-3 | First perform fragmentation at the equator tangentially, keeping the tip angled. Once the nucleus diameter has been reduced, another turn can be repeated or a croissant technique can be performed. |
| **Sector technique** | **Procedure** |
| One-handed or two-handed procedure suitable for nuclei with hardness equal to 3-4 | Approach the nucleus at the equator for one sector, removing first the superficial layer, then the intermediate part, and eventually the deep portion. Use the spatula to turn the nucleus 90 to 180° and fragment another sector. Turn again and remove a further sector, thus reducing progressively the nuclear volume. |

entire thickness, starting with the equator under the U/S tip. The operator must try to obtain a reasonably broad, crescent-shaped central excavation of the nucleus. A narrow groove may block the tip and occlude it. When this technique is performed with a modern instrument, using the parameters just recommended, the surgeon should note that occlusion causes a progressive increase of the vacuum to the maximum preset values, so that the nucleus *sticks* to the tip and follows its every movement.

On the one hand, the occlusion can be used to the operator's advantage to position the nucleus in a more favorable position. On the other hand, the operator must remember that he is working in the anterior chamber and that even a slight movement can damage the endothelium. However, under normal conditions, this technique does not make use of occlusion to move the nucleus.

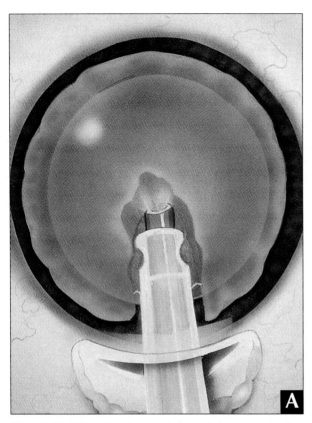
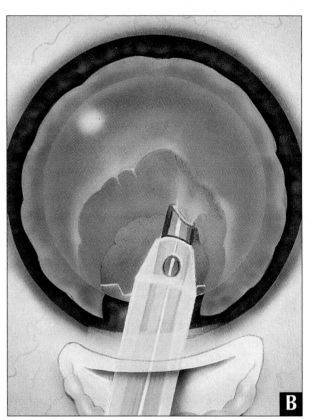

Figure 6-5A. Kelman's croissant technique of phacoemulsification in the anterior chamber. The nucleus is already luxated in the anterior chamber. The U/S tip is brought into contact with the equator of the nucleus, and one sector is emulsified. First, the superficial layers are removed, followed by the intermediate layers.

Figure 6-5B. The groove is extended on both sides and distally, and it is deepened toward the center of the nucleus, then toward the deep layers.

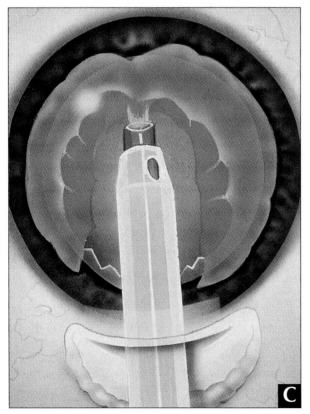
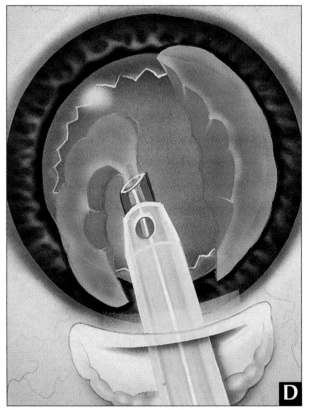

Figure 6-5C. The groove is extended and gradually deepened. The nuclear residue takes on the shape of a croissant.

Figure 6-5D. The croissant is split into two pieces that are then emulsified.

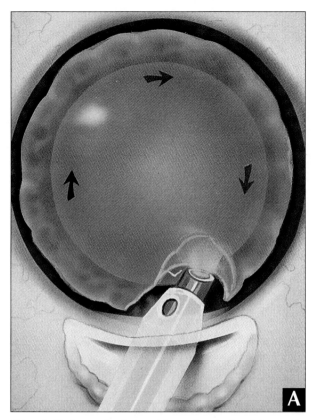

Figure 6-6A. Carousel technique. The nucleus is already luxated in the anterior chamber. The tip is introduced into the chamber and directed toward the equator with the pedal in Position 2. The U/S is then activated, and a part of the equatorial material is fragmented.

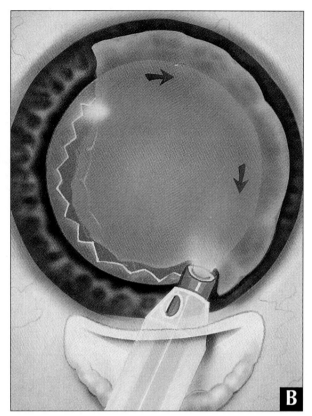

Figure 6-6B. As the equatorial material is soft, it will tend to stick to the tip under the effect of aspiration. As the material is removed, the nucleus rotates (like a carousel). The maneuver must be slow because faster movements could damage the endothelium.

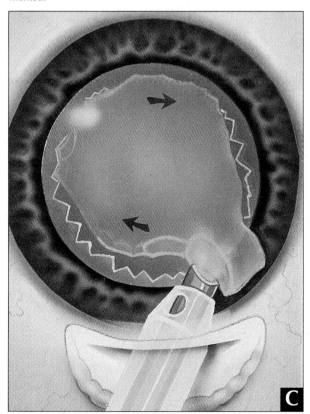

Figure 6-6C. Slowly, all the equatorial material is removed. If the residual nucleus is soft, the carousel technique can be repeated.

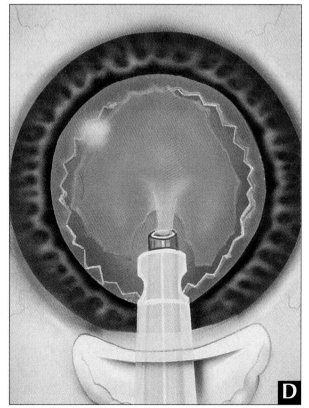

Figure 6-6D. Alternately, and particularly if the residual nucleus is hard, the surgeon should proceed with the croissant technique.

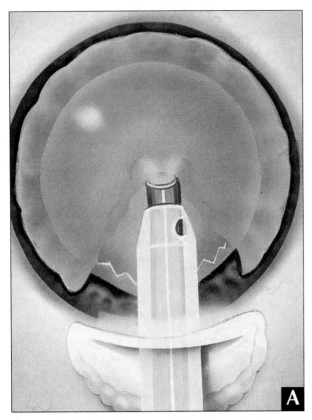

Figure 6-7A. One-handed sector technique. The nucleus is tackled at the equator near the incision and carved to remove a segment of material through the thickness.

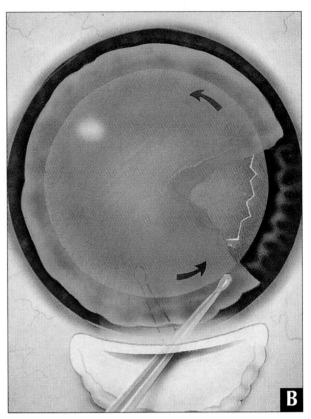

Figure 6-7B. The U/S tip is removed, and the spatula is introduced to rotate the nucleus through 180°.

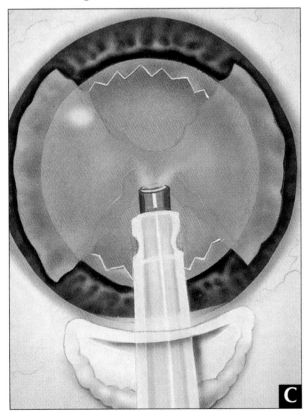

Figure 6-7C. The U/S tip is introduced once again, and another sector is carved. The equator can be tackled immediately throughout the entire thickness. Alternately, the superficial layers can be removed first, followed by the intermediate and then the deep layers.

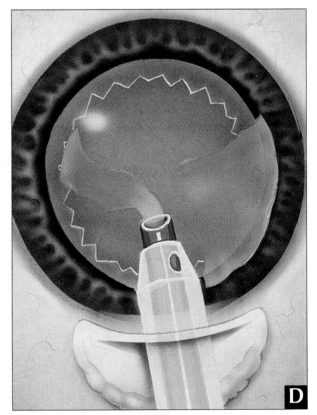

Figure 6-7D. The residual bridge between the two carved sectors is emulsified, and then the two residual pieces are tackled. Alternately, the external parts are tackled first, followed by the central parts.

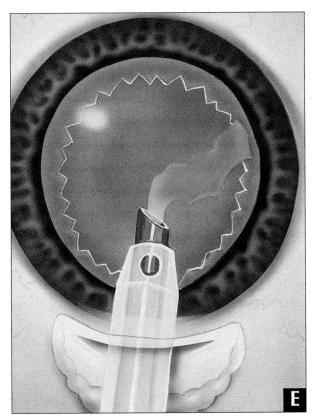

Figure 6-7E. The last piece is emulsified, taking care to prevent it from bumping into the endothelium.

Central sculpting is continued with the stated criteria until the portion of the nucleus at 6 o'clock is reached. A broad crescent in the nucleus is produced, illustrating the croissant or crescent shape.

The U/S power must be lower than in the previous phase so that the operator does not inadvertently penetrate the nucleus and find him- or herself on the iris or the posterior capsule.

Continuing fragmentation near 6 o'clock, the operator reaches the inferior equator of the nucleus; the nucleus is split into two pieces, each one then treated as described above. It is important to reduce the U/S power gradually as the fragments get smaller. Otherwise, these will be projected in all directions without being aspirated.

If this happens, apart from increasing the operating time, it can damage the endothelium and the posterior capsule.

Once phacoemulsification has been completed, it is advisable to keep the foot pedal in Position 2 for a couple of seconds to allow suitable flow of liquid to the anterior chamber. There may also be small fragments of nucleus that were not seen previously.

*Carousel technique*—This is a one-handed technique, suitable for a medium-hard nucleus (Grade 2-3) with reasonably soft equatorial material. The parameters can be the same as the previous technique.

The U/S tip is introduced to the anterior chamber with the foot pedal in Position 1; it is then moved to Position 2 to control the depth and stability of the chamber. The U/S is moved toward 3 o'clock, tangentially to the equator of the nucleus, which is engaged by the tip in this position.

The technique involves rotating the nucleus on the frontal plane, a sort of *carousel*, taking full advantage of the U/S action and the aspiration created by the U/S tip. In practice, with short bursts of U/S, the nucleus *follows* the tip and continually presents it with new pieces through the followability.

Once rotation has been completed, the volume of the nucleus is significantly reduced. At this point, it can be tackled directly with central sculpting or another carousel. The choice depends on the consistency of the nucleus; if the nucleus is hard, it should be tackled directly. Again with this technique, the progressive reduction of the nuclear volume must correspond with a reduction in the U/S power to avoid the mishaps described in the previous technique.

The surgeon should also remember to proceed from the U/S phase with the pedal in Position 3, to the pedal in Position 2 to avoid interrupting the flow. It should be noted that when the nucleus is attacked, real U/S times may be lengthy, and in addition to the total energy irradiated to the ocular structures, the question of overheating may come into play. The surgeon must take all steps to minimize surgical trauma, as there are several problems linked to overheating.

This technique requires a certain degree of familiarity with the handpiece and the U/S action for the following reasons:

- The oblique orientation of the tip may cause traction on the incision, resulting in problems of anterior chamber stability and overheating of the U/S tip through obstruction of the irrigation flow along the shaft, which tends to bend.
- U/S is performed mainly in a shallower area of the anterior chamber compared to the center with the iris closer to the U/S tip.
- The nucleus may move rapidly, sometimes unpredictably.

Situations may arise that can catch the beginning surgeon unaware. He or she should concentrate on the fact that the safe area for the U/S tip is the pupillary zone. This technique is suitable for those surgeons with moderate experience (even though the techniques in the anterior chamber were taught prior to the more complex posterior chamber techniques).

*Sectors technique*—This method can be used with one or two hands and is suitable for nuclei of moderate-high hardness (Grade 3).

The operating parameters of the U/S machine are the same as those defined for the previous techniques (simply because these were the only ones available when Kelman was developing his original technique)—vacuum 41; flow 20; U/S 70/80%; with currently available instruments, vacuum can be 80 to 120.

The rationale of this technique lies in a progressive reduction of the central portion of the nucleus. The central nucleus is tackled in portions close to the incision. First, the superficial layer is removed, then the intermediate, and then the deep layer (the same as in the croissant technique).

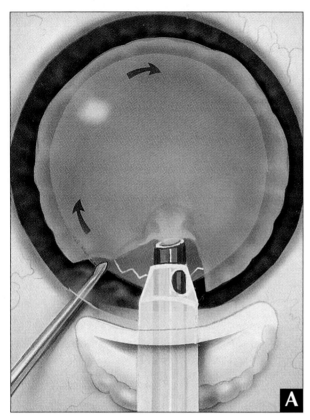

Figure 6-8A. Two-handed sector technique. The nucleus is tackled at the equator by the U/S tip. The spatula through the side port incision helps to stabilize the nucleus and better expose it to the U/S tip.

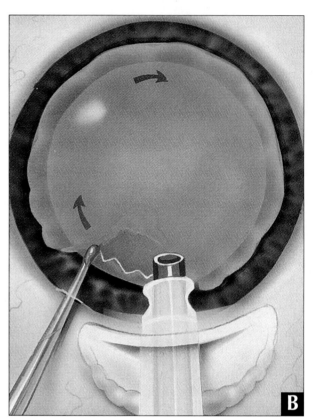

Figure 6-8B. Once one sector has been emulsified, the spatula will help to rotate the nucleus and expose another portion of the equator or help extend the previous groove.

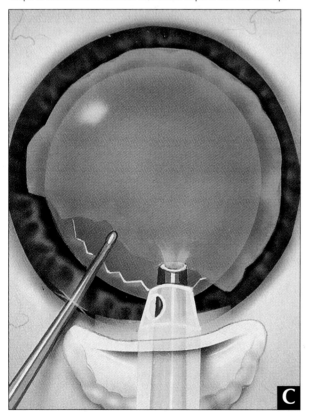

Figure 6-8C. The maneuvers with the spatula are always complementary and secondary to the use of the U/S tip.

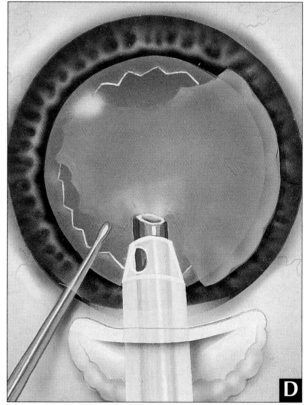

Figure 6-8D. Slowly, the nucleus is rotated through 180°, and the sector opposite the first one is tackled.

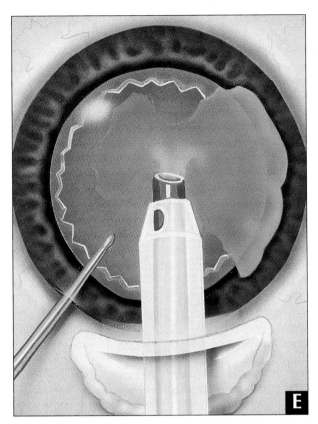

Figure 6-8E. The bridge of material is tackled, and the residual nucleus is split into two parts. The smaller portion is emulsified, followed by the larger portion.

The nucleus is then rotated through 180° using a spatula. Another sector is tackled. The bridge that unites the residual nucleus is then broken. The two pieces obtained are fragmented separately.

Again, the action of the tip must sculpt the nucleus in its entire depth. In the one-handed technique, in each sector, the U/S tip exits from the incision; a cystotome or spatula is introduced, and the nucleus is rotated through 180°.

In the two-handed technique, the nucleus is rotated gradually with a spatula introduced through a side port incision and is then fragmented by U/S.

When there is enough room in the chamber, the nucleus can also be split into two pieces, each one then fragmented separately.

Variation of the one-handed technique—The tip is inserted with the pedal in Position 1, the nucleus is engaged in the equatorial portion at 12 o'clock, and the U/S action is started. With short U/S bursts of 2 to 3 seconds each, a crescent-shaped groove of about 90° is carved in one sector of the nucleus.

It is advisable to prepare a broad groove at the beginning to prevent the tip from becoming blocked in the mass of the central nucleus, which will compromise the smooth completion of the procedure.

When the first sector is the right size, the pedal is brought into Position 1, and the U/S tip removed. A cyclodialysis spatula (or similar) is introduced through the main incision. It is positioned on the edge of the nuclear fragment toward 8 o'clock. By pushing the spatula forward, the 180° rotation of the nucleus is obtained until the phacoemulsified sector is at 6 o'clock and the sector still to be emulsified is at 12 o'clock.

The U/S tip is introduced again once the spatula has been removed, and a new sector of about 90° is emulsified to the central portion of the first sector, using the same procedure as described previously. In this way, there are two separate portions of the nucleus remaining at 3 and 9 o'clock respectively.

At this point, it is possible to engage the central portion of one of these two residual sectors with the U/S tip. It is emulsified and progressively centralized. The final sector of the nucleus is emulsified in the same way.

As pointed out in the previous pages, the U/S action on the harder central portions of the nucleus requires higher power, which must be rapidly reduced as the operator moves toward the softer peripheral areas, or when the material begins to press on the tip or make sudden, uncontrolled movements.

Once the nucleus has been completely removed, the pedal must be kept in Position 2 for a couple of seconds to remove any residual fragments. The U/S tip can then be removed from the anterior chamber.

Variation of the two-handed carousel technique—In this case it is necessary to prepare a side port incision about 70 to 90° from the entrance of the U/S tip. If the left eye is being operated, the main entrance should be at 12 or 1 o'clock, with the service incision at 3 or 2 o'clock. For a right eye, the main incision should be at 11 o'clock with the service incision at 1 or 2 o'clock. These positions generally allow good freedom of movement despite the presence of two instruments in the anterior chamber, from which one—the U/S tip—is connected to what may be a far-from-manageable handpiece.

The fragmentation with U/S begins at 12 o'clock as previously described. Nevertheless, the first sector emulsified may be smaller because once the U/S phase has been interrupted with the pedal in Position 2, the accessory spatula is introduced through the lateral incision. It rotates the nucleus and presents a new equatorial portion of the nucleus to the U/S tip to be emulsified. The presence of a second instrument in the anterior chamber is an important advantage under some aspects, but a possible source of problems from others.

Advantages:
- Stability of the nucleus and prevention of undesired movements.
- More delicate, precise, manipulation of the nucleus.
- Limited number of entrances with the U/S tip, resulting in greater stability of the anterior chamber. The operator should remember that instability and repeated fluctuations of the anterior chamber are the main causes of intraoperative miosis and complications during cataract surgery with automated instruments.
- Greater fluidity of the procedure with considerable time saving, consequently reduced circulation of liquids and materials in the anterior chamber.

Table 6-3

## PHACOEMULSIFICATION IN THE ANTERIOR CHAMBER ACCORDING TO KELMAN

|  | Kelman original technique | Updated technique |
|---|---|---|
| Incision | Limbal, on two planes | Scleral or corneal tunnel |
| Capsulotomy | Christmas tree | Wide capsulorhexis |
| Chamber filling during capsulotomy | BSS or air | Cohesive VES |
| Nucleus luxation in the anterior chamber | A typical Kelman maneuver to mobilize the nucleus | Hydrodissection/hydrodelamination, then hydro- or viscoluxation |
| Fragmentation | Croissant technique for soft nuclei / Sector technique for harder nuclei | One of the techniques described by Kelman, with the innovative use of a dispersive VES to protect the endothelium |
| Iridectomy | Yes | No |
| I/A | Yes | Yes |
| IOL implantation | In the anterior chamber | In the posterior chamber, inside the capsular bag |
| Suturing | 8-10 silk | No suturing, or single or multiple sutures in nylon 10-0 |

Disadvantages:

- The operator has to control two instruments in the anterior chamber simultaneously, which may distract his or her attention from the main instrument or require the interruption of the U/S phase in order to check the position of the spatula.
- The spatula may cause pressure and traction on the cornea or the iris when it is not being used during the action of the U/S tip, thus reducing the visibility or causing corneal or iridial lesions or iridial miosis.
- Possible contact between the instrument and the U/S tip, which can damage the tip itself and expel metal fragments into the anterior chamber, particularly during phases when the U/S is active.

From the above observations, it is clear that this technique must be tackled by a surgeon who has already acquired good dexterity with the U/S handpiece and good control of all the phases of phacoemulsification.

### Final Steps

#### Cortex Aspiration

Once the nucleus has been completely removed, a basal iridectomy is performed at 12 o'clock (in Kelman's original technique, it is done prior to aspiration of the cortex). Then the I/A tip 0.3 mm is inserted to remove the residual cortex with the usual automated methods. Material at 12 o'clock can be removed by introducing the tip through the iridectomy.

After cleaning the posterior chamber with the diamond-tipped cannula, the anterior chamber is reshaped with air. The incision is then extended for artificial lens implantation in the anterior chamber.

#### IOL Implantation

Kelman's anterior chamber lens with angular support (Tripod Omnifit or Multiflex) is chosen after having measured the corneal diameter from white to white. The lens must be about 1.0 to 1.5 mm longer than the diameter.

After having injected a miotic into the anterior chamber, the lens is fixed using a McPherson forceps. The distal support feet are inserted in the anterior chamber under air until they are positioned at the chamber angle distal to the incision. With the help of a lens hook or the tip of a 15 or 30° blade positioned in the orifice of the superior foot, the latter is allowed to slide through the incision to position itself in the corner.

Some interrupted 8-0 silk sutures are applied (Kelman always preferred silk to nylon). Finally, the air is replaced with a saline solution, and the lens position is controlled with a gonioscope.

If the positions of the support feet are not perfect, they can be corrected using a lens hook.

The operation is terminated with a posterior capsulotomy using a Ziegler knife.

#### Modernization of the Procedure

Implantation of the Kelman lens in the anterior chamber as described has now been updated by the use of a posterior chamber IOL. In this case, the incision can be chosen according to the surgeon's preference and the characteristics of the individual case.

The capsulotomy can be can opener or even a capsulorhexis. All the steps for luxation in the anterior chamber can be made easier and given better visibility by using VES.

The phacoemulsification can be made safer by injecting Viscoat into the anterior chamber both under and above the nucleus in order to protect the vital structures of the anterior segment.

The silk sutures can be replaced by nylon or the incision can even be self-sealing and sutureless.

The posterior chamber implant can be inserted according to the following technique. At the end of the phase of cortex aspiration, the anterior and posterior chambers are reshaped with VES, and the incision is extended to the size of the optic diameter of the chosen lens.

The lens is inserted in the anterior chamber, and the inferior loop is placed under the iris at 7 o'clock in the sulcus or in the bag, depending on the type of capsulotomy performed. If the lens has positioning holes, it is rotated in a clockwise direction with a lens hook, while an iris hook retracts the pupil to allow the superior loop to slide under the iris.

If the lens does not have positioning holes, the superior loop must be caught at the distal third with a McPherson forceps. The lens is rotated in a clockwise direction and pushed gently under the iris. In this case also, it is advisable to retract the iris with a hook, possibly through the side port incision at 2 o'clock to facilitate the passage of the superior loop of the lens.

It is important to have visual control of the loop position to ensure that both are positioned in the ciliary sulcus or in the capsular bag to avoid any decentering of the lens.

At the end of the lens implantation procedure, the substances that maintain the anterior chamber are removed, and a mixed suture is applied—two interrupted sutures and one continuous in 10-0 nylon.

### Comment

Kelman's technique in the anterior chamber is one of the foundation techniques of ocular surgery in that it includes the basic steps of phacoemulsification. Apart from the historical value, it is a technique that all surgeons performing phacoemulsification must learn.

Even if he or she just has to remove the nucleus, the surgeon cannot ignore the importance of mobilization and emulsification, because they may be necessary even when the surgeon has planned a different, more modern technique.

Difficulties that may arise during phacoemulsification with one of the current techniques may be one of two types:
1. Difficult mobilization of the nucleus because of its size and the cortex connections;
2. Spontaneous luxation of the nucleus in the anterior chamber because of vitreous pressure or other.

In both cases, if the surgeon has experience in the original maneuvers he or she will have the necessary skills to quickly and successfully correct a surgical condition that may be the source of some severe intraoperative complications.

Of course, there is nothing to prevent the surgeon from opting for this technique as his or her first choice while remaining within the realms of advanced surgery. However, some preoperative conditions are necessary. For example:
- A very deep anterior chamber.
- Difficulty in performing the phacoemulsification within the capsular bag.
- Difficult exposition of the globe.
- Difficult visual control of the peripheral lens structures (gerontoxon, miosis, or other).
- Doubts regarding the strength of the zonules or the integrity of the posterior capsule.
- Rupture of the posterior capsule.

One fundamental preoperative condition in the decision to perform a technique in the anterior chamber is either that the endothelium must be normal or that the surgeon has a highly adhesive VES at hand to protect the cornea from any surgical trauma.

## Phacoemulsification in the Pupillary Plane: Little's Technique (1979)

This method was the first variation of Kelman's original technique to have caught the attention of phaco surgeons. It was also the first variation that spread rapidly throughout this limited group of practitioners. Perfected separately and empirically by various surgeons, it was tackled and described by Little and Emery in 1979, and later perfected by Shearing, Sinskey, and Kratz in particular.

At that time, the use of IOLs was increasing, particularly in the United States. However, the good expectations were often frustrated by the modest functional results of the iris-fixated lenses available at that time and by the long list of complications they brought with them.

As true today as it was then, the surgical techniques for cataract removal were more advanced than the design and production procedures of the IOLs. The development of second-generation IOLs for the posterior chamber (Shearing and others) was preceded by the surgical techniques suitable for their implantation.

Phacoemulsification in the pupillary plane is the technique that best interprets this role. It was developed to reduce the disadvantages of Kelman's technique to a minimum, particularly where the endothelium was involved.

In this technique, a large part of the surgical action occurs close to the posterior capsule, so the possible risks are shifted from the endothelium to this structure.

It is extremely important that the surgeon has acquired sufficient experience and that he or she has acquired a certain degree of confidence with the various basic steps of phacoemulsification before attempting this technique. He or she should always be aware that this variation of phacoemulsification may have to be resorted to even though the surgeon may have planned a more advanced form of surgery, such as the techniques that will be described in the following chapters. For this very reason, the steps of phacoemulsification in the pupillary plane must be an integral part of the surgical armamentarium of all surgeons who use phacoemulsification as a routine instrument in cataract surgery.

The steps in the operation are:
- Preliminary steps.
- Phacoemulsification with U/S.

### Preliminary Steps

The operating field is prepared with fixing of the superior and inferior rectus.

The conjunctiva is cut at the limbus, and the episcleral vessels are coagulated with a bipolar coagulator.

A 3.1 mm incision is made with a calibrated blade in correspondence to the posterior third of the surgical limbus, parallel to the iris to allow entrance of the cystotome.

The incision, in the technique presented by Little and Emery, was an evolutionary step in phacoemulsification. It is performed in the scleral portion of the surgical limbus and produces two planes, the first orthogonal to the sclera and the second parallel to the iris.

This type of indirect incision allows better hold on the infusion liquids, facilitates access to the pupillary plane

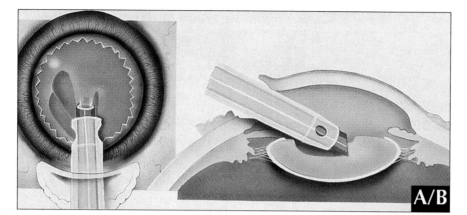

Figures 6-9A, 6-9B. Technique on the pupillary plane. The nucleus is carved to a bowl-shape in the proximal and central parts. The removal of the material must be deep and wide. The nucleus is left intact distally.

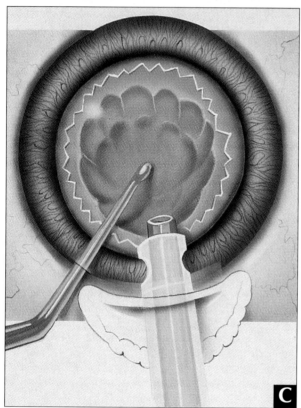

Figure 6-9C. The spatula is introduced through the side port incision, and then the U/S tip is withdrawn to the limit of the capsulotomy. At this point, the surgeon moves the pedal to Position 0 (ie, he or she closes I/A ) so the chamber will flatten and the nucleus will tend to rise in the anterior chamber.

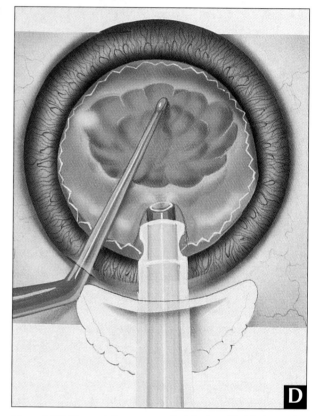

Figure 6-9D. The spatula presses at 6 o'clock and holds the nucleus in position in that area so only the proximal equator dislocates from the capsular bag and rises in the anterior chamber also due to interruption of irrigation. When the proximal equator has been brought forward sufficiently, the U/S tip is brought forward until it hooks the nucleus at the equator. At this point, the pedal is first brought into Position 1 (irrigation) and then into Position 2. Once the situation has been checked, the phaco can begin.

where the ultrasonic fragmentation takes place, and lastly reduces postoperative astigmatism.

However, care must be taken when performing the cuts to ensure they are not too deep, ie, they should not reach the base of the iris, risking a prolapse. Also the incision must be exactly the right size, because if the main incision is even slightly larger than required, the entire operation will be much more difficult. The iris tends to obstruct the incision and therefore prevent the escape of BSS. No preliminary maneuver is performed on the nucleus before staring phacoemulsification.

Finally, the stimulus of the iris brings about a tendency toward miosis with increased operating difficulties. The reduction in the outward flow also can result in a reduction of the depth of the chamber; if the tip is also in occlusion (if there is zero flow in aspiration) and the surgeon is using U/S, the tip will not be cooled, and the edges of the incision may be burnt. The reduced fluid loss

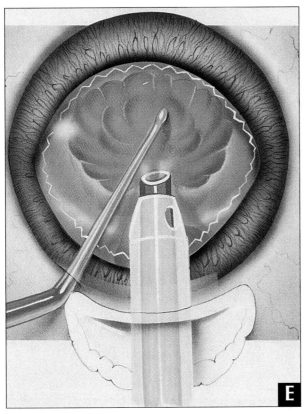 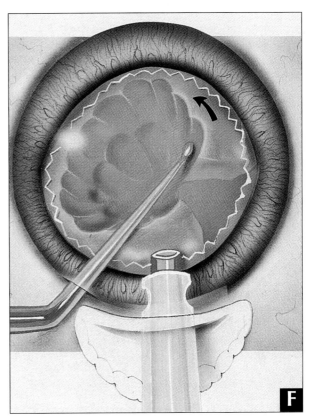

Figure 6-9E. Emulsification removes a proximal equatorial sector while the spatula stabilizes the nucleus and keeps it slightly raised, ready and waiting for the U/S tip.

Figure 6-9F. The nucleus is rotated through 20 to 40°. Another sector of the nucleus is presented to the U/S tip for emulsification.

### Table 6-4
### PHACOEMULSIFICATION AT PUPILLARY PLANE ACCORDING TO LITTLE

| | |
|---|---|
| Comment | This was the first technique in the posterior chamber. The procedure has been developed and perfected by various authors including Emery, Shearing, Sinskey, and Kratz. |
| Nucleus | It is indicated for middle hard nuclei (Grade 3). |
| Incision | Posterior limbal. |
| Capsulotomy | Can opener with various shapes like a D or H, triangular, round, wide, and narrow. |
| Central fragmentation: Phase 1 | No preliminary maneuver is performed on the nucleus before starting phaco; the parameters are those fixed by the current machines (vacuum 40, flow 20, U/S adjustable by the surgeon). Shearing, which is removal of superficial layers, engaging only one-third to one-half of the tip hole. About half or two-thirds of the nucleus is carved to make a bowl. Carving is not extended distally to leave a portion of the nucleus that will be useful as support for the spatula in the subsequent phase. |
| Mobilization of the nucleus on pupillary plane: Phase 2 | Penetration with the U/S tip close to the incision. The spatula is inserted in the lateral incision and placed at 6 distally to the U/S tip in the hollow made in Phase 1. The pedal is set on Position 0 in order to stop emission of fluid and reduce the depth of the anterior chamber. This way, the portion of nucleus proximal to the incision is lifted (whereas the distal portion is lowered by means of the spatula). The U/S tip moves forward and captures the nucleus at 12; then the pedal is operated on Position 1 and subsequently on Position 2. |
| Equatorial fragmentation: Phase 3 | Once fixation of the nucleus has been achieved, a portion of equator equal to 30 to 40° mm is fragmented. With the spatula, the nucleus is rotated, and another equatorial portion is exposed to the U/S tip. Further rotation and fragmentation follow until the whole nuclear equator is removed. The central deep portion remains. |
| Fragmentation of the central residue: Phase 4 | The spatula mobilizes the nucleus residue and exposes it to the U/S tip, which fragments it in the anterior chamber. |

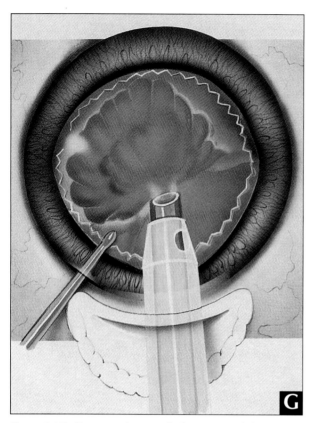 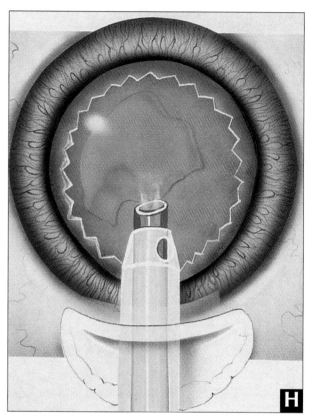

Figure 6-9G. Phaco continues with the support of the spatula, which stabilizes the material and exposes it to the tip.

Figure 6-9H. The last piece of nucleus is emulsified with or without support from the spatula; a large part of the emulsification was therefore performed on the same plane as the iris.

from the chamber may increase the internal pressure.

The anterior capsulotomy to be associated with this type of operation is the classical can opener technique. The widest range of shapes have been suggested—round, wide, narrow, D-shaped, H-shaped, triangular—to name but a few. However, most surgeons prefer the wide, round opening (ie, large cap opener).

At the end of the capsulotomy, the nucleus is not manipulated. However, it is useful to mobilize the anterior capsule to ensure that it is completely free for removal with a McPherson forceps or for aspiration in the first step using the U/S tip.

### Ultrasonic Fragmentation

Once the capsulotomy has been completed, if possible, the anterior capsule is removed and the U/S tip is introduced with the pedal in Position 1. This is a two-handed technique.

The accessory spatula can be introduced through the main incision, but it is better to cut an accessory incision 70 to 90° from the main one toward 2 to 3 o'clock (for right-handed surgeons), prior to beginning phacoemulsification.

When the U/S tip is inside the anterior chamber, the anterior capsule can be aspirated by bringing the pedal to Position 2 or by pushing to Position 3 and beginning the fragmentation. This consists of four basic stages:
- Central fragmentation in situ.
- Subluxation of the nucleus on the pupillary plane.
- Equatorial fragmentation.
- Fragmentation of the residual central nuclear material.

### Central Fragmentation

Initially, the nucleus is not mobilized and is therefore still connected to the cortex and the capsule. In order to avoid excessive pressure on the capsulo-zonular system, in the first step, the tip *shaves* the nucleus. In this first phase, the tip is held tangentially so that the central orifice is covered by material for not more than one-third to one-half of its diameter.

As the grooves in the nucleus become deeper, the tip will encounter harder layers, and it must therefore shave more firmly though more superficially. With the Cavitron/Kelman 8000 V, the parameters were standard (ie, they could not be varied). Only U/S power can be varied; vacuum is set at 41 mm Hg and flow at 20 cc/min.

With currently available instruments, the same values can be used, or they can be varied slightly depending on the surgeon's experience.

The aim of central shaving is to create a sort of concave-convex bowl with removal of about one-half or one-third of the thickness of the central nucleus.

This is obtained with 50 to 80% of U/S power depending on the hardness of the nucleus. Shaving should not extend too close to 6 o'clock, but should be slightly asymmetrical so that the residual material in this position acts as a support for the spatula in the successive step.

Table 6-5
## TECHNIQUE ON PUPILLARY PLANE ACCORDING TO BURATTO

| | Technique used between 1980 and 1987 | Updated technique |
|---|---|---|
| Incision | Sclero-corneal or limbal. | Scleral or corneal short tunnel with early entrance in the chamber. |
| Capsulotomy | Can opener under BSS. | Large rhexis with peripheral decentration close to the incision. Chamber filled with Provisc. |
| Early phase of phaco | Shaving first, then deep carving involving the proximal and central portion of the nucleus. The procedure is gradual and progressive. Carving goes deep if the nucleus is hard and is less extended if it is soft. The distal portion of the nucleus is left nearly intact. | Shaving and carving as the procedure described on the left. |
| Intermediate phase of phaco—Luxation of the nucleus | Two-handed procedure. Olive-shaped spatula at 6. Retraction of the U/S tip toward the incision behind the proximal end of the equator. Pedal on Position 0 to let the chamber flatten. Slight pressure with the spatula at 6 to induce elevation of the nucleus at 12. Advancement of the tip with impalement of the proximal equatorial nucleus. Pedal operated on Position 1 and soon thereafter on Position 2. | The same as described on the left. In addition, the protection is provided by viscoelastic in the anterior chamber. Possibility to induce or ease viscoluxation of the upper hemi-nucleus with injection of Viscoat inside the bag superiorly. Higher parameters may be used to ease capture of the nucleus at the equator. Vacuum—60-120. Flow—15-22. U/S linear control. |
| Advanced phase of phaco | Equatorial emulsification of a sector. Nucleus rotation with spatula. Emulsification of another proximal sector. | Beginning of U/S with equatorial emulsification. |
| Final phase of phaco | Emulsification of residual nucleus in the anterior chamber, which is mobilized by the spatula. | Capture of the residual nuclear material can be accomplished occluding the U/S tip. |

One critical decision is the amount of central shaving. The surgeon must be experienced enough to know when to stop and when to continue. The hardness of the nucleus can provide important information. If the nucleus is hard, the surgeon may stop earlier in order to avoid precocious mobilization (and phacoemulsification in the anterior chamber). If the nucleus is soft, the surgeon must proceed to reach the harder layers in order to have sufficient support for the spatula during luxation.

In any case, the surgeon must stop as soon as the reflex of the central nucleus changes from gray to pink, as this shows that he or she is close to the posterior cortex.

It should be remembered that the U/S tip, particularly when used at the stronger levels, brings with it mechanical energy. Its action, which may appear sufficient for the nucleus, may damage less resistant structures located just a few tenths of a millimeter away (posterior capsule).

### Subluxation of the Nucleus

Once the first step of phacoemulsification has been satisfactorily completed, the foot pedal is brought into Position 2, and the tip is stopped at 12 o'clock close to the incision. The spatula is also inserted. The accessory instrument is positioned at 6 o'clock on the edge of the previously carved concavity, and the U/S tip is gently pulled backward close to the entrance at 12 o'clock.

When the two instruments are positioned along the ideal line, which connects 12 o'clock to 6 o'clock, the pedal is brought to Position 0 to block the intake of fluid and reduce the depth of the anterior chamber. In this way, the nucleus is pushed upward, while the spatula at 6 o'clock tilts and luxates the equatorial portion alone at 12 o'clock in correspondence to the U/S tip.

Once this situation is created, the U/S tip must quickly engage the equator. This must be accompanied by a rapid shift of the pedal to Position 1 and immediately afterward to Position 2.

This combined maneuver must give a two-fold result. It must:
1. Keep the portion of luxated nucleus in the anterior chamber through contact with the instrument and aspiration.
2. Separate the cortico-nuclear adhesions in the superior sector—thanks also to irrigation.

This is a critical step as it requires considerable coordination and may be frustrating even for a highly skilled, expert surgeon. Sometimes the nucleus will not move, or it escapes when irrigation is activated.

If after repeated attempts the maneuver is not successful, the surgeon can proceed in one of two ways. He or she can either:
- Continue the central shaving and try to extend it laterally.
- Try to rotate the nucleus with the spatula to remove the cortico-nuclear adhesions. This must be done carefully as the fine instrument can come into contact with an area of lower resistance and perforate the nucleus, damaging the posterior capsule.

### *Equatorial Fragmentation*

Once the surgeon has obtained the fixation of the nucleus with the U/S tip, fragmentation begins with short bursts of U/S to remove a 40 to 50° sector of the nucleus, just enough to avoid excessive inclination of the U/S tip and keep it within the central safety zone.

Then the U/S tip is gently pulled backward and with the pedal in Position 2, the nucleus is rotated in a clockwise direction with the spatula, so as to present the U/S tip with a new equatorial portion for emulsification. Simultaneously, the last cortico-nuclear adhesions are removed.

During this phase, it can happen, through lack of control of the instruments, that the nucleus slips back into the posterior chamber and cannot be engaged by the U/S tip. In this case, the surgeon must repeat the initial maneuver of partial luxation of the nucleus with the spatula positioned at 6 o'clock and the pedal in Position 0.

If it does happen, the surgeon must avoid collapse of the anterior chamber with inevitable damage to the endothelium. It is better, therefore, to reactivate Position 1 or 2 of the pedal even if the nucleus is not engaged, rather than attempt to continue with a flattened chamber. The VES can be very useful if difficulties arise as they allow the surgeon to mobilize the nucleus without any trauma. However, as this involves a series of supplementary steps, it is best used only if there is no other way out. Viscoat is particularly useful in these situations.

Once the nucleus has been completely rotated, a small central free portion remains.

### *Fragmentation of the Central Remaining Nucleus*

With the foot pedal in Position 2, the nucleus is engaged in the anterior chamber to complete the emulsification with U/S power reduced. During this phase, the spatula is extremely useful because it mobilizes the nuclear material and brings it close to the U/S tip, stabilizing it while the tip fragments it. It protects the endothelium and the posterior capsule from any contact with the nuclear material. For best results, excellent coordination between the hand and foot movements is essential.

## **Completion of the Operation**

The pieces of residual cortex are removed with the I/A tip. The incision is then extended to implant the artificial lens. With the standard technique, which involves a wide anterior can opener capsulotomy, the implantation is scheduled for the sulcus.

In the original technique, a posterior chamber lens was used (J-loop type). The lens was grasped with a McPherson forceps and inserted in the anterior chamber under air so that the inferior loop slid over the inferior edge of the capsulotomy, under visual control.

The superior loop is caught in correspondence to the distal third; it is pushed toward the 6 o'clock position while the lens is rotated. The superior loop thus slides gently under the superior edge of the capsulotomy, again under visual control.

If the intraoperative conditions require, the maneuver can be facilitated by using a hook to retract the iris or the capsular edge. Then an iridectomy is performed, and the incision is sutured with 10-0 nylon.

## **Indications for Fragmentation on the Pupillary Plane**

The ideal conditions for this technique are a deep anterior chamber, a pupil that can be well-dilated, and a medium-hard nucleus (Grade 3).

If the nucleus is soft, the procedure may not be straightforward, as the spatula may *slice through* the nucleus without luxating it. If, on the other hand, the nucleus is hard, the procedure may require a longer time and fragments may form, which are projected forcefully toward the endothelium and the posterior capsule under the action of the U/S.

## **Updating of the Technique**

At present, this technique can be performed with a large capsulorhexis under VES protection.

Also by using a VES (Viscoat), it is possible to perform the phacoemulsification with greater endothelial protection and implant in the capsular bag.

As the instrumental parameters can be set on modern equipment, values that are more suitable to the various phases of phacoemulsification can be used.

During the central shaving, in proportion to the hardness of the nucleus, the vacuum can be set between 0 and 20 mm Hg to avoid excessive mobilization of the nucleus. The flow rate can be set between 10 and 20 cc/min for the same reason. The U/S power can be regulated with the linear control pedal. In the initial phase, the limit can be 50 to 70% and in the intermediate phase 60 to 90% in proportion to the hardness of the nucleus.

The phase of subluxation of the nucleus is facilitated by increasing the vacuum to 8 to 100 mm Hg and the flow rate to 25 cc/min in order to make it easier for the U/S tip to block the equatorial nucleus. Equatorial fragmentation can be performed with vacuum of 60 to 80 mm Hg, flow rate of 18 to 22 cc/min, and the linear U/S.

In the final step, the residual portion of the nucleus is easily attracted by the U/S tip with these parameters helped by the spatula. Phacoemulsification can be performed with short, low power U/S bursts, adjusting foot pedal to Position 3, and, if necessary, resorting to the pulsed U/S mode to make the maneuver more delicate.

## Comment

Phacoemulsification in the pupillary plane is a bridge technique between Kelman's and the techniques in the posterior chamber, which will be described in the following chapters. It is important historically, as it indicated the possibility of intervening with the U/S tip in an area that is equidistant from the endothelium and the posterior capsule.

Readers should not forget that in 1978, with the instruments and the equipment available at that time, the endothelium and the posterior capsule worried the surgeon most (and not much has changed), and this potential danger was the core of the debate forwarded by the opponents of phacoemulsification.

Today, the numerous possibilities of adjusting the instrument, the technological developments in the phacoemulsifiers, the improvements in the surgical techniques, and the use of VES have made every intraocular operation much safer. However, though some developments may appear to be taken for granted, they are really the consequence of a constant drive toward innovation, such as the method I have just described.

From a purely technical point of view, the most important step is the anterior subluxation of the superior nuclear equator with simultaneous fixing by the U/S tip, very different and much safer than Kelman's technique.

It is a technically difficult phase that can frequently give rise to problems. It is no coincidence that the more recent techniques base the evolution of the operating strategy on overcoming this step.

In practice, the surgeon should consider that with a single maneuver he or she obtains:
- Mobilization of the superior hemi-nucleus.
- Cleavage of the cortical connections.
- Access to the nuclear equator by the U/S tip.

This observation alone justifies the surgeon learning the correct way of performing this technique. Moreover, he or she may have to use it in the event other maneuvers planned for phacoemulsification cannot be continued safely during the operation.

## Phacoemulsification in the Posterior Chamber: Maloney's Technique (1988)

This was a natural step forward. The change consists in performing a greater part of the phacoemulsification phase underneath the iridial plane.

The in situ sculpting is extended to involve most of the nucleus. It saves for the final stage, following mobilization, just the equatorial and posterior portions. In this way, phacoemulsification is performed almost totally under the iris plane.

The technique is the maximum development in the two-handed techniques associated with a traditional can opener capsulotomy.

Numerous authors have contributed to this technique, which Maloney (1988) defined by summarizing the various points perfected in previous years. This technical progress was the response to the need to make phacoemulsification more accurate and more reliable, thanks also to the developments in the equipment designed to correspond to the operators' requests.

This method is also split into:
- Preliminary steps.
- Central shaving with the U/S.
- Mobilization of the nucleus.
- Emulsification of the residual plate.

### Preliminary Steps

Following the standard preparation of the operating field and the conjunctiva, an incision is made in the posterior limbal sector. This is a scleral extension of the two-plane limbal incision. The sclera is cut perpendicularly 1.5 mm from the limbus for about half its thickness. With a beveled blade, the surgeon makes a cleavage to the cornea leaving a thin diaphragm of sclero-corneal tissue in front of the Schwalbe line. This can be easily exceeded by the cystotome so that the capsulotomy is performed in a closed chamber.

If the dissection is too deep, it may mean that the entrance to the anterior chamber is too close to the base of the iris, with greater risk of a prolapse of the iris during the various surgical phases. Once the preparation of the main incision is completed, the side port incision is prepared. This must be done at 2 to 3 o'clock, in front of the limbal vascular arches, parallel to the iris plane, with a width of 1 mm.

The main entrance to the anterior chamber will vary depending on the type of capsulotomy planned. The entrance of the cystotome can be varied:

1. Direct entrance of the cystotome. The dissection must push anteriorly almost to Descemet's membrane.
   In this way, the bent tip of a 25 to 27 gauge needle can enter the anterior chamber without excessive pushing so that the capsulotomy can be performed in a closed chamber. In this case, the side port incision is created once the capsulotomy has been completed.
2. Incision just less than 1 mm (just wide enough to allow the cystotome to enter). The blade must be inserted parallel to the iris in correspondence to the end part of the sclero-corneal cleavage. If the capsulotomy does not require excessive manipulation, the depth of the anterior chamber can also be maintained with BSS but VES is preferable.
3. A 3.2 mm incision with a calibrated keratome. By anteriorizing the sclero-corneal dissection sufficiently in the cornea, the surgeon can perform an incision suitable for phacoemulsification. However, he or she must use a VES to maintain the shape of the anterior chamber during the capsulotomy.

With this technique, the can opener capsulotomy can have a variety of shapes. The surgeon can choose his or her elective shape as the successive phases are independent of the capsulotomy performed. Once the capsulotomy is completed, which I will assume is the classical wide can opener, the U/S tip is inserted with the foot pedal in Position 1. The tip must be placed in contact with the surface of the nucleus, with the beveled orifice toward the operator because the cutting action is under direct visual

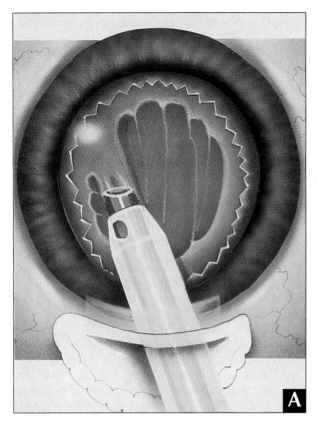

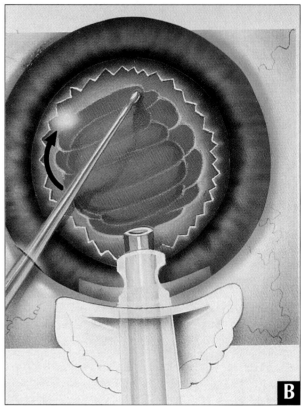

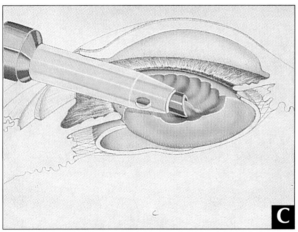

Figures 6-10A, 6-10B, 6-10C. Phaceomulsification in the posterior chamber. The nucleus is carved to a bowl shape. This is rotated through 180° using an olive-tipped spatula. The sculpting is repeated distally.

control. The U/S tip is 30 or 45° with the sleeve in the usual position.

Upon moving the pedal to Position 2, there is immediate aspiration of the anterior capsule, which must be completely free. The parameters of the instrument have the standard values.

This type of incision is more sophisticated and is also more difficult than those used previously. Nevertheless, it is an important milestone when learning self-sealing tunnel incisions.

### Central Shaving with U/S

The most suitable U/S tip has a 30° cutting surface. The U/S power is set between 50 and 80% depending on the hardness of the nucleus.

Central fragmentation begins with shaving the nucleus by placing the U/S tip tangentially to the surface. Superimposed grooves are created with the action of the U/S tip always superficial to the material. Gradually, the sculpting is deepened in each successive step.

The surgeon should always remember to return the pedal to Position 2 when the cutting phase has ended and bring the U/S tip backward toward the incision after every sculpting step.

The depth of each groove must correspond to about half the diameter of the U/S tip (or slightly less), but in soft nuclei, a depth corresponding to two-thirds to three-fourths of the diameter of the tip itself can be reached.

The extension of the sculpted area depends on the size of the capsulotomy and the degree of mydriasis. In any case, it should be as wide as possible so that the majority of phacoemulsification is performed in the posterior chamber with the nucleus in its original position. When cutting the grooves, the surgeon should allow for the biconvex shape of the lens and deepen the sculpting more in the center and less nearer the equator.

The adhesion of the nucleus to the cortex during this surgical phase is very important in that it resists the action of the U/S tip, permitting more rapid, effective emulsification.

Moving toward the periphery of the nucleus, the surgeon must pay a lot of attention to avoid any contact

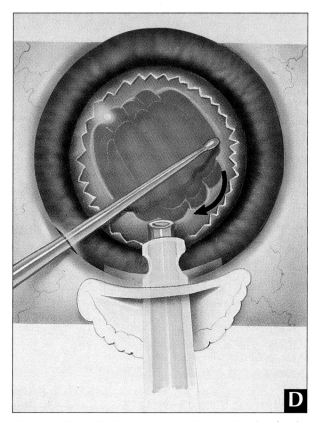
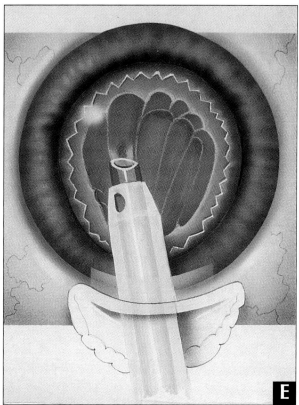

Figures 6-10D, 6-10E. The nucleus is again rotated and sculpted to produce a wide bowl and to leave a thin layer of material inside the bag.

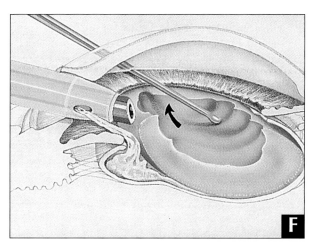

Figures 6-10F, 6-10G. The spatula introduced through the lateral opening presses the nucleus gently at 6 o'clock. This initially raises the nucleus and facilitates the capture of the equator by the U/S tip. The surgeon thus obtains emulsification of the superficial equatorial sector. The maneuver requires good coordination. The foot pedal is brought to Position 0. The U/S tip is withdrawn to the limit of the capsulotomy. The surgeon presses gently with the spatula at 6 o'clock; the tip is then brought close to engage the equator of the nucleus. Irrigation is reactivated. In this way, liquid passes underneath the nucleus, which is separated from the external cortex and/or the posterior capsule. At this point, the equatorial nucleus is emulsified.

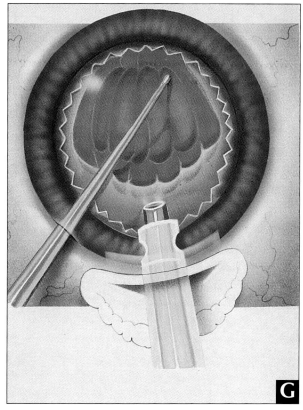

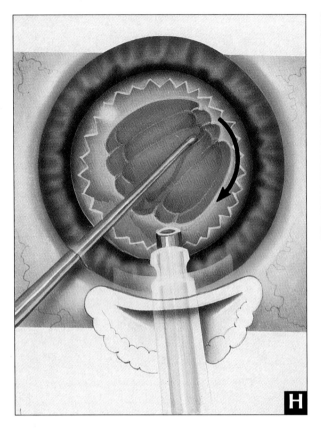

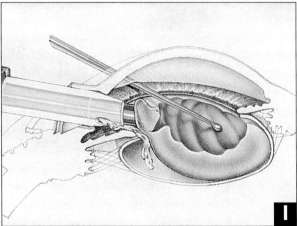

Figures 6-10H, 6-10I. The nucleus is rotated through 90°, and another portion of the equator is emulsified.

between the tip and the edges of the capsulotomy and the iris, as this can be transformed into zonular traction and possible miosis; both situations can be sources of complications as the operation progresses. Regarding the depth of the sculpting, it is better to remove as much nuclear material as possible—about 70 to 80%.

In order to evaluate the depth, the surgeon can refer to the red reflex, which deepening toward the posterior cortex changes from gray to pink. In this phase, the surgeon's personal experience is extremely important. If there is any doubt, it is better not to deepen the sculpting excessively.

In the case of soft nuclei, the sculpting must be reduced in both length and depth, so that the spatula has more material available for the subsequent phases without running the risk of slicing toward the posterior capsule.

As fragmentation proceeds, the U/S power must be adapted to the hardness of the portion of nucleus, adjusting the power of the instrument or, if possible, in real time thanks to the linear surgeon control of the pedal.

The hardest parts of the central nucleus must be tackled by proceeding slowly with the U/S tip on a large contact point between the U/S tip and the material or, better still, with a superficial contact but with repeated short bursts in the central site where the nucleus is thicker and harder.

During sculpting, the surgeon should avoid occluding the tip. This would involve:
- A vacuum increase in the tubes (up to a preset maximum if the occlusion lasts long enough).
- Interruption of the aspiration of the liquid and nuclear particles.
- Heating of the tip (due to a lack of liquid flow inside it) if the U/S continues to be used and if the power is high.
- Suction forces on the nucleus, which are transmitted to the capsulo-zonular system because there was no preliminary separation of the various cataract components (hydrodissection or hydrodelamination).

At the end of the central sculpting, the nucleus is a concave-convex bowl shape with a very wide concavity

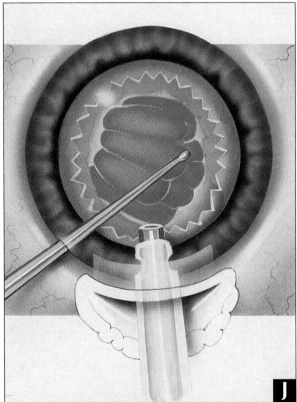

Figure 6-10J. The maneuver is repeated once more.

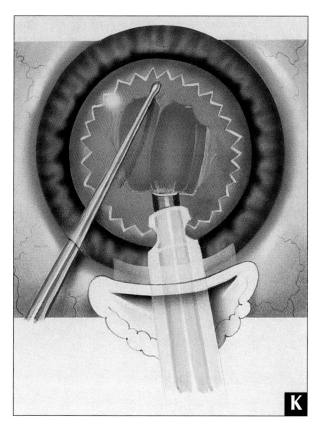
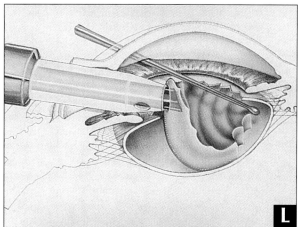

Figures 6-10K, 6-10L. Finally, the last portion of equator and nuclear plate is captured and emulsified.

extending to the limits of the pupillary edges. This material still adheres to the cortex and, indirectly, to the posterior and equatorial capsule.

### Mobilization of the Nucleus

When the central emulsification of the nucleus is extended sufficiently (about 70%), the next step is mobilization.

In order to free the nucleus from the cortico-capsular adhesions, the surgeon can proceed in one of three ways, which can also be combined depending on the requirements of the individual case.

- If the nucleus is moderately hard (Grade 3), it is partially luxated with a maneuver similar to that described already in the previous chapter.

  The U/S tip is gently pushed backward toward the 12 o'clock position just behind the pupillary edge, and the cyclodialysis spatula is positioned at the 6 o'clock position paracentrally and exerts slight pressure, which will detach the superior equatorial portion of the nucleus from the cortical adhesions. When the equator of the nucleus can be seen, the pedal is released (Position 0), and the nucleus is allowed to rise until the equator is above the iris plane. Now the spatula pushes the nucleus toward 6 o'clock once again; the U/S tip fixes the equator, while the pedal is moved to Position 1 and then immediately to Position 2.

  In this way, with a minimal lift and no further luxation of the nucleus, the infusion frees the cortico-nuclear adhesions. This maneuver is an important transition step toward the endocapsular techniques when the surgeon is still practicing the can opener capsulotomy. It can also be used if the capsulorhexis gets out of control.

  The wave of infusion, which moves posteriorly, causes a slight change in the red reflex of the fundus. The nucleus is then returned to the posterior chamber and with the pedal in Position 1, using the spatula, rotated in a clockwise direction. This will free the residual peripheral cortical adhesions without dislocating the nucleus or fragmenting it.

  The rotation must occur in two phases in order to avoid traction on the zonules and posterior capsule. Approximate or hasty manipulations with the spatula should be avoided because these can rupture the nucleus without really freeing it from the cortex.

  The ideal outcome is when there is a nuclear *bowl* rotating freely in the posterior chamber. The nucleus is then caught at 6 o'clock with a spatula and rotated to 8 o'clock to free the cortical adhesions further. The success of this maneuver depends on the hardness of the nucleus and the exactness of the previous steps.

  The greatest problem is that of fragmenting the nucleus with the spatula without succeeding in rotating it. If this happens or if the nucleus is soft or the spatula cannot obtain the desired effect, the partial luxation of the nucleus should be repeated.

- With a medium-hard nucleus (Grade 3), sometimes the cortical adhesions can be freed with a movement of push and rotation (clockwise or counterclockwise; it's not important) using the spatula introduced through the side port incision. The same maneuver can also be performed with the U/S tip, but it is more difficult. If the maneuver is successful, it is enough to depress the nucleus with the spatula in the sectors distal to the main incision, keeping the pedal in Position 2, in order to engage the nuclear equator with the U/S tip at 12 o'clock and begin the intermediate phase of nuclear fragmentation with progressive rotation.

- If the nucleus is medium-soft (Grade 2), a one-handed technique can be adopted. This is possible because the central carving of soft nuclei is reduced in size and depth. The nucleus is impaled by the tip at 6 o'clock at the edge of the central sculpting. With the pedal in Position 2, the tip is allowed to occlude. It then sinks into the nucleus with a short U/S shot. In occlusion, the vacuum increases (to the preset maximum value), and the nucleus sticks to the U/S tip. With this impalement maneuver, keeping the pedal in Position 2, it is possible to rotate the nucleus in a clockwise or counterclockwise direction with a movement of push and rotate by the U/S tip. Once this has been obtained, the nucleus is lifted and brought toward the center, and the surgeon can start emulsifying a limited 30 to 40° sector.

When this is completed, the tip is occluded once again, and the rotation maneuvers are repeated; then, the nucleus is brought above the iris toward the center, and a new sector is fragmented. The maneuver is repeated until the nucleus has been completely rotated and the central portion alone remains.

### *Phacoemulsification of the Residual Nucleus*

Depending on the type of mobilization, the residual portion of nucleus can be of different dimensions—larger if the surgeon just cleaved the cortical planes, smaller if the surgeon subluxated the nucleus, emulsifying the periphery.

If the nuclear portion is mobilized but still extended into the peripheral areas, the nucleus must be given a small lift with the spatula. The spatula is positioned against the inferior wall of the central sculpting giving the nucleus minimal movement both at 6 o'clock and slightly in the depth of the groove. In this way, keeping the pedal in Position 2, the equator is engaged at 12 o'clock with the U/S tip. Then, phacoemulsification is performed.

Fragmentation occurs from the superficial portions to the deep portions of the nuclear equator. Every subsequent portion for emulsification is presented to the U/S tip through a delicate movement of rotation and simultaneous tilting of the nucleus.

Once the circle has been completed, a small portion of nucleus remains—the plate—which is emulsified in the posterior chamber with the help of a spatula and short U/S burst. The surgeon must avoid rapid, uncontrolled movements of the nuclear fragments, which could damage the posterior capsule and the endothelium.

If the residual nucleus is small, it can be attacked directly by the tip. The surgeon can take advantage of the occlusion and bring the nucleus toward the center of the pupil. Alternately, he or she can control it with the spatula in order to emulsify with small U/S bursts.

The basic difference between this technique and that in the pupillary plane is that 80 to 90% of the phacoemulsification occurs under the iris plane.

The spatula is actively involved in the mobilization of the nucleus, which is luxated minimally on the antero-posterior plane but more so on the frontal plane. In this way, compared to the technique in the pupillary plane, the peripheral portions of the nucleus are attacked starting from the superficial portion to the deeper ones with fewer manipulations.

As the techniques become more sophisticated, it stands to reason that the surgeon must be more experienced and competent.

The advantage lies in the fact that he or she has a greater number of exit routes from potentially dangerous situations, thanks to the wide range of techniques, which can be adopted on the basis of the individual case.

### *Completion of the Operation*

Once the emulsification has been completed, the surgeon proceeds with the aspiration of the cortex using a routine I/A, followed by cleaning of the posterior capsule, if necessary.

At this point, a VES is injected into the anterior chamber, and the incision is extended to the size of the lens to be inserted. The original Maloney technique involved the implantation of a posterior chamber *C loop*. The insertion maneuvers of the lens are the same as those described previously.

A variety of sutures can be used with the incision suggested for this technique. Normally, a continuous suture is used with an oblique whip stitch in 10-0 nylon. The addition of one or two interrupted sutures may improve the hold and the control of the postoperative astigmatism.

Of course, sutureless sclero-corneal tunnels can be used with this technique but this is advisable only for expert phacoemulsification surgeons. In fact, the type of entrance incision for the U/S tip created with a tunnel incision modifies all the steps of the phacoemulsification and changes some of the fundamental concepts relative to the basic maneuvers.

It is always better to analyze them. As it may be necessary to have to discard or modify the scheduled technique, it would be better if the surgeon did not have to change the incision, too. A typical case is the formation of a radial tear in the anterior capsule as the surgeon performs a capsulorhexis. The surgeon will then have to complete the capsulotomy with a can opener technique. At this point, if a sclero-corneal tunnel has been created or the surgeon wishes to proceed with the phacoemulsification in the posterior chamber, the technique described above is the elective choice.

With the advancing penetration of the U/S tip, folds and traction are created, which make it necessary to modify the classical maneuvers as follows:

- The handpiece must be tilted upward quite considerably in order to direct the U/S tip downward on the lens.
- During phacoemulsification, the tip must also be slightly tilted laterally in order to obtain better contact with the equatorial nucleus. A larger part of the operation must be done in the posterior chamber.
- With mobilization of the nucleus, the surgeon must be very careful because, as he or she retracts the tip, the irrigation orifices may be obstructed as it pass-

Table 6-6

## POSTERIOR CHAMBER PHACOEMULSIFICATION ACCORDING TO MALONEY

| | Classic technique | Technique updated by Buratto |
|---|---|---|
| Incision | Scleral pocket. | Short scleral tunnel. |
| Capsulotomy | Can opener. | Rhexis decentered superiorly. |
| Early phase of phaco | Shaving and carving with 30° tip using 50-80% of U/S. Sulci are created to the superficial material engaging about 40-50% of the U/S tip. In small increments, carving goes deeper as it must be as extensive and deep as possible (70-80%). The nucleus still adheres to the cortex and capsule, and this has an important function. In fact, it opposes the action of the U/S tip providing a more effective phaco. At the end of carving, the nucleus must be shaped like a concave-convex bowl. No parameters are provided to operate the machine. | Carving with the same technique but protected by viscoelastic and with different parameters:<br>Vacuum—0-20.<br>Flow—10-13.<br>U/S adjustable with pedal according to hardness of the nucleus. |
| Mobilization of the nucleus | This is accomplished with spatula and U/S tip, with maneuver similar to that of the technique on pupillary plane, but with less elevation of the nucleus (which has been carved more deeply and widely in the distal portions).<br>With a combined movement of push and rotation, clockwise and reversed, with the spatula (and in necessary supported by the tip). | With U/S tip only, preceded by hydrodissection or viscodissection with Provisc. |
| Emulsification of the equator and the plate | While depressing distally with the spatula, the U/S tip engages the nucleus proximally.<br>Emulsification is performed in the proximal portion.<br>The nucleus is rotated.<br>With the spatula at 6 the plate is pushed downward. The equator is caught by the U/S tip, and emulsification is performed. Using this procedure, the whole equatorial nucleus is removed.<br>The plate is then lifted with the spatula and emulsified with short U/S low-power bursts (30-40%). | Using the parameters of the machine, the procedure is simplified:<br>Vacuum—60-120.<br>Flow—10-15.<br>U/S linear, low-power.<br>The plate is removed using the U/S tip in occlusion:<br>Vacuum—40-60.<br>Flow—10-15.<br>U/S linear. |

es through the cornea. As aspiration continues, this may result in instability or even collapse of the anterior chamber.

- Likewise, during mobilization, if the tunnel has a perfect hold, it may be difficult to reduce the chamber depth by bringing the pedal into Position 0. It will also be almost impossible to subluxate the nucleus in a single manipulation.

If these problems cannot be resolved, the surgeon should backtrack, close the tunnel, and cut a new incision that gives easier access to the nucleus.

### *Updating the Procedure*

With the knowledge that we have today and the instruments that are now available, the instrument parameters can be adapted during the various phases of the operation in order to optimize the various surgical steps. The general concept is to start with relatively low values of vacuum (0 to 20 mm Hg) and flow (10 to 15 cc/min) to avoid traumatizing the nucleus and the zonula.

After sculpting and mobilization, the vacuum can be increased to 80 to 120 mm Hg and the flow to 20 to 25 cc/min to facilitate the removal of the residual nucleus.

The U/S power, with a maximum limit of 80% in linear, can be adjusted on the basis of the hardness of the nucleus by controlling the pressure on the pedal.

### *Comment*

The above technique represents the end of the evolution of traditional phacoemulsification associated with the traditional techniques of capsulotomy. It is, undoubtedly, the method that allows the most sophisticated and precise operation and allows the surgeon to tackle a very wide range of surgical cases.

The incision with the scleral pocket itself is a very important innovative element, which leads directly to the

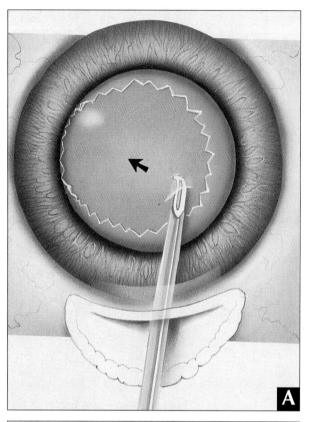

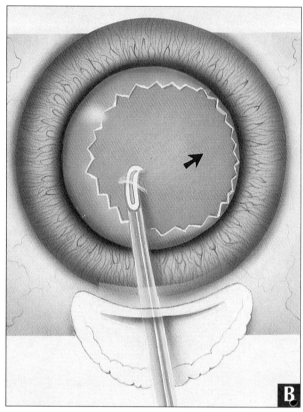

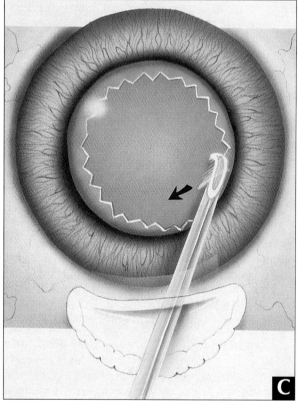

Figures 6-11A, 6-11B, 6-11C. Phacoemulsification in the posterior chamber, variation with narrow pupil. In the diagram, the pupil is left partially mydriatic so the maneuver can be seen more clearly. With the cystotome, the nucleus is moved to the left and then to the right inside the capsular bag, and as soon as the cortical adhesions have been reduced, it is rotated. This maneuver serves to free the nucleus inside the bag.

advanced sutureless techniques of phacoemulsification, dealt with in the following chapters.

In fact, this type of approach has opened the door to a whole series of comments on the control of postoperative astigmatism and on patient rehabilitation times, which have been the main objectives of phacoemulsification for the past 10 years and are the focal points of cataract surgery at present. Even the methods for nucleus removal strive for higher levels of precision and delicacy, possible also through the amazing technological developments in phacoemulsification equipment.

This type of operation, with all its special characteristics, is, therefore, extremely important and is a fundamental milestone in a surgeon's surgical training. The surgeon must learn this if he or she wishes to be in a position to tackle techniques that are even more advanced and sophisticated.

## Endocapsular Phacoemulsification

This term covers the all the various advanced techniques of phacoemulsification introduced during the second half of the 1980s.

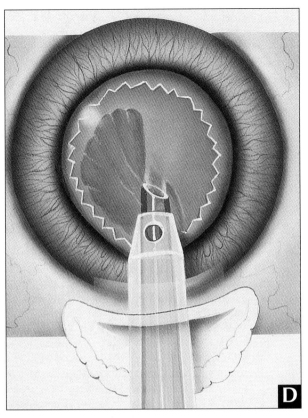

Figure 6-11D. Phaco starts with the superficial sculpting, which is then extended toward the center and then toward the equator (without reaching it).

Figure 6-11E. In this position, the tip is impaled using the U/S (foot pedal in Position 3). (The diagram shows the U/S tip too close to the posterior capsule.)

Figure 6-11F. Using the tip as an instrument (pedal in Position 2), the nucleus is raised slightly to present it inside the pupil (and inside the capsulotomy). Here, the accessible, raised portion is emulsified; the nucleus is then rotated; and the procedure is repeated in another site. Sector by sector, the equatorial nuclear mass is reduced considerably. The residual central mass is then raised, dislocated using the spatula, and then slowly emulsified.

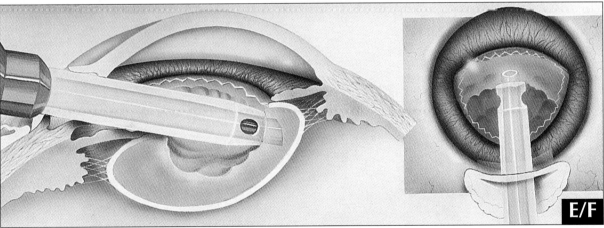

The innovation involves all the various phases of the cataract operation, which will be covered in the following chapters. I have included descriptions of some of the basic operation types and all the relative steps.

In these years, the main factors that are considered the turning point in the techniques of phacoemulsification and that rekindled interest in the technique and highlighted the advantages are:
- Capsulorhexis.
- Hydrodissection.
- Self-sealing tunnel incision.
- The technological evolution of the phacoemulsification equipment.
- The growing use of foldable intraocular lenses or those for small incisions.

Regarding the equipment, the two most important innovations were the introduction of the linear foot control and the possibility of selecting the flow rate and the vacuum to suit the needs of the surgeon during every single phase of the operation.

Technically, these characteristics have been translated into the possibility of being able to perform some of the basic steps with an U/S tip alone, and, therefore, I had the development of new one-handed techniques in addition to the classical two-handed techniques.

We have already mentioned capsulorhexis, hydrodissection, and the self-sealing or sutureless incisions, and they will be mentioned again.

IOLs are dealt with in a specific chapter.

## General Comments on the Endocapsular Techniques

The endocapsular techniques have evolved in time in the quest of the objective of making phacoemulsification safer and the least traumatic possible, an objective reached through the identification of a series of ideas to learn, rules to follow, surgical techniques to learn, and precautions to take.

### Respect for the Cornea

This objective is followed by intervening on three basic factors: spatial, mechanical, and kinetic.

- First of all, the position of the phacoemulsification. The action on the nucleus must be done in the posterior chamber with protection by the capsular bag (the smaller the diameter of the capsulorhexis, the greater the protection). In this case, the spatial factor comes into play because all the elements that are potentially traumatic are applied at a safe distance from the cornea.
- Secondly, the power and the time of U/S are reduced. The techniques of nucleofracture permit this result even with hard nuclei. In this case, the important factor is mechanical.
- The third factor is the method of phacoemulsification. The nucleus is mobilized inside the bag with the hydrodissection reducing, if not eliminating completely, the traction on the zonules.

This is where the kinetic factor comes into play relative to the total energy transmitted to the ocular structures and the turbulence that is created in the anterior chamber.

Moreover, the procedure of endocapsular phacoemulsification has a specific variation for every degree of nuclear hardness, with the objective of always using reduced U/S power for a limited effective time, compared to the traditional techniques of phacoemulsification.

The result is a greater intraoperative respect for the endothelium with consequent better corneal transparency in the immediate postoperative, but particularly in the long-term.

### Respect for the Iris

The same factors that limit the trauma to the endothelium can be called upon to reduce the negative effects on the iris.

All the preparatory and effective maneuvers for the endocapsular phacoemulsification avoid contact with the iris. The rim of the capsulorhexis acts as an important protective diaphragm for the iris. (This means not exclusively in the cases where it is possible to obtain wide mydriasis, but particularly in those cases where the pupil is difficult to dilate or that contracts during the operation.)

With respect to the iris, there is the possibility of completing the operation with the pupil still quite well dilated, and there is a marked reduction in the inflammatory response with a less problematic postoperative result.

### Respect for the Capsule and the Zonules

Some of the surgical steps that were described previously in relation to the techniques in the pupillary plane and in the posterior chamber can be elements that are potentially traumatic for the capsulo-zonular system.

The maneuvers of mobilization and emulsification inside the bag with the techniques described previously tend to transfer mechanical-kinetic energy to both the capsule and the zonules. This does not happen with the endocapsular techniques.

Numerous factors contribute in an important manner to the safety of phacoemulsification in the capsular bag.

- The first is the capsulorhexis. As it provides a continuous circular capsular rim, it provides a resistant elastic opening that allows the surgeon to free the nucleus inside the capsular bag, preventing it from sliding or escaping into the anterior chamber.
- The second is the hydrodissection, a general term that covers the various steps that allow the hydrocleavage of the lens structures, making them independent of each other from a mechanical-kinetic point of view.
  With hydrodissection, there is complete mobility of the nucleus in the bag, and the elasticity of the capsular-zonular system is maintained for the emulsification of the nucleus.
- The third factor is the technological development in the phacoemulsification equipment, which now allows the surgeon to perform extremely delicate maneuvers inside the bag. In particular, the surgeon can adapt the maneuvers to his or her own dexterity and preferences with real-time adjustment of the parameters of the machine's performance, on the basis of the various requirements that appear during the operation.

It is, therefore, unquestionable that the advanced techniques of endocapsular phacoemulsification, with or without nuclear fracture, must be the final objective of the surgeon practicing phacoemulsification.

This result can be obtained with a methodical, progressive preparation that is based on the following steps:

- Suitable theoretical training.
- Technical-practical training, also through simulated systems, in the basic maneuvers of phacoemulsification.
- Selection of cases suitable for the surgeon's capability and careful adherence to the various steps of the operation.
- Gradual progression to the more difficult techniques following a suitable amount of training with the traditional techniques.
- In the event of difficulties, the surgeon should resort to a simpler technique of phacoemulsification. If necessary, convert the procedure to a manual extracapsular technique.
- In this evolution, realize that there is no single best operation, but just the one that will give the best results in the surgeon's hands. It is in the patient's best interest that the surgeon chooses the one he or she feels most comfortable with.

## Fragmentation Using U/S

In endocapsular phacoemulsification, the U/S tip performs a variety of functions, which are the extension of those performed in the traditional techniques of the past.

| Table 6-7 |
|---|
| **CLASSIFICATION OF THE ENDOCAPSULAR TECHNIQUES** |
| 1. Shepherd's one-handed endocapsular phacoemulsification technique. |
| 2. The intercapsular phacoemulsification technique according to Michelson-Hara. |
| 3. Two-handed phacoemulsification, Davison's Cut and Suck technique. |
| 4. Fine's two-handed nuclear cleavage technique. |
| 5. Two-handed nuclear fracture technique: |
|     Nuclear fracture (cross-shaped or into four quadrants) according to Shepherd. |
|     Gimbel's Divide and Conquer nuclear fracture technique. |
|       Trench DCN. |
|       Gimbel's Crater DCN. |
|       Downslope sculpting (Gimbel's DSS). |
|     Dillman-Maloney's Fractional 2/4 technique. |
|     Crack and Flip technique according to Fine, Maloney, and Dillman. |
|     Nagahara's Phaco Chop. |
|     Stop and Chop by Koch. |

| Table 6-8 |
|---|
| **OTHER ENDOCAPSULAR TECHNIQUES** |
| Divide and Conquer—Pacifico's one-handed variation |
| Davison's minimal multiple lift |
| Separation of the nucleus according to Smith |
| Kelmen's V technique |
| Arnold's nuclear flip technique |
| Akahoshi's phaco prechop |
| Spring surgery according to Osher |
| Divide and Tilt according to Budo |
| Snap and Split according to Fukasaku |
| Phaco with inverted flow according to Kelman |
| Phaco flip according to Brown |
| Phaco Sweep sculpting according to Gimbel |

- Manipulation—The U/S tip can be used to rotate, raise, and fragment the nucleus mechanically, with or without the help of a spatula.

    These maneuvers are performed once the lens structures have been carefully defined by hydrodissection, and the nucleus can then be easily mobilized inside the capsular bag.

- Rotation of the nucleus using the U/S tip—This one-handed maneuver can be done basically in two ways.

    In the first, with the foot pedal in Position 2, the nucleus is pushed and rotated without occluding the tip. This occurs under the condition that the nucleus is sufficiently mobile after hydrodissection, because for the correct execution of this maneuver, it is necessary for the tip to exert as little force as possible for the rotation.

    The second possibility is that of occluding the tip, ie, impaling the nucleus or part of it and pulling it in the desired direction, and rotating it. This is indicated particularly in the event of incomplete mobilization, when the surgeon wishes to complete the operation despite an insufficient hydrodissection.

    The first maneuver is done more easily with the tip at 30°; the second with the tip at 45° because occlusion is obtained more easily.

    Details of the maneuvers will be described in the specific chapter.

- Nuclear fracture with the U/S tip—This is a two-handed technique where the U/S tip and spatula are used as surgical instruments.

After having created a sufficiently deep groove, the U/S tip is placed in the deep part more or less at the right side of the groove, while the spatula is placed on the left side (some surgeons actually cross the instruments to increase the separation). The instruments are progressively distanced, so that the groove opens until the surgeon sees the fracture line appear running from the peripheral area to the center of the nucleus.

The details of the maneuver and the technique are described in the specific chapter.

## Classification

The various endocapsular techniques can be classed as follows:
1. One-handed phacoemulsification.
2. Intercapsular phacoemulsification.
3. Two-handed phacoemulsification.
A. Technique of cut and suck for nuclei of moderate-low hardness.
B. Technique of cleavage for nuclei of moderate hardness (Chip and Flip by
C. Technique of nucleofracture for nuclei of moderate-high hardness.
- Shepherd's cross technique.
- Divide and Conquer by Gimbel, Nucleofractis and variations (Trench DCN and Crater DCN).
- DSS by Gimbel.
- Fractional 2/4 by Dillman and Maloney.
- Technique Crack and Flip by Fine.
- Technique of Phaco Chop by Nagahara and variations.
- Stop and Chop by Koch.
- And many other variations.

## One-Handed Endocapsular Phacoemulsification (Shepherd's Technique)

This is a one-handed technique suitable for nuclei of moderate to low hardness (Grade 1 to 2). With care, the surgeon can use it with nuclei of moderate-high hardness.

In this technique, the surgeon should not use excessive hydrodissection, as the nucleus may mobilize too early, creating problems with control of the phacoemulsification.

## Preparation

The operating field and the conjunctiva are prepared in the usual fashion.

The operation lends itself to various types of incision depending on the surgeon's preference. It is advisable, at least for the first operations with this technique, that the surgeon use a scleral incision.

An incision is made 1.5 mm from the limbus perpendicular to the sclera for about half the thickness. Scleral dissection is completed with a rounded blade (Alcon's bevel-up crescent knife) to the anterior limit of the limbal vessels, taking care to remain equidistant from the cornea and the base of the iris to avoid damaging Descemet's membrane and the iris.

A circular continuous capsulotomy is prepared using both the cystotome and forceps. If the cystotome alone is used, the entire procedure takes place inside a closed chamber. The side port incision is then prepared at 2 o'clock.

If the surgeon decides to prepare a capsulorhexis with forceps, after injecting VES, he or she enters the anterior chamber with a calibrated keratome set on 3.1 or 3.2 mm. In this case, the side port incision can be prepared prior to the capsulotomy.

Once the capsulorhexis has been completed, the surgeon performs hydrodissection with a flat 25 gauge cannula mounted on a 3 cc syringe.

Cleavage between the nucleus and the cortex varies according to the position in which the fluid is injected and on the extension of the nucleus itself.

In the advanced cataract, the central nucleus corresponds largely to the size of the crystalline lens so it can only be separated from the external cortex. In softer cataracts or those of recent onset, the nucleus may be quite small. In this case, it is possible to create a separation between the central nucleus, epinucleus (hydrodelineation), and the peripheral cortex.

A successful hydrodissection must free the nucleus from all the cortical adhesions so that it can rotate freely in the capsular bag without being luxated. At the end of hydrodissection, the surgeon must rotate the nucleus to make sure it is mobile. He or she can use the tip of the cannula or a hook, such as a Sinskey-Buratto hook.

The surgeon enters the anterior chamber with the 30° U/S tip (I often use a 45° tip) and the pedal in Position 1. Moving the pedal to Position 2, the surgeon aspirates the anterior capsule (if it has not already been removed with the capsulorhexis forceps), and central phacoemulsification of the nucleus is started with the pedal in Position 3.

When using the U/S, the surgeon must check that the edge of the capsulorhexis does not come into contact with the U/S tip.

Emulsification is split into three phases:
1. Central sculpting—this removes a large part of the nucleus inside the capsulorhexis.
2. Rotation of the nucleus to reach the para-equatorial portions beyond the capsulorhexis.
3. Removal of the residual central and deep nucleus.

## Central Sculpting

In the first phase, I prepare the instrument as follows (Shepherd does not actually specify the parameters):
- Vacuum—0 to 20 mm Hg.
- Flow rate—15 to 20 cc/mm.
- U/S power—70%.

The surgeon carves the anterior cortex and the epinucleus first with short U/S bursts at low power at a depth of slightly less than half the diameter of the U/S tip.

If there is good visual control, the nucleus can be emulsified in the peripheral portions too (ie, under the rim of the anterior capsule), taking care not to carve too far toward the posterior capsule or the equator of the lens.

If the surgeon goes in deeper toward the central part of the nucleus, the U/S power is increased simply because the material is usually harder. This progression ensures a smooth operation with minimal stimulation to the iris, the capsule, and the zonule.

When the surgeon observes a clear red reflex of the fundus, the U/S power is reduced, particularly if the surgeon intends, to go in deeper. As he or she comes closer to the posterior capsule, the diaphragm that separates it from the posterior chamber consists only of the peripheral cortex.

The extension and depth of the central carving should be carefully controlled. The surgeon should deepen as much as possible without coming too close to the posterior capsule and the equator of the capsular bag.

The degree of central carving must be proportional to the hardness of the nucleus. The harder the nucleus, the wider and deeper the carving. At this stage, the nucleus has a concave groove in it, which is slightly decentered toward 6 o'clock; it has a thin floor and thicker equatorial edges.

## Rotation of the Nucleus

The U/S tip is positioned on the edge of the groove at 9 o'clock (or at 3 o'clock—depending on the surgeon's preference), and the nucleus is pushed and rotated through 90° toward 6 o'clock.

This maneuver should ideally be performed with the pedal in Position 1 (this facilitates the distention of the posterior capsule and the rotation of the nucleus). If the pedal is in Position 2, the surgeon must avoid occluding the U/S tip. Otherwise, under the effect of vacuum, the movement of the nucleus will be radial instead of along the circumference.

If it is difficult to mobilize the nucleus, rotation can also be performed in occlusion. The vacuum value allows the surgeon to obtain occlusion easily and therefore rotate the nucleus without excessive traction. In order to respect the rules of the procedure, mobilization must follow the direction of the circumference.

The nucleus can also be rotated with the two-handed technique using the U/S tip and a spatula inserted through a lateral side port incision, with the foot pedal in Position 1 or 2.

Another alternative is to fill the anterior chamber with VES and rotate using an olive-tipped spatula alone. At this point, the peripheral material is emulsified at 6 o'clock.

The rotation is repeated to expose another equatorial

Table 6-9

## ONE-HANDED ENDOCAPSULAR PHACOEMULSIFICATION: SHEPHERD'S TECHNIQUE

| | |
|---|---|
| Nucleus | For nuclei of Grade 1-2 hardness. |
| Incision | Scleral pouch or scleral or corneal tunnel. |
| Capsulotomy | Capsulorhexis. |
| Viscoelastic | Viscoat. |
| Hydrodissection | Must be complete in order to free the nucleus inside the bag. |
| Superficial and central sculpting | Parameters:<br>　Tip—30° or 45°.<br>　Vacuum—0-20.<br>　Flow rate—5-15.<br>　Linear U/S—50-60%.<br>The anterior cortex and the epinucleus are shaved. The sculpting is deepened toward the central part of the nucleus, slightly increasing the U/S power. The depth of the sculpting depends on the hardness of the nucleus. The harder the nucleus, the deeper the sculpting must be. The bowl-shape that results must be decentered distally. |
| Rotation of the nucleus | The U/S tip is used to rotate the nucleus through 90°. It should be positioned at about 3 o'clock with the foot pedal in Position 1. The nucleus is pushed and rotated through about 90°. |
| Fragmentation of the distal portion | Parameters:<br>　Vacuum—80-100.<br>　Flow rate—15-18.<br>　U/S—30-40%.<br>The distal equatorial portion of the nucleus is fragmented.<br>Further rotation and fragmentation until just the nuclear plate remains. |
| Fragmentation of the plate | Parameters:<br>　Vacuum—60-80.<br>　Flow rate—12-15.<br>　U/S—40%.<br>At 6 o'clock, the last portion of the equatorial nucleus is captured, which is attached to the plate. This is then brought to the level of the pupil and fragmented. |

portion. In this phase, the parameters of the equipment are changed as follows:
- Vacuum—100 mm Hg.
- Flow rate—15 cc/min.
- U/S 40%.

Fragmentation of the peripheral portions below the capsulorhexis must be done very carefully, even though correct setting of the parameters goes a long way to guaranteeing the necessary safety.

Once the entire peripheral nucleus has been removed, a thin shell remains, which consists of the deep and posterior portions of the nucleus.

## Removal of the Residual Nuclear Plate

This is the final phase. The parameters for this phase are:
- Vacuum—80 to 100 mm Hg.
- Flow rate—20 cc/min with linear U/S.

The portion at 6 o'clock is captured with the U/S tip directed to obtain occlusion so that the equatorial nuclear portion is pulled gently into the pupillary field to be emulsified with gentle U/S bursts. Bit by bit, all the nuclear equator is gradually removed. When all the peripheral nuclear edges have been removed, a small portion of the posterior nucleus remains.

With the pedal in Position 1 (ie, with just irrigation active), it may happen that the residual nuclear plate moves spontaneously toward the pupillary plane where it can be easily captured by the U/S tip. Capture is performed with the pedal in Position 2, ie, with irrigation and aspiration active.

Once the plate has been fixed, the material is emulsified with low U/S power. In this phase, the surgeon can also use U/S bursts, which makes the maneuvers of phaco even less traumatic. If intraoperative conditions make capturing the nuclear residue at 6 o'clock difficult or dangerous, the surgeon can proceed in a number of ways.

- The nucleus is fixed in a central position with a U/S tip and pushed toward 6 o'clock. In this way, it folds over on itself, and the equator is exposed through capsulorhexis in the pupillary field. This facilitates emulsification and is a maneuver indicated for very soft nuclei.
- The nucleus is captured with the U/S tip bevel-down. The foot pedal is moved to Position 2 to obtain brief occlusion. It is a maneuver indicated if the nucleus is not too hard and is free from cortical adhesions. As soon as the nucleus is captured, it is brought to a safe position and emulsified using low power U/S.

  All the steps must be executed very carefully; the surgeon must make slow, deliberate movements using minimum U/S power yet strong enough to obtain the emulsification.
- A third method involves injecting VES under the

nuclear plate so that it can be moved and positioned in a more suitable position for the action of the U/S tip. Alternately, emulsification can be completed using a combined U/S-I/A tip or a 0.5 mm I/A tip.

### Completion of the Operation

Correct phacoemulsification in the capsular bag will normally leave just a small amount of cortex that is relatively easy to remove—if I exclude the portion positioned at 12 o'clock.

In this position, the rim of the capsulorhexis may create some difficulty. In order to facilitate this part of the operation, the surgeon can use a bent I/A tip, which provides a number of interesting advantages over the others. It works particularly well if the surgeon performs a slightly off-center capsulorhexis toward 12 o'clock. Alternately, he or she can use two separate irrigation and aspiration cannulas (Buratto's technique) introduced through two separate side port incisions (usually at 10 and 2 o'clock).

Once the capsular bag has been cleaned, the incision is extended to accommodate the implant. Endocapsular phacoemulsification lends itself to the implantation of a variety of IOLs: three-piece, one-piece PMMA and foldable, acrylic, silicone, or hydrogel.

Once the IOL has been implanted, the VES is removed by aspiration, the anterior chamber is reshaped, and a suture is applied if traditional incision techniques have been used. If the surgeon had prepared a self-sealing tunnel incision, the operation will terminate with a control of the check of the water tightness of the incision and the sealing of the conjunctiva.

### Comment

Endocapsular phacoemulsification leads us into the realms of the so-called advanced techniques of phaco.

The term is justified because of the innovative steps introduced (if I compare it to the classical technique in the posterior chamber), but also because of the updated technical and instrumental requirements for the correct completion of this type of operation.

The advantages in terms of precision, efficiency, safety, gentleness, and surgical speed are considerable and deserve some comments.

- *Incision*—Self-sealing, sclero-corneal tunnel incisions are an enormous step forward in the evolution of cataract surgery and are ideal in the endocapsular techniques.

    The perfect seal of the incision helps keep the depth of the anterior chamber as uniform as possible, so that all the steps are performed with the ideal amount of space and the correct anatomical relationship between the structures of the anterior segment.

- *Small self-sealing incisions*—With phacoemulsification and foldable lenses, in addition to the minimal surgical trauma, these incisions allow better control of the postoperative astigmatism and permit a more rapid functional recovery.

- *Capsulotomy*—With the capsulorhexis, a uniform resistant capsular bag is created. This provides an excellent support for the maneuvers of mobilization and emulsification of the nucleus, which is fragmented and mobilized completely inside the bag, so the entire operation is suitably isolated from the surrounding structures.

    The implantation in the bag is greatly facilitated, and the lens is isolated in a physiological site, all to the advantage of the centering and the reduction of the postoperative inflammation.

- *Hydrodissection*—Cleavage and the mobilization of the nucleus are performed gradually and delicately without dislocating the nucleus or part of it outside the bag.

    The separation of the lens structures means that phacoemulsification can tackle them selectively. In turn, this means that the total amount of U/S energy used is reduced, as is the stress on the capsulo-zonular apparatus.

- *Phacoemulsification*—This is performed almost entirely inside the capsular bag at a safe distance from the corneal endothelium, which is subjected to only a minimal amount of stress. The posterior capsule is also protected for two reasons:

1. The nucleus has been separated from the epinucleus by the fluid injected. As a result, vibrations are not transmitted.
2. The nucleus is attacked from the center to the periphery in all the phases of emulsification with direct action of the U/S tip on the material to be emulsified. This is possible thanks to the more modern machines, which allow linear control of the U/S power and the selection of flow rate and vacuum values suitable for every situation.

    It differs from the traditional phacoemulsification techniques in that it is the machine that adapts to the needs of the surgeon and not vice versa.

3. *I/A*—Thanks to hydrodissection, hydrodelineation, and controlled phacoemulsification, when removal of the nucleus has been completed with the endocapsular techniques, very little cortical material remains.

    This advantage should not be ignored, in a phase of the operation generally considered to be critical for the integrity of the posterior capsule.

    At present, a number of specific accessories are available to optimize the I/A phase, which follows capsulorhexis and endocapsular phacoemulsification, instruments such as angled tips and separate irrigation and aspiration cannulas.

- *The implant*—The surgeon can choose almost any type of lens, from the more traditional three-piece to the more recent foldable lenses in acrylic or silicone. The choice location would be implantation in the capsular bag. Nevertheless, if the intraoperative conditions are difficult, the surgeon can obtain excellent results by implanting in the sulcus.

- *Suture*—In addition to the possibility of sutureless, self-sealing, sclero-corneal tunnels, there are a large number of suture-types associated with sclero-corneal tunnels and endocapsular phacoemulsifi-

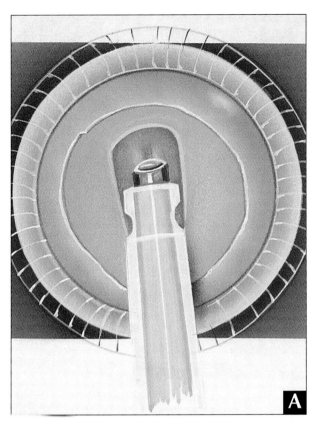
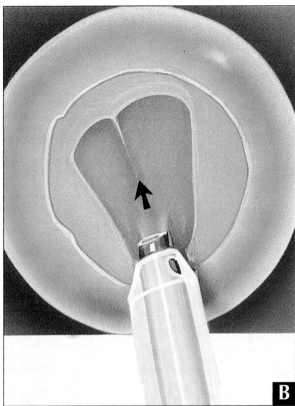

Figures 6-12A, 6-12B. One-handed endocapsular phaco. Rhexis and careful hydrodissection have already been completed. The surgeon now performs central carving, which is deepened progressively, while remaining inside the rhexis edges. The surgeon emulsifies without occlusion.

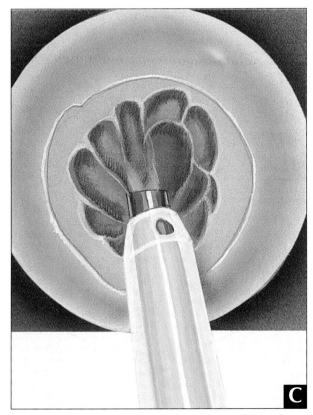
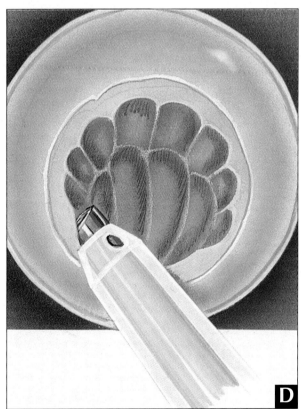

Figure 6-12C. Carving is deepened gradually using short U/S bursts. In this way, the surgeon removes all the central and distal nucleus.

Figure 6-12D. With the U/S tip applied laterally at the extremity of the carved portion, the nucleus is rotated to distally expose a portion which has not been emulsified to any great extent.

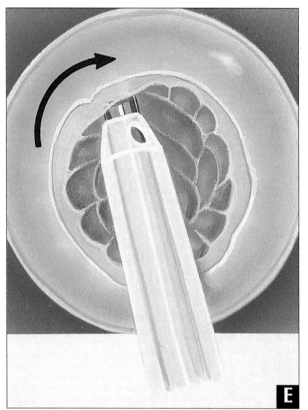
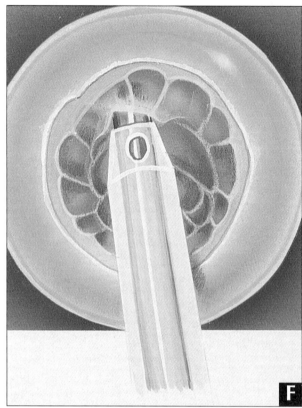

Figures 6-12E, 6-12F. The distal portion is now captured in occlusion, pulled gently toward the center, and emulsified with short bursts of U/S.

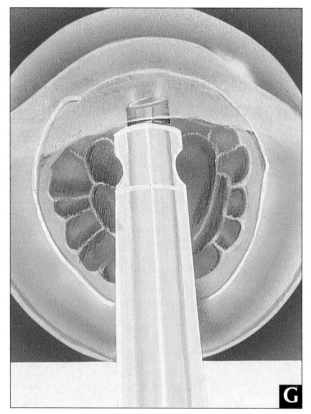
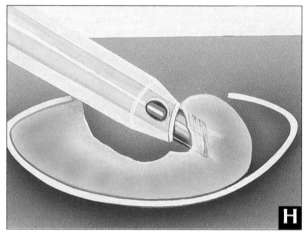

Figures 6-12G, 6-12H. The surgeon performs further rotation, and then he or she looks for occlusion with U/S. When the edges of the nuclear equator are mobilized (ie, it moves toward the center), it is emulsified.

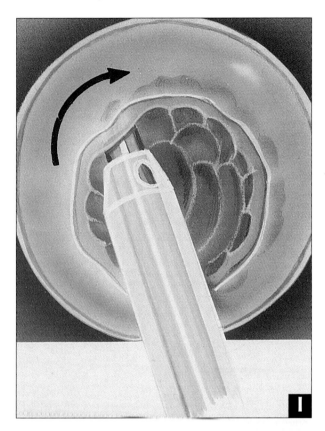

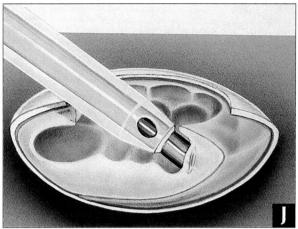

Figure 6-12I. The nuclear shell is rotated again.

Figure 6-12J. Another equatorial portion is tackled. The surgeon looks for occlusion until he or she obtains traction toward the center. The sector is then emulsified at the center of the capsular bag.

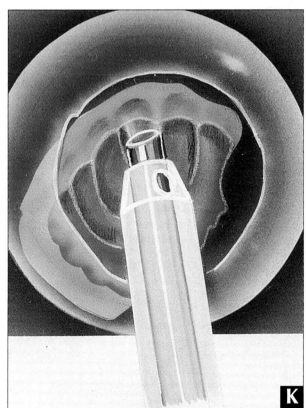

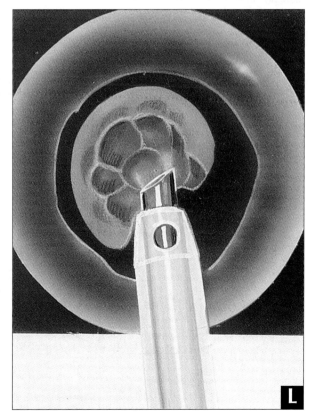

Figures 6-12K, 6-12L. The residual portion of the nucleus, the plate, is then emulsified at the center of the capsular bag.

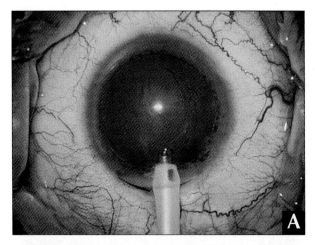
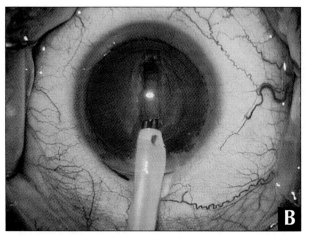
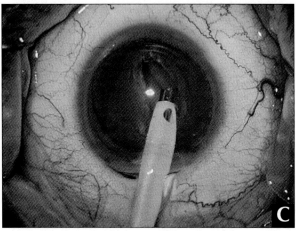

Figures 6-13A, 6-13B, 6-13C. Shepherd's one-handed technique. The U/S tip attacks the nucleus to the proximal edge of the rhexis. The surgeon then carves the groove from the entrance to the distal limit of the endonucleus to rotate it.

cation. The latter must respond to standard criteria that have been developed in cataract surgery for quite some time.

## Intercapsular Phacoemulsification According to Michelson and Hara

The development of intercapsular phacoemulsification is largely due to the studies and experience of Hara and Michelson.

It is a technique where a large part of the anterior capsule is left intact during the initial phases of the operation, so that the phacoemulsification occurs entirely within the capsular bag. It is suitable for nuclei of moderate-low hardness (Grade 2) and eyes with well-dilated pupils.

Intercapsular phacoemulsification aims to obtain the following results, with the added advantages of safety and reduced trauma of the phacoemulsification:
- The procedure is completely isolated and is done under the protection of the capsule, which acts as an efficient barrier between it and the adjacent structures.
- The fluid exchange in the anterior chamber is minimal so turbulence is reduced.
- The flow is concentrated around the U/S tip without creating turbulence in the anterior chamber and keeping the circulation of the nuclear fragments toward the corneal endothelium to a minimum.
- The VES that fills the anterior chamber is not affected by the circulation of BSS, so it is always present and is not altered in terms of volume, transparency, and protective capacity.

### Technique

The technique consists of a series of steps that must all be performed correctly in order to obtain the desired results.

### Preparation

The operating field is prepared as normal and a two-plane. Sclero-corneal incision is performed at about 2 mm from the limbal vascular arcades.

The entrance in the anterior chamber is done initially with instruments for about 1 mm in order to inject a VES. The opening can then be completed at 3.0 to 3.2 mm with a precalibrated blade.

### Capsulotomy

This is the first important step in performing the technique planned. The surgeon must obtain a mini-capsulorhexis at 12 o'clock, close to the iris edge without touching the zonular fibers. The ideal shape is an oval opening with the larger diameter of 4 to 5 mm and the smaller diameter of 0.5 to 1 mm.

The incision of the anterior capsule is obtained with a 25 G needle that has been bent at the tip; then the needle is moved horizontally for 3 to 4 mm and then brought downward 0.5 to 1.0 mm to create a small flap.

The surgeon then enters with the capsulorhexis forceps, and the capsulorhexis is completed.

The opening must be wide enough to allow the entrance and the movements of the U/S tip without any traction being created on the anterior capsule.

A small opening on the edges of the mini-capsulorhexis can be corrected by catching the larger part of the flap and slightly extending the capsulotomy in a direc-

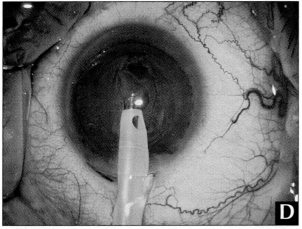

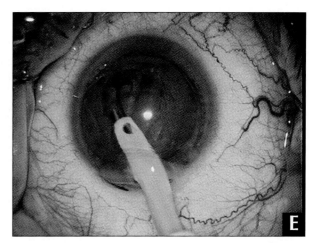

Figures 6-13D, 6-13E, 6-13F. A small portion of the endonucleus, which is soft, is pulled toward the center and emulsified. Another portion of central hemi-nucleus is rotated, captured, and brought to the center.

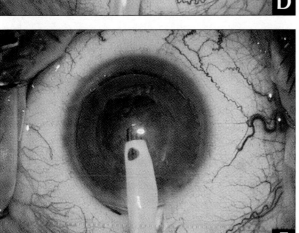

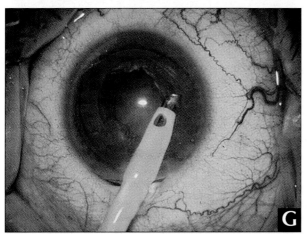

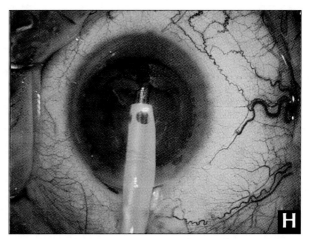

Figures 6-13G, 6-13H, 6-13 I. The U/S tip is brought into contact with the epinucleus in the left lateral sector and the surgeon tries to rotate the material. The epinucleus, which was at 3 o'clock, is now at 6 o'clock. It is pulled toward the center and fragmented.

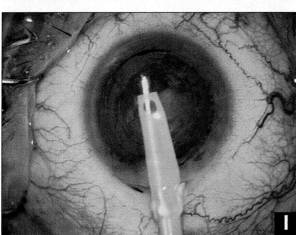

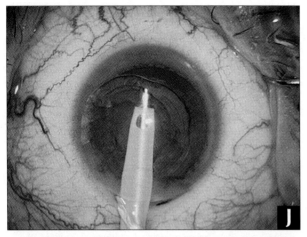
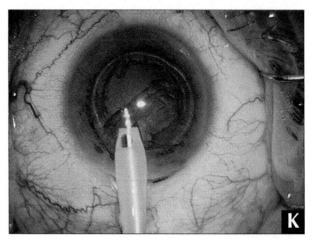
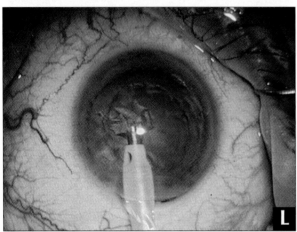

Figures 6-13J, 6-13K, 6-13L. The residual epinucleus is captured at 6 o'clock and brought to the center and emulsified until completely removed.

tion opposite to that of the tear. If the tear is wide, the surgeon should convert to another method and perform a wider capsulotomy.

### Hydrodissection

As the capsulotomy is small, the injection of BSS under the anterior capsule allows the surgeon to free the cortico-capsular adhesions accurately and completely. Hydrodissection must be followed by hydrodelamination to separate the epinucleus from the endonucleus.

If the cleavage of these planes is not sufficient, during the phacoemulsification procedure, the surgeon runs the risk of aspirating the peripheral capsule with the U/S tip.

### Central Sculpting

As the anterior chamber is formed with the VES, the U/S tip can be introduced with the pedal in Position 0. In this way, the VES will not escape from the wound and will remain in position for the majority of the operation.

After having inserted the tip into the mini-capsulorhexis, a work-space is created in the anterior cortex and in the epinucleus through aspiration or fragmentation with low power U/S.

The mean values are the following:
- Vacuum—0 to 15 mm Hg.
- Flow rate—15 cc/min.
- Power—70%.

The carving maneuvers must be restricted to the central portion of the nucleus, leaving the epinucleus intact. At least until 60 to 70% of the nuclear thickness is emulsified.

In the initial phases, the carving must never exceed the peripheral epinuclear limit, ie, the area of cortical demarcation, highlighted by the hydrodelamination.

The persistence of the epinuclear ring absorbs the action of the U/S tip and prevents an equatorial portion of the posterior capsule being aspirated with the epinucleus, with possible capsular rupture or zonular dialysis.

Step 1—The nucleus is sculpted to two-thirds of its depth mainly in the center. The surgeon must limit the lateral movements of the U/S tip as much as possible and leave about half the nucleus to the left of the U/S tip untouched.

Step 2—With the foot pedal in Position 2, the U/S tip is partially retracted toward the capsular opening and positioned in correspondence to the left-hand edge of the sculpting to engage the nucleus and rotate it 90° in a clockwise direction.

At this point, the remaining cortico-capsular adhesions are freed so the surgeon can safely proceed with the removal of the material beyond the epinuclear limit.

Step 3—The surgeon completes the sculpting of the half of the central nucleus that had been brought to the 6 o'clock position.

The surgeon should ensure that during the backward movement, the silicone sleeve of the U/S tip does not exit from the capsulorhexis and that the tip is not bent in relation to the entrance to the capsulorhexis. These two possibilities carry with them the risk of a mini capsulorhexis opening.

Step 4—Removal of the nuclear plate. At the end of phacoemulsification of the equatorial nucleus, a nuclear plate covered in epinucleus remains.

The vacuum is increased to 80 to 100 mm Hg, the flow rate is unchanged, and power is at 40%.

The residual nucleus can be distanced from the posterior capsule with the U/S tip and emulsified with short bursts of U/S.

Table 6-10
## ENDOCAPSULAR PHACOEMULSIFICATION: MICHELSON'S-HARA'S TECHNIQUE

| | |
|---|---|
| Type of nucleus | Grade 2-3 hardness. |
| Incision | Sclero-corneal or limbal. |
| Viscoelastic | The technique involves filling the chamber with a viscosubstance that will stay in position. Viscoat is the most suitable to reach this objective. |
| Capsulotomy | Mini oval-shaped capsulorhexis close to the incision: 4.5 x 1.0 mm. |
| Hydrodissection/ hydrodelamination | It is easy to perform also because of the small size of the capsulorhexis. It should be associated with careful hydrodelamination, which will separate the central nucleus from the peripheral. |
| Central carving: Phase 1 | The tip is introduced directly into the rhexis with the foot pedal in Position 0. A working space is created just inside the rhexis with some short bursts of U/S. Sculpting is then done on the central portions and the areas to the right of the nucleus, while trying not to exceed the limits of the golden ring obtained with hydrodelamination. The parameters are vacuum 0-15, flow rate 15, U/S 70%. |
| Rotation of the nucleus: Phase 2 | Using the U/S tip and the foot pedal in Position 2 (with or without occlusion depending on the degree of nuclear mobility), the nucleus is captured in the left sector, which remains after Phase 1, and the nucleus is rotated through 90° to expose the inferior parts of the material that were previously lateral. |
| Final central sculpting: Phase 3 | The portion of the nucleus that is distally following rotation is emulsified. |
| The removal of the plate: Phase 4 | The residual nucleus, now reduced to the inferior portion, is mobilized by the U/S tip and fragmented. The epinucleus attached to it is captured simultaneously and removed. |
| I/A of the cortex | This part is usually done easily as there is usually only a small amount of material present. |
| Injection of VES | The anterior chamber and the capsular bag are filled with Viscoat. |
| Extension of the rhexis | Vannas scissors are used to perform two cuts on the rhexis. Then, using suitable forceps, the opening is extended and the IOL chosen is inserted in the capsular bag. |

If the epinucleus still adheres to the residual nucleus and detaches from the posterior capsule, together the residual nucleus is emulsified sector by sector.

However, if the epinucleus and the residual nucleus are separated, the latter can be captured with the U/S tip with the pedal in Position 2 and brought into a central position where it is emulsified. The epinucleus can then be captured at 6 o'clock and progressively distanced from the posterior capsule.

Alternately, the U/S tip can be positioned on the epinuclear rim toward 12 o'clock, and with the pedal in Position 2, the material is raised and pushed toward 6 o'clock so that the epinucleus folds on itself to reach a central position where it can be emulsified and aspirated in complete safety. In these final steps, the vacuum can be set on 50 to 80 mm Hg in proportion to the hardness of the material. The flow rate can be set at 15 to 20 cc/min and the U/S power 40%, taking care to use the pedal properly to regulate the power actually used.

With effective power of 10 to 30%, there are no risks for the posterior capsule.

If the surgeon follows this procedure accurately, at the end of phacoemulsification, a small quantity of cortical material will remain, and the capsular bag will be almost completely intact.

### Comment

This is an extremely sophisticated technique, but it is not used much as it is so difficult to perform.

However, the technique has a number of important advantages that are appreciated at present and will be more interesting in the future.

The current advantages involve the optimal use of the technological potential available today, with the result that there is very little surgical trauma to the cornea in particular.

Having an anterior chamber that is isolated for the entire turbulent step of the operation means minimizing the effects of the phacoemulsification on all the eye structures, as fluid exchange, turbulence, and heat variations are of little importance.

The VES is used throughout the entire operation and contributes to reducing the stress in the anterior chamber and mobilizing the nuclear material. Moreover, this is a one-handed technique with fewer entrances in the anterior chamber.

In addition to these advantages, which can already be obtained with available equipment, endocapsular phacoemulsification provides an excellent starting point for future developments. In particular, the procedure would appear to be extremely interesting in the preparation of the eye for injectable lenses and the preparatory treatment of the nucleus with laser machinery.

However, the technique does have some disadvantages that should be mentioned.

First of all, the incision: the self-sealing sclero-corneal tunnel makes it quite difficult, if not totally impossible, to perform the mini capsulorhexis at 12 o'clock, at the entrance point of the U/S tip.

In addition, the difficulty of operating on hard nuclei with two-handed techniques is largely conditioned by the reduced size of the capsular opening and the pro-

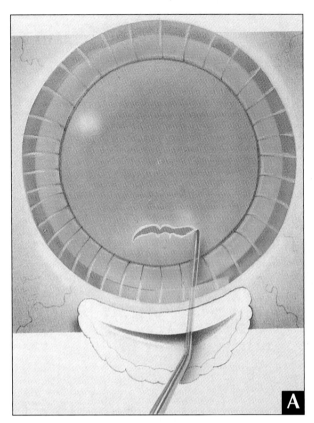

Figure 6-14A. Intercapsular phacoemulsification. A straight capsular incision is created just inside the corneo-scleral opening in front of the zonular attachment, with the formation of a capsular flap.

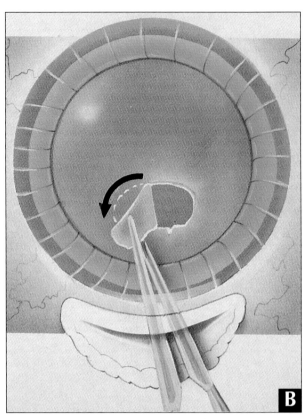

Figure 6-14B. A small, oval-shaped rhexis is created horizontally, close to the corneal incision.

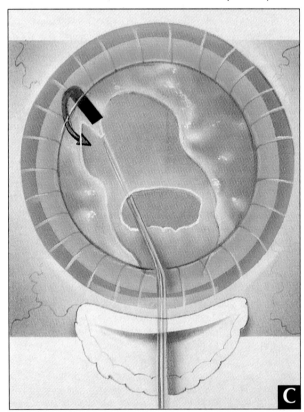

Figure 6-14C. Accurate hydrodissection is more complete through a small rhexis. Accurate hydrodelamination is also done to separate the central nucleus from the epinucleus.

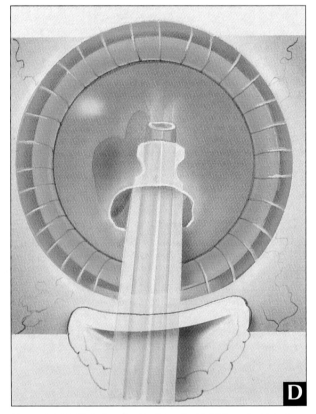

Figure 6-14D. The chamber is shaped with VES so the tip enters with irrigation closed. Once just inside the rhexis, the surgeon creates a small amount of space by removing a small amount of nuclear material with U/S.

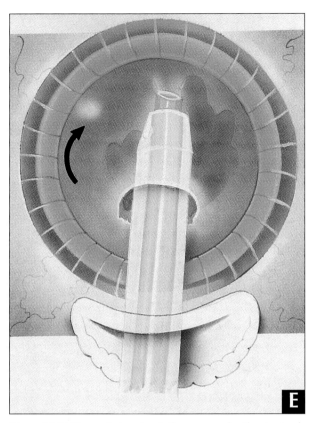

Figure 6-14E. The central portion is then removed without extending beyond the area marked by hydrodelamination.

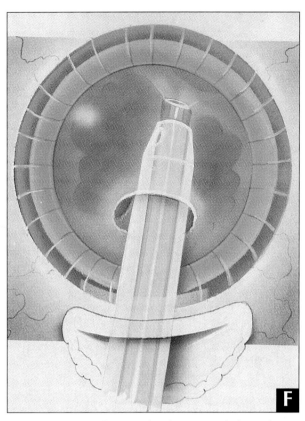

Figure 6-14F. Once the space has been created, the nucleus is rotated and emulsified once again. The nucleus is gradually removed.

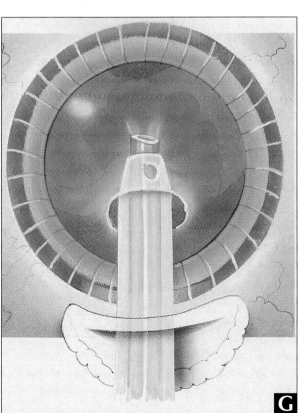

Figure 6-14G. The surgeon looks for occlusion with the epinucleus, which is removed at the end. The cortex is aspirated with the traditional method.

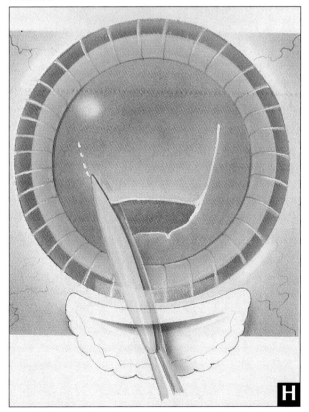

Figure 6-14H. With the chamber and the bag shaped with VES, the capsule is cut on the left side and then on the right of the rhexis, using scissors.

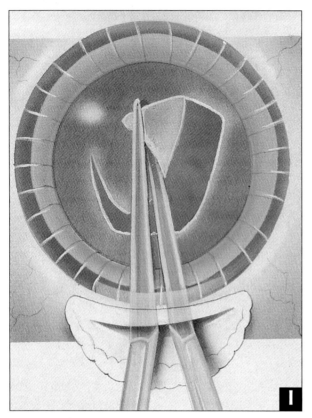

Figure 6-14I. The capsulectomy is completed through a distal continuous capsulotomy by tearing. Endocapsular IOL implant follows.

longed fragmentation inside the bag—a procedure that is made more difficult because of the poor visibility of the anterior capsule, characteristic of hard nuclei.

This method should only be used once the patients have been carefully selected. At a later stage, it may be possible to extend this patient group.

## Two-handed Endocapsular Phacoemulsification or Cut and Suck Technique

This method can be used with nuclei of moderate-low hardness (Grade 2 to 3). A 30° U/S tip is recommended; however, some surgeons prefer to use the 45° tip. The surgeon should perform the incision he or she prefers.

The surgeon then completes a capsulorhexis of 4.5 to 5.5 mm depending on the type of lens he or she wishes to implant, and hydrodissection is completed.

The appearance of an obvious wave of fluid indicates good cortico-capsular cleavage. If the surgeon does not see the fluid wave, he or she should inject liquid into the four quadrants and attempt to rotate the nucleus using the cannula inside the capsulorhexis. This maneuver should be done only if the nucleus puts up sufficient resistance to the cannula, ie, if the nucleus is at least moderately hard. If the nucleus is soft, it will be more difficult to rotate.

Once good hydro-cleavage has been obtained, the U/S tip is introduced with the foot pedal in Position 0 (under VES) or alternately with the foot pedal in Position 1.

### Central Sculpting

The parameters for this phase are as follows:
- Vacuum—0 to 20 mm Hg.
- Flow rate—10 to 20 cc/min.
- U/S power—80%.

The U/S tip creates superimpositioned grooves (shaving) on the anterior cortex and then on the superficial nucleus, to then go down deeper into the nucleus with sculpting.

The peripheral edges of the sculpting push beyond the limits of the capsulorhexis; in this maneuver, the U/S tip must be directed laterally so that the aspiration opening points toward the edge created by the sculpting. With this sweeping maneuver, the surgeon obtains the following advantages:
- The concavity obtained is regular, definitely better than that obtained through the simple up-down movement of the U/S tip.
- Occlusion of the tip is not possible because the direction of the aspirating orifice follows the margin of the carving.
- The action of the U/S tip can be observed clearly, so the surgeon is completely aware of the amount of material emulsified, particularly as he or she moves closer to the posterior cortex.
- The nuclear material immediately underneath the edges of the capsulorhexis can be aspirated without risking the capture of the anterior capsule and possible opening of the edge of the capsulorhexis.

### Rotation of the Nucleus

After having sculpted the central part of the nucleus to the right depth, and for a width just slightly greater than the diameter of the capsulorhexis, an accessory spatula is inserted. Its apex is placed on the edge of the sculpting on the opposite side to the entrance incision. The surgeon rotates the spatula to completely free the nucleus from the cortico-capsular adhesions. When the nucleus is soft, the surgeon must ensure that the spatula does not sink in too deeply and penetrate beyond the cortical layers.

### Removal of the Equatorial Portion of the Nucleus

The parameters for this phase are as follows:
- Vacuum—60 mm Hg.
- Flow rate—15 cc/min.
- U/S power—60%.

In fact, the foot pedal controls fluctuate the real value if the U/S is between 20 and 30%.

The U/S tip is positioned at 2 to 3 o'clock in correspondence to the peripheral edge of the anterior nucleus. The surgeon looks for occlusion (which is not always easily obtained given the angulation of the tip), then the nuclear material is brought toward the center of the pupillary field where it is emulsified with short bursts of low power U/S.

Toward the periphery, the nuclear material is softer. In order to aspirate it, it is normally sufficient to occlude the tip, bring the sector captured toward the center, and fragment it with short bursts with the foot pedal in Position 3.

After having removed one portion, the nucleus is

rotated with a spatula to bring another portion of the nuclear equator into a position that is easily accessible to the U/S tip and repeat the fragmentation.

The volume of the cortical mass is gradually reduced by the U/S tip, while the spatula continues to present the remaining larger fragments of the residual nucleus.

With two or three rotations, the peripheral volume of the nucleus is reduced, and a plate-like portion of the posterior part of the nucleus remains.

### *Removal of the Residual Nuclear Plate*

This can be captured by occluding the U/S tip or by bringing the piece toward the tip with the spatula to complete the emulsification.

### *Comment*

The secret of this technique lies in alternating the use of occlusion—traction toward the center—low power emulsification.

The use of moderate vacuum to obtain occlusion and shift the nucleus is possible because of the softness of the material. However, it is also crucial to perform optimal hydrodissection in the initial phase.

## Chip and Flip According to Fine or the Technique of Nuclear Cleavage

This technique is ideal for cataracts of moderate-low hardness (Grade 2 to 3).

### *Preparation*

The scleral tunnel is prepared using a diamond blade. The anterior chamber is formed using Viscoat.

Following a capsulorhexis of 4 to 4.5 mm, hydrodissection is completed with a small quantity of liquid injected underneath the capsule and toward the periphery. The surgeon must try to leave the thinnest possible layer of cortex attached to the peripheral capsule.

The cannula is retracted slightly and inserted deep into the nucleus, injecting BSS tangentially to obtain the hydrodelineation. The cleavage between the nucleus and the epinucleus can be seen as a golden ring that corresponds to the demarcation zone. Hydrodelamination must be performed prior to hydrodissection. This allows a better evaluation of the degree of hydrodelineation and a better delimitation of the central nucleus from the peripheral. It is very important that the central nucleus is well-separated from the epinucleus and just as important that the nucleo-epinuclear complex is well-separated from the external cortex through hydrodissection.

### *Sculpting*

The epinucleus is sculpted, followed by the central nucleus using the methods described previously for the other procedures. The surgeon must try to obtain a nuclear bowl that is as concave as possible.

The parameters in this step are as follows:
- Vacuum—10 to 50 mm Hg.
- Flow rate—10 to 15 cc/min.
- Maximum power set—70%.

Using a spatula (Fine uses the Bechert nucleo-manipulator), the nucleus is gently moved toward 12 o'clock keeping the U/S tip in a central position so that the internal edge of the nuclear equator is brought into contact with it at 5 to 6 o'clock. It is then emulsified. The movement of the nucleus toward 12 o'clock, while phacoemulsification is being done at 5 and 6 o'clock, protects the capsule distally. In fact, part of the nucleus involved in the emulsification is distanced by the capsular fornix and the iris, even when the pupil is narrow.

Emulsification is performed just underneath the anterior capsule close to the center of the rhexis, ie, in the safer areas.

The nucleus is lightly rotated in a clockwise direction to emulsify a new equatorial portion inferiorly, keeping the U/S tip in a central position. In this way, the whole edge of the equatorial border of the endonucleus is removed, ie, the internal nucleus around 360°.

The spatula is then inserted into the cleavage plane obtained with hydrodelamination. This passes under the residual chip (under the internal nuclear residue) and raises it, bringing it to the center of the bag or to the same level as the rhexis for emulsification. Under the control of the spatula, the chip is easily removed, preferably using U/S bursts.

The epinuclear bowl is now pushed out of the capsular fornix at 5 to 6 o'clock by pushing the epinuclear edge from 12 to 6 o'clock (for a superior incision). Alternately, the same result can be obtained with another maneuver, by pushing the center of the bowl toward 5 to 6 o'clock to allow it to slide out of the fornix and under the distal flap of the anterior capsule.

When using the U/S tip (with the foot pedal in Position 2, using I/A alone), the epinuclear bowl is pulled from 5 to 6 o'clock toward 12 o'clock, toward the main incision. With the help of the spatula, which pushes toward 5 to 6 o'clock, the epinucleus is flipped over.

This maneuver is not always successful on the first attempt. The surgeon will often have to repeat the move several times before it is successful; and he or she must rotate the bowl with every attempt.

The spatula or the U/S tip must fold the epinucleus over on itself and then overturn so that the equatorial portion, distal to the incision, will be found at the center of the posterior capsule. Once the bowl has been flipped over successfully, it will be far from the capsule and able to be removed safely.

The parameters in this phase are:
- Vacuum—100 to 150 mm Hg.
- Flow rate—20 cc/min.
- Power—50%.

### *Comment*

With this technique, the surgeon never sculpts in depth close to the posterior capsule, or in the capsular fornix or under the iris. All the work is done at the center of the pupil in the central part of the capsular bag, within the *safety zone*.

The emulsification is performed easily within a zone called the *circle of hydrodissection*.

With the emulsification of the internal nucleus, a *pad* remains, which consists of epinucleus and peripheral cor-

| Table 6-11 | |
|---|---|
| **PHACOEMULSIFICATION WITH THE CUT AND SUCK TECHNIQUE** | |
| Type of nucleus | For Grade 2-3 hardness. |
| Incision | Scleral or corneal tunnel. |
| Capsulotomy | Capsulorhexis. |
| Viscoelastic | Viscoat. |
| Hydrodissection | Must be complete to completely free the nucleus inside the capsular bag. |
| Shaving, carving, and brushing | Removal of the superficial layers.<br>Removal of the deeper layers.<br>Brushing of the lateral areas. |
| Parameters | Vacuum—0-20.<br>Flow rate—10-20.<br>U/S power—80%.<br>Tip—30°-45°. |
| Rotation of the nucleus. | Is done with a spatula applied distally to the entrance point of the carving. |
| Removal of the equatorial portion of the nucleus | Vacuum—60.<br>Flow rate—15.<br>U/S power—The maximum preset value is 60%. In actual fact, it is used in linear at 20-30%.<br>Capture in occlusion of the distal equatorial edge of the nucleus, the traction toward the center, and the fragmentation. Rotation.<br>The maneuver is repeated until all the equatorial nucleus is removed; only the nuclear disc remains. |
| Removal of the residual plate | The parameters remain unchanged.<br>Capture in occlusion or through the use of the spatula and then perform phacoemulsification. |

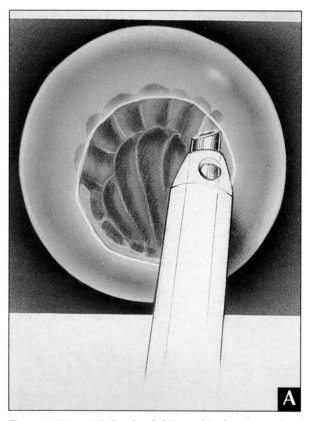
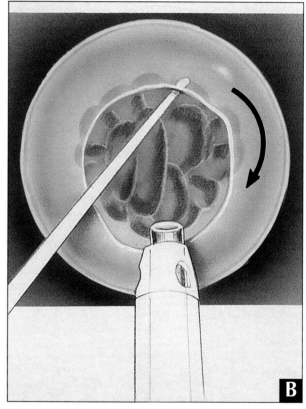

Figures 6-15A, 6-15B. Two-handed Cut and Suck endocapsular phaco. After capsulorhexis, hydrodissection, and predominantly distal central sculpting, the nucleus is rotated using the spatula.

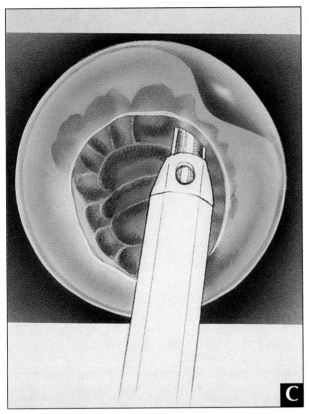

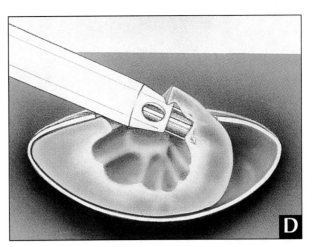

Figures 6-15C, 6-15D, 6-15E. The surgeon looks for equatorial occlusion (the equator is detached from the capsule) and the preequatorial portion of material is fragmented. The nucleus is then rotated in the bag to present another portion of the equatorial edge to the U/S tip.

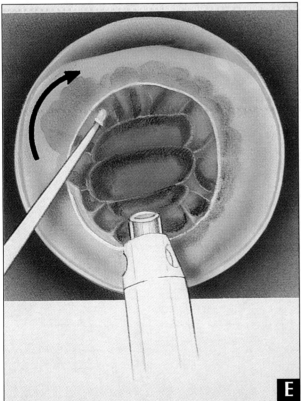

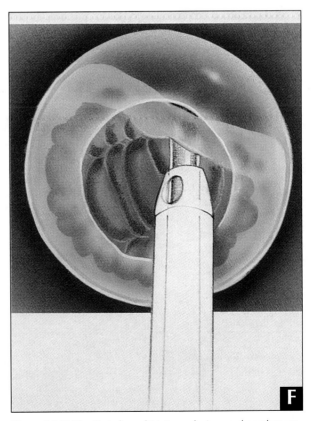

Figure 6-15F. The tip is brought into occlusion, and another preequatorial portion is fragmented.

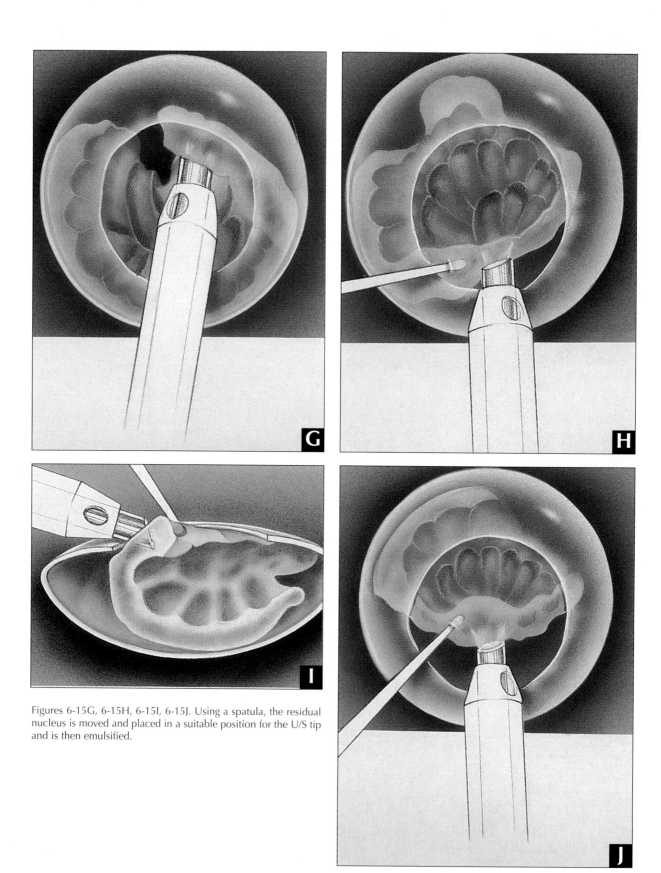

Figures 6-15G, 6-15H, 6-15I, 6-15J. Using a spatula, the residual nucleus is moved and placed in a suitable position for the U/S tip and is then emulsified.

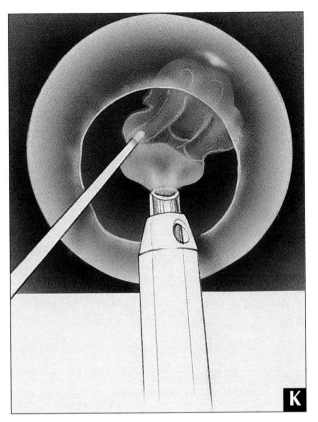

Figures 6-15K. End of phacoemulsification.

tex, which protects the capsulo-zonular structures. This protection is particularly useful when the central nucleus is not extensive but is very dense (the *hard core* typical of severe myopia).

The shock-absorbing effect of the epinucleus limits the amount of mechanical energy transmitted to the posterior capsule and the zonules even when the amount of U/S power necessary to emulsify the central nucleus is high.

Therefore, this technique can be used to remove moderately hard nuclei because the surgeon can safely create the demarcation zone using hydrodelamination.

## Techniques of Nucleofracture

### General Rules

The techniques of nucleofracture have been developed to split the nucleus into pieces and to emulsify the large pieces of nucleus that cannot be extracted through the opening in the capsulorhexis of 4.5 to 5.5 mm, ideal for the correct implantation of the IOL in the bag.

The techniques of nucleo-fracture also have the common objective of phacoemulsifying nuclei of moderate-high hardness (Grade 3) or very hard (Grade 4) inside the bag without having to use excessively high ultrasound power for prolonged times.

The nucleus in practice is split into separate sectors that can be emulsified in a suitable position (in the bag or in the pupillary plane) with U/S power reduced, compared to the amount the nucleus would require if it were whole.

Nucleofracture allows the surgeon to shorten U/S and surgical times. Generally speaking, it makes phacoemulsification safer in that the U/S tip is always used in the center of the pupillary field.

All the techniques have the following steps in common:

*Capsulorhexis*—This must be continuous.

*Hydrodissection*—This must be complete and accurate to allow the nucleus to rotate freely inside the capsular bag, in order to facilitate the various maneuvers of mobilization and nucleofracture.

Therefore, the surgeon must check that the nucleus is free from the cortico-capsular adhesions prior to starting the procedure. He or she can do this by rotating the nucleus once or twice inside the capsular bag.

*Sculpting*—The objective of sculpting is to create one or more grooves in the nucleus. They must be wide and deep enough to allow the surgeon to fracture the nucleus with a two-handed maneuver.

- Width—The groove must be slightly wider than the U/S tip, including the silicone sleeve. In that way, the formation of the groove is easy because the sleeve does not come into contact with the barrier of the walls. Moreover, if the groove is wide enough, there is enough space for the U/S and the accessory instrument. The fracture is then easier, even if the groove is wide. It also means that a certain amount of hard nuclear material has been removed.
- Length—The sulcus must extend just below the capsulorhexis. The extension depends on the hardness of the nucleus and the type of hydro-cleavage (dissection) done during the preparation.

If the hydrodissection has separated the nucleus from the epinucleus, ie, hydrodelamination has been performed, the groove must be extended to the limits of the hard nucleus. In the event that the nucleus also involves the peripheral portions of the lens (when the endonucleus and the epinucleus have not been separated), the groove can be lengthened but must not extend as far as the equator. If there is no hydrodelamination, the groove should extend inside the rhexis.

- Depth—This is a fundamental element for the success of the procedure. The depth of the groove must be 80 to 90% of the nuclear thickness for its entire length. The surgeon must allow for the convexity of the lens.

The most reliable criterion is the visual control of the color of the lens material. The change from gray to red indicates that the surgeon is approaching the cortex.

The surgeon should remember that in hard nuclei, the cortex may be very thin, and the color change may indicate a very dangerous proximity to the posterior chamber. One way that can help evaluate the depth of the sculpting consists of comparing it with the diameter of the U/S tip.

As the thickness of the nucleus is 3.5 to 4.0 mm and the diameter of the tip (including the sleeve) is 1.0 mm, the groove must not exceed (in depth) two and a half times the diameter of the tip (sleeve included).

Table 6-12
# CHIP AND FLIP PHACOEMULSIFICATION TECHNIQUE ACCORDING TO FINE

| | |
|---|---|
| Nuclei | Suitable for nuclei with hardness 2-3. |
| Incision | Corneal tunnel. |
| Capsulotomy | Rhexis with small diameter. |
| Hydrodissection/ hydrodelamination | Both are required to be correctly performed. It is important that hydrodelamination adequately separates the central nucleus from the epinucleus and that the whole nucleus rotates easily. |
| Phaco carving | Vacuum—10-50; flow—10-15; U/S power—70%. The anterior portion is carved as usual. |
| Phaco shifting of the nucleus | Shifting the nucleus upward with the spatula and exposition of the lower nucleus lip. The aim of the maneuver is to move the portion being emulsified away from the distal posterior capsule. Emulsification of the border inside the equator at 6. |
| Nucleus rotation with the spatula | The maneuver is made to bring another portion of nuclear rim to 6. Aim of the capture of the border at 6 and then phacoemulsification. The operation is repeated until the whole rim has been emulsified. |
| Nuclear chip phaco | The residual nucleus (chip) is lifted with the spatula from below and taken to the middle of the bag and then fragmented. |
| Epinuclear flip | Tip occlusion distally in the epinucleus. Combined maneuver of spatula and U/S tip to elevate, rotate, and position the epinucleus inside the rhexis. Phacoemulsification of the epinucleus at a safe site. |
| Flip parameters | Vacuum—100-150. Flow—20. U/S—50%. |

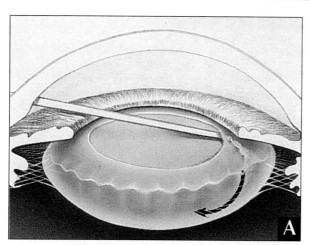

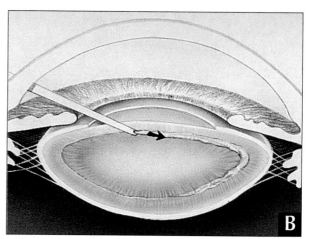

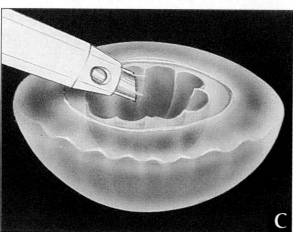

Figure 6-16A. Chip and Flip technique. Following rhexis, the surgeon performs an accurate hydrodissection.
Figure 6-16B. The surgeon performs an accurate hydrodelamination to define the central nucleus clearly from the epinucleus, almost to mobilize it.
Figure 6-16C. The portion of the central nucleus is sculpted. This is rotated and emulsified uniformly at the center.

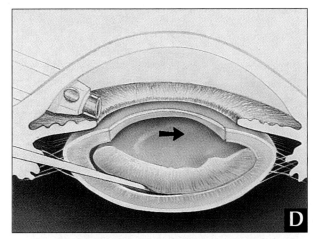

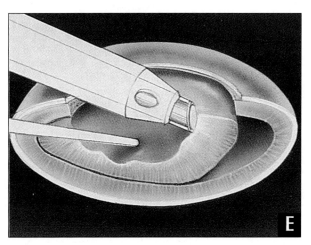

Figures 6-16D, 6-16E, 6-16F. With a spatula inserted to the side, the nucleus is moved toward the incision, and the U/S tip captures the equatorial nuclear edge distally and emulsifies it. The nucleus is rotated once again, and the procedure is repeated. With the U/S tip in occlusion, applied to the distal portion of the endonucleus, using the spatula, the nucleus is rotated from below upward to be brought into the center of the rhexis.

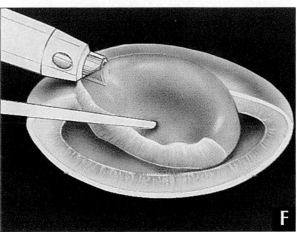

The following parameters are used to sculpting the groove:
- Vacuum—0 to 20 mm Hg.
- Flow rate—15 to 20 cc/min.
- U/S power—60 to 80%.

When the right-sized groove is created, the surgeon can proceed with nucleofracture.

### Nucleofracture

The fracture of the nucleus is obtained largely by separating the two edges of the groove using the U/S tip on one side and a spatula on the other.

A 45° U/S tip is most suitable because of the greater surface area available on the longer edge. The second instrument can be a common nuclear-spatula. In the event of soft nuclei, a spatula with a greater surface area may be useful (eg, a Koch spatula). This will not slice into the nucleus. The two instruments can be placed parallel to each other on the edges of the groove or crossed over. Their depth in the groove is very important.

The ideal depth is two-thirds of the groove depth because an excessively superficial or deep position will not allow for optimal leverage necessary for nucleofracture.

The two instruments must be placed distally inside the groove so that fracture can begin at the periphery. It then proceeds toward the center gradually as the separating force increases.

On separation of the groove edges, the surgeon must be able to see a fracture line on the floor of the groove, which continues from the equator toward the center of the lens. During fracture, the parameters of the machine are not changed, and the surgeon can intervene in a number of ways:

- Irrigation closed (pedal in Position 0)—This technique can be useful in those cases with a very deep anterior chamber, or if the lens is voluminous in order to reach the right depth easily with the two instruments. Closed irrigation may be useful for another reason: the posterior capsule relaxes. This will reduce the risk of it tearing during the maneuvers of nucleofracture.
- Irrigation open (pedal in Position 1)—This can be useful if the anterior chamber is reduced or the pupil tends to miosis.
- Irrigation and aspiration open (pedal in Position 2)—This is the usual condition for maintaining the spaces.
- Use of VES—This allows the surgeon to tackle both vitreal pressure and miosis, thanks to the possibility of maintaining the spaces dilated. It improves visibility, reduces the stress required for fracture—particularly when it is more difficult than usual. It reduces or eliminates any anterior chamber instability.

With VES, the tip is used without irrigation, that is with the foot pedal in Position 0. Alternately, a nucleofracture forceps can be used.

- The nucleus can also be split into pieces using a nucleofracture forceps introduced into the groove with the arms closed. It is then opened to separate the edges. In this case, the U/S tip must be removed and the anterior chamber and groove should be filled with VES.

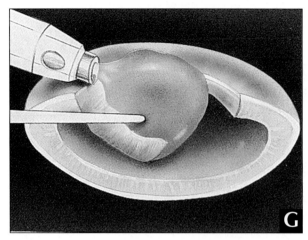
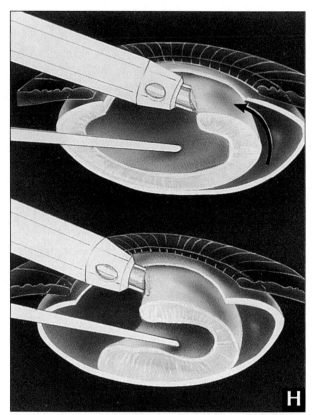

Figure 6-16G. The nucleus is then fragmented at the center of the rhexis inside the capsular bag. The epinucleus protects the posterior capsule.

Figure 6-16H. All that remains is the epinucleus, which is captured with the tip in occlusion and rotated with the spatula (flip) to bring the captured portion to the center of the capsular bag.

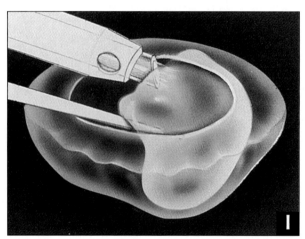
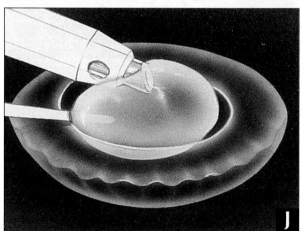

Figures 6-16I, 6-16J. The epinucleus is aspirated and emulsified gradually inside the rhexis.

A different technique of nucleofracture involves using a hook, which creates a crack in the nucleus even without the preliminary creation of a groove (see Phaco Chop).

### Capture and Emulsification of the Nuclear Fragments

With nucleofracture, the nucleus is split into two to four or more portions that will be emulsified.

The surgeon must therefore increase both the tendency of the nucleus to approach the U/S tip (high flow rate) and the capacity of tip to hold on to the nucleus (holding power—ie, high vacuum) to emulsify and be aspirated. This can be obtained by increasing the vacuum to 100 to 120 mm Hg, the flow rate to 20 cc/min, and reducing the mean power of the U/S to 50 to 70%. The parameters can be modified in proportion to the hardness of the nucleus.

For soft nuclei, the vacuum can be set at 60 to 80 mm Hg, whereas for very hard nuclei it should be 160 to 180 mm Hg.

The flow rate can vary between 16 and 22 cc/min in proportion to the vacuum use. As the vacuum increases, it would seem normal to reduce the flow rate, ie, reduce the speed BSS is removed from the chamber. This involves a drop in the speed of the operations in the anterior chamber with equal vacuum and U/S. In actual fact, when the vacuum is increased, the flow rate is also increased. This occurs when high vacuum is used and the surgeon is faced

### Table 6-13
### FLOW RATE AND VACUUM IN THE PHACO FRACTURE TECHNIQUE IN MACHINES FITTED WITH A PERISTALTIC PUMP

The modern phaco techniques are not traumatic because they use low levels of U/S. This considerably reduces the turbulence in the anterior chamber. If U/S power is reduced but surgical times are not to be prolonged, the fragmentation ability must be increased. This is obtained by increasing the contact between the nucleus and the U/S tip. Let's take a look at how this is done.

The flow rate is the quantity of fluid that is aspirated in unit time. It has the important task of mobilizing the residual lens fragments and drawing them toward the aspiration orifice. So the value of the flow rate determines the speed with which the masses are drawn or removed. During the fragmentation phase, the higher the flow rate, the greater the capacity of the tip for attracting the material toward the U/S tip. A high flow rate will therefore accelerate the tip's ability to fragment, with equal U/S and vacuum values. Higher flow rate also means greater turbulence in the chamber.

The vacuum is the depression that is created in the tubes for the effect of the rotation of the pump. The vacuum allows the tip to maintain contact with the material (and to draw it, after fragmentation by the U/S, beyond the orifice and into the tube). Clinically, increasing or decreasing the vacuum means increasing or decreasing the force with which the material is aspirated. The higher the vacuum, the more firmly the material is held.

**Other important information**

During the operation, the flow rate must be sufficient to mobilize and capture the pieces. Once this has happened, the vacuum must be sufficient to keep the material stuck to the tip until it is fragmented and aspirated (during occlusion, the flow rate will decrease despite the fact that the vacuum increases). After removal of the piece that has been captured and that obstructs the tip, the vacuum returns to the previous values so that the flow rate is reestablished. A pump with a low flow rate provides a greater safety margin even though a low flow rate involves longer operating times. The ideal situation is to have the flow rate that is suitable for the needs of that particular moment.

The rising time of the vacuum measures how quickly the vacuum increases when the orifice is occluded. It decreases with an increase in the rotation speed of the pump, ie, with an increase in the aspiration flow rate. A decrease in the rising time brings about an increase in the speed the vacuum increases in the aspiration line once occlusion has been obtained.

When the surgeon asks the machine for zero vacuum, he or she asks for something that does not actually exist, at least not when there is an irrigation flow rate and the pump still rotates occasionally or slowly or until vacuum is formed in the tubes (silicone=elastic). In practice, a high flow rate produces a slight vacuum even without occlusion. When the orifice is occluded by the material, the flow rate is zero (ie, there is no movement of the liquid to the aspiration, and vacuum comes into action) and the vacuum present in the aspiration line.

---

with a hard nucleus, which requires stronger fluid movement (a stronger flow rate to move the nucleus and bring it closer to the tip). The U/S are varied between 30 and 70 in relation to the hardness of the nucleus—ie, the harder the nucleus, the greater the level of U/S. However, the surgeon should remember that if the piece of nucleus is free, it is often counter-productive to use high ultrasound.

Each fragment must be captured by the U/S tip. The tip should be brought into occlusion.

The tip engages the material. The surgeon activates the aspiration while he or she waits for the contact with the material and also waits for the vacuum to reach the maximum value set. If the material is soft, aspiration is sufficient for obtaining occlusion.

If the material is hard, spontaneous occlusion is more difficult; it is facilitated by short bursts of low-power U/S. With these bursts, the tip will adhere better to the nuclear material and will occlude better. Then, the surgeon must wait for a few seconds to allow the vacuum to increase in the tip thus increasing the holding power.

The fragment is then brought into the pupillary field and emulsified. The traction toward the center must be slow and gradual and must be supported by the spatula, which must free the quadrant from the nearby material. Emulsification must be done with short bursts with the material constantly controlled with the spatula.

Capture of the last fragment with the U/S tip can be facilitated by using the pulse mode of the ultrasound.

The most suitable site for attempting occlusion in a sector of the nucleus to be emulsified differs in relation to the size and the hardness of the nucleus and to the size of the capsulorhexis.

Generally speaking, the superficial portion of the nucleus is usually softer. The central and deeper part is usually harder.

### Table 6-14
### THE VACUUM AND THE FLOW RATE IN THE TECHNIQUE OF NUCLEAR FRACTURE INTO FOUR QUADRANTS

| | Vacuum | Flow rate |
|---|---|---|
| Superficial shaving | Low | Medium-low |
| Sculpting of the grooves | Low | Medium-low |
| Fracture into quadrants | Not needed | Not needed |
| Capture of the quadrants | High | Medium-high |
| Fragmentation of the quadrants | High | Medium-high |
| Capture of the epinucleus | Medium-low | Medium-low |
| Emulsification of the epinucleus | Medium-low | Medium-low |
| I/A | Medium-low | Medium-high |

### Table 6-15
### PHASES OF THE OPERATION OF NUCLEAR FRACTURE INTO FOUR QUADRANTS AND EMULSIFICATION

| | |
|---|---|
| Shaving of the cortex and the epinucleus and sculpting to produce the grooves | This occurs by engaging the tip for at least half of its surface, without total occlusion. Optimal results are obtained with low vacuum, high flow rate, and high U/S. |
| Division of the nucleus into pieces | This occurs with the two separating instruments with the foot pedal in Position 2, ie, with I/A. The orifice of the U/S tip is not occluded. |
| Capture of the pieces at the equator | This occurs under occlusion with strong vacuum, moderate flow rate, and no U/S. |
| The pieces are pulled to the center | This occurs in occlusion with strong vacuum, moderate flow rate, and no U/S. |
| Phacoemulsification of the pieces | This occurs with high vacuum, reduced flow rate, and low U/S. |
| Capture of the epinucleus and its removal | This occurs in occlusion with intermediate vacuum (a value that lies somewhere between the initial and final values). The flow rate is lower than that used in the previous phases. U/S values are also very low. |

### Table 6-16
### THE GROOVES IN THE TECHNIQUES OF NUCLEOFRACTURE

| | |
|---|---|
| Length | If hydrodissection alone has been used, the groove can be extended just slightly beyond the rhexis. If hydrodelamination has also been performed, the groove can extend to the limits of the endonucleus. |
| Width | It is just slightly wider than the tip and its sleeve (one and a half times). |
| Depth | About 80% of the nuclear thickness, if only hydrodissection has been performed. Maintain this depth both at the center and toward the equator. Adapt the shape of the groove to the original shape of the posterior surface of the nucleus. If hydrodelamination has been performed, the groove can be carved for the entire thickness of the endonucleus (which is separate from the epinucleus). |

If the nucleus is not very hard and the capsulorhexis is wide, the U/S tip can be placed in correspondence to the length of the groove so that the orifice comes into contact with the material. The surgeon should then wait until the orifice is occluded and the material is engaged, and then bring it toward the pupillary center.

If the nucleus is hard and the quadrants have sharp corners, it is advisable to raise the deep portion of the quadrant with a second instrument (the spatula). The spatula is placed superficially to raise the deep portion of the quadrant; the apex is raised and can be engaged with the U/S tip to obtain occlusion. The quadrant is then brought to the center of the bag and emulsified.

If the U/S tip is positioned in a portion of the fragment that is too superficial, it will rotate on its axis so that the apex of the nucleus moves in the direction of the posterior capsule. This may, of course, cause the posterior capsular rupture.

The action of the spatula is important in the capture of the quadrants because these are mobilized (thus facilitating the transport toward the center). They are positioned in an optimal position (thus facilitating a good relationship between the tip and the material, which in turn makes successful occlusion easier). It serves to maintain the contact between the quadrant and the tip if one of the fragments escapes or in the event the vacuum is not sufficient to maintain contact. It is used to protect the endothelium and the posterior capsule from free sharp pieces rotating in the anterior segment.

### Comment
The techniques of nucleofracture represent an enormous step forward in the procedure of phacoemulsification. They are easy techniques to learn and give excellent results.

In order to be used correctly, they must be properly understood. The surgeon must also gradually gain confidence with the various operating steps; he or she should be prepared to cope with any difficulties that may arise during the operation by applying the variations of the techniques.

## Cross Nucleofracture According to Shepherd or Quartering Technique or In Situ Fracture (1989)

Even though this is a variation of Gimbel's original technique, it has become the most commonly used technique of nucleofracture to the point of being considered Divide and Conquer par excellence.

Table 6-17
## TYPE OF U/S TIP FOR THE NUCLEOFRACTURE

| Angulation tip | Sculpting of the grooves | Traction of the quadrants (ie, occlusion) | Emulsification of the quadrants | Capture and removal of the epinucleus |
|---|---|---|---|---|
| Zero | — | ++++ | ++ | ++ |
| 15° | ++ | +++ | +++ | +++ |
| 30° | +++ | ++ | ++ | + |
| 45° | ++++ | + | + | — |

+ indicates a positive effect.

Table 6-18
## PARAMETERS OF THE VARIOUS PHASES OF THE TECHNIQUES OF NUCLEOFRACTURE

| | Shaving of the nucleus | Capture of the quadrants | Emulsification of the quadrants | Capture and removal of the epinucleus |
|---|---|---|---|---|
| Tip | 45°-30° | 15°-0° | 15°-0° | 15°-0° |
| Vacuum | 0-20 | 60-180 | 60-180 | 40-80 |
| Flow rate | 10-20 | 16-22 | 10-16 | 10-16 |
| U/S | 50-100% | 0-30% | 30-50% | 20-40% |
| Occlusion | No | Yes | Yes | Yes |

## Preparation

Once the surgeon has prepared the main incision and side port incisions, he or she injects VES into the anterior chamber and completes a capsulorhexis with a diameter of 4.5 to 5.5 mm.

Hydrodissection is done through the main incision, using a suitable cannula. The hydrodissection must be performed very accurately to obtain the complete mobilization of the nucleus, which must be free to rotate inside the capsular bag. The mobility of the nucleus is checked by rotating it with the hydrodissection cannula.

## Sculpting

A 30 or 45° U/S tip is preferable.

This phase can start in one of two ways in proportion to the hardness of the nucleus.

- If the nucleus is moderately hard, the surgeon starts by shaving the superficial cortex and the epinucleus to expose the nucleus. Then he or she can directly create a central groove directed from 12 to 6 o'clock to the inferior edge of the capsulorhexis.
- If the nucleus is hard, the surgeon shaves superficially and then creates a central groove as wide as the capsulorhexis. He or she then starts the creation of the grooves.

The depth of the groove must reach about 90% of the nuclear thickness. The width must correspond to twice the diameter of the U/S tip (ie, one and a half times the width of the sleeve).

The groove must follow the shape of the posterior capsule. It must be shallower at the beginning, become deeper at the center, and then return to the surface at 6 o'clock.

Table 6-19
## PARAMETERS FOR THE CAPTURE OF THE QUADRANTS AND THE EPINUCLEUS IN RELATION TO THE HARDNESS OF THE MATERIAL

| Nucleus | Vacuum | Flow rate | U/S |
|---|---|---|---|
| Soft | 60-80 | 16-18 | 30-40% |
| Medium | 80-120 | 18-20 | 40-50% |
| Hard | 120-180 | 20-22 | 50-70% |
| Epinucleus | Vacuum | Flow rate | U/S |
| Soft | 30-40 | 12-14 | 20-30% |
| Medium | 40-50 | 14-16 | 30-40% |
| Hard | 60-80 | 16-18 | 30-40% |

The grooves should be extended within the limits of the rhexis. If the surgeon wishes to extend further, he or she can expose the superior hemisphere of the nucleus by pushing the nucleus gently toward 6 o'clock with the spatula. Then, the nucleus is moved toward 12 o'clock to extend the groove further toward 6 o'clock.

When the first half-groove (first arm) has been completed at the right depth and width, the nucleus is rotated through 90° in a clockwise direction with the spatula. A new half-groove is cut, perpendicular to the first (second arm).

In the rotation phase, the pedal must be in Position 1 so that the capsule is distended and the nucleus can move more freely. In this phase, the spatula is also used to stabilize the nucleus to obtain more regular grooves.

A new half-groove is created (a continuation of the

Table 6-20
# ANGULATION OF THE TIP IN ENDOCAPSULAR PHACO

45° tip     The circumference of the orifice and the theoretical surface area of the orifice are large. With equal aspiration and flow rate, there is a low tendency to go into occlusion. It is a tip suitable for shaving and sculpting. It should therefore be used in the initial phase of the phaco to:
- Remove the anterior cortex.
- Remove the epinucleus.
- Create the grooves in the nucleofracture techniques.

Apart from anything else, the angulation of the tip allows the surgeon to have an excellent view of the various phases of groove formation and to be able to evaluate the depth correctly.

15° tip     The circumference of the theoretical surface of the orifice is reduced, so with equal vacuum and flow rate, the tip will tend to move into occlusion very easily. It is a tip suitable for:
- Capturing the pieces at the equator and transporting them to the center.
- Fragmenting the free pieces of the nucleus.
- Normal use with strong vacuum and low U/S. The surgeon takes full advantage of the contact between the tip and the material, and the U/S power.

30° tip     This is a compromise tip, halfway between the 15 and 45°. It has some of the advantages of one and some of the other. It is ideal for the techniques of nucleofracture into quadrants.

0° tip     This is ideal for anyone who wishes to perform the operation using occlusion alone. It is the ideal tip for the Phaco Chop. With this tip, the initial phase of the operation is not very easy (ie, the phase of shaving). The compromise tip for a Phaco Chop is 15°.

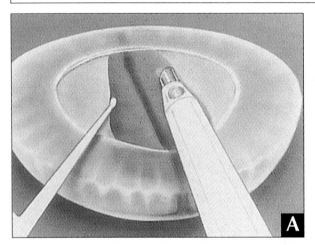

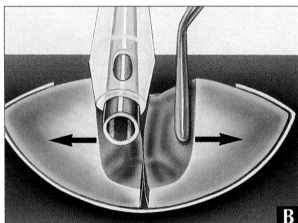

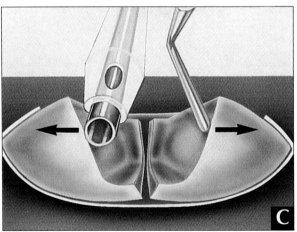

Figures 6-17A, 6-17B, 6-17C. How to split the nucleus. The nucleus is split using two instruments; the U/S tip pushes to the right while the spatula pushes to the left. The two instruments must be positioned at the same depth (about two-thirds of the depth of the nucleus) inside the groove, in the distal third of the groove (after rupture, they can be moved into the central third to extend the split). The movements used for separation must be coordinated.

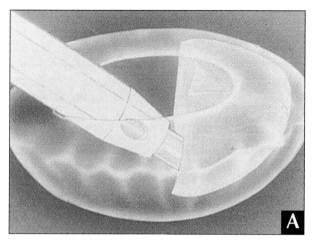 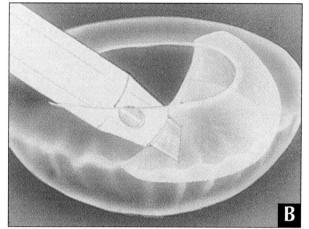

Figures 6-18A, 6-18B. How to occlude the U/S tip. The hemi-nucleus is distal. Occlusion and capture of the hemi-nucleus, which is then attracted to the center to be emulsified or split.

Table 6-21
**COMPARISON OF VARIOUS INSTRUMENTS**

|  | Alcon Legacy | Alcon Master | Alcon Universal II | Allergan Prestige | OMS Diplomat | Optikon P400 | Storz Premiere |
|---|---|---|---|---|---|---|---|
| Pump | Peristaltic | Peristaltic | Peristaltic | Peristaltic | Peristaltic | Peristaltic | Venturi |
| Loading | Cassette | Cassette | Tubes | Cassette | Tubes | Tubes | Cassette+Tubes |
| Handle | Piezoelectric 40 KHZ | Piezoelectric 40 KHZ | Piezoelectric 40 KHZ | Piezoelectric 47 KHZ | Piezoelectric 40 KHZ | Piezoelectric 55 KHZ | Piezoelectric 28 KHZ |
| Flow rate in U/S cc/min | 12-60 | 15-40 | 15-40 | 4-40 | 0-44 | 0-50 | Continuous |
| Vacuum in U/S mm Hg | 0-400 | 0-400 | 0-200 | 0-500 | 0-55 | 0-500 | 0-120 |
| Vacuum in I/A mm Hg | 0-500+ | 0-400+ | 0-400+ | 0-500 | 0-55 | 0-500 | 0-600 |
| Flow rate in I/A cc/min | 0-60 | 0-40 | 0-40 | 12-40 | 0-44 | 0-50 | Continuous |
| Pulsed U/S | 1-15 sec | 1-15 sec | 1-15 sec | 2-18 | 33-50-66% | 1-10 | 0-50 |
| Memory | 24 program with 4 memories each | 3 memories | 3 memories | 31 memories | 4 memories and 3 submemories | 20+3 subprograms in U/S and I/A | 20 |

first arm) perpendicular to the previous, then on to the fourth in order to form a cross. The second groove is usually slightly deeper than the first. Once every half-groove is created, the nucleus is rotated 90° so that a new arm is accessible at 6 o'clock. Rotation after rotation, the groove can be gradually deepened to reach the desired depth. Once the cross has been completed at the right depth and extension, the surgeon proceeds with the procedure of nucleofracture.

In order to obtain a uniform fracture line without creating excessive traction forces, the U/S tip and the spatula should be positioned quite deeply in an intermediate portion of one arm of the cross positioned at 6 o'clock.

Normally, the U/S tip is placed on the right-hand wall of the groove with the spatula on the left. However, in order to obtain greater separation of the two edges, the instruments should be crossed over. This way, the U/S tip passes on the left deep down while the spatula, crossing over and above it, puts pressure on the right-hand edge.

With the pedal in Position 0, so that the posterior capsule is relaxed, the instruments are pushed in opposite directions in order to separate the walls of the groove. A fracture line will appear from the periphery toward the center of the posterior nuclear wall.

Once this first groove has been obtained, the nucleus is rotated through 90°. The maneuver is repeated for each quadrant until the nucleus has been split into four wedges.

It is important that each wedge is completely detached from the others, ie, the fracture must go through the entire thickness of the material. Once the four segments have been obtained, the surgeon will often rotate the nucleus once again to check that the fracture has reached the posterior portions of the nucleus and that there are no residual bridges of material between the wedges.

Table 6-22
## COMPARISON OF VARIOUS INSTRUMENTS

|  | Alcon Legacy | Alcon Master | Alcon Universal II | Allergan Prestige | OMS Diplomat | Optikon P4000 | Storz Premiere |
|---|---|---|---|---|---|---|---|
| Remote control | Yes, infrared | Yes, by cable | No | Yes, by cable | Yes | Yes, by cable | Yes, optional |
| Computerized control | Yes | Yes | Yes | Yes | Yes | Yes | Yes |
| Self-diagnosis | Yes | Yes | Yes | Yes | Yes | Yes | Yes |
| Auto-tracking | Yes | Yes | Yes | Yes | Yes | Yes | Yes |
| Venting | Yes (liquid)[2] | Yes (liquid) | Yes (air) | Yes | Yes (air) | Yes (air and liquid) | Yes |
| Reflux | Yes (liquid) | Yes (liquid) | Yes (inversion pump) | Yes | Yes (liquid) | Yes | Yes |
| Audible confirmation of the function | Yes | No | No | No | No | Yes | No |
| Vitrectomy | Yes (ant) | Yes (ant) | Yes (ant) | Yes (ant) | Yes (ant) | Yes (ant-post) | Yes |
| Vacuum mm Hg | 0-500+ | 0-400+ | 0-400+ | 0-500 | 0-550 | 0-500 | 0-600 |
| Flow rate cc/min | 0-60 | 0-40 | 0-40 | 12-40 | 0-44 | 0-50 | Continuous |
| Cut rate/min | 50-400 | 50-400 | 50-400 | 180-400 | 100-600 | 60-700 | 30-750 |
| Bipolar cautering | Yes | Yes | Yes | Yes | Yes | Yes | Yes |
| Free flow | Yes | Yes, separate | Yes[3] | No Yes, if the program is upgraded (memory card) | Yes | Yes | Yes |
| Adjustable foot pedal | Yes | No | No | Yes | No | No | Yes |
| Bottle height can be adjusted electrically | Yes | Yes | No[4] | Yes | Yes |  | Yes |

2 Liquid- a sterile solution from an infusion bottle.
3 For the Universal 1, free flow is optional.
4 Can be obtained with the specific trolley.

When the two perpendicular fracture lines have been completed, the nucleus is split into four wedge-shaped segments that can be fragmented individually. The main technical problem common to the various forms of nucleofracture is the creation of the fracture line in the posterior of the nucleus.

In particular, if the nucleus is hard, the peripheral material will put pressure directly on the capsulo-zonular system because there is no suitable bumper effect of the epinucleus. The separating force is transmitted to the capsulorhexis, and this can rupture. If escape lines appear, these can extend dangerously toward the equator and then toward the posterior capsule, particularly if the surgeon is not aware of them immediately.

### *Fragmentation*

If the nucleus is moderately hard, the surgeon should remove the central apices of the wedges by shaving with the U/S tip. In this way, the tip has a broad support for occluding under the action of short U/S bursts. It is then possible to bring the nuclear quadrant toward the center of the capsular bag to complete the fragmentation.

In his original paper that described the technique, Shepherd actually proceeds in a different manner. The spatula is used to push the apex of the quadrant posteriorly until the equator of the fragment rotates centrally. The quadrant is then emulsified.

If the hardness of the nucleus is moderate-high, the surgeon can act in one of two ways.

With the foot pedal in Position 2, the inferior apex of the wedge is raised with the spatula, and the deep portion of the quadrant is captured with the U/S tip. The quadrant is then brought toward the center of the capsular bag.

Alternately, the surgeon can leave the pedal in Position 0 so the capsular bag is relaxed and the depth of the posterior chamber is reduced. In this way, the central part of the quadrant is raised thanks to the use of the spatula and because of the vitreal pressure. When the quadrant is in a favorable position, the pedal is moved to Position 2 to attempt occlusion. If this is not successful,

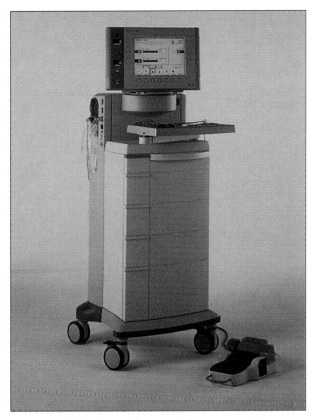

Figure 6-19. Alcon Legacy Phacoemulsifier.

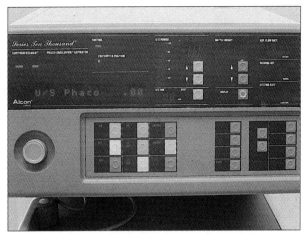

Figure 6-20. Alcon's Master 10,000 Phacoemulsifier.

the surgeon uses short bursts of low power U/S to facilitate the contact between the tip and the material.

The quadrant is brought into the pupillary field to be emulsified. It must always be emulsified when it is in a central position. The site (in the bag, on the pupillary plane, or in the anterior chamber) depends on the sizes of the quadrant and the capsulorhexis.

A small quadrant often moves spontaneously into the anterior chamber. A section of moderate size can be processed either in the bag or brought into the anterior chamber.

A large quadrant must initially be kept in the bag with the spatula and reduced in volume, particularly if the capsulorhexis is small. Then, it can be brought into the anterior chamber. If, on the other hand, the capsulorhexis is wide, a large quadrant can be emulsified in the pupillary plane.

The spatula controls the movements of the nuclear wedge to avoid turbulence or contacts.

The maneuver is repeated for the other three sectors of nucleus until the nucleus has been completely removed.

If the nucleus is not hard and the surgeon would prefer to avoid using high aspiration, the nuclear quadrant can be subluxated by depressing the base or lower part with the spatula toward the posterior capsule to expose the apex to the U/S tip for emulsification.

If the nucleus is hard, this may be a risky procedure for the posterior capsule. In this case, it is preferable to engage the quadrant in the center, sinking the U/S tip in with a short shot of U/S. Once occlusion has been obtained, with the vacuum constant, the quadrant is brought to the center of the bag and emulsified.

The last remaining quadrant can be slightly more difficult because is it no longer restrained in the capsular bag by the other quadrants and will tend to wander. In this case, the spatula is very useful in controlling the movements of the remaining quadrant bringing it toward the U/S tip.

The operation is completed in the normal fashion with the removal of the residual cortex, the implantation of the artificial lens, and sutures if required.

## The Divide and Conquer Technique According to Gimbel (Divide and Conquer Nucleofractis [1986])

This technique has two variations: the Trench technique for moderate-hard nuclei (Grade 3) and the Crater technique for hard nuclei (Grade 4).

### *Introduction*

This is the parent technique of nucleofracture techniques. Since its original description in 1986, it has been constantly improved by the author and numerous variations have developed.

The initial observation was made using the two-handed phacoemulsification techniques in the posterior chamber according to Kratz (Minimal Lift). Gimbel noted that it was possible to obtain radial cleavage lines in the nucleus, according to the anterior and posterior Y-suture planes. In practice, while the spatula stabilized the nucleus, the U/S tip was used to detach portions of the nucleus.

The procedure started with sculpting of the right portion of the nucleus, in the normal manner, while the spatula stabilized the left portion. The latter was then tackled directly by sinking the U/S tip in and detaching the various sectors one at a time.

In the harder nuclei, sculpting was extended both in width and in depth to create a central crater that would weaken the nucleus and permit its fracture into a number of pieces.

Table 6-23

# FOUR QUADRANTS NUCLEOFRACTURE TECHNIQUE ACCORDING TO SHEPHERD

| | |
|---|---|
| Nuclei | Hardness 2-3 and sometimes 4. |
| Tip 45° | |
| Parameters | Low vacuum in the early phase, middle-high in the capture phase, and medium in the later phases. U/S high at the beginning and low toward the end. |
| Incision | Scleral or corneal tunnel. |
| Emulsification—early stage | Shearing of cortex and epinucleus inside the rhexis without occlusion. |
| Formation of the first hemisulcus/groove and its characteristics | Emulsify starting from the proximal limit of the rhexis and going toward the distal end. Sulcus/groove width is equal to one and a half diameter of the sleeve. Deeper in the middle and less deep in the periphery. Contained within the limit of capsulorhexis. |
| Formation of the second hemisulcus/groove | The nucleus is rotated 90° with the spatula. Formation of the second hemisulcus/groove slightly deeper than the first; further rotation. |
| Formation of the third and fourth hemisulci/grooves | Direct prosecution of the first and second hemisulci/grooves. |
| Deepening the first, second, third, and fourth hemisulci/ grooves | The four hemisulci/grooves are deepened to reach three-fourths of the nucleus depth |
| First nucleofracture | With the spatula on one side and the U/S tip on the other, fracture of the distal sulcus is accomplished. |
| Second, third, fourth nucleofracture | 90° rotation, then further fragmentation. 90° rotation and fracture. Again 90° rotation and then another fracture. |
| Capture and fragmentation of the quadrants | Occlusion-capture of the quadrant with the pedal on Position 2. Shifting out of the equator toward the middle and then emulsification. |

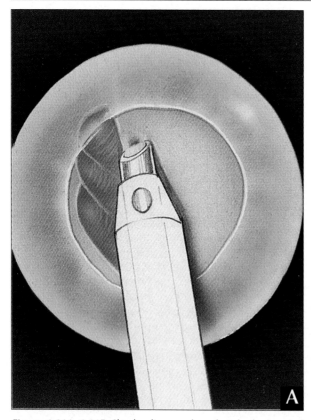 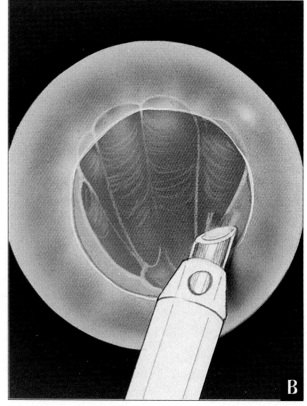

Figures 6-21A, 6-21B. Shepherd's cross-shaped nucleofracture technique or quartering technique. Rhexis and hydrodissection have been completed. The U/S tip used to shave the cortex and the epinuclear material in the area enclosed by the rhexis.

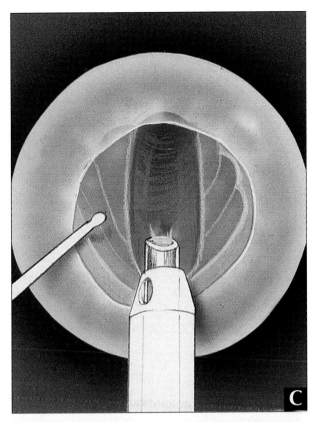

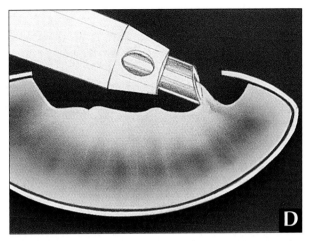

Figures 6-21C, 6-21D. A first hemi-groove is created at 12 and 6 o'clock. It must have a diameter that corresponds to 1.5 times the width of the sleeve.

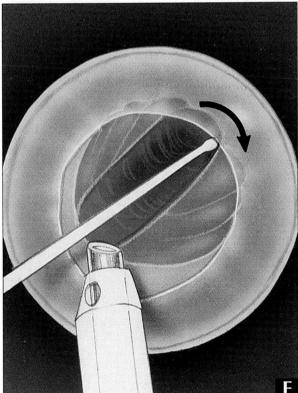

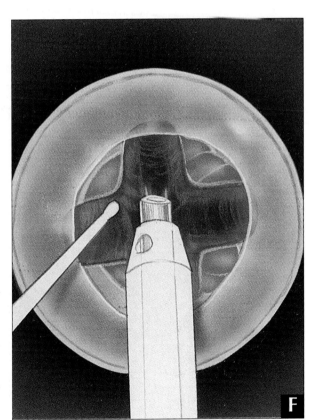

Figure 6-21E. The nucleus is rotated through 90° with a spatula. Then another hemi-groove is created, and two perpendicular grooves are created in a cross shape. Initially, they are neither deep nor extensive.

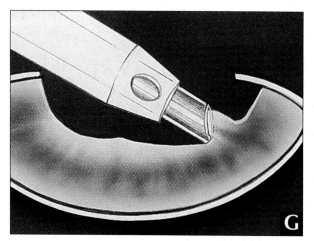

Figure 6-21G. The grooves must be deepened gradually.

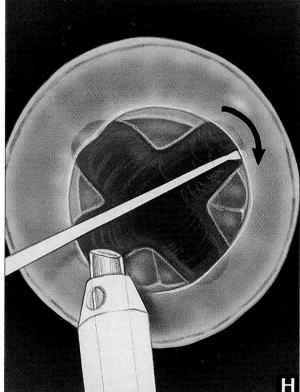

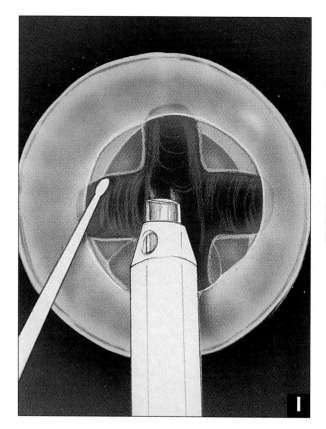

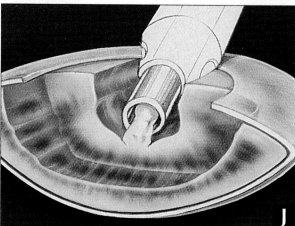

Figures 6-21H, 6-21I, 6-21J, 6-21K, 6-21L, 6-21M. The nucleus is therefore rotated further, and the grooves are deepened distally and in the center of the nucleus. Gradually, the residual material inside the grooves is reduced, and the red reflex becomes increasingly evident.

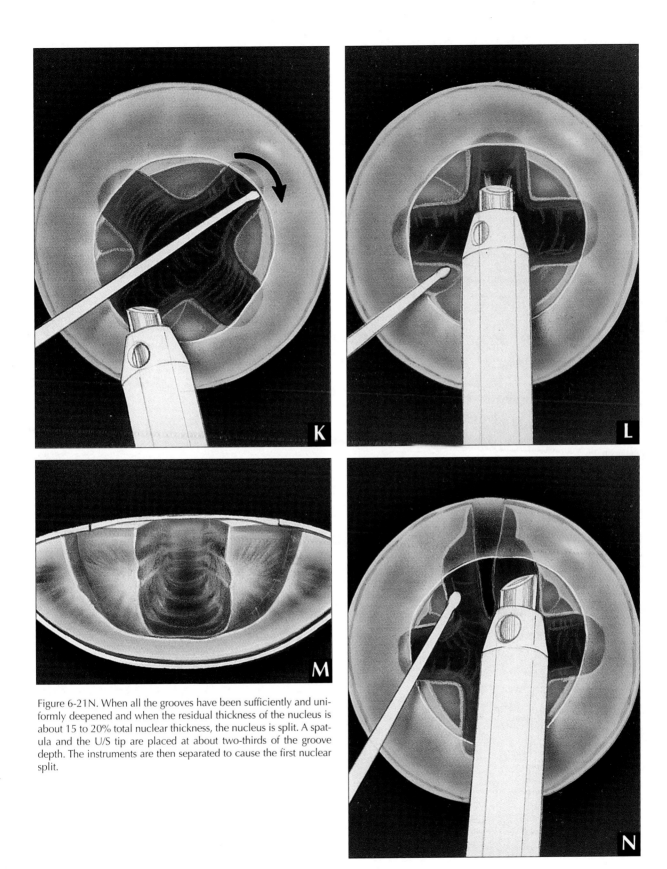

Figure 6-21N. When all the grooves have been sufficiently and uniformly deepened and when the residual thickness of the nucleus is about 15 to 20% total nuclear thickness, the nucleus is split. A spatula and the U/S tip are placed at about two-thirds of the groove depth. The instruments are then separated to cause the first nuclear split.

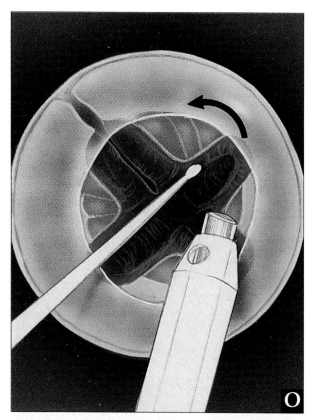

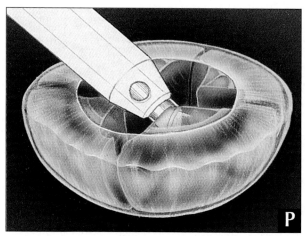

Figures 6-21O, 6-21P, 6-21Q, 6-21R. The nucleus is rotated and fractured distally again. All four fractures are obtained in the same way. The fractures must reach the deep layers of the nucleus

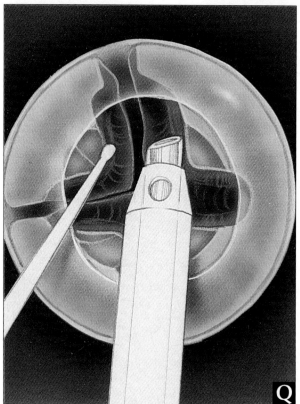

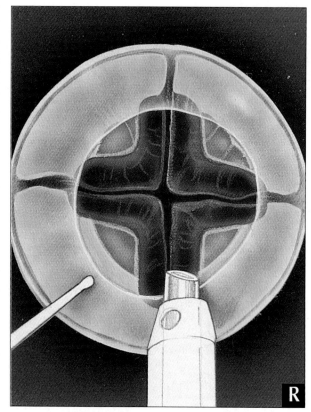

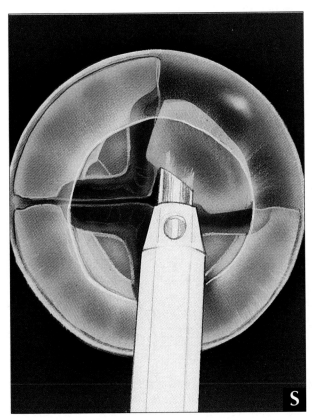 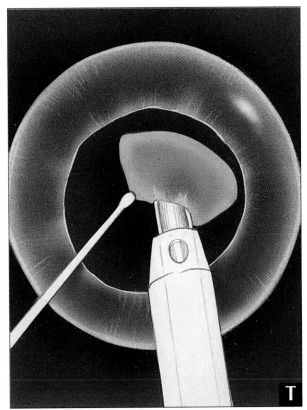

Figure 6-21S. At this point, the parameters on the machine are changed. Vacuum is brought to 100 to 180 mm Hg depending on the hardness of the material, flow rate to 18 to 22 cc/min, and U/S is reduced to 50 to 60%.

Figure 6-21T. The tip is brought into contact with one quadrant, and the surgeon waits for occlusion. If this does not occur spontaneously, he or she uses a short burst of U/S. Under occlusion, the material is dislocated from the equator and brought toward the center of the capsular bag.

The technique of in situ Divide and Conquer nucleofractis is split into four steps:
1. Deep central sculpting of the nucleus until a thin posterior disc of material remains.
2. Fracture of the disc (nucleofractis).
3. Rupture of a wedge-shaped section and its emulsification.
4. Rotation of the nucleus so that another wedge-shaped portion can be detached and emulsified.

*Central sculpting*—The nucleus is stabilized with a spatula while the 30° U/S tip removes the material along the line that runs from 11 to 7 o'clock. U/S is set in linear control, and the tip works on the surface without going into occlusion; a trench is then carved. It must be wide enough to receive the U/S tip and its sleeve. The groove must proceed to the deep layers of the nucleus, that is until the surgeon observes the red reflex of the fundus.

*Fracture of the disc and rupture of the wedge*—The U/S tip is embedded into the edge of the sulcus under the effects of a short U/S burst. The surgeon waits until occlusion causes the vacuum to increase to the preset values. With a spatula, the nucleus is pushed to the left while the U/S tip is pushed to the right to cause the fracture of the nuclear edge, which runs from the periphery toward the center. The U/S tip is fixed in the largest part of the nucleus, and while the tip stabilizes the material, a portion of the nucleus is detached.

*Rotation of the nucleus*—The nucleus is rotated in a clockwise direction, and the phacoemulsification is repeated to obtain a wedge of nuclear material that can be emulsified in the pupillary plane.

This sequence is repeated in a systematic manner until the nucleus is completely removed. The number of segments formed by nucleofracture depends on the hardness of the material; the harder the nucleus, the greater the number of pieces produced (from four to eight).

Let's take a more detailed look at the original technique.

### Preparation

A small conjunctival incision is performed to prepare the sclero-corneal field in the normal way.

The main incision is performed. It is usually a two-plane posterior limbal incision. The first is perpendicular to the sclera, 2 mm from the limbus. The second plane is parallel to the iris along a cleavage line that reaches the limbal arches.

Alternately, the surgeon can perform a sclero-corneal tunnel with a self-sealing corneal flap. However, the surgeon should remember that the maneuvers with the U/S tip in this technique can create a considerable number of corneal folds that can make the visibility of the intraoperative procedures somewhat difficult. Before extending

Table 6-24
# FOUR QUADRANTS NUCLEOFRACTURE TECHNIQUE ACCORDING TO BURATTO

## Corneal temporal incision
Vertical preincision in clear cornea just before the vascular arcades, 250-300 μm deep, about 4.0 μm wide.
Formation of a tunnel about 2.0 mm long.
Two lateral incisions are made 60° superiorly and inferiorly to the main port (30° knife Alcon).
Penetration in the chamber inside the tunnel with a 30° knife, careful selection of the entrance site; particular care in the creation of the inside valve of the incision.
Widening of the main port to 2.8 with precalibrated blade.

## Capsulorhexis
The chamber is filled with Viscoat.
Capsulorhexis forceps (Buratto) is introduced. In the center of the capsule, the jaws are opened and placed so as to touch the surface of the anterior capsule.
The jaws are closed causing capsular break and therefore formation of a lip.
The base of the lip is grasped by the forceps, and capsular opening is performed by tearing for a quarter of a turn. The opening under the tunnel is made first.
The lip is grasped again, and the opening is widened 40-50° further. The base of the lip must be grasped again at least four to five times.
The opening is completed from the outside toward the inside. It must be centered with continuous borders, round and about 5.0-5.5 mm wide.

## Hydrodissection
A glass 3.0 mL syringe filled with BSS is used. An Asico-Buratto hydrodissection cannula is used.
Entrance through the main port.
Go distally under the rhexis toward 5 under the capsule.
The anterior capsule is gently lifted by the cannula, and a small amount of BSS is quickly injected toward the equator.
Using the cannula, the center of the nucleus is compressed, causing the injected BSS to leak around the equator (decompression).
Hydrodissection procedure is repeated at 1 and decompression is again performed.
The nucleus is rotated inside the bag. A quarter- or half-turn, clockwise and reverse, is sufficient.
The nucleus is ready for phaco.

## Phaco: first phase

| | |
|---|---|
| Shaving and formation of sulci | Vacuum: 10; flow: 10-15; U/S: 70-80%; instrument Legacy by Alcon with 30° tip. |
| | Removal of the cortex and the epinucleus within the limits of the rhexis. |
| | Start just beyond the proximal border of the rhexis and stop just before the distal border. |
| | Carve, without occlusion, a sulcus with a width equal to 1.5 diameter of the sleeve. |
| | Depth equal to diameter of the sleeve. |
| | Enter the spatula in the lateral incision. |
| | Rotate the nucleus 90°. |
| | Perform another hemisulcus following the scheme described above. |
| | Extend the first hemisulcus. This part of the sulcus is a bit deeper than the former. Lengthen the second hemisulcus as was done for the first. |
| | Deepen the former hemisulcus in the middle (remember that nucleus thickness is greater in the middle than in the distal portion, where the tip tends to carve more). |
| | Nucleus rotation with the spatula. |
| | Deepen the latter hemisulcus following the scheme previously described as well as all other sulci until good depth is reached. |
| | Control whether each sulcus is deep enough in the middle and follows the theoretical curve of the posterior capsule. |
| | The reflex coming from the fundus must be sufficiently red (when the reflex is very obvious, the sulcus is too deep, whereas when the reflex is less obvious the sulcus is superficial). |
| | Check the sulcus width. It must be equal to 1.5 the diameter of the sleeve. |
| Nucleofracture | Position the spatula just beyond half the depth of the sulcus. |
| | Position the tip at the same level on the other side of the sulcus. |
| | Irrigation open or I/A open. |
| | Separate the two instruments until the nucleus splits from 6 to the area directly after the middle of the sulcus. |
| | Rotate the nucleus 90°, and repeat the procedure. |
| | Rotate again 90°, and repeat the maneuver. |
| | Rotate again, and repeat the maneuver. |
| | The nucleus is now divided in four sections. To confirm, repeat one full turn and check that the fracture extends to the deepest portions of the nucleus. |

Table 6-24 (cont)

| | |
|---|---|
| Capture and removal of the quadrants | Parameters are changed. Vacuum: 80-180 according to nucleus hardness; flow: 12-18 according to nucleus hardness; U/S: 50-70%. |
| | With the spatula applied to the upper part, lift the lower apex of the quadrant. |
| | With the U/S tip, start contact. If occlusion is likely to occur, wait. If the nucleus is cornered and hard and no occlusion follows, discharge small amount of U/S to excavate a small hollow favoring the occlusion. |
| | Once the occlusion has been achieved, wait until the vacuum reaches the set levels. |
| | Then pull the nucleus toward the middle. |
| | Fragment the nucleus with small discharges, keeping it under control with the spatula. |
| | Repeat the procedure for the other quadrants. |
| Removal of the epinucleus | Mobilize the epinucleus with the U/S tip and the spatula. |
| | Occlude the tip with the epinucleus using aspiration and/or short U/S bursts. Remove the epinucleus. |
| | Parameters—vacuum: 50-80; flow: 15-118; U/S 30-40%. |
| Cortex | The Buratto bimanual system is employed. |
| | Parameters—vacuum: 400; flow: 20; aspiration tip with 0.3 hole. |
| | The irrigation cannula is inserted through one of the two lateral incisions while the aspiration tip is introduced through the other. |
| | While the irrigation cannula remains immobile just inside the incision, the aspiration tip is introduced in the bag, placed on a portion of cortex with no aspiration. |
| | The pedal is operated to aspirate. The cortex edge occludes the tip. |
| | When vacuum has increased enough, the cortex edge is detached and brought to the middle. |
| | At this point, the pedal is pressed further thus increasing the vacuum. The material is removed a small amount at a time. |
| | The procedure is repeated as many times as necessary to remove the cortex from one-half of the bag. |
| | The two cannulas are inverted, and the cortex is removed from the other half of the bag. |
| Preparation of the bag and the anterior chamber | The capsular bag is filled with Provisc. |
| IOL implantation | The foldable IOL AcrySof MA60 by Alcon surgical is used. |
| | The lens is placed longitudinally on the folding forceps by Asico-Buratto. The forceps is then released, and the lens is folded. |
| | The lens is taken with the insertion forceps by Asico-Buratto and checked that the lens has been folded correctly. |
| | The anterior lip of the incision is lifted with atraumatic tweezers. |
| | The lens is inserted with the folded part of the lens on the left. |
| | The distal loop is introduced in the capsular bag along with a part of the lens distal portion. |
| | The forceps is rotated 90°. |
| | The forceps is opened, and the lens unfolds in a slow and controlled way. |
| | The forceps is extracted. |
| | The proximal loop is grasped with McPherson's tweezers and introduced in the bag while the spatula introduced laterally depresses the optic disc toward the capsular bag. |
| Removal of viscoelastic | The viscoelastic is removed by two-handed technique. |
| | Parameters—vacuum: 400; flow: 25. |
| | The two cannulas are introduced through the two lateral incisions; the material is removed first from the anterior chamber and then from the capsular bag. |
| Check of incision tightening | With the cannula of the syringe filled with BSS, the cornea is edematized at the three incision (two lateral and the main cut). |
| | Then globe tension is increased with BSS injection. |
| | With a dry sponge, the sclera is pushed about 2.0 mm posteriorly to the incision. The same maneuver (now with wet sponge) is performed in clear cornea. If the incision is not leaking, the intervention is thus completed. Alternatively, radial suture of nylon 10-0 is applied. |

Table 6-25
**PARAMETERS SET BY BURATTO ON ALCON'S LEGACY 20,000**

| Memory | Bottle height | U/S power | Flow rate cc/min | Vacuum mm Hg |
|---|---|---|---|---|
| | | Linear Control | Pedal in 2 | Pedal in 3 |
| Soft nuclei in the U/S phase | | | | |
| 1 | 75 cm | 40% | 24   16 | 0 |
| 2 | 75 cm | 40% | 22   12 | 50 |
| 3 | 75 cm | 40% | 22   12 | 76 |
| 4 | 75 cm | 40% | 22   12 | 100 |
| Moderately hard nuclei in the U/S phase | | | | |
| 1 | 75 cm | 70% | 24   16 | 0 |
| 2 | 75 cm | 60% | 20   14 | 60 |
| 3 | 75 cm | 60% | 20   14 | 100 |
| 4 | 75 cm | 60% | 20   14 | 140 |
| Hard nuclei in the U/S phase | | | | |
| 1 | 75 cm | 90% | 24   16 | 0 |
| 2 | 75 cm | 90% | 18   12 | 120 |
| 3 | 75 cm | 90% | 18   12 | 160 |
| 4 | 75 cm | 90% | 18   12 | 200 |
| Soft, moderate, and hard nuclei during the I/A phase | | | | |
| 1 | 75 cm | | 18 | 200 |
| 2 | 75 cm | | 22 | 400 |
| 3 | 75 cm | | 30 | 500 |
| For cleaning the posterior capsule | | | | |
| 1 | 50 cm | | 11 | 15 |
| 2 | 50 cm | | 16 | 20 |
| 3 | 50 cm | | 16 | 25 |

the incision to 3.2 mm, a 1 mm paracentesis is performed 70 to 90° from the center of the main incision with 30° bent knife.

The surgeon enters the anterior chamber with a 3.2 mm precalibrated blade. The 4.5 to 5.5 mm capsulorhexis is performed with the cystotome under VES. The presence of a resistant, uniform capsular margin is a basic requisite for the correct performance of this technique. In addition, this procedure should only be done with an intact rhexis. The surgeon must also do a hydrodissection.

The instrument is prepared by fitting a 30° tip.

Emulsification of the nucleus involves the following steps:

### Central Sculpting

The parameters are:
- Vacuum—0 to 20 mm Hg.
- Flow rate—15 cc/min.
- Maximum power—should not exceed 50% of the available power (reference value Alcon 10.000 Master).

A groove is created in the nucleus along an ideal line, which runs from 11 to 7 o'clock. The spatula introduced through the side port incision stabilizes the nucleus while the surgeon proceeds with linear power control of the U/S.

The width of the groove must be at least as wide as the U/S tip and sleeve, while the depth must be regulated on the basis of the color of reflex observed in the depth of the groove. A red reflex indicates that the posterior cortex is close and still kept under tension by the residual portion of the nucleus.

Table 6-26
**PARAMETERS SET BY BURATTO ON ALCON'S MASTER 10,000**

| | |
|---|---|
| Phaco sculpting | Maximum U/S power—80% for hard nuclei, 60% for moderate nuclei and for soft nuclei; linear control. Flow rate—25 cc/min. Vacuum—5 mm Hg. |
| Capture and removal of the quadrants | When the nucleus has been split, the surgeon moves to Memory 1, 2, or 3 depending on the hardness of the nucleus (Memory 1 for soft nuclei, 2 for moderate nuclei, and 3 for hard nuclei). |

| Memory | Bottle height | U/S power | Flow rate cc/min | Vacuum mm Hg |
|---|---|---|---|---|
| 1 | 75 cm | 50% | 18 | 81 |
| 2 | 75 cm | 60% | 22 | 121 |
| 3 | 75 cm | 80% | 25 | 171 |
| **I/A** | | | | |
| 1 | 75 cm | | 17 | 250 |
| 2 | 75 cm | | 21 | 350 |
| 3 | 75 cm | | 30 | 400 |
| **I/A cap vac** | | | | |
| 1 | 50 cm | | 11 | 11 |
| 2 | 50 cm | | 15 | 15 |
| 3 | 50 cm | | 20 | 20 |

Table 6-27
**DIFFERENCE IN THE OPERATING PARAMETERS FOR THE CAVITRON-KELMAN 8000 AND THE LEGACY DURING THE U/S PHASE**

|  | Cavitron-Kelman 8000 | Legacy 20,000 |
|---|---|---|
| U/S | All or nothing Manual tuning Manual selection of the required U/S power | Variable from 0 to 100% Continual self-tuning Linear selection of the U/S power with the foot pedal |
| Vacuum | Fixed at 41 mm Hg | Variable between 0 and 400 mm Hg |
| Flow rate | Fixed at 20 cc/min | Variable between 12 and 60 cc/min |

Table 6-28
**PARAMETERS SET BY BURATTO ON ALCON'S MASTER 10,000 ALTERNATIVE**

| Function and memory | Bottle height | U/S power | Flow rate cc/min | Vacuum mm Hg |
|---|---|---|---|---|
|  |  | Linear control | Pedal in 2 | Pedal in 3 |
| Phaco |  |  |  |  |
| 1 | 60 cm | 30% | 18    18 | 61 |
| 2 | 60 cm | 50% | 21    16 | 131 |
| 3 | 60 cm | 70% | 24    14 | 201 |
| I/A |  |  |  |  |
| 1 | 60 cm |  | 20 | 200 |
| 2 | 60 cm |  | 30 | 300 |
| 3 | 60 cm |  | 40 | 400 |
| Cap vac I/A |  |  |  |  |
| 1 | 60 cm |  | 7 | 15 |
| 2 | 60 cm |  | 9 | 19 |
| 3 | 60 cm |  | 11 | 25 |
| AVIT |  | Cut rate |  |  |
| 1 | 15 cm | 150 | 9 | 300 |
| 2 | 15 cm | 250 | 12 | 300 |
| 3 | 15 cm | 350 | 15 | 300 |

Table 6-29
**PARAMETERS SET BY BURATTO ON OPTIKON'S P4000**

|  | Vacuum | Flow rate | U/S power in linear |
|---|---|---|---|
| 1. Sculpting | 10 | 25 | 80% |
| 2. Capture of soft quadrants | 80 | 23 | 80% |
| 3. Capture of moderate hard quadrants | 120 | 21 | 80% |
| 4. Capture of hard quadrants and Phaco Chop | 180 | 18 | 80% |
| 5. Epinucleus | 60 | 15 | 40% |
| 6. I/A | 400 | 18 | 40% |

Table 6-30
**PARAMETERS SET BY BURATTO WITH ALLERGAN'S PRESTIGE**

**31 MEMORIES ARE AVAILABLE**

| Sub-memory | Vacuum mm Hg | Flow rate cc/min | U/S power in linear |
|---|---|---|---|
| 1. Phaco sculpting (low position) | 10 | 26 | 70% |
| 2. Phaco capture of hard quadrants (high position) | 180 | 22 | 50% |
| 3. I/A | 350 | 26 (30 for Viscoat) | — |

Table 6-31
**PARAMETERS USED BY BURATTO WITH THE STORZ PREMIER PHACO**

|  | U/S | Vacuum |
|---|---|---|
| Phaco 1 | 80% fixed | 30 mm Hg |
| Phaco 2 | From 5-70% in linear | Fixed 90 |
| Phaco 3 (alternative to Phaco 2) | From 5-30% possibly from 6 to 10 pulses per second | Fixed 70 |
| Phaco aspiration 4 | 30% fixed | Linear from 0 to 60 |
| I/A of the cortex |  | From 0 to 550 in linear |

The parameters—Flow rate does not exist in the machines with a Venturi pump. It is tightly correlated to the preset vacuum.

### Nucleofracture and Creation of the First Nuclear Sector

This maneuver aims to create a fracture line on the floor of the groove that was prepared in the previous phase. This line follows the radial cleavage planes between the nuclear fibers.

The U/S tip is fixed in the peripheral part of the nucleus on the right of the groove. While on the left, the cyclodialysis spatula is inserted in the anterior chamber through the side port incision at about 70° from the main incision.

With the foot pedal in Position 2, the U/S tip is pushed to the right, and the spatula is pushed to the left. The fracture line is obtained by exerting slight pressure, and it extends from the periphery to the center of the nucleus.

Once the first fracture-line has been obtained, vacuum is increased to 80 to 120 mm Hg, and the U/S tip is

> **Table 6-32**
>
> ## PARAMETERS OF THE LEGACY INSTRUMENT FOR PHACOEMULSIFICATION USING THE TECHNIQUE OF NUCLEOFRACTURE, ACCORDING TO BURATTO
>
> **In a nucleus of moderate hardness**
> **Shaving and sculpting**
>
> That is the removal of the cortex and the epinucleus within the limits of the rhexis and the creation of the grooves. It is normally performed using a tip engaged to about 30-50% (in absence of occlusion). So the surgeon needs to have:
>
> - Low or zero vacuum—A high value is of no use because, as there is no occlusion in the line, the vacuum will be low or zero in the tubes. By using low or zero vacuum, if the surgeon accidentally goes into occlusion, he or she will avoid the tip becoming trapped in the nucleus, or capturing the iris or pulling the posterior capsule toward the orifice if the sculpting is particularly deep.
> - Moderate-high flow rate—In excess of 10 cc/min. The higher it is, the more it produces a rapid liquid exchange in the anterior chamber and rapid removal of the nuclear fragments. Moreover, as high aspiration flow rate is equivalent to a high irrigation flow rate, the tip is cooled better (which may be extremely useful with high U/S power).
> - High U/S—This allows the surgeon to fragment the nuclear material very rapidly.
>
> The use of low U/S during sculpting will make progression of the tip very difficult. It will scrape the nucleus and push it rather than fragment it.

> **Table 6-33**
>
> ## CAPTURE AND TRANSPORT OF THE QUADRANTS
>
> The quadrants are captured with the tip 100% engaged (ie, the tip is occluded), and it occurs in I/A, ie, without using U/S (foot-pedal in position 2). So the surgeon needs to have:
>
> - High vacuum (80-120-180 depending on the hardness of the nucleus). In this way, the pieces captured will remain firmly attached to the tip and can be transported to the equator of the bag at the center of the chamber.
> - Moderate flow rate (between 18 and 22) to provide perfect control of the maneuvers of approach and capture of the material.
>
> **Fragmentation of the quadrants**
>
> In order to optimize the use of the U/S, the procedure should be completed keeping the quadrant in good contact with the tip. So the surgeon should have:
>
> - High vacuum (60-120-180 depending on the hardness of the material) to keep the pieces in contact with the tip and to improve the fragmentation power. This adhesion also prevents the pieces rotating in the anterior and/or posterior chamber and causing endothelial or capsular complications.
> - Moderate-low flow rate (10-18 cc/min) reduces the turbulence in the anterior chamber and controls the approach of the material to the tip. In addition, when the orifice disoccludes with low flow rate, there is a lower risk of collapse or minicollapse and therefore the capture (rupture) of the capsule or other structures.
> - Low U/S (30-60% depending on the hardness of the nucleus) because with high aspiration, there is good contact between the tip and the material, and the fragmentation ability is optimized.
>
> **Capture and removal of the epinucleus**
>
> In this phase, the surgeon must detach the peripheral layer of the nucleus (the epinucleus) from the capsule, if possible in a single bowl-shaped piece without aspirating the underlying capsule. The foot pedal is in Position 2 for this procedure, and the surgeon must have:
>
> - Low vacuum (30-80 mm Hg) fundamental to engage the epinucleus firmly without removing any small pieces.
> - The flow rate must be low (10-18 cc/min) because, as this is a delicate stage, it must be performed slowly.
> - Once the material has been captured, it can be removed with I/A alone and the foot pedal in Position 2 or with short low power U/S shots (20-40%).

applied to the nucleus to the left of the fracture line. With a short U/S shot, it is brought forward to achieve occlusion. A new fracture line is created perpendicular to the first using the spatula; a wedge of nuclear material is obtained.

With the pedal in Position 2, the sector is fixed to the tip with the U/S tip and brought toward the pupillary center to be emulsified.

### Rotation and New Phaco Fracture

After emulsification of the first nuclear sector, the remainder is rotated in a clockwise direction, and the maneuver of nucleofracture is repeated to obtain a new wedge of nuclear material for emulsification according to the procedure described previously.

Normally, the nucleus is fragmented into four quadrants that are then emulsified. However, depending on the

| Table 6-34 | |
|---|---|
| **DIVIDE AND CONQUER NUCLEOFRACTIS: ORIGINAL TECHNIQUE BY GIMBEL (FOUNDER OF NUCLEOFRACTURE TECHNIQUE)—1986** | |
| Nuclei | Hardness 3-4. |
| Incision | Limbal, posterior on two planes. |
| Capsulotomy | Capsulorhexis is mandatory; diameter 4.5-5.5. |
| Hydrodissection | Accurate, until rotation of the nucleus is achieved. |
| Carving | 30° tip. Nucleus stabilized with the spatula. Formation of a sulcus from 11 to 7. Sulcus width equal to one and a half the diameter of the sleeve and deep enough to significantly increase the red reflex. |
| Nucleofracture | Pedal on Position 2, U/S tips on the right side of the sulcus, and the spatula stabilizing the left side. Separation of the nucleus in the lateral portion formed with the sulcus. |
| Emulsification of the first fragment* | Vacuum is increased to 80-120. Capture of the fragment followed by emulsification. |
| Creating the second fragment | The U/S tip is occluded in the large sulcus portion on the left side of the first fragment (that has now been removed). Stabilizing the nucleus with the spatula, further fracture is induced along with formation of a moving piece. The piece is brought to the middle and emulsified. |
| Completing the procedure | Nucleus rotation; new engagement. New fracture and emulsification of a new wedge until the procedure has been completed. |

* In the original article, the author provided no phaco settings in the description of this technique. The values found in the above description are suggested by the author of the present chapter.

hardness of the nucleus and the mydriasis possible, there can be a larger number of sectors for fragmentation. These will be smaller in size to facilitate the emulsification.

In this way, the entire procedure of phacoemulsification occurs in the bag at a neutral point that is equidistant from the endothelium, the capsule, and the iris.

### Removal of the Epinucleus

At the end of nuclear removal, a large amount of epinucleus may persist, but this can also depend on the hydrodissection technique used.

This material can be aspirated using the U/S tip and fragmented with short bursts of low power U/S once the material has been brought to the center of the pupillary field. Alternately, it can be mobilized with a spatula if there are still marked adhesions with the peripheral cortex.

This is a very delicate phase, and the surgeon should tackle it very cautiously as the capsule is more relaxed because of the absence of the nucleus. A relaxed capsule can easily come into contact with the U/S tip.

The operation ends with aspiration of the residual cortex, implantation of the IOL, and sutures if necessary using the standard methods described previously.

## Trench DCN and Crater DCN

For nuclei with Grade 2 to 3 hardness, the original technique described previously is replaced by a trench technique, which involves the creation of a central groove. In the treatment of harder nuclei, the technique has been replaced with the crater technique.

- In nuclei of moderate-low hardness, the central groove must be narrow, central, and not too deep so that the instruments are positioned at the center of the groove. The nucleus is fractured from 6 to 12 o'clock.

In this phase, the instrument parameters setting must be low. The sculpting can be deep, and with the groove the surgeon can push deep down toward the epinucleus with no risk of capturing the capsule. The power of the U/S is controlled with the linear pedal. In the periphery and near the capsule, the power level should not exceed 20 to 30%.

When the nucleus has been split into two hemispheres, the U/S tip is impaled in the median portion of the left hemi-nucleus. While the spatula stabilizes the nucleus, the U/S tip pushes the nucleus, detaching a segment of the hemisphere. This segment is brought into the pupillary field and emulsified with short bursts of U/S.

The maneuvers are repeated on the right hemi-nucleus and finally on the segments that are found in the superior hemisphere. This technique does not involve any successive rotation.

- In hard nuclei (Grade 3), the central groove must be wider, deep, and the nucleus is rotated through 180° to allow the completion of the central groove. In this case, nucleofracture is obtained more easily by positioning the instruments inferiorly in respect to the center of the nucleus. This will create a split that extends from the peripheral areas to one-half or three-fourths of the nucleus diameter.

In order to complete the fracture, the instruments are then positioned superiorly to the center of the nucleus, toward the incision.

Table 6-35

# DIVIDE AND CONQUER NUCLEOFRACTIS (DNC) TRENCH TECHNIQUE ACCORDING TO GIMBEL

| | |
|---|---|
| Type of nucleus | Hardness 2-3. |
| Incision | Limbal, angled. |
| Rhexis | Absolutely necessary. |
| Hydrodissection | Significant aspect. |
| Shearing and carving (Phase 1 according to Gimbel's procedure) | Nucleus stabilized with the spatula.<br>Formation of a sulcus from 12 to 6 wide enough to allow the U/S tip and its sleeve to slide easily inside (for main incision cut at 12).<br>Linear power of U/S about 50%.<br>Tip engaging only 30-50% of the lumen. |
| Nucleofracture (Phases 2 and 3 according to Gimbel's procedure: fracture of the plate+fragmentation of a wedge-shaped piece of nucleus) | The plate, the portion of nucleus left over in the sulcus depth, is broken so that the nucleus is split in two.<br>The break must be made in the thinner portion (toward 5-6) with two instruments.<br>The U/S tip is pushed into the right side of the peripheral nucleus, and the spatula is placed on the left of the trench.<br>While the tip is operating suction, the nucleus is pushed to the right and the spatula to the left. Distal division of the equatorial border and the deep portion is achieved.<br>The U/S tip is engaged in the left portion of the nucleus and introduced with a short U/S discharge.<br>Stabilizing with the spatula and exerting slight pressure-push with the U/S tip, a wedge-shaped sector of nucleus is detached. This is brought to the middle and emulsified. |
| Rotation (Phase 4 according to Gimbel's procedure) | Once the first sector has been removed, the nucleus is rotated, and the procedure of impalement and fracture is repeated.<br>Another piece of nucleus is brought to the middle and emulsified one piece at a time until the whole nucleus is removed. |
| Removal of the epinucleus | The U/S tip and the spatula can be easily aspirated. |

Table 6-36

# DIVIDE AND CONQUER NUCLEOFRACTIS (DNC) CRATER TECHNIQUE ACCORDING TO GIMBEL

| | |
|---|---|
| Type of nucleus | Hardness 4. |
| Incision | Limbal, angled. |
| Rhexis | Absolutely necessary. |
| Hydrodissection | Absolutely necessary. |
| Carving (Phase 1 according to Gimbel's procedure) | The groove is made between 12 and 6.<br>Starting from the early sulcus wide and deep, carving of the nucleus is performed (formation of a crater) with repeated shearing maneuvers.<br>The spatula is used to shift the nucleus inferiorly to extend shearing superiorly.<br>Then, the nucleus is moved to the left in order to extend shearing on the right, until no more material is available for the tip.<br>Clockwise rotation of the nucleus is induced, and further shearing is performed.<br>The procedure is repeated until the entire hard core has been carved. A portion of peripheral material must be left. |
| Plate fracture and formation of sectors (Phase 2 and 3 according to Gimbel's procedure) | The spatula is placed on the rim of hard residuals on the left, while the U/S tip does the same on the right. The first fracture, followed by the second, is made with formation of the first sector.<br>Removal of the first sector. |
| Rotation, formation, and emulsification of the other sectors (Phase 4) | Rotation of the nucleus and production of other sectors.<br>The harder the nucleus, the smaller the sectors, so that they can be managed and emulsified easily.<br>Only the first sector is removed to create space inside the capsular bag. The other sectors are left in situ to keep the bag stretched and to allow subsequent maneuvers of nucleofracture to be performed more easily.<br>In this way, sectors are created until the whole nucleus is broken. One at a time they are brought to the middle and emulsified. |

Table 6-37

## GIMBEL'S DOWNSLOPE SCULPTING—1992

| | |
|---|---|
| Nucleus | Hardness 4-5. |
| Incision | Scleral tunnel. |
| Rhexis | Indispensable. |
| Hydrodissection | Necessary. |
| Sculpting (Phase 1) | With a 30° tip. |
| | Formation of a superficial groove slightly to the right while the spatula stabilizes the left-hand portion of the nucleus. |
| | The nucleus is shifted slightly inferiorly with the spatula in order to perform the sculpting with an inferior slope of the nucleus. In this way, the U/S tip will always be found parallel with the surface to be sculpted. |
| | In this way, the sculpting can be done very deeply. |
| Fracture (Phases 2-3) | The fracture occurs under I/A alone without U/S. The surgeon pushes the phaco tip toward the right and the spatula toward the left. |
| | Normally the nucleus opens from the center right down to the inferior edge in a single maneuver (if the two instruments have been positioned quite deeply and at the center of the sculpting). |
| | With the two instruments still deep inside the sculpting, the surgeon carves in depth just beside the fracture and then with a spatula. A second fracture is produced, which on intersection with the first produces a quadrant that is brought to the center and emulsified. |
| Rotation (Phase 4) | The remaining nucleus rotates to present distally more material for fracture. The tip is impaled with a short U/S burst. The surgeon pushes downward and right with the U/S tip and left with the spatula to produce another piece. |
| Advantages of the technique | The surgeon can sculpt in depth while staying parallel to the material and distant from the capsule. |
| | This technique reduced the possibility of rupturing the posterior capsule. |

Nuclear fracture with the segment formation proceeds as previously described, except that the number of segments increases in proportion to the hardness of the nucleus (six to eight pieces) and the nucleus is rotated on itself to facilitate the impalement of the tip.

- In very hard nuclei (Grade 4), the trench is extended to the right and to the left by shaving. The U/S tip can be helped by the spatula to move the nucleus inferiorly to thin-down the superior part. When the central part is no longer accessible to the U/S tip, the nucleus is rotated, and further shaving is performed.

Bit by bit, the hard core of the nucleus is removed to leave a crater (crater technique). Some hard material must be left around the equator to allow the spatula and the U/S tip to engage the edge and fracture the nucleus into fragments. In addition, in order to facilitate the maneuvers of nucleofracture, the surgeon might find it useful to create a small groove on the edge of the crater so that the instruments have a support for the *crossed* maneuver on the nuclear edge. In this case, the spatula pushes to the right, and the U/S tip pushes to the left, to exert greater pressure.

With large, hard nuclei, it can happen that the segment produced by the fracture is very large. In this case, the surgeon brings it into the pupillary field, and he or she splits it into two with a spatula, after having engaged it with the U/S tip.

In ambroid cataracts, the surgeon should perform nucleofracture leaving the segments produced in their original position so that the posterior capsule remains distended. Alternately, the first segment is removed to allow sufficient space for the manipulations of the nucleus inside the bag, and those produced as nucleofracture proceeds are left in position.

The harder the nucleus, the smaller and more numerous the pieces; this will make them more manageable. Initially, they are left in position to keep the capsular bag well distended.

In extremely hard nuclei, the crater must be brought as deep as possible. However, the surgeon must be careful not to confuse the ambroid reflex of the nucleus with the red reflex of the fundus.

The fragments are produced as previously described.

## Downslope Sculpting (DSS) by Gimbel

For nuclei of Grade 4 to 5 hardness, Gimbel developed a further variation of nucleofracture—downslope sculpting (DSS). This procedure is particularly useful when, in addition to the hard nucleus, the patient has a narrow pupil.

The technique involves pushing the nucleus downward toward 6 o'clock or, better still, distally to the incision with the spatula while sculpting is done (DSS). The groove runs parallel to the posterior capsule for its entire length.

The advantage of this technique is that the surgeon can create deeper grooves and obtain a more rapid, effective nucleofracture.

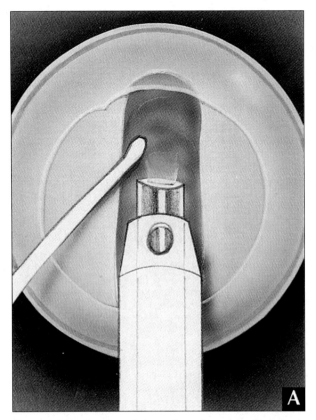

Figure 6-22A. Trench technique. Formation of a distal hemigroove, which is quite deep; rotation of the nucleus through 180°; and completion of the groove.

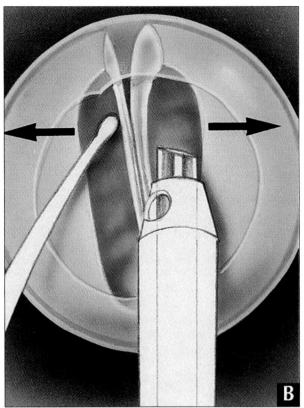

Figure 6-22B. Distal split of the nucleus.

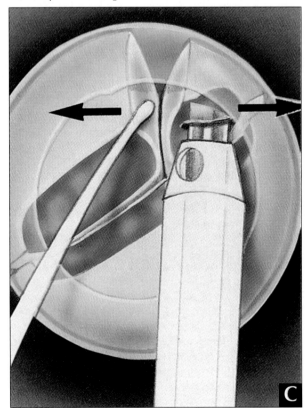

Figure 6-22C. The U/S tip is brought into occlusion in one heminucleus. The spatula is then used to split a fragment of nucleus.

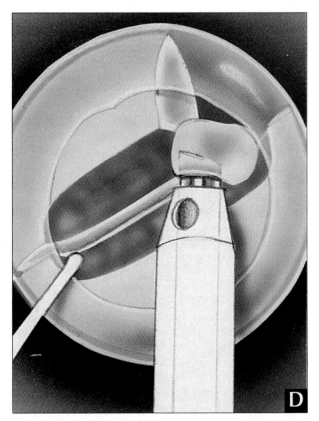

Figure 6-22D. The piece is brought to the center and fragmented.

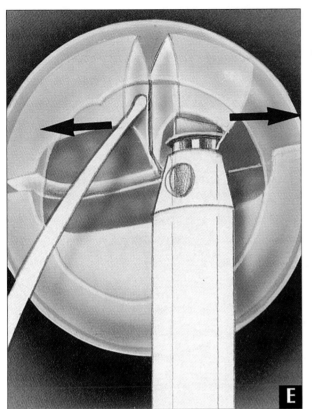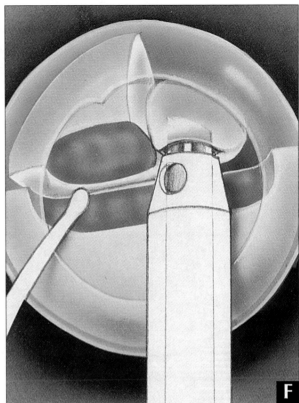

Figures 6-22E, 6-22F, 6-22G. The maneuver is repeated. Another piece is created and fragmented; in this way, the first hemi-nucleus is therefore removed.

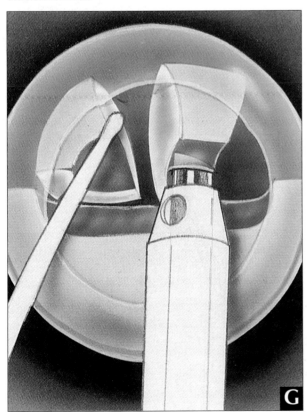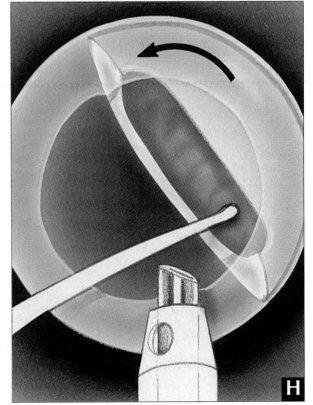

Figure 6-22H. The remaining hemi-nucleus is rotated and positioned distally.

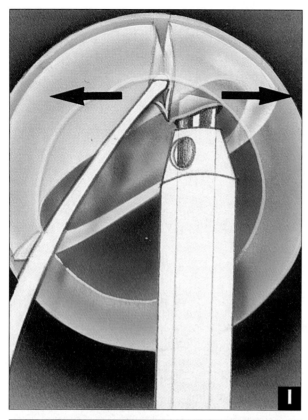
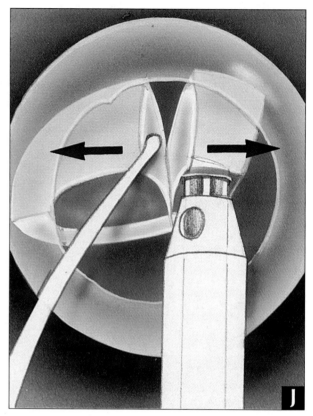
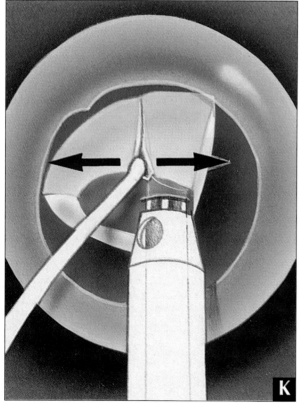

Figures 6-22I, 6-22J, 6-22K. The tip is brought into occlusion, and a portion of the nucleus is removed. The maneuver is repeated until the second hemi-nucleus has been completely removed.

At this point, thanks to the greater depth of the first sculpting, the surgeon can create a larger number of fracture lines depending on how many are needed by the individual case without having to sculpt other grooves. This variation is suitable for very expert surgeons. If it is used incorrectly or imprecisely, it can induce a radial opening of the distal edge of the capsulorhexis. This can then extend to the equator and the posterior capsule.

## Dillman-Maloney's Fractional 2/4

This is a further variation of the DCN technique and is suitable for nuclei of Grade 2 to 3 hardness.

### Preparation

After capsulorhexis, hydrodissection is performed to separate the external cortex (immediately below the capsule) from the deep cortex, which is in contact with the nuclear material.

Then, inserting the cannula more centrally and deeper, hydrodelamination is performed. When the luminous ring appears, the surgeon separates the internal nucleus and the epinucleus.

### Central Sculpting

A groove is created from the center of the nucleus toward 6 o'clock. The groove is as wide as the sleeve of the U/S tip and is deep as much as possible toward the posterior capsule. As the nuclear material is thinner

Table 6-38

## DILLMAN-MALONEY'S FRACTIONAL 2/4 (BURATTO'S VARIATION)

| | |
|---|---|
| Nucleus | Hardness 2-3. |
| Incision | Scleral tunnel, corneal tunnel, limbal incision. |
| Rhexis | Indispensable. |
| Hydrodissection and hydrodelamination | Indispensable. |
| Sculpting and formation of the first groove | Parameters—vacuum: 0-20 mm Hg; flow rate: 15-20 cc/min; U/S: 70%; tip: 30°. Formation of a distal groove. Rotation of the nucleus through 180° with the spatula and completion of the groove. |
| Nuclear fracture | With the spatula and the U/S tip crossed over each other, the nucleus is split into two halves with a single movement (without having to rotate the nucleus completely). |
| Rotation | Rotation through 90°. |
| Formation of the first two quadrants | Formation of another distal groove in the first hemi-nucleus. |
| Fracture into two quadrants | Emulsification of the first two quadrants. |
| Increase of vacuum to 80-120 mm Hg | Capture in occlusion and emulsification of the two quadrants at the center of the pupil. |
| Rotation | Rotation of the second hemi-nucleus to place it at 6 o'clock. |
| Formation of the third and fourth quadrants | Formation of a groove in the middle. Fracture into two quadrants. Capture and emulsification of the two quadrants. |
| Epincleus | This is removed under lower power I/A and U/S. |

toward the equator, the surgeon should take care when extending the emulsification toward the periphery and remember that, in the bag, the lower limit of the nucleus is closer to the posterior capsule and remember that the resistance of the posterior capsule in the semiperiphery is less than at the center.

The parameters I suggest are as follows:
- Vacuum—0 to 20 mm Hg.
- Flow rate—15 to 20 cc/min.
- U/S power—70%.

Using a cyclodialysis spatula, the nucleus is rotated 180° in a counterclockwise direction. Sculpting continues with extension of the previous sulcus for the entire length of the nucleus. In order to perform the technique correctly, it is important that the central part of the groove is deep and narrow.

### Fracture and Emulsification

The 30° U/S tip and the spatula are positioned on the two edges of the central and deep part of the groove. Each one makes a movement across each other in a downward and lateral direction to create a central fracture and split the nucleus into two halves (so there is no 180° rotation to complete the split).

The nucleus is then rotated through 90°, and a groove is carved in the first half, with characteristics similar to the initial central groove. Again using the U/S tip and the spatula, a fracture of the nucleus is created with a lateral movement to produce two quarters of the nucleus, which are then emulsified in the center of the pupil. The parameters are changed. Vacuum is increased to 80 to 120 mm Hg in proportion to the hardness of the nucleus; the flow rate and the U/S remain unchanged.

The remaining half of the nucleus is rotated through 180°, pushing it toward the capsular fornix and bringing it to the inferior half of the field. The surgeon once again separates the half into two quarters, which are then removed in the deep central area of the capsular bag.

## The Crack and Flip Technique According to Fine, Maloney, and Dillman (1992)

This is a variation of the Chip and Flip technique described previously. Nucleocleavage is replaced by nucleofracture of the central nucleus.

It is a technique that is suitable for nuclei of Grade 3 to 4 hardness. It can be used when hydrodelamination can be used, ie, the separation of the epinucleus from the central nucleus.

In this procedure, I aim to achieve a circumferential division of the nucleus through hydrodelamination and successive manipulations. I want to free the central nucleus from the surrounding material not just through the fluid wave but also mechanically by moving it, rocking it, and rotating it with the tip of the hyrdodelamination cannula.

In this way, the sculpting is less peripheral. Smaller sectors are produced, the capsular bag is kept well-distended by the remaining material, and the peripheral material absorbs all the mechanical forces, reducing the risk of lesions to the posterior capsule to a minimum.

### Sculpting

The surgeon performs a first superficial *shaving* and then the grooves are carved as in the other phaco techniques. The surgeon proceeds to create a cross as described. The sculpting must remain at the center of the hard mass and should not reach the golden ring of the hydrodelamination.

After the first groove has been created, the nucleus is rotated through 90° and so on. The sculpting must just exceed the central hard portion of the nucleus and must not extend too deeply. The spatula should be used to exert a countering force to stabilize the nucleus during the tip's action; this reduces the U/S time quite considerably.

In this phase, the machine is set as follows:
- Vacuum—0 to 10 mm Hg.
- Flow rate—15 to 20 cc/min.
- U/S power—maximum 80%, in linear mode.

### Fracture

This is achieved through the combined spatula-U/S tip action with the pedal in Position 1 or 2 in relation to the size of the lens and the anterior chamber.

The quadrants obtained are mobilized and emulsified at the center of the capsular bag, as described for the Cross technique.

After cracking, the pieces are removed under pulse mode (10 pulses per second). This allows the tip to exert a good attraction force on the material. Vacuum is 115 to 125 mm Hg, and the flow rate is 20 to 25 cc/min.

### Removal of the Epinucleus

The epinucleus remains in its original site following the removal of the quadrants of the central nucleus. It is aspirated and emulsified with the flip maneuver done with a spatula or with the U/S tip facing downward toward the center of the epinucleus with the pedal in Position 1.

The epinuclear edge is captured at the extremity of the capsulorhexis by the U/S tip with the pedal in Position 2. It is pulled toward the center on the same plane as the capsulorhexis. The superior portion, which has been captured, is removed with a short burst of low-power U/S, and the epinucleus is allowed to fall into the bag. It is rotated through 180° with spatula, and the same maneuver is then performed distally. In this way, the epinuclear shell has been converted to a rectangle.

The material is rotated to present it with the greater axis according to the incision.

The distal portion is captured with the U/S tip in Position 2 and pulled toward the incision, while the spatula is placed in the center, with the traction of the U/S tip and the thrust of the spatula toward 6 o'clock. The epinucleus rotates easily (flipping); it is freed on the same plane as the rhexis and is then removed.

With suitable cortical cleaving hydrodissection at the beginning of the operation, there is very little cortical material left; this can be aspirated with the VES once the IOL has been inserted.

## Phaco Chop by Nagahara

### Introduction

This is the most recent technique of nucleofracture (developed by Nagahara and presented in Seattle in 1993 at the ASCRS meeting and in Milan in 1994 at Videocataract).

After capsulorhexis and hydrodissection, the U/S tip removes part of the superficial cortex and the epinucleus and is then sunk into the superior portion of the nucleus as close as possible to the incision.

The chopper in inserted through the side port incision. It is a modified lens hook that has a longer, stronger terminal part (about 1.5 mm). The hook is positioned at 6 o'clock below the anterior capsule, as far peripheral and as deep as possible.

While the U/S tip holds the nucleus steady, the hook scores and cracks the nucleus. When close to the U/S tip, the hook is moved to the left, while the tip is moved to the right to split the nucleus into two parts.

The action can be compared to an ax that splits a trunk (chop). The whole procedure occurs with no sculpting or preliminary grooves. After having split the nucleus into two parts, it is rotated about 90° so that the crack is now horizontal.

The fixation and cracking of the nucleus is repeated in the lower half of the nucleus, which is also split into two pieces.

Each segment can then be brought into the pupillary field to be emulsified one at a time. This method was developed in order to tackle extremely hard nuclei (Grade 4 to 5) or nuclei that are difficult, if not impossible, to treat with the phacoemulsification techniques available to date.

Nevertheless, if a very hard nucleus is split into four quadrants with the above method, the four nuclear fragments are difficult to remove from the capsular bag as there is not enough room for the various manipulations. For this reason, Koch suggested a variation of the technique called Stop and Chop.

### Preparation

A 3 mm sclero-corneal tunnel is prepared, of width to suit the lens the surgeon has selected for insertion.

Prior to entering the anterior chamber with an angled 3.2 mm tip, two paracenteses (about 1 mm) are performed at 10 and 2 o'clock with 15° instruments. VES is injected through the left paracentesis, and a cystotome for the capsulorhexis is introduced through the right one. Hydrodissection is performed with a 25 G angled cannula, and the nucleus is mobilized. The anterior chamber is reformed with Viscoat, and the U/S tip is introduced.

Fifteen or 30° tips are preferable with a sleeve that is retracted more than usual, to leave the tip exposed for about 1.5 mm.

The parameters are:
- Vacuum—at least 120 mm Hg.
- Flow rate—25 cc/min.
- U/S power—100% with linear control.

With two to three superficial passages using the U/S tip, the surgeon removes the superficial cortex and the epinucleus to reach the nucleus. The chopper is then inserted; the special hook is used to crack the nucleus.

While the hook stabilizes the nucleus, the U/S tip impales it, with a U/S shot that is sufficient for occlusion. The maneuver can be done in a position somewhere between the center and the superior third exposed by the capsulorhexis (or between the center and the proximal third of the incision).

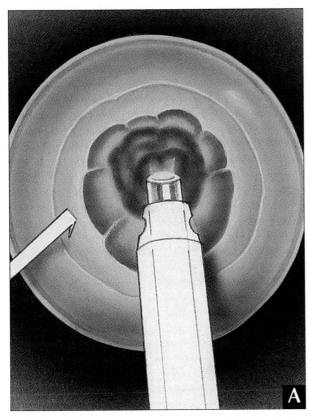

Figure 6-23A. Phaco Chop. The cortical material and the anterior epinucleus are removed.

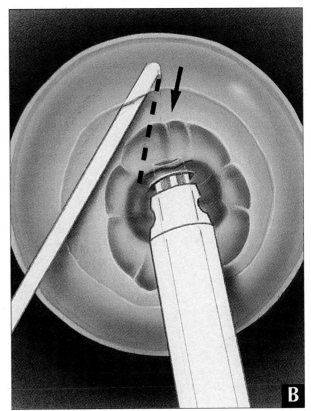

Figure 6-23B. Insertion of the U/S tip in the nuclear material proximal to the incision. Try to push it deep down in the center of the nucleus for occlusion, and wait until the vacuum reaches the maximum preset value. Insert the chopper under the rhexis, deepening it horizontally and then making it vertical.

The surgeon moves the pedal into Position 2 and impales the nucleus with the U/S tip (U/S is not required in this phase). The hook is positioned on the equator distal to the U/S tip under the edge of the capsulorhexis and the rim of the epinucleus obtained with the initial shaving. The hook is sunk firmly into the nucleus and retracted in the direction of the tip.

Just before it reaches the U/S tip, the hook is moved to the left while the tip is moved to the right; cracking is obtained. The surgeon should continue the maneuver until the opening involves the entire nuclear thickness and until it extends to the equator, below the U/S tip.

The nucleus is then rotated with a hook of about 60° in a counterclockwise direction, and the U/S tip is sunk in a central position, in correspondence to the inferior edge of the crack obtained with the previous maneuver. The surgeon looks for occlusion once again.

The hook is again placed peripherally and then retracted centripetally to obtain a second crack in the nucleus with the help of the U/S tip as described before.

What results is a wedge of nuclear material that can be engaged by the U/S tip (at this point, the vacuum can be increased to as much as 150 to 180 mm Hg if the nucleus is very hard—Grade 4 to 5), then with occlusion, it is moved toward the center of the rhexis to be emulsified just outside the bag.

With five to six cracks, it is usually possible to remove a Grade 3 to 4 nucleus. However, if the nucleus is very

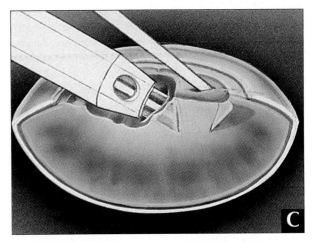

Figure 6-23C. Keeping the nucleus steady with the U/S tip, move the chopper toward the tip, separating the cortical and nuclear material along the route.

large and the portion of the epinucleus only moderate or absent, it is better to produce a greater number of segments, all smaller in size.

The most critical moment of the operation is when the partially-fractured nucleus is still inside the capsular bag and it has to be manipulated to obtain further cracks. In order to simplify the procedure, the surgeon should

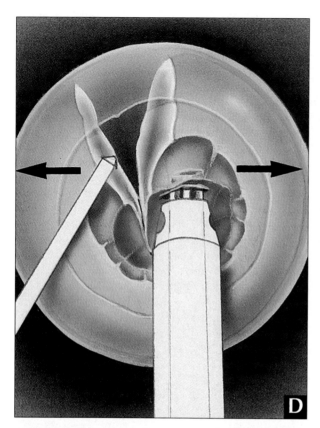

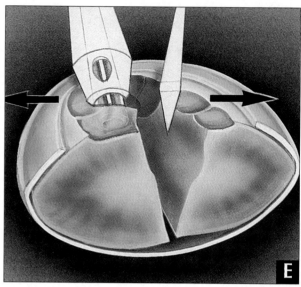

Figures 6-23D, 6-23E. When the two instruments are about to come into contact, separate them. In this way, a deep split will be created in the nucleus. Widen the split by pushing the U/S tip to the right and the chopper to the left. Try to obtain a fracture that reaches the deepest layers of the nucleus.

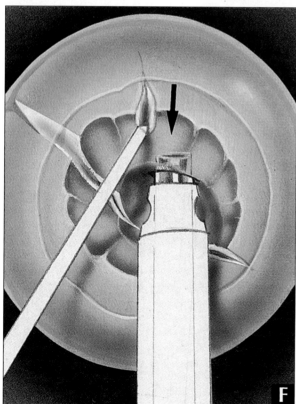

Figure 6-23F. Look for stable occlusion once again (inside the groove previously created, if necessary) and then with the chopper to separate a piece of nucleus.

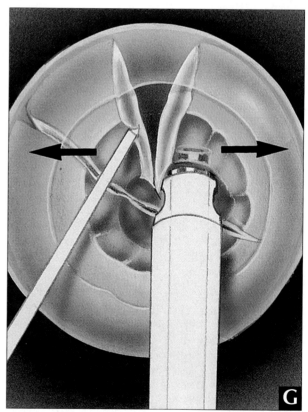

Figure 6-23G. Further rotation through 30 to 40° with the chopper.

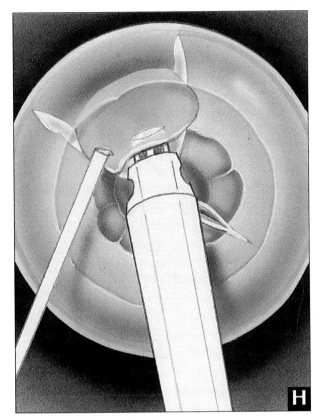

Figure 6-23H. Capture of another segment.

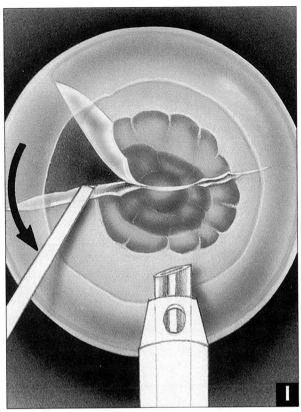

Figure 6-23I. More rotation and fracture.

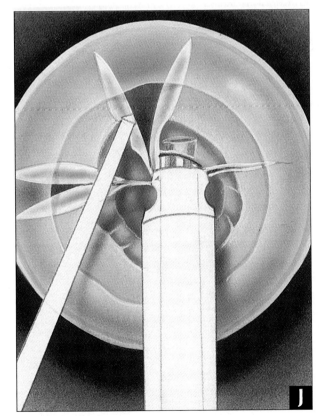

Figure 6-23J. Further occlusion and nucleofracture.

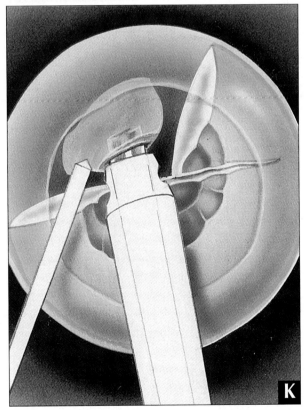

Figure 6-23K. Occlusion, and when the material has been firmly blocked, free emulsification.

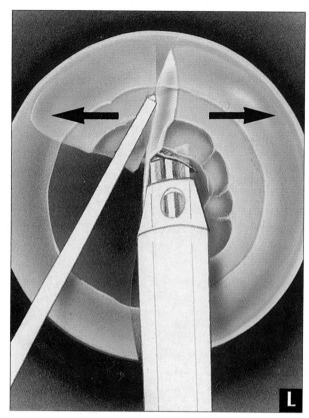

Figure 6-23L. Ulterior occlusion and production of a sector with the chopper.

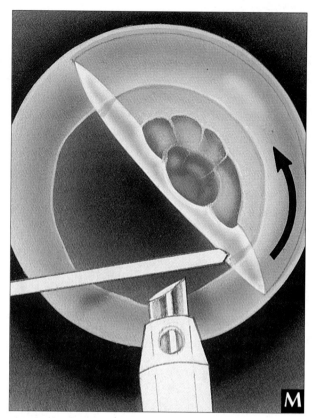

Figures 6-23M, 6-23N. Rotation of the residual nucleus.

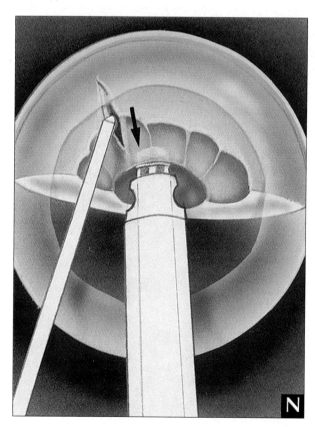

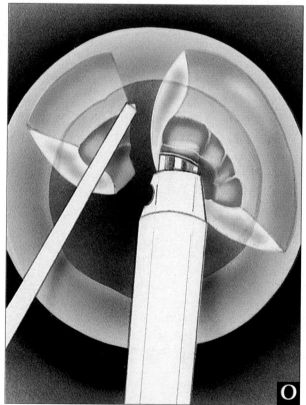

Figures 6-23O. Rotation of the remaining nucleus. Occlusion and, when the material has been firmly blocked, chopping with the creation of a further fragment until all the nuclear material has been removed. The last piece of nucleus is captured and divided; the two pieces are fragmented in the pupillary area.

Table 6-39
## CRACK AND FLIP
## ACCORDING TO FINE-MALONEY-DILLMAN

| | |
|---|---|
| Incision | Scleral tunnel, corneal tunnel, limbal. |
| Nucleus | Hardness 3-4. |
| Rhexis | Yes. |
| Hydrodissection and hydrodelamination | Hydrodissection and hydrodelamination with cortical cleaving hydrodissection. Hydrodelamination is very important. In fact, it produces a covering of soft material that surrounds the central nuclear mass (circumferential splitting of the nucleus). Before starting phaco, try to mobilize the central portion with the cannula in order to eliminate adhesion of the central nucleus and the surrounding cortex. |
| Early carving | Vacuum: 0-10; flow: 15 mL/min; maximum U/S: 80%. Formation of the sulci as described for the other procedures without exceeding the golden ring; regarding the depth, it is the limit of the nucleus center. |
| Emulsification of quadrants | Follow the modalities formerly described for other procedures. |
| Removal of the epinucleus | The distal portion is captured in occlusion, pulled toward the middle, and emulsified; 30-40° rotation and further distal removal. Then 180° rotation so that another lateral portion of epinucleus can be removed; rotation; place the epinucleus rectangle with the main axis parallel to the U/S tip. The distal rim is captured with the U/S and pedal in Position 2. Push toward 6 with the spatula and flip maneuver. Aspiration and fragmentation follow. |

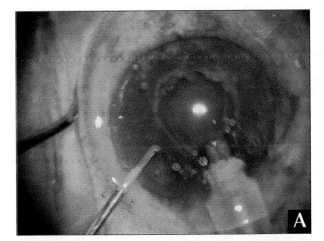

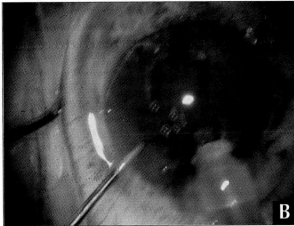

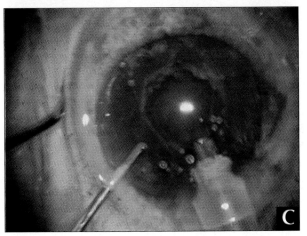

Figures 6-24A, 6-24B, 6-24C. Phaco Chop. The epinucleus and the anterior cortex are removed. The U/S tip is placed at the center of the nucleus and goes into occlusion.

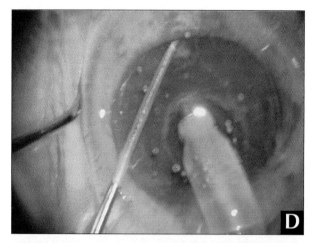
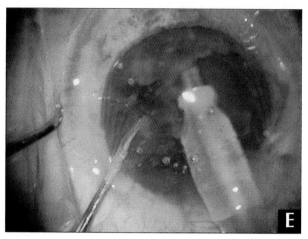
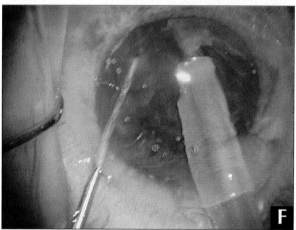

Figures 6-24D, 6-24E, 6-24F. The surgeon moves the chopper to the edge of the equator and brings it toward the U/S tip. He or she separates the two instruments. In this way, the first fragment is created. The tip is occluded again.

remove the first fragment immediately, at least a small nuclear segment. This will leave the surgeon with an adequately formed bag and enough space to position the nucleus ideally for the successive phases of the procedure.

In the final phases of the technique, the surgeon may find that he or she is left with a large piece of material in the center of the capsular bag. If this is too big, it will have be to split into another two or three parts with the chopper before it can be tackled directly. This will make the emulsification procedure faster and simpler.

When the nucleus has been removed, the operation continues as usual.

## Stop and Chop by Koch

This technique begins with a groove, as though the surgeon was preparing for Shepherd's cross nucleofracture. This produces a space for the U/S tip and the hook, which will be able to fracture the nucleus into two parts. At this point, the surgeon stops, he or she rotates the nucleus through 90°, fixes the lower half of the nucleus with the U/S tip, and a crack is created with the hook.

A number of fragments result, which can be easily mobilized from the capsular bag to be emulsified in the pupillary field according to the methods described for the other techniques of nucleofracture.

It is undoubtedly much simpler than the Phaco Chop and is slightly more difficult than the technique of nucleofracture into four quadrants. It is a very interesting procedure, which can be preliminary to the Phaco Chop. It opens new possibilities to apply the advantages of phacoemulsification in those cases that were excluded in the past.

The procedure is simple. However, the various surgical steps must be completed accurately and carefully.

- Hydrodissection, for example, must be extremely accurate. Depending on the clinical case, it is sometimes associated with hydrodelineation of the nucleus. The nucleus must be completely mobile, so before beginning the phacoemulsification, the surgeon should rotate the nucleus a couple of times inside the bag.
- The formation of the groove allows the formation of the space inside the nucleus. The space is useful for easily obtaining occlusion. This also permits the surgeon to free the sectors easily and to remove them from the capsular bag and bring them forward.

In this phase, it may be useful to use high U/S power (60 to 70% of Legacy 20,000 Alcon), as the surgeon is working at a safe distance from the endothelium and the capsule is protected by the posterior cortex.

When the surgeon has reached a good depth, he or she should attempt to fracture the nucleus. Normally, it is very easy to split the nucleus into two parts—also because the chopper separates the nucleus better than the classical olive-tipped spatula. If the typical centripetal fracture line does not appear, the groove can be deepened, but the surgeon must pay great attention to the color of the red reflex.

The fracture of the nucleus into two parts is the key moment of the operation. This step will allow the surgeon to produce free segments by cracking with the chopper.

Cracking with the chopper depends largely on the instrument insertion depth. Normally, the maneuver is simple because the U/S tip can provide strong occlusion

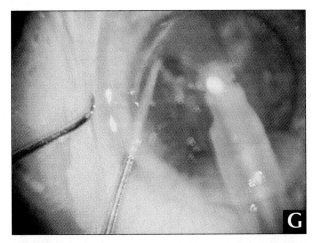
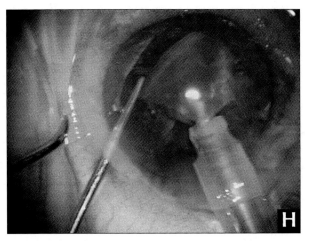
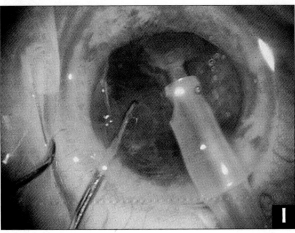

Figures 6-24G, 6-24H, 6-24I. A second fracture is induced with the chopper. The piece is brought to the center, and the tip is occluded again.

inside the groove. But also, as the surgeon has removed part of the cortex, the action of the chopper is easier to perform.

Once the nuclear fragments have been formed, the procedure can continue with the classical maneuvers of phacoemulsification. At the end of nucleus removal, in most cases, there is a small quantity of residual material.

- The technique provides excellent stabilization of the nucleus. It differs from other endocapsular techniques because the chopper has an active, important role in the procedure. The two-handed action extends for the entire duration of the phacoemulsification and is constantly involved in the phase of nucleofracture and removal of the nuclear sectors.

This means that the surgeon should pay close attention to the accessory instrument, which must be controlled as carefully as the U/S tip.

- Throughout the entire procedure, the energy transmitted to the nucleus, freed from connections to the epinucleus and the cortex, is not passed on to the capsule and the zonules thanks to the absorption by the external cortex and the separation induced through hydrodissection.

## Comment on the Techniques of Nucleofracture

Howard Gimbel's DCN is the original technique which gave rise to the proliferation of many variations of the nucleofracture technique, the most famous being that of John Shepherd. Nagahara's Phaco Chop and its numerous variations have recently been stirring a lot of interest.

Nucleofracture is a very elegant, versatile method of tackling a broad range of clinical cases. It has the undoubted advantage of having widened the indications for phacoemulsification.

The procedure has one enormous advantage; it is safe and precise and has well-defined rules that lend themselves perfectly to being taught and learned. This has allowed the technique to spread so rapidly.

Thanks to nucleofracture, extremely hard nuclei can now be tackled without having to resort to very high power levels and long U/S times. This means less surgical trauma, better postoperative comfort, and more rapid recovery.

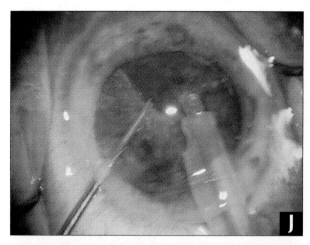
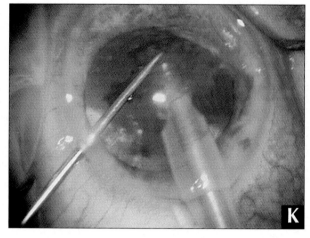

Figures 6-24J, 6-24K, 6-24L. Another fracture. A piece is brought into the center, it is fractured again and removed.

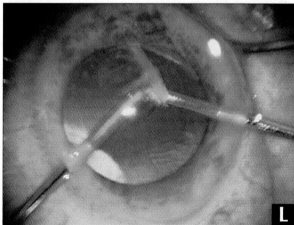

| Table 6-40 | |
|---|---|
| **INSTRUMENTS NEEDED FOR THE PHACO CHOP** | |
| Chopper | This instrument must be: |
| | Curved to adapt to the curvature of the nucleus. |
| | With a blunted end to reduce the risk of posterior capsule tearing. |
| | Sharp or thin on the inside. |
| | Long enough to cover the entire nucleus from the equator toward the center. |
| | Strong enough to exert enough pressure to fracture hard nuclei. |
| U/S tip | This instrument must be: |
| | More exposed than normal with respect to the sleeve in order to penetrate the nucleus easily. |
| | Only slightly angulated so that it can go into occlusion easily. |
| | Used mainly in occlusion with high-level vacuum. |

Table 6-41
## INCISION AND CAPSULORHEXIS IN THE PHACO CHOP
Incision: Scleral or corneal tunnel with precocious entry in the anterior chamber so that the U/S tip can find the correct slope in order to go into occlusion immediately through impalement.

In the Phaco Chop, the capsulorhexis must be quite wide (5.0-5.5 mm):

In order to facilitate the penetration of the chopper under the capsule and at the equator of the nucleus.

To split the nucleus right through in complete safety. In order to do this, the maneuver must be firm and obvious. The rhexis must be quite wide to avoid excessive traction on the edges of the capsular opening.

It is useful also when the first piece is captured at the equator and brought to the center.

It facilitates the access of the U/S tip to the piece to be extracted.

It facilitates the extraction of the piece itself. This is normally difficult to detach and bring to the center of the chamber. However, this has irregular margins because the entire nucleus is still inside the bag and because frequently there are still some small adhesions with the remaining nucleus. A wide rhexis facilitates the procedure of separation and capture-transport.

Table 6-42
## PHACO CHOP: ROLE OF HYDRODISSECTION
Any hydrodissection cannula can be used, provided that it achieves the fixed aim. However, it is preferable to use a bent-tipped cannula. At the end of the procedure, check nuclear mobility by mechanical rotation.

It is fundamental that, before starting a chop technique, the nucleus is able to rotate freely inside the bag. This is because:

When it is caught with the tip in occlusion, it must be pulled gently toward the incision. This enables the chopper to reach the equator more easily while being separate from the capsule.

When the chopper reaches the equator, it must not pull, break, or lacerate the posterior capsule. This will not be the case if the nucleus has not been freed completely from cortical adherence and is not split from the capsule.

If the fixation procedure with the U/S fails, the nucleus shall be rotated free and a more suitable site selected.

Once the fracture has been accomplished, the broken piece must be free to move from the equator toward the middle.

To break the second or third piece, the nucleus must be rotated to be placed in the right position for fracture.

Hydrodissection is sometimes performed with hydrodelamination. This provides greater safety for whole procedure. In fact, it separates the central nucleus from the epinucleus. This enables the maneuver to be performed with the chopper only on the endonucleus and to achieve occlusion with the U/S tip keeping the nucleus protected.

Table 6-43
## PHACO CHOP: ROLE OF SHAVING
To perform chop safely and correctly, the U/S tip must be firmly occluded in the hard material. For this purpose, the overlying soft material must be removed.

The cortex.

The superficial layer of the nucleus (epinucleus). To accomplish this task, the U/S tip is used with a few quick passages to remove all the soft material inside the rhexis. Vacuum parameters may be high or low. This is not important as no occlusion is present. Because this surgical phase is short, it is preferable to use the same parameters as used for the following phase.

Removing soft material eases the procedure because:

It allows better assessment of nucleus hardness.

It improves visibility and therefore where and how deep the U/S tip can be inserted can be determined.

It allows the chopper to be inserted with greater safety as the nucleus and its equator can be visualized better (ie, the working planes improve).

Table 6-44
## PHACO CHOP: EMULSIFICATION TECHNIQUE

### Performance of the first fragmentation

Parameters—high vacuum value: 100-250 mm Hg; medium flow: 15-25 mL/min; U/S: (60-100%).

The tip is directed toward the middle of the nucleus on the rhexis border lying closest to the entrance in the chamber.

When cortex and epinucleus have been removed, it is useful to excavate a small hollow in the hard material. This will ease occlusion, which is used to perform the first chop.

With a small U/S discharge, the tip is stabbed in the nuclear material.

The U/S tip must penetrate deep toward the center of the nucleus in order for the chopper to be able to divide.

Once the tip is in place, the nucleus is slightly shifted to the right and then the left to assess the level of attraction on the U/S tip (ie, the state of occlusion). Should the phaco tip not fixate the nucleus it is because:
  1. The tip is not sufficiently directed toward the center of the nucleus.
  2. The U/S tip is not engaged enough by the material (there is no occlusion).
  3. The nucleus is too soft.
  4. There is not enough aspiration.
  5. The tip is not correctly oriented toward the center.

With the U/S tip, the nucleus is slightly pulled toward the incision to create space distally to the chopper.

The chopper is introduced under the rhexis (not over). The instrument is inserted horizontally or at a slight incline so that it hardly touches the anterior capsule. Then, the chopper is rotated until it is placed vertical to the equatorial periphery of the hard nucleus.

The hook is pulled toward the U/S tip to form a full-thickness sulcus in the nuclear material.

When the U/S tip comes close, the hook is shifted to the left (if the surgeon holds the phaco handle with his or her right hand).

Both instruments make a splitting movement to divaricate the two pieces of the nucleus.

Particular care must be taken so that full-thickness splitting is achieved. The nucleus must open completely, until the posterior capsule is seen.

### Performance of the second fragmentation

Once splitting has been accomplished, the nucleus, which is still attached to the U/S tip, is rotated about 30-45° with the U/S tip.

The tip is disoccluded and fixed 30-40° to the right, then occluded again.

Splitting tasks are repeated with the chopper. Thus a sector about 30-45° is created.

The splitting maneuver must be accomplished such that the sector is completely emptied from all connections with the remaining nucleus.

The U/S tip is disoccluded.

Table 6-45
## CHOP

### Removal of the first sector

Once the first segment is made, it must be removed immediately. If other segments are made, the volume inside the bag increases, and motility of the first segment is reduced.

For this purpose, the U/S tip is placed touching the emptied sector, and occlusion is attempted and reached.
  As soon as the piece has been fixated, it is pulled toward the center. To accomplish this task easily, the segment must be completely free.

Should even the slightest difficulty arise, the chopper must intervene to mobilize the segment, complete separation from the remaining nucleus, and support the action of the tip.

When the segment is free, it should be emulsified as close as possible to the nuclear surface (far from the endothelium), at the center of the chamber and the center of the pupil.

### Final part

A very hard nucleus can be split in to 12-16 pieces; a less hard nucleus can be split into 4-6 segments.

Each large segment must be further fragmented with the chopper. The task is accomplished when the sector is out of the capsular bag.

The piece is fixated by occlusion and divided with the chopper in two or more smaller pieces that are quickly emulsified.

The smaller the pieces, the easier they are to emulsify with short, quick U/S discharges.

When there is no more material to divide, extract the chopper and replace it with an olive-shaped spatula.

Complete the removal of the epinucleus.

### Table 6-46
### ADVANTAGES AND DISADVANTAGES OF THE PHACO CHOP

| Advantages | Disadvantages |
| --- | --- |
| It permits emulsification of very hard nuclei. | The penetration of the chopper under the capsule is a critical phase. |
| It reduces the amount of time the U/S are used. | Bringing the chopper close to the U/S tip is a critical phase. |
| It permits efficient use of the U/S. | The rupture of the nucleus through its thickness to the posterior capsule is also critical, both for the rhexis and for the posterior capsule. |
| It reduce surgical time. | The capture and transport of the first piece from the periphery to the center of the anterior chamber is also critical. |
| It uses first aspiration (occlusion) and then the emulsification. | It is very critical the fact that the entire procedure is performed under high vacuum. |
| As the surgeon is working in occlusion, he or she can bring the U/S immediately to a maximum. | It is also critical having fragments of nucleus that are floating around in the chamber toward the end of the procedure. |

### Table 6-47
### THE DIFFERENCE BETWEEN THE PHACO CHOP AND NUCLEAR FRACTURE INTO FOUR QUADRANTS

| Phaco chop | Nuclear fracture into four quadrants |
| --- | --- |
|  | Low parameters are used at the beginning, and high values are used at the end once fracture has been obtained. |
| High vacuum must be used throughout the procedure. | High vacuum is only used to extract the pieces from the equator. |
| The nucleus is split, but the division is predominantly centrifugal-radial. | The two instruments are used to separate and distance the two hemi-nuclei. |
| The division occurs from the equator to the center. | The fracture occurs from the center to the equator. |
| The emulsification is always (or almost always) in occlusion, ie, under aspiration; U/S is used less for less time. | The central sculpting involves emulsification without (or with just a little) aspiration (ie, without occlusion). This involves time loss and dispersion of energy. |
| There is no space created for the mobilization of the sectors. | The grooves create space, which allows the pieces to detach easily and to be mobilized very easily. |
| In the chop, the high vacuum (ie, occlusion) is used to rupture. The tip therefore performs a mechanical action and not just the emulsification. | The division occurs without involvement of the U/S tip. The tip is used as a normal spatula. |

### Table 6-48
### STOP AND CHOP ACCORDING TO KOCH

| | |
| --- | --- |
| Nucleus | Hardness 3-4. |
| Incision | Sclero-corneal, scleral, or corneal tunnel. |
| Rhexis | Absolutely necessary. |
| Hydrodissection | Absolutely necessary. |
| Carving | Parameters—tip: 15°; vacuum: 0-10; flow: 10-15; U/S: 60-70%. Formation of a distal sulcus. 180° rotation of the nucleus. Completing the sulcus distally. Splitting the nucleus in two hemi-nuclei with chopper and U/S tip. |
| Chop | 90° rotation of the nucleus to place it perpendicular to the U/S tip. Parameters—vacuum: 80-180; flow: 15-22; U/S: 40-70%. Occlusion of the U/S tip inside the carving perpendicular to it. The distal hemi-nucleus is divided by the chopper in two quarters or in three to four quarters, and then fragmented. |
| Completing emulsification | The residual hemi-nucleus is rotated and placed distally. Occlusion and fragmentation by the chopper. Emulsification of the residual pieces. |

Table 6-49
# STOP AND CHOP ACCORDING TO BURATTO

| | |
|---|---|
| Preliminary | The pure chop procedure according to Nagahara is a difficult technique that must be learned step by step. The Stop and Chop technique is simple and an introduction to pure chop phaco. |
| First part | Parameters—tip: 15°; vacuum: 10; flow: 18; U/S: 70%. |
| | A hemisulcus is formed that crosses the nucleus in the direction from proximal to distal. To complete the hemisulcus, the nucleus is rotated 180°. |
| | The sulcus should have a depth greater than half the nucleus thickness and a width exceeding the diameter of the sleeve. |
| | The nucleus is broken by the chopper and U/S tip to obtain two separate pieces. It is important that these are completely separated. In the following phase, when the chopper divides the hemi-nucleus in pieces, they should not be connected with the remaining material. |
| Second part | The sulcus is placed perpendicular to the U/S tip. This position can be comfortably attempted and occlusion easily obtained. |
| | Parameters are changed—vacuum: 150-200; flow: 18; U/S: 50%. |
| | Occlusion, the vacuum is left at a high setting. |
| | The chopper passes under the rhexis and reaches the equator, creates the first segment of one-eighth to one-sixth of the nucleus or simply one-fourth (half hemi-nucleus). |
| | The segment is easily freed; the splitting line will be found in the middle. It is easily mobilized because, during creation of the sulcus, some space has been formed inside the nucleus. |
| | The first sector obtained is captured in occlusion and taken to the middle of the rhexis. If small, it can be emulsified; otherwise, it is split in two by the chopper. |
| | The same procedure should be used for the second quadrant. |
| | The second hemi-nucleus is placed distally, captured in occlusion, divided, and fragmented. |

Table 6-50
# MODIFIED STOP AND CHOP ACCORDING TO BURATTO

| | |
|---|---|
| Preliminary statement | This is an intermediate procedure between Stop and Chop and pure Chop. It is suitable as intermediate step for pure chop learning. |
| Nucleus | Hardness 2-3-4. |
| Incision | Corneal tunnel, scleral tunnel, limbal, incision. |
| Capsulorhexis | Yes, rather wide. |
| Hydrodissection | Yes, complete, so the nucleus is able to rotate inside the bag. |
| Carving | Formation of a distal sulcus. |
| | 180° rotation of the nucleus. |
| | Completion of the sulcus distally. |
| Rotation | 90° rotation. |
| Second stage | The sulcus is used to visualize where the tip goes and to achieve good occlusion. |
| | The tip is placed in the middle of the sulcus. The pedal is operated in Position 2 and then, with a short U/S discharge (Position 3), nuclear material is entered. Position 2 is then restored, and the vacuum is allowed to rise within the aspiration line (occlusion). |
| | Ongoing occlusion is maintained, while checking that the nucleus is held by slightly pulling it toward the incision. |
| | The chopper is inserted under the rhexis, and the equator is reached. |
| | The chopper is pulled toward the U/S tip, and close to it both tools are separated. |
| | The first fracture must reach the deepest fundus layers, so that a deep and sharp splitting can be achieved. |
| | The nucleus is rotated 30-40°, and the procedure is repeated, freeing about one-eighth of nucleus. This must be mobile inside the bag |
| | It must be captured by the U/S tip, pulled toward the center, and fragmented. |
| | The procedure now becomes easier as more space is available. |
| | Pieces in size equal to one-fourth are fragmented first, and then the remaining material is emulsified. |
| | Big pieces can be split in two. |
| Comment | This technique is slightly more complex than Stop and Chop (there is no division of the nucleus into two hemi-nuclei). Nevertheless, it is easier than Nagahara's Phaco Chop, because of the sulcus, which easily occludes the tip. Furthermore, the space created enables parts of the nucleus to be detached without problems. It is an intermediate technique between Stop and Chop and pure chop, and therefore should be used when learning pure chop. |

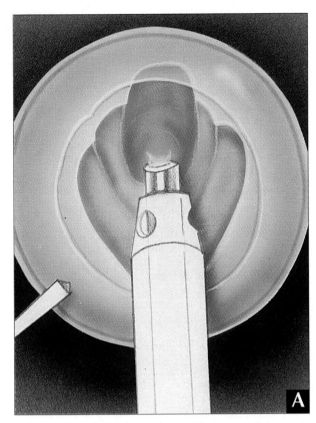

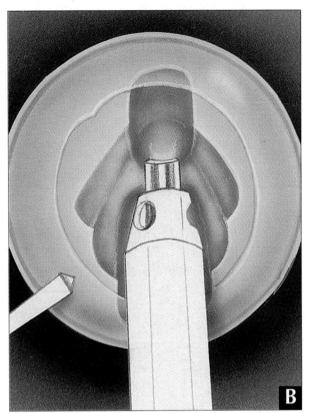

Figure 6-25A. Stop and Chop technique. The cortex and the anterior epinucleus are removed. A groove is created from the center of the nucleus toward its periphery. If the surgeon is sure that he or she will not come into contact with the anterior capsule, the surgeon can exceed the limits of the rhexis. The groove does not have to be deep, at least initially.

Figure 6-25B. Rotate the nucleus through 180°, and complete the groove. If necessary, repeat the rotation, and deepen the first groove. The depth of the groove must be at least half the nuclear thickness.

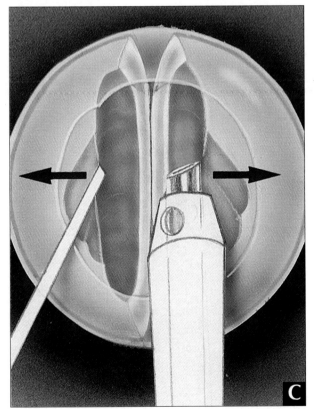

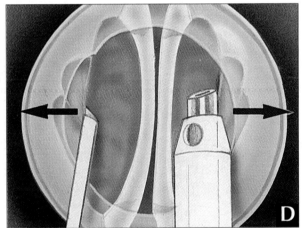

Figures 6-25C, 6-25D. Introduce the chopper inside the groove proximally to the side port incision. With the U/S tip, split the nucleus into two hemi-nuclei. Check that the fracture reaches the deep layers of the nucleus.

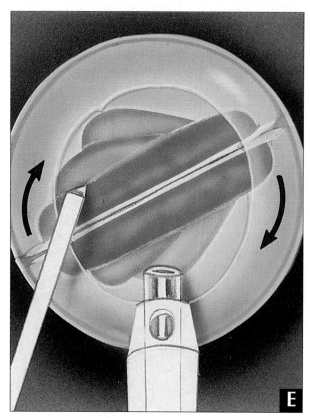

Figure 6-25E. Rotate the nucleus through 90° in order to present the groove transversally, ie, perpendicularly to the U/S tip.

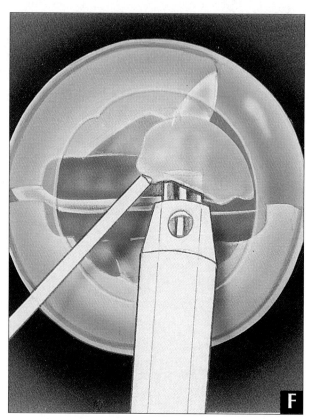

Figure 6-25F. Place the U/S tip inside the groove, and occlude under appropriate parameters. Keeping it horizontal, insert the chopper under the rhexis. Proceed almost to the equator, bring it into a vertical position, and pull it toward the U/S tip. Prior to moving into contact with the U/S tip, move it toward the left. In this way, a segment of nuclear material is produced which detaches from the residual hemi-nucleus.

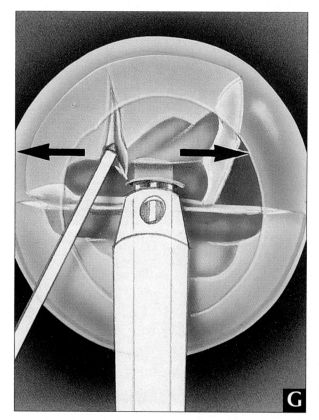

Figure 6-25G. Repeat the occlusion and fracture procedure, then emulsification of the fragment created.

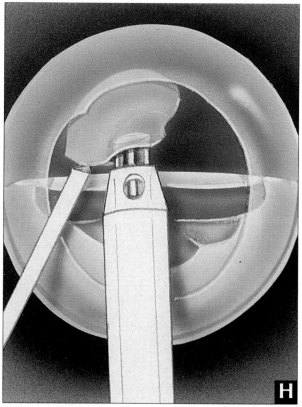

Figure 6-25H. Once the segment has been obtained, pull it toward the center using occlusion and fragment; then emulsification begins. Continue until the first hemi-nucleus has been completely removed.

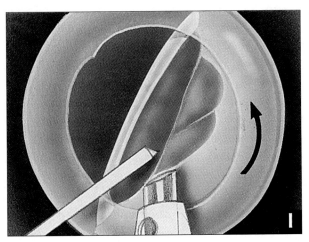

Figure 6-25I. Rotate the second hemi-nucleus, and present it distally to the U/S tip.

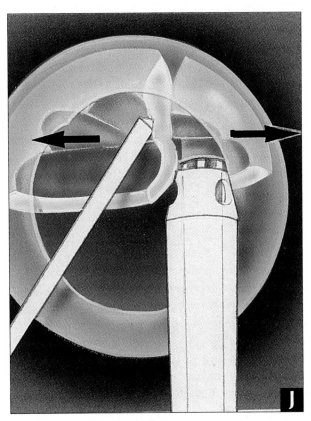

Figure 6-25J. Occlude the U/S tip and use the chopper to produce a segment. The U/S tip is used in the opposite direction to the chopper.

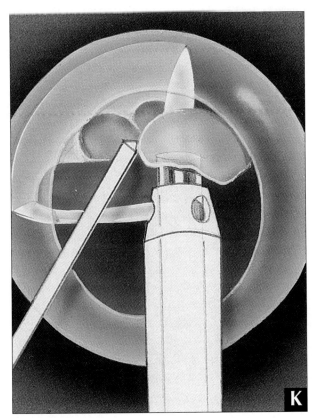

Figure 6-25K. Two pieces are produced; removal of the piece attached to the U/S tip.

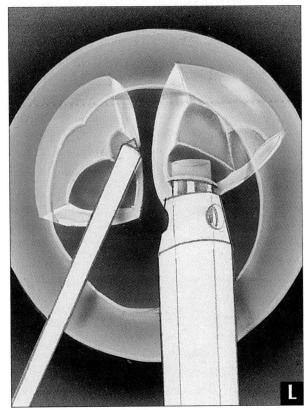

Figure 6-25L. Capture of the last piece of nucleus with U/S tip. Occlusion, division, and emulsification until the nucleus has been completely removed.

Table 6-51
## ELECTIVE TECHNIQUE FOR PHACOEMULSIFICATION OF GRADE 1 NUCLEI

**With an intact capsulorhexis**

| | |
|---|---|
| Incision | Surgeon's choice. |
| Hydrodissection/hydrodelamination | These are extremely useful. |
| Removal of the nucleus with emulsification | One-handed in situ phacoemulsification. Direct aspiration with the I/A tip. Aspiration with the I/A tip with U/S; low vacuum and flow rates, and reduced U/S power. |
| Removal of the cortex | The traditional methods are used. |

**In the event of a can opener or rhexis escape**

| | |
|---|---|
| Incision | Depending on the surgeon's choice. |
| Hydrodissection/ hydrodelamination | No. |
| Mobilization of the nucleus | No, because the nucleus is soft. |
| Phacoemulsification | With the in situ technique. |
| Removal of the cortex | With the traditional technique. |

Table 6-52
## ELECTIVE TECHNIQUE FOR PHACOEMULSIFICATION OF GRADE 2 NUCLEI

**With an intact capsulorhexis**

| | |
|---|---|
| Incision | Depending on the surgeon's choice. |
| Hydrodissection | Indispensable. |
| Mobilization | Yes. |
| Technique of nuclear removal | Fractional 2/4. Chip and Flip. Cut and Suck. One-handed phacoemulsification. |
| Emulsification | With low U/S power. |
| Removal of the cortex | With the traditional techniques. |

**In the event of a can opener or rhexis escape**

| | |
|---|---|
| Incision | Depending on the surgeon's choice. |
| Hydrodissection/hydrodelamination | No. |
| Mobilization | No. |
| Phacoemulsification technique | Minimal lift. Technique in the posterior chamber. Technique in the anterior chamber. |
| Removal of the cortex | According to the traditional methods. |

Table 6-53
## ELECTIVE TECHNIQUE FOR PHACOEMULSIFICATION OF GRADE 3 NUCLEI

### With capsulorhexis

| | |
|---|---|
| Incision | Depending on the surgeon's preference. |
| Hydrodissection | Yes. |
| Mobilization | Yes. |
| Phaco technique | 1. Endocapsular technique, in situ, one or two-handed; for relatively young patients (40-50 years) and recent cataracts (Nucleus 3a). |
| | 2. Two-handed technique Chip and Flip, Crack and Flip; for patients of between 50-60 years with a slightly amber-colored cataract (Nucleus 3b). Possibility of cleavage between the nucleus and the epinucleus (hydrodelamination): |
| | 3. Technique of nuclear fracture: In situ fracture, Trench Divide and Conquer, Stop and Chop for elderly patients with mature cataracts, large nucleus (Nucleus 3c). |
| Cortex | Removed using normal techniques. |

### In the event of a can opener or rhexis escape

| | |
|---|---|
| Incision | According to the surgeon's preference. |
| Hydrodissection | No. |
| Mobilization | No. |
| Phacoemulsification | Technique in the posterior chamber. |
| | Technique in the anterior chamber. |

Table 6-54
## ELECTIVE TECHNIQUE FOR PHACOEMULSIFICATION OF GRADE 4 NUCLEI

### With capsulorhexis

| | |
|---|---|
| Incision | Depending on the surgeon's preference. |
| | A limbal incision is advisable, which will facilitate the maneuvers in the event of a conversion. |
| Hydrodissection | Indispensable. |
| Mobilization | Indispensable. |
| Removal | Endocapsular techniques of cross-shaped nucleofracture or related variations; use of moderate-high U/S. |
| | Phaco Chop or relative variations. |

### In the event of a can opener or rhexis escape

| | |
|---|---|
| Incision | Limbal. |
| Hydrodissection/ hydrodelamination | No. |
| Mobilization | No. |
| Phacoemulsification | Technique on the pupillary plane. |
| | Technique of minimal lift. |
| | Conversion. |

Table 6-55
## ELECTIVE TECHNIQUE FOR PHACOEMULSIFICATION OF GRADE 5 NUCLEI

**With intact capsulorhexis**

| | |
|---|---|
| Incision | Depending on the surgeon's preference. If the procedure is expected to be difficult, a limbal incision is advisable. |
| Capsulotomy | Wide capsulorhexis. |
| Hydrodissection | Yes, with the usual techniques. |
| Mobilization | After hydrodissection. |
| Removal | Technique of Phaco Chop or related variations. Conversion in the event of difficulties during phaco. Planned extracapsular. |

**In the event of a can opener or rhexis escape**

| | |
|---|---|
| Incision | Limbal or sclero-corneal. |
| Hydrodissection/hydrodelamination | No. |
| Mobilization | No. |
| Removal | Phaco in the posterior chamber. Planned extracapsular. |

Table 6-56
## TABLE SUMMARIZING THE PHACO TECHNIQUES ON THE BASIS OF THE HARDNESS OF THE NUCLEUS

| Hardness of the nucleus | Endocapsular techniques to use with an intact rhexis only<br>Suggested technique | Other techniques to be used with open rhexis and/or can opener or Christmas tree<br>Suggested technique |
|---|---|---|
| Grade 1 | I/A alone.<br>I/A with the U/S tip.<br>One-handed in situ. | Phaco as it happens. |
| Grade 2 | Fractional 2/4.<br>Chip and Flip.<br>Cut and Suck.<br>One-handed in situ phaco. | Carousel technique in the anterior chamber. |
| Grade 3 | In situ one- or two-handed.<br>Chip and Flip.<br>Crack and Flip.<br>In situ fracture.<br>Trench Divide and Conquer.<br>Stop and Chop. | Minimal lift.<br>Technique in the posterior chamber.<br>Carousel technique in the anterior chamber. |
| Grade 4 | Crack and Flip.<br>Phaco Chop.<br>Crater Divide and Conquer. | Technique on the pupillary plane.<br>Minimal lift technique.<br>Sector technique in the anterior chamber.<br>Conversion.<br>Extracapsular. |
| Grade 5 | Phaco Chop. | Conversion. |

Table 6-57
# REMOVAL OF THE EPINUCLEUS

| | |
|---|---|
| Epinucleus intact around 360° | Flip Technique.<br>Parameters—vacuum: 60-70; flow rate: 15-18; U/S: 30-40%.<br>Place the tip in contact the internal parts of the material, distally.<br>Activate the aspiration to look for occlusion.<br>Once occlusion has been obtained, move the tip slightly toward the incision, and use the spatula to help rotate the epinucleus toward the center of the bag, trying to overturn the bowl and free it by transporting it to the level of the rhexis.<br>Activate the U/S and remove the material. |
| Epinucleus Intact around 360° | Rotation technique.<br>Parameters as above.<br>Place the tip in occlusion distally with the anterior edge just below the rhexis. Wait until the vacuum reaches the maximum preset values.<br>Detach the interested area of the epinucleus from the capsule, and fragment it with a short burst.<br>Rotate the epinucleus using the spatula, using the U/S tip to help if necessary to distally expose another portion of the epinuclear edge.<br>Repeat the maneuvers of occlusion, detachment, and emulsification.<br>During occlusion, try to mobilize the nucleus by moving the U/S tip from right to left and back again.<br>If it is sufficiently mobilized, fragment it at the center of the capsular bag. |
| Partial epinucleus | If it is hard:<br>Mobilize it with an olive-tipped spatula, and place it close to the U/S tip.<br>Position it in a favorable position for the U/S tip, and capture it with low vacuum (60-80 mm Hg) and fragment it with low U/S (30-40%).<br><br>If it is soft:<br>Use the U/S tip with the above-mentioned parameters, and look for occlusion. Mobilize the nucleus and then luxate it inside the bag; aspirate.<br>If mobility is poor:<br>Inject Provisc between the capsule and the epinucleus to separate the two structures; then capture the epinuclear edge separated with the U/S tip.<br>Repeat the hydrodissection (inject BSS between the epinucleus and the capsule). Capture the piece with the U/S tip.<br>Turn the U/S tip very carefully downward. With the first signs of occlusion, withdraw the tip (do not use U/S).<br>Use the I/A tip with an orifice of 0.3 or 0.5; vacuum—200-300; flow rate—15-20. The procedure will be longer but safer. |

Table 6-58
## FUNCTION OF THE SPATULA DURING PHACO

### In the preliminary phases
Detach the iris synechiae.

Retract the iris for the capsulorhexis in the event of a narrow pupil.

### During phaco
Stabilize the nucleus during the formation of the grooves (counteract its tendency to move distally under the action of the U/S tip).

Rotate the nucleus or pieces of it.

Split the nucleus into quadrants.

Raise the quadrants to facilitate occlusion.

Rotate the quadrants to expose them to the tip.

Place the fragments of nucleus in a position suitable for the U/S tip.

Keep the nuclear fragments in contact with the U/S tip.

Protect the posterior capsule or the endothelium if there is excessive movement of a mobil fragment in the anterior chamber.

Block the fall of the material inside the vitreal chamber in the event of posterior capsule rupture.

Keep the iris far away from the U/S tip.

### During I/A
Retract the iris in the event of miosis.

Mobilize the hard fragments of cortex from the capsular bag.

Facilitate aspiration of the material engaged by the tip through a movement of rubbing.

### During implantation
Facilitate the passage of the IOL through the incision counteracting the pressure exerted on it.

Depress the lens toward the bag (with tunnel incisions, it will tend to move toward the internal apex of the cornea).

Facilitate the penetration of the lens in the rhexis.

Retract the iris to control the position of the IOL.

# Chapter 7

# IRRIGATION/ASPIRATION

*Lucio Buratto, MD*

## INTRODUCTION

Once the removal of the nucleus has been completed, the cortical material must be aspirated. It can be free (ie, mobile in the anterior chamber) or attached to the posterior capsule and the residual anterior capsule. The free cortex has a fluffy appearance. It is almost always soft and located mainly in the anterior chamber in front of the iris plane. The attached cortex is sometimes stratified (like onions), or it can be fluffy. Sometimes it is soft and easily aspirated or it can be harder and require considerable aspirating power.

The phase of irrigation/aspiration (I/A) removes all the remaining soft cataract residue. It is a procedure that occurs almost totally in the posterior chamber and more precisely inside the capsular bag.

I/A must satisfy certain requirements:
- Safety—This means that the maneuvers necessary for the removal of the material must not damage the eye structures. In particular, they must respect the integrity of the posterior capsule and the zonules as well as the endothelium and the iris.
- Progression—The removal must be in small steps, with small portions of cortex removed each time. This way, reduced traction forces are applied to the cortex, the capsule, and the zonule.
- Gradual—The aspiration of the cortical material must be gradual. In order to obtain this, the vacuum level set on the instrument must not be excessive and the mass must be detached from the posterior capsule before being aspirated. These are important factors to reduce traction forces on the zonules and avoid capsular detachment.
- Rapidity—If the maneuvers in the anterior chamber are lengthy, repetitive, and slow, there is a greater possibility that the pupil will contract, the endothelium will be damaged, etc. Aspiration of the cortical material must therefore be rapid. However, safety and the gradual removal or the progression must not be compromised in any way.
- Efficacy—The orifice of the aspiration tip must be large enough to aspirate any size of mass, irrespective of whether it is small or large, soft or hard, fluffy or thread-like, and the correct amount of aspiration power must be used.
- Complete aspiration—Modern surgery does not allow for any remaining cortical material in the anterior chamber or the capsular bag. The I/A process must therefore produce fine, accurate cleansing throughout the anterior segment. This way, postoperative inflammation is limited, the degree and quality of functional recovery is improved, further operations are avoided, and the posterior capsulotomy is delayed. However, a residual cortex left in the eye is preferable to a ruptured capsule or the vitreous mixing with the cortex. The surgeon must realize when to stop at the right moment and allow a small complication to prevent a more serious one.

## THE I/A CYCLE

Using a pump fitted with a peristaltic pump there are three similar ways of removing the cortical material.

### Simplified I/A Cycle
- The assistant sets the minimum I/A on the machine (ie, vacuum levels of 65 to 70 mm Hg).
- The aspiration orifice is brought close to a cortical mass or clump with only the irrigation open.
- The pedal is pushed into Position 2 and aspiration is activated; the mass sticks to the tip.
- Let aspiration continue for an instant. The orifice becomes obstructed by the mass and with the

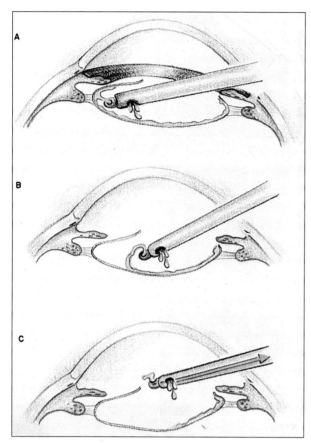

Figure 7-1. (A) Capture of the cortex with low aspirating power. (B) Detach the material slowly. (C) Transport it to a safe place, outside the capsular bag.

pump functioning, the vacuum increases (inside the cannula) thus engaging the mass further. Aspiration can begin.
- The tip is moved toward the center of the chamber gently detaching the cortex captured.
- In this position (ie, in the center of the chamber) the assistant selects vacuum on maximum I/A (300 to 400 mm Hg) and the mass is rapidly absorbed.
- The vacuum selector is returned to minimum I/A and the cycle is repeated.

### Intermediate I/A Cycle

The intermediate I/A cycle or cycle in linear suction consists of the following steps:
- Maximum vacuum is preset at around 400 mm Hg and the machine is set at linear aspiration. In this case, the aspirating power increases as the pedal is pushed and the orifice is occluded (if the orifice is open, the vacuum is low because the fluid present in the anterior chamber does not provide sufficient resistance).
- The orifice is brought close to a cortical fragment with irrigation only open in order to deepen the spaces.
- The pedal is pushed into Position 2 and after the click, the pedal is pushed slightly to activate a moderate aspiration. The mass sticks to the orifice.
- The orifice is allowed to occlude.
- The probe is then gently moved toward the center of the anterior chamber while the pressure on the pedal is gradually increased. This way, the piece of cortex captured will be gently detached and aspiration can begin.
- When the probe is at the center of the anterior chamber, the operator pushes the pedal to its limit and waits until the mass has been completely absorbed by the aspiration line. He or she interrupts the process using the pedal and goes into venting (cutting out the aspiration within the line). This prevents an excessive amount of liquid from being drawn into the line.
- The orifice approaches a cortex fragment adjacent to the one removed previously. Once contact has been made, aspiration is reactivated, the mass is captured, and the procedure is repeated.

### Advanced I/A Cycle

The operator uses the option of linear vacuum and preselects a maximum limit of 400 or 500 mm Hg.
- The surgeon brings the orifice to the mass and immediately activates a high level of suction.
- Once occlusion has been obtained the tip is moved toward the center of the chamber and the cortex is detached.
- The pedal is pushed to its limit to obtain the complete removal of the cortex fragment involved in the maneuver.
- The procedure is repeated as often as necessary.

## GENERAL PRINCIPLES OF ASPIRATION OF THE CORTEX MATERIAL USING AN INSTRUMENT FITTED WITH A PERISTALTIC PUMP

For the I/A cycle to be performed correctly, some important rules must be followed:
- Examination of the probe—Before introducing the I/A tip into the anterior chamber, the assistant must ensure that it works properly. He or she must examine the patency of the cannula, check that the level of irrigation is adequate, check that the sleeve is positioned correctly, and check if the aspiration is working at the required level.
- Test of the artificial anterior chamber—The assistant can also use a *chamber test*; ie, he or she can check the balance between incoming and outgoing liquid on an artificial silicone anterior chamber.
- The equilibrium of the anterior chamber—The I/A tip must be introduced through a corneal incision with the irrigation open to shape the chamber immediately (foot pedal in Position 1). As soon as the liquid flows into the anterior chamber, it expands in order to avoid excessive dilatation of the internal spaces. The pedal should be brought into Position 2 to activate the aspiration. The tip is

Table 7-1
## I/A USE OF THE TIPS

|  | Vacuum range mm Hg | Flow mL/min | Material | Tip |
|---|---|---|---|---|
| 0.2 tip | 0-500 | 15-40 | Suitable for threadlike material or small masses | Straight |
| 0.3 tip | 0-500 | 15-30 | Any kind of cortical material | Straight or angled |
| 0.5 tip | 0-100 | 15-20 | Wide dense cortical masses | Straight |
| 0.7 tip | 0-100 | 10-15 | Wide dense cortical masses or epinucleus or soft nucleus | Straight |

then moved to the center of the anterior chamber and in this position, with irrigation and aspiration active, the operator observes whether:

- The anterior chamber is a suitable depth. If it is too shallow, he or she must raise the bottle until the desired depth is obtained. The opposite applies if the chamber is too deep.
- The anterior chamber remains at a constant depth after just a few seconds of I/A. This means that the balance between incoming and outgoing liquid is correct.

The equilibrium between infusion liquid and aspirated liquid will oscillate during aspiration of the cortical material. In fact, when the cortex obstructs the orifice there will be a reduction in the aspiration of the liquids and as the introduction will still be active, the anterior chamber will deepen in proportion to the length of time the orifice remains obstructed (some of the excess liquid escapes from the incision) and in proportion to the height of the bottle. As soon as the mass is aspirated there will a momentary increase in liquid aspirated, a surge (due to the accumulation of vacuum in the aspirating line following the obstruction of the orifice), with partial reduction in the chamber depth. The balance of the situation will be redressed after just a few seconds.

- The anterior and posterior chambers must be deep. The ideal situation is to have a chamber that is just slightly deeper than the physiological depth which will keep the pupil well-dilated. The spaces are wide and therefore the safety margins are wider. With the deep chamber the tip is not obstructed by the iris, the posterior capsule is distended and distant, and contacts with the endothelium and damage to Descemet's membrane are avoided. In practice, the large spaces allow the operator to move with confidence throughout the posterior chamber.

The wide space also separates the iris and the posterior capsule and the anterior and posterior capsules. This facilitates the placement of the tip under the iris and inside the capsular bag and provides excellent access to the cortex.

With deep spaces, the posterior capsule is placed under tension and is distended. The operator will find this way easier and he or she will have more control in detaching the cortex.

The depth of the anterior chamber depends basically on two factors: the amount of irrigating flow and the degree of fluid loss. The former depends on the diameter of the tube, the diameter of the connections, and the size of the orifices in the tip. With equal diameter of the above, the flow rate depends on the height of the bottle. The other element that determines the chamber depth is the fluid loss through the aspiration orifice and partly through the main and side port incisions. The latter depends on the type of incision, the traction exercised by the operator during the maneuvers, etc. The loss from the aspiration orifice depends on its diameter and the level of vacuum set on the machine (with equal velocity of the peristaltic pump and until the orifice is obstructed).

The losses can be compensated by greater flow (by raising the bottle). A simple method to give the operator wider spaces when he or she is ready to aspirate a mass is to suspend the aspiration and let irrigation prevail.

- Wide mydriasis facilitates I/A. This is because the cortex is more visible and because every maneuver is under the direct visual control of the operator. In addition, there is a better red reflex of the fundus which allows the surgeon to make a correct evaluation of the mutual relationships between the various structures. In particular the operator can give a more accurate evaluation of the adhesion of the cortex to the posterior capsule. He or she can safely and accurately locate the residues and distinguish their arrangement on the capsule.

When there is poor mydriasis at the beginning of the operation, 0.5 cc of 1/1000 adrenalin (preservative-free) for intracardiac use can be added to the 500 cc bottle of saline solution (anesthesist permitting). If this does not produce sufficient dilatation, some special maneuvers must be used (see the relative article).

- The aspirating orifice of the instrument must always be under the visual control of the operator. This avoids snagging the anterior capsule and the iris, but above all it avoids capturing and tearing the posterior capsule.

In the event of miosis, the operator can introduce the tip of the cannula under the iris and aspirate *blindly*. This must be done quickly, keeping the time necessary to capture a fragment of the cortex to a minimum, and positioning the orifice to avoid damaging the posterior capsule, using a low or moderate aspirating power. Once the mass has been captured the operator must bring it to the pupillary area where, under direct visual control, he or

| Table 7-2 |
|---|
| **ASPIRATION CYCLE** |
| Step 1 — Place the hole near the material with the pedal in Position 1 (only irrigation). |
| Step 2 — Go with pedal in Position 2 (irrigation and aspiration) and press it until sufficient vacuum has been reached (linear aspiration) to engage the material in the hole. |
| Step 3 — Wait a few seconds until the occlusion of the hole is achieved and the vacuum rises in the line until the set value is reached. |
| Step 4 — Pull the tip toward the middle of the capsular bag. The suction will detach the capsular material. |
| Step 5 — In the middle of the capsular bag wait until the material is aspirated and the hole disoccluded. |
| Step 6 — Repeat the operation as many times as necessary to complete removal of the cortex. |

she can aspirate, increasing the vacuum in the line if necessary.

- The diameter of the I/A tip orifices can be 0.2, 0.3, 0.5, or 0.7 mm.

The tips with 0.2 to 0.3 mm orifices are designed to be used with maximum vacuum (300 to 400 mm Hg), as they are more selective with regard to the material to be aspirated. They allow very small pieces of cortex to be aspirated thanks to the greater ease of occlusion.

The 0.5 to 0.7 mm orifices should be used with minimum vacuum (about 60 to 100 mm Hg) to aspirate the larger pieces of cortex. If the operator uses higher values there is a risk that the anterior chamber will collapse and he or she may aspirate the iris or the posterior capsule.

The 0.3 mm orifice is ideal:

- It easily captures all types of cortex, all parameters being equal. It can therefore remove both the small and large masses, the stratified and the fluffy cortex.
- The operation is faster because it can aspirate all the mass types rapidly.
- Good balance between irrigation and aspiration is maintained in the anterior chamber, and consequently the spaces are maintained with sufficiently constant depth.
- A small orifice will not tear the posterior capsule if it is accidentally snagged (naturally as long as the surgeon operates properly and sees the capture in time) because only a minimal part of the capsule surface penetrates the orifice.
- A silicone sleeve is preferable. The aspiration cannula is covered by a sleeve. The irrigation liquid flows between the sleeve and the tip.

Though the sleeves are available in silicone or metal, silicone is preferable for number of reasons:

- First of all, as it is soft, it adapts better to the shape of the incision. This allows the anterior chamber to maintain a homogeneous, stable depth irrespective of the position of the tip because very little liquid escapes from the incision. As the metal sleeve is rigid, it gapes the edges of the opening with greater loss of liquid particularly when the aspiration occurs in the superior and lateral sectors, when the tip moves vertically or laterally. It raises or separates the anterior edge of the incision from the posterior one.
- It does not reflect the microscope light which can disturb the surgeon.
- As it is transparent, it permits a better general view of the anterior chamber.
- It can be advanced or retracted in relation to the aspiration cannula allowing the operator to adapt its position to the surgical needs. The metal sleeve in most cases is fixed, that is, one with the I/A tip. In some cases the handle, the tip, and the sleeve are all one.
- The silicone sleeve, as on the U/S tip, must be positioned with the aspiration orifice toward the operator and the irrigation orifices oriented laterally.
- To do aspiration with the tip at the center of the anterior chamber, the safer point. The free cortex can be engaged in every sector of the anterior segment. The cortex attached to the capsule must be captured at the adhesion point with the edges of the anterior capsule. It must then be gently pulled toward the center of the pupil through a slow, delicate detachment of the equatorial capsule. Then it should be detached from the posterior capsule and when it is at the center it is aspirated.
- The basic rule of aspiration involves capturing the cortical material in the peripheral areas and aspirating them in the center of the chamber. The foot pedal must always be in Position 1 during the approach to the cortical material. This way, irrespective of the phacoemulsification technique used, spaces are created for optimizing the cortical capture by the I/A tip.

When the tip is in contact with the cortical material, the pedal is moved to Position 2 to occlude the aspiration orifice and allow an increase of the vacuum level to the maximum levels preset on the machine.

Once the cortical material has been captured (occlusion), the tip is gently moved toward the pupillary center to detach the triangular wedge of cortex progressively from the periphery toward the center.

First aspirate the free material, then the stratified material, and then finally remove the material attached to the posterior capsule. Aspirate first in the more accessible sectors, that is, in the temporal, nasal, and inferior sectors, and then proceed to those that are more difficult to reach (ie, those close to the incision).

- The aspiration of the cortex must be complete. This will avoid the onset of inflammation, allow a better and more rapid visual recovery, allow better centering of the artificial lens, and reduce the possibility of the posterior capsule becoming opaque in the postoperative.
- During I/A, the surgeon should avoid capturing the anterior capsule because the traction forces created may detach the zonules or weaken it at any rate. If the capsule is captured, the operator should not pull but should try to release it immediately

(activating venting and reflux if necessary).
- The surgeon should quickly recognize the presence of folds on the posterior capsule. These appear in most cases because the capsule becomes trapped in the aspiration orifice.

It is of the utmost importance that the surgeon immediately recognizes that the capsule has been captured and to do this he or she needs to have a good red reflex of the fundus, and perfect, continual focus on the posterior capsule. If the focus is trained on the posterior capsule, the surgeon will realize immediately if anything is wrong (ie, he or she will see lines or folds starting from the point of capture with radial extensions caused by the crumpling of the capsule around the orifice).

The view of these folds is better and more immediate when the capsule is captured in the central part. It is more difficult to see when this happens in the peripheral area where the surgeon will only perceive the folds that extend toward the center of the capsule.

The involuntary capture of the posterior capsule is seen particularly with the tips with a large orifice and it occurs with greater frequency when the chamber is shallow and the margins of maneuver are limited or when there is a vitreal pressure. It happens when the equilibrium between I/A is unsuitable. As a result, the chamber flattens easily. This happens more frequently in the terminal phases of I/A (ie, when the cortex has been removed for the most part and the posterior capsule is transparent as the surgeon may not be able to identify it clearly).

The capture of the posterior capsule is often related to the type of capsule. When the anterior capsule has proved to be easily cut, is thin, etc, the posterior capsule is likely to have the same characteristics and therefore is easier to capture. It also depends on its relationship with the vitreous. If it is not attached to the hyaloid, it is more likely to be captured; the same applies to fluid vitreous.

Nevertheless, behind every capture, there is a human operating error. The aspiration orifice will have been placed too close to the capsule thus causing the aspiration.

As soon as the capsule is captured, its rupture must be prevented at all costs. Therefore it is necessary that the surgeon:
- Avoid any movement or traction with the tip.
- Interrupt aspiration immediately.
- Activate venting (move the foot pedal into position 0 to block the vacuum inside the aspiration tube).

If the machine is not fitted with the venting option or alternately this option does not activate, or again if the capture occurred with high depression and the capsule has penetrated the aspiration orifice (even without tearing), the reflux must be activated. Some instruments are fitted with this device which, by using the pedal, inverts the direction of the aspirating flow and allows the captured capsule to be freed.

Alternately, the surgeon can clamp the bulb or the aspiration tube to produce a certain degree of reflux in the anterior chamber. The maneuver is performed as follows: as soon as the operator realizes that he or she captured something that shouldn't have been captured with the aspiration orifice, he or she should move the pedal from Position 2 to Position 1 (from I/A to irrigation alone). The assistant squeezes the aspiration tube or bulbs about 30 cm from the I/A tip between his or her thumb and index finger. This way he or she provokes a moderate reflux in the tube. This is normally sufficient to obtain the desired effect.

In the event of a serious adhesion, a double clamping may be necessary (ie, repeat the compression with the thumb and index finger of the right hand just behind the previous with the left hand). This way there will be a strong reflux of liquid in the tube which will push the material captured by the tip back into the eye, freeing it.

- Avoid the introduction of air to the anterior segment. During I/A, air bubbles may appear in the anterior chamber which block the surgeon's view and interfere with the correct aspiration procedure. The bubbles are due to the air in the infusion tubes. In this case the tube should be detached from the handle and abundant saline solution should be introduced. The tube should then be controlled to ensure the absence of any bubbles inside it.
- Use a good automated I/A machine (ie, the surgeon should use an I/A machine able to provide rapid safe aspiration of the cortex material). Use a modern, versatile, reliable, modular instrument (our preference lies with the Legacy, the Alcon 20,000 series).
- The instruments fitted with a peristaltic pump are easier to use and they are safer—particularly for the surgeon who does not perform many of these operations.
- The peristaltic pump allows the operator easy capture of the cortical material. Its rotation creates an increasing depression which, depending on its speed, reaches the machine's maximum preset values from the zero starting point in a short or moderate length of time. A progressive negative force is created around the orifice (moderate until the orifice is partially or completely obstructed). The progressive action is one of the biggest advantages of this device.
- It allows easy penetration of the cortical material to the lumen of the probe and then to the silicone tube. The continual rotation of the peristaltic pump, when the orifice is obstructed, allows a progressive increase of the vacuum in the tube and in the cannula which permits a progressive aspiration of the material.
- Adaptability to current needs—The cortex must be removed by aspirating forces and with different flow rates depending on the needs of the moment. A strong aspirating force may be necessary at some points; at others the surgeon may prefer a lower one. This can be obtained easily with a good machine fitted with a peristaltic pump which varies the degree of depression by changing the pressure on the pedal. Sometimes it may be neces-

sary to speed up the process (high flow rate); sometimes it may be necessary to slow it down (reduction of the flow rate).

In conclusion, a good quality machine will aspirate the cortex in a rapid yet controllable fashion that is efficacious yet safe.

## I/A AND CAPSULOTOMY

Removal of the cortex differs depending on the type of capsulotomy performed.

### Aspiration with Can Opener

The phacoemulsification techniques associated with the can opener capsulotomy and the limbal incision, not a tunnel incision, normally leave a significant quantity of cortex, particularly if the cataract is not very mature.

The I/A tip with the aspiration orifice toward the operator is positioned distally to the incision site (at the 6 o'clock position if the incision is at the 12 o'clock position) in contact with a fragment of cortex with the foot pedal in Position 1. This way, the iris and the edges of the anterior capsule are distanced from the aspirating orifice. Then with the pedal in Position 2, the operator can occlude the orifice with cortex only.

The wedge of cortex engaged by the tip is brought toward the pupillary center to be detached from the capsule and aspirated. The maneuvers are repeated for the various sectors until the fornix of the capsule is reached while keeping the aspiration orifice visible. For the subincisional position, it may be necessary to resort to other maneuvers.

The I/A tip is positioned with the aspiration orifice placed laterally. Once the fragment has been captured, the tip is rotated toward the operator again and directed distally to progressively detach the cortex.

This maneuver—the ice cream scoop—can be facilitated by the mobilization of the cortex. One of the following three methods can be used:

1. The iris is massaged with the I/A tip below the incision, with the foot pedal in Position 0. The cortex is mobilized with lateral movements until a fragment of material becomes accessible to the aspiration orifice. With this procedure the pupil will tend to contract.
2. With the accessory spatula, the cortex is mobilized under the I/A tip while the chamber is kept deep with irrigation alone.
3. The I/A tip is extracted and a cannula connected to a syringe containing balanced salt solution (BSS) is inserted through the side port incision to mobilize the residual cortex at the 12 o'clock position.

In each phase of aspiration of the cortex, the surgeon must take care not to capture fragments of the anterior capsule and the iris with the aspiration orifice. If this happens, as in the case of capture of the posterior capsule, the surgeon must release the pedal immediately to activate venting or alternately he or she should activate reflux (if the phacoemulsifier is fitted with this device).

If a delicate cortical material is attached to the posterior capsule, the surgeon can reduce the vacuum (5 to 15 mm Hg with a flow rate of 5 to 10 cc/min) to aspirate the material directly or to pass the tip over the posterior capsule with the aspiration orifice turned toward it (the vacuum cleaner maneuver).

The cortex layer attached to the posterior capsule can also be mobilized using a sandblasted irrigating cannula, mounted on the irrigation handle.

Using circular movements, the diamond tip of the cannula detaches the cortex residues gently and safely thus minimizing the risk of rupturing the posterior capsule.

The same maneuver can be performed in the capsular fornix to mobilize the harder material that was not removed with the I/A tip. The I/A tip can be inserted again to aspirate the material that has been mobilized.

The special conditions described in this paragraph can be tackled using specific instruments that are part of the instrument kit for advanced phacoemulsification techniques. How they are used will be described in the following paragraph.

### Aspiration Inside the Capsulorhexis

Aspiration of the cortex following capsulorhexis and phacoemulsification in the capsular bag differs considerably from the previous method.

First of all, the quantity of cortex is usually smaller, because the cortex is partly mobilized during hydrodissection and part of it escapes with the epinucleus.

The method of hydrodissection actually determines the quantity of residual cortex. Cortical cleaving hydrodissection allows the surgeon to aspirate a large quantity of the cortical material along with the epinucleus, leaving just a fine layer attached to the capsule. This can be removed with the vacuum cleaner maneuver.

The capsulorhexis facilitates the approach to the cortex quite considerably:
- There are no flaps of the anterior capsule.
- The edge of the capsulorhexis prevents the iris from being captured.
- The capsular bag is always formed so that the tip can be positioned in the capsular fornix under the protection of the anterior capsule.

The surgeon should proceed as follows. The I/A tip is inserted with the aspiration orifice upward and the pedal in Position 1. Once the I/A is in contact with the cortex, the material is captured by moving the pedal to Position 2. It is aspirated detaching it progressively from the posterior capsule according to the aspiration cycle described in the previous paragraphs.

Remember that with modern instruments, fitted with a peristaltic pump and linear pedal control, the vacuum level can be varied by pushing the foot pedal. The flow rate can also be varied on the computer to suit the surgeon's needs. This way, the procedure can be adapted in real time to suit the individual clinical situation.

## REMOVAL OF THE SUBINCISIONAL CORTEX

One of the problems with the phacoemulsification operation undoubtedly is the aspiration of the cortex

Table 7-3
# POSSIBLE TECHNIQUES TO ASPIRATED SUBINCISIONAL CORTEX

## Technique of tip verticalization

| Technique | Drawbacks |
|---|---|
| Lift BSS bottle. | The posterior capsule can be captured easily. |
| Turn the hole toward the material and attempt occlusion. | Tension on the rhexis. |
| Rotate the tip by 180°. | Abnormal pressure on the incision lips. |
| Take the tip to the middle and detach the cortex. | Formation of corneal folds. |
| Wait for removal induced by the effect of aspiration. | Reduced visibility. |
| Divarication of the incision with BSS leakage and imbalance of flow in the anterior chamber. | Possible sleeve retraction or constriction inside the tunnel with subsequent stop or decrease in irrigation. |

## Widening the incision

| Technique | Drawbacks |
|---|---|
| Widen the tunnel to 4-5 mm and insert the tip at the ends. | Most of the problems described above remain, especially if the tunnel is long. |
| Use the right end to aspirate in the left sectors and vice versa. | As leakage increases, the chamber depth decreases. |

## Mobilization of masses with cannula and syringe

| Technique | Drawbacks |
|---|---|
| Capture the capsule with the hole. | The cannula must be thin; otherwise imbalance may be induced in the anterior chamber. |
| Traction toward the center and detachment. | Long and difficult procedure. |
| Mass release. | |
| Repeat the procedure. | |
| Once masses have been accumulated use automatized I/A. | |

## Mobilization of masses with the IOL

| Technique | Drawbacks |
|---|---|
| Leave the masses and insert the IOL. | Stress on the zonules and the equatorial capsule. |
| Rotate the lens inside the bag and free the masses. | Incomplete mobilization. |
| Aspirate while removing the viscoelastic. | Incomplete removal. |
| | Difficult IOL rotation. |

## 180° bent cannula by Binkhorst

| Technique | Drawbacks |
|---|---|
| Introduce the cannula in flat position. | The cannula is big and bulky. |
| Rotate to place it vertically. | It induces lip distortion with BSS leakage and consequent reduction of space inside the bag. |
| Introduce the hole in the fornix. | It is likely to cause capture of the posterior capsule and rupture of the rhexis. |
| Capture the mass. | Aspiration and/or cortex capture in blind position. |
| Aspirate the mass. | |

## Bent and angled coaxial cannulas

| Technique | Drawbacks |
|---|---|
| Insert the cannula. | A certain verticalization of the tip inside the tunnel is required. |
| Rotate it until the hole touches the material. | Difficulties persist in case of small rhexis and/or miosis. |
| Capture the material and aspirate it. | |

## Two-handed technique by Buratto

| Technique | Drawbacks |
|---|---|
| Two separate cannulas are used: one for irrigation and one for aspiration. | Two lateral incisions are required. |

material from the sectors underlying or surrounding the incision. This is particularly true with a tunnel, corneal, or scleral incision, and in concomitance with a rhexis particularly if it is small or decentered distally, (ie, with anterior capsule persisting in the sectors close to the incision).

Access to the material is obstructed by the tissue of the tunnel floor, by the iris, by the anterior capsule, and by the fact that any verticalization of the coaxial I/A tip will induce a series of problems that will be examined later.

Now take a look at the various methods used to mobilize, capture, and aspirate the material in these particular situations and then I will suggest how to resolve the problems.

### Table 7-4
### I/A OF SUBINCISIONAL CORTEX: TWO-HANDED TECHNIQUE BY BURATTO

**Advantages**

| | |
|---|---|
| Both cannulas can be alternatively introduced through both side port incisions to reach easily the entire 360° of the capsular bag. | Thus the entire capsular bag can be thoroughly cleaned. |
| Closed chamber technique. | The tunnel incision is closed by the internal pressure. The two lateral incisions are too small to allow a significant amount of fluid to leak out, and besides, they are obstructed by the cannulas. |
| Positive pressure technique. | The increased internal pressure causes stretching of the cornea, of the posterior capsule and the iris (which induces mydriasis). |
| Corneal stretching. | Reduction or absence of fold with consequent improved visibility. |
| Stretching of capsular bag and posterior capsule. | Erases folds, increases access to the masses, and improves visibility. It widens working spaces for the cannula. |
| It permits moving one cannula against the other. | It eases aspiration of hard masses or masses difficult to aspirate. |
| Iris retraction. | The irrigation cannula can be used to retract the iris in case of miosis and facilitate working with the other cannula. |
| Quick, easy, and safe technique. | It reduces the risk of rupturing the rhexis and/or the posterior capsule. |
| Checking eyeball motility. | Especially with topical anaesthesia or under Tenon's capsule, the bimanual technique provides very good control of ocular motility. |

**Drawbacks**

| | |
|---|---|
| Two lateral incisions. | Greater corneal trauma. |
| Occasional instability of the chamber depth. | During occlusion phases, the chamber tends to widen, as no leaks are present. |

### Table 7-5
### REASONS FOR DIFFICULTY WHEN ASPIRATING SUBINCISIONAL CORTEX IN THE TUNNEL

- Long pathway of the tip inside the tunnel
- Difficult verticalization of the tip as well as access to the capsular equator
- Increase in fluid leakage and decrease of chamber depth due to divarication of incision lips
- Small rhexis
- Distally decentralized rhexis
- Possible miosis
- Corneal folds

A first maneuver could be the verticalization of the coaxial I/A tip. In an operation without a tunnel incision, in order to perform the maneuver of verticalization correctly, it is necessary to raise the irrigation bottle in order to widen the capsular space. Then the capture of the material is performed with low aspiration placing the aspiration orifice directly in contact. Following capture, the handle is rotated through 180° to direct the aspiration orifice upward (distant from the posterior capsule). Then the vacuum is increased until all the cortex mass has been completely aspirated.

It is obvious that during verticalization abnormal pressure is being exerted on both edges of the incision, centripetal on the anterior and centrifugal on the posterior. The former causes formation of corneal folds with consequent reduction in the visibility, while the latter can exert abnormal pressure on the iris tissue.

Both cause gaping of the incision with a resulting increase in the loss of BSS and changes to the I/A balance.

With a tunnel, scleral or corneal incision, and in the event of poor mydriasis and small rhexis, it is impossible to perform this technique because of the difficulty in reaching the material.

An attempt can be made by retracting the I/A tip, with respect to the silicone sleeve, but this will not have any great effect. On the contrary, it can cause further problems. While the aspiration orifice approaches the cortex, the two lateral irrigation orifices will find themselves inside the tunnel. Some irrigation liquid will flow into the anterior chamber and some will escape outside. All this brings about an unbalance between irrigation and aspiration, with a relative increase in the latter and consequent flattening of the anterior chamber.

A second technique involves widening the incision to the size necessary for the implant (assuming that the implant requires an incision in excess of 4.0 mm) and inserting the I/A tip through the extremity of the incision. Entrance at the 1 o'clock position is needed to aspirate the material at the 11 o'clock and 12 o'clock positions. Entrance at the 11 o'clock position is needed to aspirate the material at the 12 o'clock and 1 o'clock positions.

This is a difficult technique because the incision is large and allows the escape of a large quantity of liquid resulting in a flattening of the posterior chamber. Access to the material is therefore difficult, particularly if the rhexis is small or there is poor mydriasis, even if a spatula introduced through a side port incision is used to retract the iris.

A third technique involves mobilizing the cortical material with a cannula connected to a syringe containing BSS (manual I/A to the point of mobilizing the mass) and then aspirating it with a coaxial I/A handle.

With this technique, in the first stage the material is mobilized and in the second stage it is easily captured and aspirated.

The maneuver allows the surgeon to obtain the desired results, however, it requires a lot of time, particularly if the cortical material is large or strongly attached. Moreover, it is not always an easy technique to perform.

Another technique involves inserting the intraocular lens (IOL) in the capsular bag without having completed the aspiration of the subincisional cortical material. Therefore, with the clockwise rotation of the lens, the surgeon can take advantage of the mechanical action exerted alternately by the two loops to mobilize the material which is then aspirated by the coaxial I/A cannula along with the VES. The technique sometimes has rapid success. In other cases rotation and the mobilization of the cortical material is difficult so the technique is not completely risk-free and should be treated with necessary caution. It can cause zonular stress in some sectors, which can be aggravated by the prolonged IOL rotation in the presence of the cortical material. This method is neither rapid nor safe, and does not always result in the complete removal of the residual cortical material.

Another method involves the use of a straight I/A tip curved 180° at the end (Binkhorst type). It allows the surgeon to reach the equator of the capsular bag behind the main entrance incision. Theoretically, it should work well because this type of tip does not require any major tilting to reach the cortical material. However, in practice it causes several problems because the cannula must have a greater-than-normal diameter in order to have a sufficiently large internal lumen for aspirating the cortex. So, if the chamber depth is reduced for some reason or another, the cannula will come into easy contact with the posterior capsule.

Moreover, given its size, this type of cannula causes gaping of the incision edges with a consequent reduction of the space of the capsular bag. The movement of the posterior capsule toward the aspiration orifice, which is already closer because the tip is curved, results in easier capture and rupture of the posterior capsule.

Also, in the event of poor mydriasis, or if the rhexis is small, the surgeon risks exerting excessive traction on its edge.

A huge step forward was the invention and production of angled or curved I/A cannulas. These normally are angled between 45° and 90° with a slight, smooth curve at the tip. This allows easier access to the equator of the capsular bag near the main incision.

These cannulas should replace the straight cannula during the I/A of the cortical material.

To avoid this inconvenient replacement, many surgeons have stopped using the straight cannula and use the angled one for the entire I/A phase. Though, with the latter, aspiration of the distal sectors is slightly more difficult.

However, even the angled cannulas must be tilted to a certain degree inside the incision in order to obtain good aspiration of the cortex. If the incision is small, it will be subjected to continual distortion of the margins and the edges.

The difficulty with a small rhexis or a narrow pupil still remains, even though the surgeon may resort to using a spatula to retract the iris.

Faced with these problems, in 1992 I started using an I/A device with two separate cannulas. One for irrigating and keeping the shape of the chamber, the other for aspirating the cortical material. Initially, the former was a Kratz scratcher and the latter was a common sleeveless aspiration cannula, with the irrigation closed. Later an improved system was developed.

Now the two cannulas are both slightly curved along the shaft. The irrigation cannula has two 0.5 mm preterminal orifices (ie, they are situated on two opposite sides of the cannula along an axis perpendicular with the curvature of the cannula).

The aspiration cannula has a single 0.3 mm orifice, located on the concave side about 1.0 mm from the end.

The two cannulas can be introduced alternately through two side port incisions. In the two-handed phacoemulsification techniques, there is only one side port incision so a second one has to be cut lateral to the main entrance. In the two side port incisions the entrance to the cornea is immediately in front of the limbal vascular arches, at about 90° from the primary incision. The blade must be directed almost tangentially in the corneal stroma, with an internal width of about 1.0 mm.

The I/A is performed in two steps which differ only through the position of the cannulas. They are passed from one hand to the other in order to reach the full-circle equator of the capsular bag, to include the sectors below the primary incision.

With these cannulas, all the maneuvers are performed in a completely closed chamber. As the main incision is a tunnel and free from any instruments, it is closed hermetically under the effect of the internal pressure created by irrigation. The side port incisions are just wide enough to allow the entrance of each of the two cannulas and permit a moderate escape of irrigation liquid.

Overall, the increase in intraocular pressure (IOP) determines a distention in the areas of least resistance: the cornea, the posterior capsule, and the iris. The distention of the cornea reduces or eliminates the folds and provides better visibility of the underlying structures. The distention of the capsular bag eliminates the folds in the posterior capsule so it is more unlikely that it will be snagged or captured by the aspiration cannula. Thus visibility is

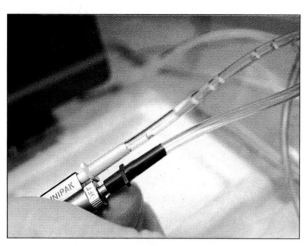

Figure 7-2. Air bubbles in the aspiration line reduce the aspiration power of the instrument. Those in the irrigation line introduce air into the anterior chamber. They should both be avoided.

improved. Above all the distention of the posterior capsule widens the capsular bag and increases the space available for the cannulas facilitating their access to the cortex. The distention of the iris widens the pupil and this is an enormous contribution to better visibility of the entire capsular equator.

Overall, the distention of all these structures provides an overall extension of the anterior and posterior chambers (in particular the capsular bag) and their communication (the pupil), with an increase in space available for the surgical maneuvers that are subsequently more precise and safer.

The complete independence of the two cannulas allows full-circle access to the capsular bag so it is easy for the surgeon to reach all the sectors including, and most importantly, the subincisional sectors or from one or another of the side port incisions.

Moreover, the aspiration of the harder material can be facilitated by *scratching* the end of the irrigation cannula against the mass that occludes the aspirating orifice of the second cannula.

In the event of poor intraoperative mydriasis, it is possible to use the irrigation cannula as though it were a spatula, in order to widen the pupil in a particular sector and then aspirate the cortical material with the second cannula.

At the end of the operation, the complete closure of the two side port incisions is spontaneous. In the event of slight loss, the incision edges can be swollen by injecting BSS through a sterile disposable syringe attached to a 25 G cannula.

In conclusion, the technique of I/A of the cortical material using two separate cannulas, while requiring a second side port incision, is easy, safe, and rapid. It gives the surgeon greater freedom of movement inside the capsular bag and allows complete full-circle cleaning of the equator. The surgeon is also working in a completely closed chamber. So, it is most definitely the elective procedure every time the subincisional cortex, for one reason or another, is difficult to remove. It is also recommended as a routine procedure for removing the whole cortex from the capsular bag.

# ASPIRATION OF THE CORTEX UNDER SPECIAL CONDITIONS

There are special conditions that may appear during aspiration of the cortex, if the material is trapped under the iris or when there are residues from the anterior capsule and numerous other situations. In these cases the surgeon will have to modify his or her aspiration technique.

## Material Under the Iris

After having aspirated all the visible cortical material, the surgeon should check whether any cortical material persists at the equator, particularly if mydriasis is not at a maximum. This can be done by moving the iris with a push-pull spatula. This maneuver often will show any residues, which can sometimes be a considerable size. They can be aspirated while the iris is held back with the spatula. If the operator has sufficient experience, he or she can introduce the aspiration tip *blindly* under the iris even when the cortical material is hidden. In this case, the aspiration orifice is directed toward the internal surface of the anterior capsule, where the cortical material is attached to a greater degree. The tip must reach this point with only the irrigation active in order to create sufficient space for access.

Once the orifice has approached the probable position of the mass, aspiration begins with low vacuum. The material is captured and the tip, with the piece of cortex attached, is moved gently toward the center of the anterior chamber. At this point, the vacuum is increased and aspiration is completed.

The aspiration of the cortex is simpler and efficacious with miosis but it requires the two-handed technique described previously. In extreme cases, the surgeon can apply iris retractors.

## Material in the Presence of Capsular Residues

If for various reasons a mobile portion of the anterior capsule remains, it becomes somewhat difficult to remove the cortex. The movement is more complicated because the free edge of the anterior capsule tends to stick easily to the aspiration orifice obstructing the cortex removal.

In these cases, it is necessary to have a deep posterior chamber that distances the aspiration orifice from the posterior capsule and the iris and to improve the separation of the free capsular fragment from the cortex, thus reducing the risk of involuntary capture. At the same time the tip has more room to maneuver. The surgeon might find it useful to use a spatula in his or her other hand to retract the mobile capsular fragment from the cortex and the cannula. It is nevertheless important to aspirate carefully and under moderate aspiration power

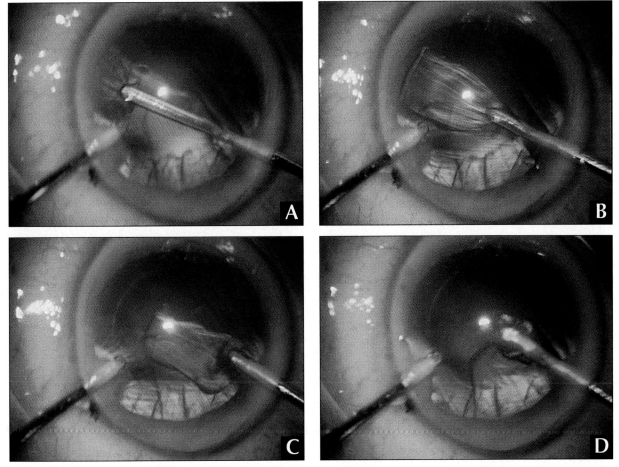

Figures 7-3A, 7-3B. Removal of the cortex with Buratto's two-handed technique. The cannula on the left is the one which irrigates; the cannula on the right is the aspirating cannula. The latter is inside the capsular bag and removes a fragment. With occlusion, it detaches from the posterior capsule and pulls it toward the center.
Figures 7-3C, 7-3D. The cortex is detached from the capsule and therefore can be completely removed and aspirated.

to avoid further damage to the capsule or the zonule in the event of involuntary capture of the capsular flap. Another solution is to interrupt the procedure, inject Healon, and then cut away the piece of capsule with microscissors. The aspiration of the cortex can continue as scheduled.

## Hard or Large Fragments

If the cortical material proves difficult to aspirate, the operator can choose one of three alternatives:

- Laterally to the tip the surgeon can insert a cyclodialysis spatula with a spherical end to fragment the cortex which will not enter the aspiration orifice spontaneously. The spatula mobilizes the mass and creates a rapid open-close mechanism which ultimately increases the aspiration capacity (potato masher technique).
- The surgeon can retract the tip from the anterior chamber and remove the attached piece of material with a dry sponge.
- The surgeon can increase the aspiration power and wait until the material is aspirated.

## Material in the Angle

Occasionally some fragments of nuclear or cortical material become stuck in the camerular angle especially in the superior sectors in correspondence to the corneal incision where the outgoing liquid carries the mobile material to the anterior chamber. In this case, the fragment can be aspirated directly by bringing the aspiration orifice into contact with the mass, changing the tip's entrance point if necessary.

Alternately, the material can be mobilized with a spatula or a current of BSS can be created in the anterior chamber. This is obtained by positioning one of the two irrigation orifices near the angular material. A semicircular current is obtained that will run along the camerular angle, flow toward the center of the anterior chamber and then toward the aspiration orifice. The fragments behave in the same way as they are flushed out and then captured.

## Difficulties with Aspiration

Imperfect aspiration of the cortex may be due to poor function of the central instrument or the peripheral aspiration line (tubes, connections, cannulas).

### Flaws in the Instrument
- Blockage of the rotation or function of the peristaltic pump.
- Incorrect application of the aspiration tube around the peristaltic pump (the tube might be too tight, too loose, etc). Incorrect insertion of the aspiration box in the instrument.
- The aspirating power is too low.
- The aspirating speed is too low.

### Flaws in the Tube or the Cannula
- Use of a closed tube—whether a flaw in the manufacture or acquired through sterilization under excessively high temperatures, or tubes that are too soft (for the instruments fitted with reusable tubing).
- Broken tube (air will enter the line so there will be no negative pressure of the orifice).
- Use of damaged connectors between the tube and the handle (whether obstructed, too small, or because they do not provide an airtight connection).
- Use of cannulas that are blocked by cortical material through careless cleaning, rust, etc.
- Cannulas that have not been properly screwed in.

In the event of inadequate aspiration, the surgeon must remove the cannula from the anterior segment and identify the problem.

# DIFFERENTIAL INTRAOPERATIVE IDENTIFICATION OF THE VARIOUS STRUCTURES OF THE ANTERIOR SEGMENT

## Between the Mobile Flap of the Anterior Capsule and the Cortex

The cortex has a ragged often fluffy appearance. For the most part it is situated deep in the chamber and equatorially. It is often attached to the posterior capsule and rarely deforms the pupil.

The capsular flap, which is thin and layered, has a more geometrical shape (triangular, rectangular, etc). It is mobile and under the effect of BSS circulation in the anterior chamber it tends to fold and lie in the anterior surface of the iris thus deforming the pupil. If it is captured by the aspiration orifice, it is not removed. On the contrary, it becomes an obstruction that the expert surgeon will be able to feel.

## Vitreous and Cortex

The vitreous is dense and tends to obstruct the aspiration orifice without being aspirated. It will tend to form an umbilical cord between its original site and the tip. It easily deforms the pupil, is not easy to see, and is not very mobile with liquid currents. It can appear in a number of zones, and it appears following capsular tear or an equatorial disinsertion, or other incorrect movement.

The cortex is a stronger color, is less thread-like, can be mobile or attached to the capsule, and is easily aspirated. It rarely deforms the pupil. The cortex mainly appears at the equator of the capsular bag.

## Vitreous and VES

VES is usually not used during I/A of the cortex. If it is used it is usually because the capsule and/or the hyaloid membrane have ruptured. In this case the VES is injected into the anterior and more into the posterior chambers where the complication has arisen. VES can be distinguished from the vitreous because it is more homogeneous, because it tends to form a single mass that remains distinct from the vitreous even though the two liquids are in contact with one another. VES may be cord-like depending on the size of the injecting cannula. Occasionally it contains microscopic air bubbles which facilitate its identification.

However, if there is free vitreous, the surgeon should use yellow Healon or Viscoat as they are easily recognizable.

## Between the Anterior Capsule and Descemet's Membrane

When there is a mobile tissue fragment in the anterior chamber, the surgeon may be unsure of whether it is the anterior capsule or Descemet's membrane. For a certain diagnosis, the surgeon should increase the magnification and the luminosity of the microscope. The surgeon should focus well first on the posterior surface of the cornea, and then on the iridial plane. One should also suspend any surgical maneuver until what is there has been clearly identified.

Descemet's membrane is likely to tear near the corneal incision where the instruments enter and exit from the anterior chamber. It can be seen as a thin, straight, or triangular line that appears on the deep corneal strata. If the surgeon focuses correctly, he or she will be able to locate the origin or site correctly. There is also a point of attachment to the deep corneal strata so it can be caught with a hook and returned to its original position.

The fragment of anterior capsule is usually deeper inside the chamber. It appears at the pupillary edge and is therefore in contact with the iris which it sometimes deformed producing a pear-shaped pupil. It can appear in all sectors of the anterior chamber, laterally, or distally where it is difficult to tear Descemet's membrane. It appears either on the can opener capsulotomy or with rhexis escape, not with an intact rhexis.

# Chapter 8

# POSTERIOR CAPSULE
*Lucio Buratto, MD*

## INTRODUCTION

In a certain percentage of cases, between 30 and 50% according to some authors, the posterior capsule in the short or long term becomes opaque after a phacoemulsification operation. Treatment of this opacity can be preventive (intraoperative capsulotomy) or secondary (postoperative capsulotomy). Nowadays very few surgeons perform the primary capsulotomy. The capsule should be kept intact, particularly in some patients such as severe myopes, in patients who have already had an operation for retinal detachment, or those who have had prophylactic treatment for retinal rupture. The capsule should also be kept intact in patients who have had cystoid macular edema in the other eye, and in glaucomatous patients where a fistolizing operation is a possibility in the future.

The intraoperative primary posterior capsulotomy can be performed using a variety of instruments, the most common is the insulin needle with a bent tip.

For the secondary capsulotomy, that is the postoperative, almost all surgeons use the Nd:YAG laser. This allows the surgeon to open the capsule in a short space of time with an almost total lack of surgical trauma. This undoubtedly is an enormous advantage and one of the more spectacular applications of the YAG laser. The procedure is completely painless, it removes the need for the patient to go into an operating room, and it avoids any type of anesthesia. Above all, it reduces the risks of possible complications with the surgical technique.

Nevertheless, during the operation the surgeon must try to:
- Make the capsule completely transparent to favor maximum functional recovery.
- Remove all the cortex material to reduce the spontaneous reabsorbance processes. Otherwise, the operator can be responsible for severe or minor inflammation and occasionally capsular fibrosis.
- Remove all the VES from the anterior chamber and the capsular bag at the end of the operation.
- Eliminate as many proliferative cells as possible to avoid secondary opacification of the posterior capsule.

Cleaning the capsule can be done in one of two ways:
1. With the sandblasted or diamond-tipped irrigating cannula.
2. With an aspirating cannula. In this case the irrigation/aspiration (I/A) tip is used set on a very low level of aspiration power (vacuum cleaner technique).

## Kratz Cannula

The Kratz cannula is a common irrigation cannula which has a slightly bent tip and is rough in the end part.

There are various models that differ largely because of quality and the type and extension of the sandblasting. The cannula is mounted on an irrigation handle, and under a high power of the microscope, is rubbed gently on the posterior capsule, particularly in the areas where there are small residues or cells.

## Cannula I/A

The 0.3 mm I/A cannula, mounted on an I/A handle, is an excellent instrument for cleaning the posterior chamber. It is used with the so-called vacuum cleaner technique.

A very low vacuum is set, about 5 to 15 mm Hg, with very low flow rate of 5 to 10 cc/min. The orifice is then oriented on the capsule and while aspirating the tip is moved continually from one sector to another, backward and forward, just like a vacuum cleaner. This way, all the fragments present on the surfaces are removed.

| Table 8-1 | |
|---|---|
| **VACUUM TECHNIQUE FOR POSTERIOR CAPSULE CLEANING** | |
| Microscope | High magnification is required. |
| Tip | 0.3 with moderately retracted sleeve. |
| Parameters | Vacuum 5-25; flow 5-15; bottle low. |
| The cornea | Must be clear reflecting and well-stretched. |
| The anterior chamber | Formed but not deep; otherwise it is difficult to put the tip at the right angle (and the posterior capsule becomes too convex posteriorly). |
| Technique | The hole is placed touching the capsule. |
| | The pedal is operated in Position 2. |
| | The tip hole is occluded (considering the parameters used, it is a moderate occlusion). |
| | The tip is moved continuously in various directions (if it is kept immobile the vacuum will have time to increase in the hose and thus the capsule may be firmly trapped inside the hole). |
| Cleaning mechanism | The capsule is aspirated inside the hole. Moving the tip continuously, the capsule is taken inside the hole and cleaned. |
| | Cleaning is accomplished by scratching on the opening rim. |
| Bottle | Placed low, so as to reduce the flow and avoid excessive chamber deepening. |

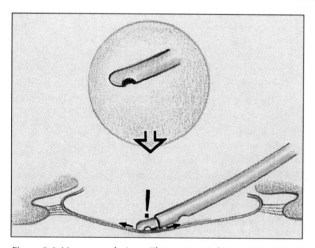

Figure 8-1. Vacuum technique. The vacuum is low (5-15 mm Hg), the flow rate is low (5-10 cc/min), and the orifice is directed toward the posterior capsule. Always keep the cannula moving in order to avoid the orifice making contact with the capsule for too much time. There is the risk of capsular rupture if the orifice becomes occluded.

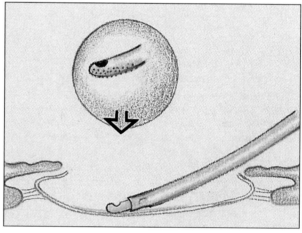

Figure 8-2. Cleaning of the posterior chamber with a rough tip.

Cleansing occurs partly because of the aspirating action, partly because of the scratching/rubbing of the edge of the orifice on the capsule, and partly through the mechanical action of the cannula. The secret of this technique is to use low aspirating power and keep the tip in continuous movement.

## RULES OF CAPSULAR EMULSIFICATION

Avoid cleansing if it is difficult to see the capsule. With the initial experiences of phacoemulsification, it is not always easy to identify this thin membrane because in the majority of cases it is transparent. So the cleaning maneuvers should be avoided at all costs. However, the surgeon must practice a lot so that he or she recognizes the capsule, using a suitable microscope magnification and suitable focalization. This way, small deposits of cortex, small areas of opaque capsule, and small traction folds, etc, can be identified on the surfaces.

In many cases, the capsule may be completely transparent (ie, there are no residues or cortical fragments) and it may be so thin that it is invisible to the surgeon. It is therefore useless to attempt to clean it.

In other cases, the vitreal pressure is such that it pushes the posterior capsule forward and puts it under tension. In this case, the integrity is at risk if it is cleaned. Every maneuver of cleansing can compromise the good result of the operation and should therefore be avoided.

Moreover, every procedure on the posterior capsule must be avoided when the corneal transparency, through epithelial abrasions, disepithelialization, and preexisting opacity, is such that it obstructs correct visual perception of the capsule.

Table 8-2
## POSTERIOR CAPSULORHEXIS WITH INTACT CAPSULE: INDICATIONS AND TECHNIQUE

### Indications
Remove central capsular opacity.

Remove the newborn's clear capsule (in order to perform anterior vitrectomy and implant the IOL in the bag).

Prevention of secondary opacity in adult and elderly patient.

### Technique
Fill the anterior chamber and the capsular bag with Healon GV. Avoid overfilling; attempt to achieve a flat posterior capsule, or slightly convex posteriorly.

Make a hook out of an insulin 30 G needle, bending it about 110-120° on the hole end (this way, when injecting viscoelastic, this will pas through the capsular opening).

Mount the cystotome on the syringe for Healon GV.

Take the cystotome just 1 mm beyond the middle of the capsule (distally with respect to the entrance in the chamber) or just beyond the opacity.

Withdraw the cystotome and introduce Utrata's or Corydon's or Buratto's forceps. Hold the lip and perform capsulorhexis, taking care that the chamber is always well-filled and making an opening not larger that 2-3 mm.

If the chamber becomes shallow inject more Healon GV. Inject Healon GV just before the opening to prevent the vitreous from going into the capsular bag.

Continue cautiously and avoid both lacerating the hyaloid and extending the opening too much (that would mean higher risk of hyaloid opening and greater difficulty to place correctly the IOL in the bag).

Table 8-3
## POSTERIOR CAPSULORHEXIS WITH OPEN CAPSULE

### Open capsule and intact vitreous
**Aims**
Avoid uncontrolled widening of the capsular opening.
Avoid hyaloid lacerations.
Allow safe implantation in the bag.

**Technique**
Inject Healon GV in the chamber and the bag until the posterior capsule has regained its physiological shape.

Inject a small amount of viscoelastic inside the opening to push the vitreous back.

Inject Healon GV under the opening to push forward the broken lip.

With the forceps hold the broken lip and perform capsulorhexis in a circular motion, trying to make it as small as possible. If possible, include the central area; should any problem occur, limit the opening to the area involved by the capsular break.

Insert the lens in the bag if the posterior rhexis is limited and/or central, otherwise place it in the sulcus. Preferable IOLs with the optics exceeding the posterior rhexis should be used.

PMMA IOL with wide haptics (LX90 by Alcon Surgical) should preferably be implanted.

### Open capsule and open vitreous
**Aims**
Allow safe anterior vitrectomy.
Prevent uncontrolled widening of the capsular opening.
Enable implantation in the bag.

**Technique**
Inject Viscoat in the chamber and the bag. It is important not to widen the opening by excessive injection. Perform anterior vitrectomy in dry conditions.

Continue slowly and very carefully, and avoid widening the capsular opening.

Remove only the vitreous before the opening and inject more Viscoat to push back residual vitreous and to visualize/push forward the capsular lip.

Hold the lip with a rhexis forceps and perform continuous capsulotomy (if creating a posterior rhexis appears difficult, do not persist, leave the opening as it is).

Complete removal of the vitreous present inside the posterior rhexis.

Fill the bag with viscoelastic.

Implant the lens in the bag if the anterior capsulorhexis is intact, and the posterior capsulorhexis is limited and/or central; otherwise implant in the sulcus.

Preferably implant a PMMA IOL with optic disc exceeding the posterior capsule opening (LX90 by Alcon Surgical). If the sulcus is to be implanted use a 13.0 mm lens with a 6.0 mm optics (MC 60BD by Alcon Surgical).

The pressure exerted with the cleaning instrument must be such as to encourage the blunt dissection and the abrasion of the material deposited in the capsule and the cells but not lacerate the capsule. Observe the capsular halo that forms around the cannula-capsule contact point (circular reflex). This must have a diameter of 2 to 3 mm maximum, it must be uniform and regular, and above all it must be free from folds. These signs will indicate that the pressure is suitable (this reflex is visible more with Kratz' cannula that with the I/A cannula).

The surgeon must see if the cleansing instrument meets any obstruction to movement or if it forms any folds. Once he or she has a certain amount of experience, the surgeon's sensitivity will allow perception of difficult running of the cannula on the capsule.

The maneuvers of cleaning consist of a backward and forward movement of the cannula. It can be done in any direction (circular, vertical, horizontal). What is important to remember is that every sector of the capsule is involved, but above all, that the cannula is moved continually. This favors better cleaning, reduces the risk of capsular tears, etc.

Keep the posterior capsule under moderate tension. In order to perform accurate cleaning without any risks of laceration, the capsule should not have too many folds. It is necessary that the anterior and posterior chambers are well-formed but not too deep.

Using active irrigation favors the cleaning of the fragments which are detached by the rubbing movement. It keeps the chamber well-formed, distends the capsule, and avoids close contacts between the instrument and the capsule.

# Chapter 9

# INTRAOCULAR LENSES
*Lucio Buratto, MD*

## INTRODUCTION

Once phacoemulsification of the cataract has been completed, the operator must insert the artificial lens, possibly in the posterior chamber and preferably inside the capsular bag. The lens to be inserted must have the following characteristics:
- Well-tolerated—The material must be perfectly accepted by the eye structures and not cause any uveal reactions or other inflammation.
- Extremely stable—There must be no change in its chemical, physical, or optical characteristics long-term.
- Light—The intraocular lens (IOL) must always have a specific weight inferior to the original weight of the cataract. In this case, even if part of the zonular fibers are damaged during the operation, or if the capsular bag loses some of its support, the lens will remain in position.

The IOL can be classified in a variety of ways. It can be based on fixation, the position of the optic, and the lens material, to name a few.

## CLASSIFICATION OF IOLS BASED ON FIXATION

### Angle Fixation

The lens supports or feet rest on two, three, or four points of the camerular angle. These are lenses for the anterior chamber (such as Kelman's, etc). The optic always remains in the anterior chamber. These lenses are becoming less frequently used, except in secondary implantation or complicated cases.

### Iris Fixation

The lens is supported by the iris; some rest on the anterior surface, others on the posterior, and others on the collarette. This category includes the Worst medallion and Worst's Lobster Claw lens. The optic is usually in the anterior chamber but can sometimes be in the posterior (Severin's lens). These lenses are no longer used.

### Mixed Fixation

This category includes the irido-capsular fixated lenses. The Binkhorst lens is the most famous of this group. It has two loops that are partially supported by the iris sphincter and partly by the capsular bag. These lenses have not been used for many years.

### Posterior Ciliary Sulcus Fixation

The loops of this lens are supported by the ciliary groove. The group includes the Shearing, Sinskey, Kratz, and Simcoe lenses, etc. The optic is always located in the posterior chamber behind the iris but external to the capsular bag.

### Capsular Fixation

The loops rest inside the lens capsule. The optic of these lenses remains inside the posterior chamber. Surgeons usually prefer insertion inside the capsular bag.

### Scleral Fixation

The loop and the optic are positioned behind the iris but do not have a physiological or anatomical support. They are held in position by transcleral sutures.

## CLASSIFICATION OF THE IOL BASED ON THE POSITION OF THE OPTIC

There are lenses suitable for:
- The anterior chamber.
- The posterior chamber.

The former, in theory, can be inserted after both intracapsular cataract extraction (ICCE) and extracapsular

Table 9-1A
## EVOLUTION OF POSTERIOR CHAMBER IOL

| Optic | Advantages | Disadvantages |
| --- | --- | --- |
| Flat-convex | Easy to hold with the forceps. Huge population with long follow-up. | High percentage of capsular opacification. |
| Meniscus | The edge acts as a separator to keep the posterior capsule separate from the IOL. | Increased percentage of capsular opacity. |
| Biconvex | Reduced percentage of capsular opacification. | More difficult to hold with the forceps and position in the bag. |
| Round | Low possibility of provoking glare at the edges. | Requires an incision which is slightly larger than the diameter of the lens to be inserted. |
| Oval (5 x 6) | It can be inserted through an incision which is smaller than that required for a round IOL. | It can cause glare at the edges. |
| Laser ridge | The posterior capsule remains separate from the lens in the central area. | It is difficult to hold with forceps. It increases the peripheral thickness of the lens. It is inefficient in preventing capsular opacification. |
| Modified surface | Reduced inflammation in the immediate postoperative. | Poor follow-up. |
| With prolene loops | Flexibility. Easy to manage. Resistant. | Poor memory of the loop. Decentering. Biodegradation in the long-term. Irregularity at the attachment point of the IOL. |
| One-piece in PMMA | Low possibility that the loop will break. Easy positioning—rotation of the loop in the bag. Reduced postoperative inflammation. | Loops are slightly rigid. |
| Foldables | Can be inserted through very small incisions. | Difficult to enter the capsular bag. Shorter follow up than the PMMA. |
| Multifocal | The patient can avoid using spectacles in some cases. Alternately, he or she can use monofocal lenses. | Loss of contrast sensitivity. Occasional glare and/or diplopia. Some patients request explants. |

Table 9-1B
## EVOLUTION OF THE POSTERIOR CHAMBER IOL

| Loop | Advantages | Disadvantages |
| --- | --- | --- |
| J loop | Follow-up is extremely long. Easy to insert. | Can ovalize the bag or the posterior capsule. Can erode the ciliary body. |
| C loop and modified | Distributes the pressure from the loops over a larger area. Low possibility to erode the capsular bag and/or the ciliary body. It is rotated in position very easily. | It is more difficult to insert than a J loop. |
| Closed loop | Produced to be inserted through a small incision and through a very small anterior capsulotomy. | Difficult to rotate and manage inside the eye. There are some problems with centering. |
| Loops which are angled anteriorly | Positions the optic disc more posteriorly. This results in less contact with the iris and less iris chafing and more contact with the posterior capsule with consequence low secondary capsule opacification. | Requires the correct insertion technique and suitable angulation. |
| End of the loop is looped | Easy to manage. | More difficult to explant. |
| Placement holes | Allows easy manipulation of the IOL when it is in the eye. It is useful for rotating the lens inside the bag or in the sulcus. | Possible source of inflammation. If one of the holes appears in the optic zone, it may cause visual disturbances—halos, diplopia. |

### Table 9-2
### IOL FOR PHACOEMULSIFICATION: RECENT PROGRESS

Lenses in PMMA with reduced diameter for small incisions
Foldable lenses
Various types of multifocal lenses
With treated surfaces
Toric
For phakic patients
Teledioptric

### Table 9-3
### PMMA IOLS FOR PHACO AND IMPLANTATION IN THE BAG

Material: CQ Perspex PMMA
Refraction index: 1.49
Optics: 5.0 mm, 5.5 mm
Loops: PMMA (one-piece IOL)
Overall length of the IOL: 12.0-12.5 mm
The most commonly used, the easiest to place
Cause the smallest amount of stretching of the incision
Longest follow-up

#### Advantages
Standard material
100% biocompatible
More than 40 years of experience
Hydrophobic
Good resistance to YAG
Sterilization with ETO
Optical resolution >250
Can be used as one-piece

### Table 9-4
### 1996 OVERALL IOL MARKET

|  | USA | Europe | Japan |
|---|---|---|---|
| One-piece PMMA IOLs | 38% | 60% | 50% |
| Three-piece PMMA IOLs | 16% | 10% | 30% |
| Foldable lenses | 46% | 30% | 20% |

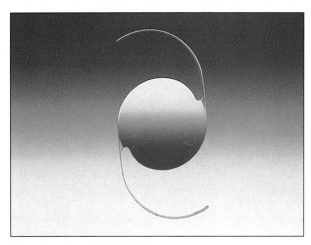

Figure 9-1. Alcon's MZ60 DB lens.

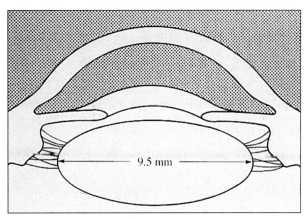

Figure 9-2. Size of the capsular bag with the human lens intact.

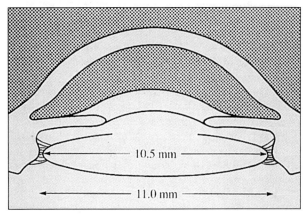

Figure 9-3. Size of the capsular bag with the anterior capsule removed.

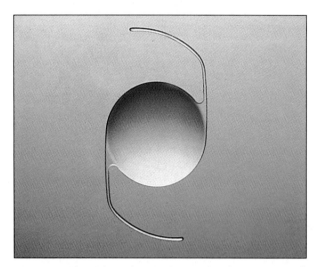

Figure 9-4. Alcon's LX90 lens (optic 5.75 mm, biconvex, overall length 12.0 mm, one-piece, no holes, loops at an angle of 5°).

Table 9-5
**FOLDABLE IOL TECHNOLOGICAL ACHIEVEMENTS**

| | |
|---|---|
| 1984 | Silicone IOL developed |
| 1984 | Hydrogel developed |
| 1990 | First silicone IOL approved by FDA |
| 1991 | First one-piece silicone IOL approved by FDA |
| 1994 | First acrylic IOL approved by FDA |

cataract extraction (ECCE). In practice they are used for primary or secondary implants particularly after ICCE, or following ECCE complicated by capsular rupture or vitreous loss.

The latter can only be used after ECCE or phacoemulsification. In very special cases, they can be used in the absence of the posterior capsule particularly as a secondary implant with scleral fixation.

## CLASSIFICATION OF THE IOL BASED ON THE LENS MATERIAL

These lenses can be split into:
- One-piece lenses—The lenses that are more avant-garde for a number of reasons are those in polymethylmethacrylate (PMMA) (there are no joints, no material that is even partially biodegradable, the manufacturing quality is good, etc). However, there can be difficulties during insertion because the flexibility and the twisting capability of the loops are still somewhat limited.
  The one-piece lenses can also be made from acrylic, silicone, Hema, etc. These foldable materials are expanding rapidly.
- Two- or three-piece lenses (or made from two different materials)—These are lenses that have an optic in PMMA or silicone, and the loops in prolene or extruded PMMA, etc.

## OTHER CLASSIFICATIONS

- The shape of the loops (open, closed, with pointed or flattened supports).
- The angulation of the loops (10, 15, or 20°).
- The diameter of the optic (5.0, 5.5, 6.0, 6.5, or 7.0 mm).
- The shape of the optic (plano-convex, convex-plano, biconvex, meniscus, round, oval, etc).
- The capacity to filter ultraviolet rays.

Without going into much detail on the construction, sterilization, shape, and size of the lenses, and without devising other classifications that could be never-ending and of little real use, cataract surgeons are generally more interested in lenses for the posterior chamber which can be:
- One-piece.
- With a biconvex optic.
- With ultraviolet protection.
- Free from orifices.
- With wide contact loops (C loop).
- With a length variable between 11.50 and 12.00 mm (lenses for the bag) and 13.00 to 13.50 mm (lenses for the sulcus).
- With an optic diameter between 5.0 to 6.5 mm (the 5.5 mm lenses are the most popular).
- With a loop angled at 10°.

Regarding the shape of the optic, the current tendency points toward biconvex lenses. Nowadays the plano-convex and the meniscus lenses are almost obsolete.

Biconvex lenses exist because they:
- Provide a very high standard of vision.
- Provide tight IOL-capsule contact at the pole of the posterior capsule, thus reducing the migration of the epithelial cells toward the center.
- Keep the capsule taut and avoid the formation of folds.
- Permit a certain amount of capsular distention which induces some degree of support of the vitreous even though it makes a subsequent laser capsulotomy more difficult.
- The shape of the disc makes penetration of the anterior and posterior chambers easier.

Multifocal lenses are continually being improved. However, they still cannot provide high standard image quality and should therefore be used in special cases only.

Lenses in acrylic, silicone, and Hema are increasingly popular and are likely to increase rapidly with the popularity of phacoemulsification and the sutureless tunnel techniques.

## IDEAL LENSES FOR THE POSTERIOR CHAMBER

The ideal lenses must provide:
- Maximum duration and tolerance over time. The material must resist for many decades in the patient's eye.
- The lens must be made from a single piece, (a one-piece). This is the most expensive and difficult part of production, but it is the only procedure that gives the lens its high standard of quality. As the

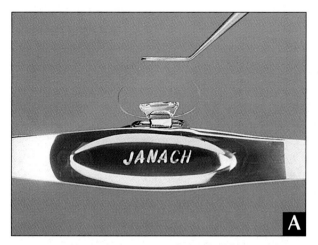
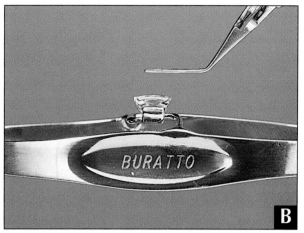

Figure 9-5A. The Cross Bow, a new device for folding soft lenses. Device for foldable lenses designed by Buratto with the silicone 920 IOL by Pharmacia folded longitudinally.

Figure 9-5B. The IOL is now folded transversally.

### Table 9-6
### COMPARISON BETWEEN FOLDABLE LENSES

| Silicone | Acrylic | Hydrogel |
|---|---|---|
| Material: silicone SLM-1, SLM2, RMX-2 | Material: acrylic/methacrylate | Material: hydrogel with water % |
| Refraction index: 1.41; 1.43; 1.46 | Refraction index: 1.48; 1.55 | Refraction index: 1.43; 1.47 |
| Hydrophobic | Hydrophobic | Hydrophobic |
| Possible damage with YAG | Possible damage with YAG | Resistant to YAG |
| Good biocompatibility | Highly biocompatible | Highly biocompatible |
| Sterilizable in autoclave | Sterilization with ethylene oxide | Sterilizable in autoclave |
| Optical resolution >100 | Optical resolution >250 | Optical resolution >170 |

### Table 9-7
### CHARACTERISTICS OF THE IDEAL FOLDABLE MATERIAL

Highly biocompatible
Easily flexed and folded
Slow and controlled unfolding
Chemically and physically stable
Mechanically resistant
100% memory
Transparent
High refractive index
Resistant to YAG laser

loops are the same material as the optic, degradation is avoided.

- The lens must be produced to the very highest standards of quality and top precision, with no physical variation due to heating, liquefaction, or distortion.
- The finish of the optic and the loops must be perfectly smooth.
- The loops must be flexible, resistant, and have a memory. The loops in one-piece lenses have an excellent memory. Prolene is being abandoned because it is subject to decay—admittedly in the long-term. The lenses are sometimes found to be irregular at the loop attachment point
- Sterilization must be dry and there must not be any ethylene oxide residue on the lens surface as these could provoke intraocular reactions.
- The optic must act as a filter for ultraviolet light.
- The optic must be a biconvex shape like the natural lens as this provides excellent image quality.
- The optic must be large enough to cover the entire pupillary area even in conditions of photopic light. With the current lens implantation techniques, the more interesting lenses measure 5.5 mm for the bag and 6.0 mm for the sulcus.
- The total length must be 11.50 to 12.00 mm for the bag implants and between 13.0 to 13.5 mm for the sulcus implants.

## GENERAL RULES FOR THE CORRECT INSERTION OF A POSTERIOR CHAMBER IOL

Always use a VES. It prepares the eye for a correct implant, it simplifies the procedure, it makes the whole operation safer and faster, it reduces complications, and it allows the surgeon to place the IOL in the desired position.

### Table 9-8
### COMPARISON BETWEEN ACRYLIC AND SILICONE LENSES

| Acrylic | Silicone |
|---|---|
| Greater refractive index and therefore thinner for equal dioptric power; an AcrySof MA60 lens of 21 D is 0.75 mm thick. | A 21 D silicone lens is 1.82 mm thick while PMMA is 0.93 mm and Hema is 1.27 mm. |
| Controlled folding and unfolding. | Difficult to fold the lens accurately. Difficult to open the lens gradually when it is inside the eye. |
| Excellent control of folding and unfolding. | Poor control of folding and unfolding in particular. |
| Smaller incision. | As the silicone is thicker, the incision must be larger. |
| Excellent optical transparency. | The transparency of the new silicone lenses is very close to that of the acrylic lenses. |
| Excellent mechanical stability. | The silicone lens is more elastic and will tend to move rapidly under even modest pressure. |
| Easy to manipulate. | As the lens is elastic, it tends to escape; the surgeon should use forceps with a strong hold to prevent the lens escape from the arms of the forceps. |
| Can be manipulated even under BSS or VES. | When the silicone lens is damp, it is no longer controllable. |

### Table 9-9
### DISADVANTAGES OF SILICONE LENSES

Insertion system poses some problems
Low refractive index
Stretching and damage to the incision
Prolene or PMMA loops (three pieces)
Uncontrolled unfolding
Hydrophobic
Decentering and tilt
Damage with YAG
Discoloration
Expensive

### Table 9-10
### INSERTION OF THE FOLDABLE LENSES WITH THE INJECTOR

This procedure is suitable particularly with the one-piece lenses.

#### Technique
Apply of VES in the open arms of the cartridge and inside the channel.
Position the lens in the cartridge, taking care to insert both sides into the grooves.
Close the cartridge.
Place the cartridge in the injector.
Insertion of the end part of the cartridge in the incision and then just underneath the distal limits of the rhexis.
Tighten the screws of the injector until the lens starts to come out.
When the lens starts to come out, and the surgeon is certain that the direction is correct, ie, that it enters the bag. The surgeon retracts the injector slightly just before the lens exits completely.
Complete the tightening to position the end part of the lens in the proximal bag.

#### Pros
Insertion through a very small incision.

#### Cons
The lens may be badly damaged through the loading and unloading movements in the injector.
If the injector is used with lenses fitted with open loops; the loops and/or the lens can be damaged.
VES is consumed in the cartridge.
Each lens model requires a different injector.
Poor quality finish of the cartridge.
Stretching of the incision edges with the injector.
Poor control of how the lens exits from the cartridge.

The anterior chamber must be well-formed, but above all the capsular bag must be deep enough to allow the loop and the optic to reach their destination easily. This will avoid damage to the posterior capsule and the other structures. The depth of the bag is particularly important for foldable IOLs. The depth can be maintained only by using a high molecular weight VES.

Avoid damaging the tissue during insertion, in particular avoid:
- Detaching Descemet's membrane.
- Touching the endothelium.
- Damaging the iris.
- Rupturing the posterior capsule.
- Lacerating the rhexis.
- Lacerating the zonular fibers.

The surgeon should perform all the intraocular maneuvers with precision, gentleness, and caution.

During the operating steps prior to the implant, avoid every maneuver that may reduce mydriasis. For a simple insertion the pupil must be wide. This gives the surgeon a clear view of the posterior capsule and the flap of the anterior chamber.

### Table 9-11
### INSERTION TECHNIQUE FOR FOLDABLE IOLS WITH OPEN LOOPS

Two forceps are necessary:
- One to fold the lens.
- One to insert it.

Two basic techniques are currently used:
1. Longitudinal insertion:
   - With rotation of the internal loop.
   - With rotation of the external loop.
2. Transverse insertion.

### Table 9-12
### LONGITUDINAL TECHNIQUE FOR THE THREE-PIECE FOLDABLE IOL

Carefully put the lens in the folder so that the loops are along the greatest axis of the instrument.

Carefully control the exact, symmetrical position of the IOL and then fold the lens.

Catch the lens using the insertion forceps not halfway but slightly closer to the folded part of the lens; the proximal loop must stay between the arms of the forceps.

At this point, the surgeon can proceed in one of two ways:

1. Insert the loop with the closed part on the left. In this case, when the lens unfolds, there is rotation through 90° of the external loop (the simpler technique).

2. Insert the lens with the folded part (the closed part) on the right. In this case, when the lens unfolds, there is rotation through 90° of the loop inside the bag but the external loop does not rotate.

Raise of the edge of the incision.

Insert of the lens horizontally, taking care not to damage the loops.

Insert of the distal loop into the bag.

Rotate through 90° of the forceps and the lens so that the folded part of the lens ends up towards the corneal dome.

Open the forceps and the lens. The lens opens slowly or rapidly depending on the material of the IOL and VES present in the capsular bag. There is rotation of the external loop if the lens is inserted with the closed part on the left.

Insert the spatula through the side port incision and depress of the optic disc toward the capsular bag while a McPherson forceps catches the proximal loop, introduces it in the incision, into the anterior chamber, and finally into the bag.

The distal loop can be folded inside the optical disc prior to insertion (tucking of the loop). This may facilitate the insertion because the loop is one with the optical disc and not free in the chamber or in the bag.

### Table 9-13
### ACRYSOF MA60

The only material with a refractive index superior to that of PMMA (1.49)

The only non-silicone lens approved by the FDA

Controlled folding and unfolding

6.0 mm optic disc (5.5 for the MA30)

Loops in PMMA

The lowest percentage of YAG capsulotomies reported

Low postoperative count of cells free in the chamber (low *flare*)

### Table 9-14
### SOME ADVICE FOR CORRECT INSERTION OF THE ACRYSOF MA60

At the beginning, use a 4.1 mm incision.

Once the surgeon is more experienced, he or she can use a smaller incision (3.6-3.8 mm) depending on the power of the lens and the type of the incision.

Avoid forcing the lens through the incision.

Use longitudinal insertion.

Do not fold the loop inside the optic disc (tucking).

Prepare a well-formed bag and chamber with suitable VES.

Handle the lens and the loop with extreme care.

Treat all the instruments which come into contact with the IOL with U/S before sterilization.

Always use clean instruments.

Fold the lens symmetrically.

The lens does not require excessive pressure from the insertion forceps to remain folded.

Always aspirate all the VES from the anterior chamber and the capsular bag.

### Table 9-15
### REFRACTIVE INDEX OF THE IOLS

| | |
|---|---|
| AcrySof (Alcon) | 1.55 |
| PMMA (various companies) | 1.49 |
| Acrylens (Ioptex) | 1.47 |
| Memory lens (ORC) | 1.47 |
| Silicone (various companies) | 1.41-1.46 |
| HydroSof (Alcon) | 14.3 |
| Hydroview (Storz) | 1.47 |

The surgeon must take care to choose the lens with the right dimensions for that particular eye. For example, the surgeon should avoid inserting a 12 mm lens in the sulcus or a 13.50 to 14.00 mm lens in the bag of a patient affected by microphthalmus.

In the event of the implantation of a hard lens use an incision that is just slightly larger than the diameter of the IOL. In the event of a foldable IOL, use a minimal incision which will allow easy implantation. Avoid excessive pressure on the incision.

The IOL must be manipulated and inserted in such a way as to avoid scratching or other damage to the optical

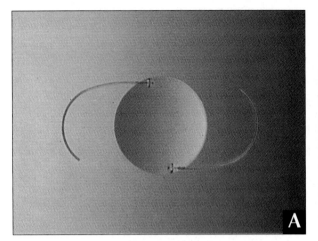

Figure 9-6A. Alcon's AcrySof MA60 IOL.

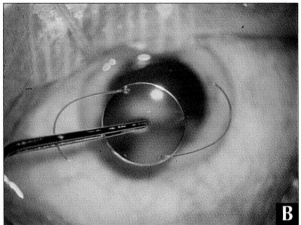

Figure 9-6B. The IOL is caught with blunt forceps.

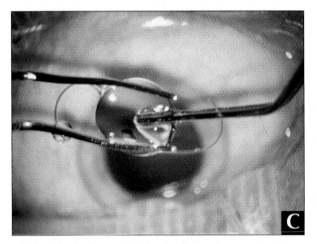

Figure 9-6C. The IOL is folded with insertion forceps.

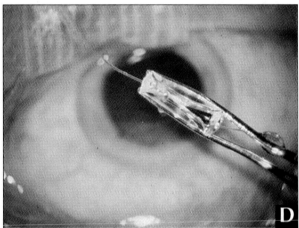

Figure 9-6D. The folding can be observed.

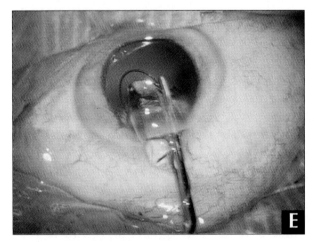

Figure 9-6E. The IOL is entering with the folded part toward the left. The loop still has to enter the bag.

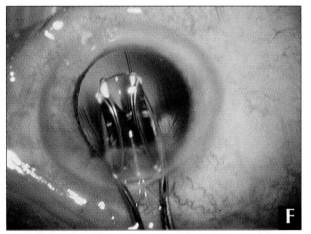

Figure 9-6F. The loop is in the bag and lens can be slowly unfolded outside the bag.

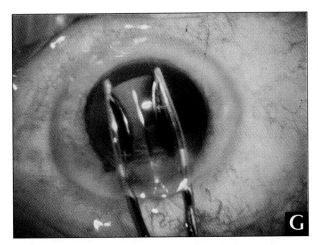

Figure 9-6G. The IOL is almost completely unfolded.

lens or the loops. The surgeon should use forceps, spatulas, and hooks that have been specially designed for this purpose.

Place both loops in the bag or both in the sulcus. Avoid a mixed insertion, as this will encourage decentering of the optic and the lens in general. Once the insertion has been completed, ensure that the optic is well-centered and that the loops have been positioned symmetrically.

## PMMA IOLS

Despite the fact that the interest of the surgeons, the patients, and the manufacturers is increasingly focused on foldable lenses, many surgeons still use PMMA in practice. This is because it can guarantee more than 20 years of excellent tolerance but it is also easy to manipulate and insert. Another factor that should not be underestimated is the low cost of these lenses.

They can be inserted easily following phacoemulsification or ECCE, in the bag or in the sulcus. They can be one-piece or three-piece. The current trend is to insert them in the bag following capsulorhexis and phacoemulsification through a tunnel incision. However, a VES must be used to reduce ocular trauma and make the procedure easier.

### Bag or Sulcus

The vast majority of surgeons agree that the capsular bag is the optimal site for implanting the IOL. This is because there is:
- Internal isolation of the IOL—The lens remains completely isolated within the eye. The loops rest on the capsular equator and do not come into contact with blood vessels, nerves, or other structures. So, they cannot alter the physiology of the eye or be responsible for complications even long-term. Only the optic, under particular conditions, can come into contact with the posterior surface of the iris. However, there is no friction between the two surfaces and no secondary effects will result.
- An IOL can be safely inserted in the bag of young

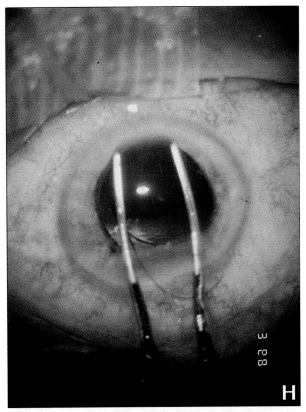

Figure 9-6H. The IOL is now open and has entered the bag.

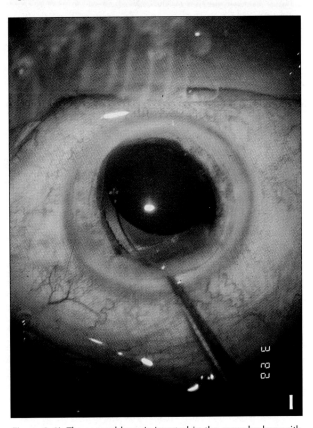

Figure 9-6I. The second loop is inserted in the capsular bag with forceps.

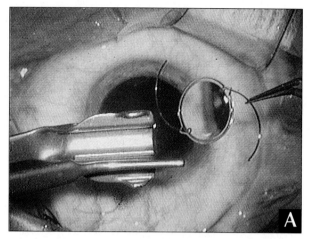

Figure 9-7A. Technique for folding and insertion of Allergan's SI40 IOL. Three-point contact folder designed by Christophe Buratto, and Allergan's SI40 IOL.

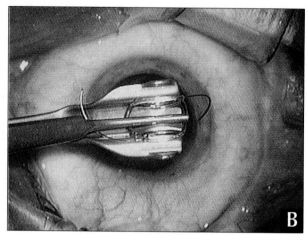

Figure 9-7B. The lens is turned over on the folder.

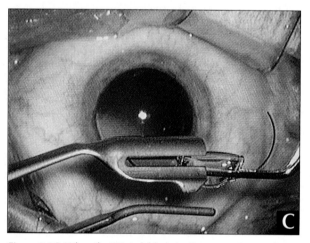

Figure 9-7C. When the IOL is folded, the instrument is turned over and the IOL is removed with insertion forceps.

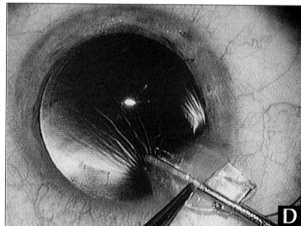

Figure 9-7D. The IOL is introduced into the incision.

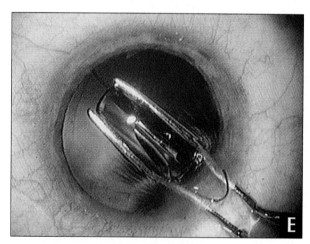

Figure 9-7E. The loop then enters the bag.

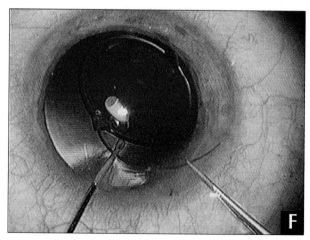

Figure 9-7F. After the lens has been opened, the second loop is positioned inside the bag.

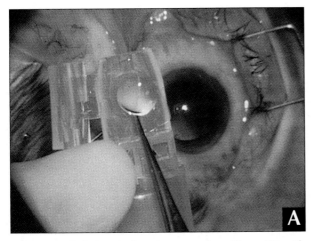

Figure 9-8A. Technique for inserting a one-piece silicone IOL with Chiron's Passport Injector. Chiron's one-piece silicone IOL is already on the surface of the cartridge.

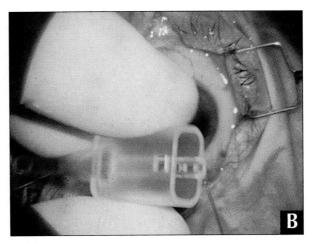

Figure 9-8B. The end of the device is coated in VES.

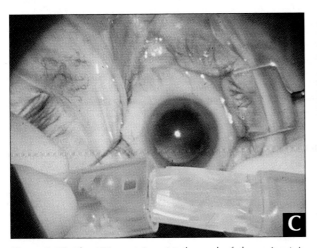

Figure 9-8C. The IOL container (at the end of the syringe) is applied to the device, the end of which will enter the eye.

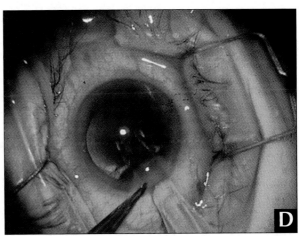

Figure 9-8D. The haptics can be seen inside the incision.

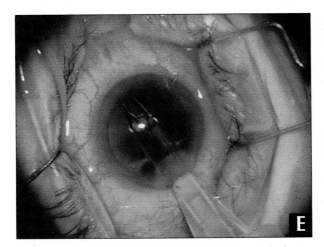

Figure 9-8E. The IOL is starting to open inside the capsular bag.

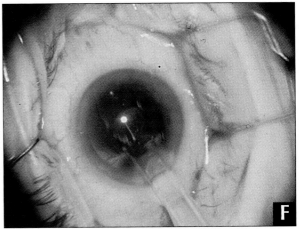

Figure 9-8F. The IOL is almost completely opened and is ready to enter the capsular bag completely.

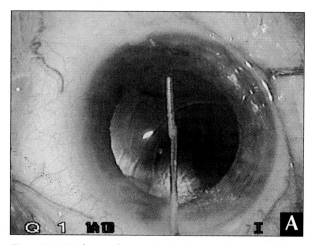

Figure 9-9A. Technique for inserting the Storz Hydroview lens. The anterior chamber and the capsular bag are formed with VES.

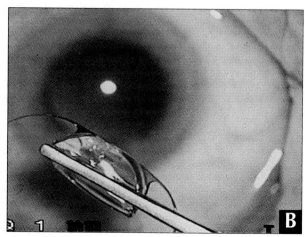

Figure 9-9B. The IOL has already been folded by insertion forceps.

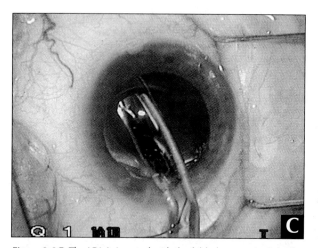

Figure 9-9C. The IOL is inserted with the folded part to the left. The distal loop is introduced to the capsular bag; the optic disc is outside the capsular bag.

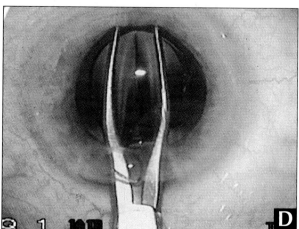

Figure 9-9D. The lens is unfolded.

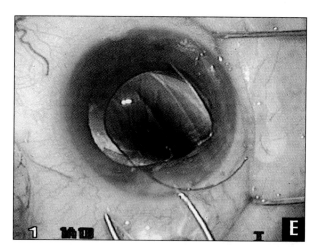

Figure 9-9E. The second loop is caught with forceps and gently guided inside the capsular bag.

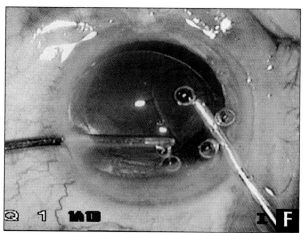

Figure 9-9F. The surgeon must carefully remove all the VES from the anterior chamber and from the capsular bag.

patients, in eyes with glaucoma or other pathologies of the anterior segment (excluding chronic uveitis and rubeosis of the iris).
- External isolation of the IOL—The lens supports rest on the capsular equator and as this is separated from the external tunic of the eye. The endocapsular lens is protected from the continual micro and macro stresses that constantly affect the eye (rubbing, contact during sleep, etc).
- Inhibition of capsular opacity—Numerous studies have shown that capsular opacity through proliferation of germinal cells is less frequent when the optic adheres to the posterior capsule and when the peripheral remnants of the anterior capsule, adhering to the posterior capsule, create a mechanical barrier to the progression of the cells toward the center of the capsule.
- Insertion in the bag using IOLs with wide loops and suitable sizes (total length 12.0 to 12.5 mm)—This involves an optimal adaptation of the lens to the capsular bag. This allows a uniform distribution of the forces on the equator and reduces or avoids variations on the zonules and maintains the capsule uniformly distended thus avoiding the formation of capsular folds.

The endocapsular fixation of the IOL offers better results in the short- and the long-term. It has one drawback. It involves a reduced-size capsulotomy so a significant portion of the anterior capsule stays in its original position. It may cause some problems in the postoperative period and hinder the observation of the peripheral retina.

## IOLS IN PMMA: INSERTION TECHNIQUES IN THE CAPSULAR BAG

Two conditions allow the safe insertion of an IOL in the capsular bag:
1. The presence of an intact rhexis. This capsulotomy allows the preparation of a capsular bag that is sufficiently snug to suitably contain the IOL and to prevent the loops from escaping.
2. The availability of a VES that can maintain the shape of the capsular bag.

---

Table 9-16

### TRANSVERSE INSERTION OF ACRYSOF MA60

Prepare the eye by injecting Provisc in the anterior chamber and inside the capsular bag until the posterior capsule is well stretched.

Position the lens on the folder so that both loops are placed transversely.

Be sure that the lens borders are perfectly positioned inside the folder; check also that the lens is well centered and the loops are placed symmetrically.

Fold the lens.

Grasp it with the insertion forceps in the third-fourth closest to the folded part (dividing half of the lens in four parts).

Lay both loops in the opening and then rotate the forceps and the lens 90°, making the loop enter in the incision and simultaneously the lens.

Insert the IOL in the incision with the folded part either on the right or the left. If the loop opens toward the chamber pass inside the tunnel with no obstacles, it must appear immediately in the anterior chamber.

Rotate forceps and lens 90° so that the folded part of the IOL is turned towards the cornea.

Be sure that both loops go inside the rhexis, lowering lens and forceps toward the posterior capsule.

Open the forceps slowly and check that the loops open correctly and the lens is positioned in the bag.

With an IOL hook, check whether the optic disc is inside the rhexis and both loops are in the bag.

Suggested instruments:
　Folder by Asico.
　Insertion forceps by Asico.

---

What follows is a description of the insertion of a one-piece lens with a 5.25 mm optic and loops angled at 5°, overall length of 12.00 mm, biconvex LX10 BD by Alcon Surgical. The technique can be used for any other type of lens with similar features. The incision should be about 5.50 mm. In this case, a direct limbal incision was done.

The insertion allows the capsular bag to be filled with Provisc. This product keeps the anterior capsule separate from the posterior capsule and allows the loop to pass

---

Table 9-17

### PROS AND CONS OF TRANSVERSE AND LONGITUDINAL TECHNIQUES

| Longitudinal technique | Transversal technique |
|---|---|
| **Pros** | **Pro** |
| Easy insertion | IOL insertion with one maneuver only |
| Good control of folding, insertion, and unfolding | Good control of folding and unfolding |
| **Cons** | **Cons** |
| Some difficulty with folding and gripping with the insertion forceps | Difficult insertion through the incision |
| Some difficulty in rotating the loop (outside or inside, according to the planned procedure) | Stronger likelihood of loop damage |
| | More difficult positioning of the optic disc in the anterior chamber |
| | Difficult to insert both loops inside the rhexis |
| | Higher risk of either posterior capsule and/or rhexis rupture |
| | More likely to result in endothelial damage |

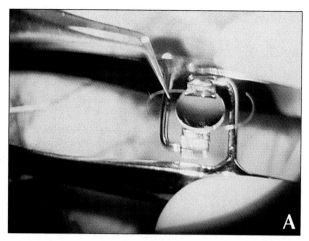

Figure 9-10A. AcrySof IOL folded with the Cross Bow and the longitudinal insertion technique. The IOL is placed longitudinally between the arms of the Janach-Buratto device.

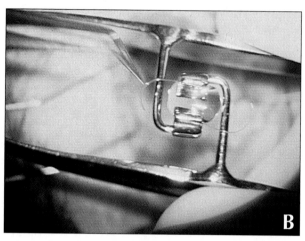

Figure 9-10B. Folding is started and is then completed correctly.

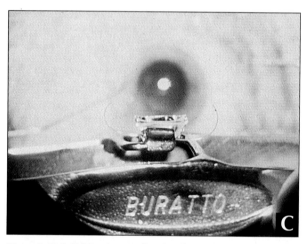

Figure 9-10C. Folding is started and is then completed correctly.

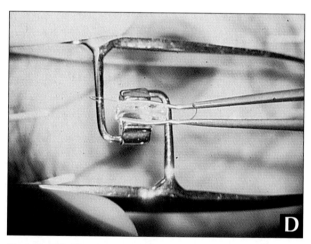

Figure 9-10D. The IOL is caught with Buratto insertion forceps and introduced to the incision with the folded part to the left.

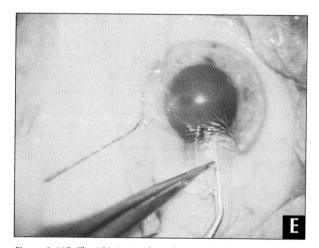

Figure 9-10E. The IOL is caught with insertion forceps and introduced to the incision with the folded part to the left.

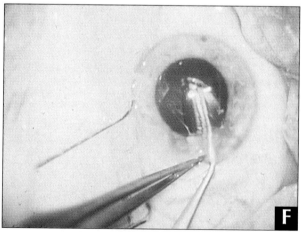

Figure 9-10F. The distal loop is introduced in the capsular bag.

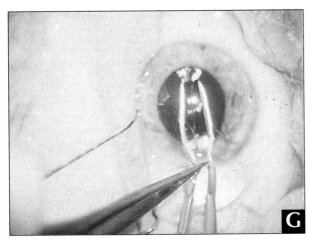

Figure 9-10G. The IOL and the forceps are rotated through 90° so that the folded part of the IOL is directed toward the corneal dome.

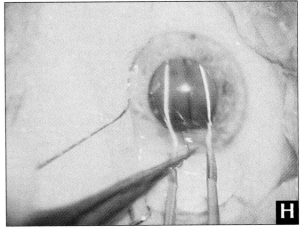

Figure 9-10H. The forceps is opened, allowing the IOL to open gently and under perfect control.

between the two capsular flaps. The product is then injected in the anterior chamber to prevent contact of the IOL with the endothelium and to keep the eye well-formed.

The lens is grasped with a lens-forceps, close to where the loop is attached. The first loop is then introduced into the incision, penetrating the anterior chamber at an angle of about 45° to enter directly under the inferior flap of the anterior capsule. The optic then slowly penetrates the anterior chamber under steady progressive pressure directing the inferior loop toward the equator of the capsular bag. The disc then enters the posterior chamber and passes under the iris.

A McPherson forceps is used to position the superior loop. The forceps catches the loop distally in order to take advantage of its elasticity and it enters the anterior chamber, beyond the superior limits of the optic of the lens. The hand holding the forceps is pronated slightly to produce moderate torsion of the loop so that when it is released, just under the superior border of the anterior capsule, it positions itself correctly inside the bag.

The lens is therefore positioned with both loops inside the capsular bag. The surgeon then controls if the lens is centered correctly and whether it is really located inside the bag.

## Alternative Technique to Implant a One-Piece PMMA IOL in the Bag

The surgeon chose a one-piece biconvex lens with an optic of 5.5 mm and an overall length of 12.0 mm, angled at 5° (Alcon MZ30 BD). The incision in this case is a scleral tunnel. The chamber and the bag are well-formed using Provisc. Some product is also injected into the tunnel to help the lens slide in. As an alternative to the total filling of the chamber and the bag, the surgeon can choose the technique of visco glide. In this case the bag is only filled distally while in the superior and lateral portions it is only marginally shaped. The chamber is moderately shaped.

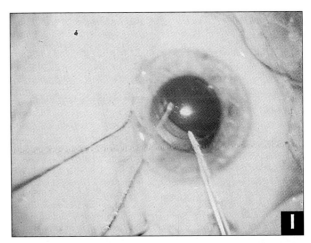

Figure 9-10I. The second loop is positioned inside the capsular bag.

The lens is grasped with Buratto's universal lens-holding forceps (Asico) which is introduced to the tunnel. Because of the shape of the tunnel the distal loop tends to move toward the internal apex of the cornea. A spatula must be introduced through the side port incision to push the loop and the optic toward the capsular bag. When the first loop and the optic are inside the bag the second loop is introduced into the tunnel with a Kelman-McPherson long-armed forceps and then positioned inside the bag.

In this case, the proximal portion of the rhexis and the viscoelastic deposited on it act as a glide which helps position the IOL.

## Technique for Inserting a PMMA Lens in the Sulcus

Following a wide can opener capsulotomy or when the rhexis has opened and is not suitable for safe IOL implantation, the IOL should be inserted with the loops in the ciliary sulcus. The posterior chamber IOL that should be used in this case is biconvex with C loop and loops at a 10° angle, an optic of 6.0 mm with no holes, an

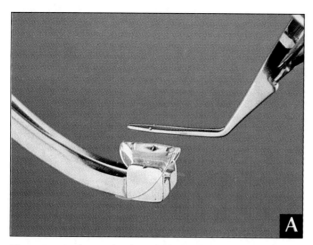

Figure 9-11A. The IOL has been folded with the Asico self-folding forceps.

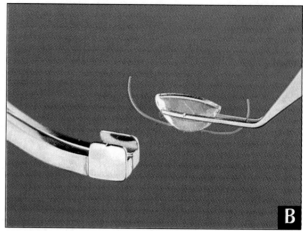

Figure 9-11B. The IOL is removed from the forceps and is ready for insertion.

overall length of 13.5 mm, and an angulation of the loop of 5° (Alcon MC60 BD).

The VES facilitates the insertion, allowing the IOL to be positioned in the sulcus with the certainty that the positioning of the loops is correct. This is a considerable help particularly for the operator who is performing the very first operations of implantology.

In order to prepare the anterior segment for the implant of the IOL, the Provisc cannula is introduced into the right lateral sector of the anterior chamber or distally and the VES is injected to deepen the anterior chamber while the liquid in the chamber is allowed to escape. The cannula is then inserted under the iris in front of the remaining portion of the anterior capsule and some more product is injected. This way, the anterior capsule adheres to the posterior and an adequately large space is created between the posterior face of the iris and the two attached capsules. If one proceeds this way around the entire 360° of the posterior chamber, an ample space is created for the safe insertion of the lens in the sulcus. The optic is grasped with Buratto's lens-holding forceps (or other similar instrument) close to the insertion point of the superior loop keeping the open part of the loop toward the right. With Bonn forceps held in the left hand, the operator raises the anterior edge of the incision very slightly (tenths of millimeters) and the inferior loop is inserted through a scleral corneal opening and then into the anterior chamber. During these maneuvers, all contact with the endothelium should be avoided.

The loop is then pushed under the iris at the 6 o'clock position.

The curved part of the distal loop will now be more or less on a plane parallel with the iris and the posterior capsule. The surgeon must raise the more distal part of the loop to come almost in contact with the posterior face of the iris. In order to do this, the surgeon must push gently downward toward the proximal part of the lens disc. This way, the loop will position itself in the sulcus.

At this point the surgeon should let go of the lens-holding forceps with his or her right hand and, using an angled McPherson forceps, he or she should catch the curved part of the superior loop and bring it just inside the incision. The surgeon continues gently under the iris bending the loop toward the optic with a movement of rotation-pronation to lower the portion of the optic close to the insertion of the loop and assist the passage of the loop under the iris.

The lens is then centered and rotated clockwise with a Sinskey-type hook, placing the two loops horizontally. The correct position of the lens is evaluated by performing suitable control tests. The incision is then closed with one or more sutures.

## FOLDABLE LENSES

The possibility of inserting IOLs through an incision the same size as those used to introduce the ultrasound (U/S) and irrigation/aspiration (I/A) tips, and therefore maintain the advantages of a smaller amount of surface cut and fewer modifications induced to the cornea, has opened a new chapter in the story of implantation of IOLs in phacoemulsification.

The limitations applied to hard lenses have always been necessitated by the need to have a sufficiently large optic to avoid refraction, glare, or ghost images. The minimum diameter is 5.0 mm. It nevertheless requires the extension of the incision performed for the phacoemulsification (on average 5.2 mm). The attention has shifted to foldable lenses which allow the use of smaller incisions.

The first to be introduced were silicone lenses. The one-piece models normally involve the use of an injector that contains the folded lens. The injector is introduced into the incision and the lens is pushed out by a piston or an adjustable screw. With this system, the incision can be limited to 3.0 mm to 3.4 mm.

The biggest problem is the fact that the lens sometimes unfolds somewhat abruptly in the anterior-posterior chamber and this does not always allow good control of the maneuver and suitable positioning.

It is also important to consider that the one-piece plate-haptic models, which are the more common, do not have fixing loops. This raises some questions about the long-term position, particularly after a posterior capsulotomy.

The latest generation of silicone lenses has morphological features which are superimposable on the traditional lenses, with an optic and fixing loops. The lens is folded using special forceps or a specific device (a three-piece may also be injected)—a folder—and then fixed and inserted with a special forceps with crossed arms. In order for this maneuver of folding and fixing to be successful, the lens must be dry and accurately positioned on the support.

If these conditions are satisfied, the lens can be inserted through an incision of 3.4 to 3.8 mm. It is then opened in the anterior chamber by releasing the forceps after having inserted the inferior loop under the capsulorhexis (in exactly the same way as a traditional lens). The superior loop is then inserted in the normal fashion.

If the maneuver is smooth and delicate and if the chamber and the bag are formed with high molecular weight viscoelastic, the lens will unfold gently. Nevertheless, if the surgeon is inexperienced or the insertion forceps are not suitable or are used incorrectly, the lens may unfold suddenly causing capsular lacerations or damage to the endothelium.

The three-piece silicone lenses, as with the one-piece, have various problems. In addition to the thickness and the difficulty in maintaining the physiologic-optical characteristics of the loop material long-term, the surgeon must also ensure that the intraoperative characteristics of the implant are maintained long-term (ie, that the centering and the positioning of the optic will not change with possible retractions of the capsular bag [adhesions, fibrosis, opacity]).

An alternative to the silicone lenses is currently offered by the foldable acrylic lenses (AcrySof, Alcon), made from PMMA with a modified polymeric structure. Originally the material was heat-sensitive, (ie, it had to be heated to be folded). Now the problem of foldability has been resolved with the development of new materials and is no longer dependent on the temperature.

The lens looks like a traditional model; it has an optic and open modified C-shape fixation loop with an elevated refractive index—it is thinner, for equal diameter and dioptric power, than any other lens. The lens can be wet without changing its easy-to-handle features. It is easily folded using simple forceps. Once the lens has been folded, it enters the anterior chamber through a 3.2 to 4.0 mm incision (depending on the diameter and power of the optic) sliding the inferior loop under the capsulorhexis and at the same time releasing the forceps to allow the lens to open in the capsular bag. The superior loop is placed under the capsulorhexis in the usual manner.

With AcrySof, the maneuver is delicate and the lens opens slowly and gradually. The foldable acrylic lenses with a traditional design, ie, with an optic and open fixation loops, are easily positioned and remain well-centered long term.

At the time of this printing, the acrylic lenses are the main option for the best results without having to extend the incision of the phacoemulsification.

For further details on the techniques of implantation of foldable IOLs, please refer to the chapters that deal specifically with this subject.

# Chapter 10

# SUTURES
*Lucio Buratto, MD*

## INTRODUCTION

Modern cataract surgery using phacoemulsification and the implantation of a foldable intraocular lens (IOL) through a scleral or corneal tunnel does not require the application of sutures in the vast majority of cases.

If one starts from the assumption that not all surgeons are capable of performing these procedures and some cases will be treated with classical techniques, this chapter will cover the placement of sutures.

Generally speaking a suture must have the following objectives:
- It must bring the two edges of the incision together in their original position with no superimposition of the tissues and no horizontal displacements.
- It must be aqueous proof (ie, it must completely seal the wound and prevent abnormal filtrations which may give rise to complications such as hypotony, prolapse of the iris, and formation of a conjunctival bleb).
- It must allow the patient to enjoy a rapid recovery of everyday functions. The suture must be strong enough and placed in a suitable position to allow the patient to undertake moderate physical exertion.
- It must avoid the onset of irritating astigmatism, particularly against-the-rule astigmatism which is difficult to correct. With-the-rule astigmatism is acceptable when temporary. This means it has a low value, which lasts a short time, and if possible, it can be reduced in the postoperative period by selective removal of some of the sutures.

Nylon suture thread is used in cataract surgery for the following reasons:
- It is strong. It can therefore be tightened as needed. It has an excellent immediate hold allowing the incision to be closed permanently.
- It is elastic. This allows the edges to be brought close together with slight relaxation of the sutures in the postoperative period. This property allows the surgeon to adjust the tension to the needs of each individual case.
- It is a single filament. The thickness is therefore homogeneous, regular, and uniform.
- It is easy to handle and is ductile.
- It can be used even in minimal thicknesses.
- It is smooth and totally compatible with the surrounding tissues, sliding through the transition canal very easily.
- Tolerance is excellent and reabsorption is very slow. It does not interfere with the normal healing processes.
- It is thin. It does not produce a foreign body sensation or occupy a lot of space in the operated area.
- The suture knots are tiny and are embedded easily. This prevents the onset of local irritations which can induce pain, a foreign body sensation, and itching.
- It can be cut easily through the conjunctiva even using a laser beam. This reduces postoperative astigmatism without any manipulations taking place in the surgical zone.
- It is mounted on thin needles so the entrance and exit orifices are small resulting in a low possibility of postoperative filtration.
- The nylon suture thread completely fills the transition channel left by the needle (which is very similar in size to the thread).
- It can be used for all types of incisions—scleral, limbal, corneal, tunnel or not, for either interrupted or continuous sutures.

However, nylon also has some disadvantages:
- It tends to stick to the instruments and to the tissue, particularly if the operating field is damp.

- It does not always do exactly what the surgeon wants it to do.
- If it is pulled too tight, it tends to lose its elasticity and get tangled, losing the original characteristics of resistance.

Nylon must be mounted on a good microsurgery needle which must:
- Be resistant. It shouldn't break under the forces in the tissue that oppose the sutures. It must not change during the entire suture process.
- Produce as little friction as possible.
- Have a high penetrating capacity, which depends on how sharp it is, its curvature, and which metal is used.
- Be elastic to support the surgeon's action.
- Be atraumatic, which depends on the thickness and the shape.

The point is the most important part and it plays a role of considerable importance in the type of trauma caused to the tissue. For cataract surgery, the spatulate form is the best.

## INTERRUPTED SUTURES

With interrupted nylon 10-0 sutures:
- The sutures must be equidistant. In order to perform a regular suture, the surgeon can use some simple aids. Mark the reference points with sterile methylene blue when preparing the incision. Apply provisional sutures prior to placing the final suture. Introduce a large air bubble into the anterior chamber and then apply the first suture exactly halfway along the incision. Then others on the two sides and so on, being careful to avoid any asymmetry. The observation and the control of the incision are improved by the air bubble in the chamber.
- The sutures must be radial to provide a uniform distribution of the traction forces over the entire cornea and to reestablish the original geometry of the anterior segment. All the sutures applied must produce forces that converge toward the center of the cornea.
- The sutures must be under the same tension. They must have a uniform closure tension.
- The sutures must be tightened with the same degree of tension to ensure the exact same closure of the two sides of the incision. The air bubble in the anterior chamber will show if the suture is very tight through the formation of corneal folds. If the sutures are too tight, not only will they cause severe astigmatism to develop, they can also squeeze the edges causing the appearance of localized folds and poor adhesion of the deeper portions of the incision. There is also the possibility of filtration. If the suture is too loose, aqueous humor will filter from the anterior chamber. It also causes against-the-rule astigmatism to develop which is difficult to correct. Healing times are prolonged.
- The sutures must be placed at the same depth in the tissue.
- The hold on the tissue must be adequate. It must not be too near the edge or superficial otherwise the suture will erode through the tissue and the closure will be insufficient. However it should not go in too deeply either or it will perforate the interested tissue and adhesion of the two edges will be poor. The ideal depth is three-fourths of the tissue depth.
- The length of the suture must be suitable. The suture must not be placed too far forward on the anterior edge or too far backward on the posterior edge. A distance of about 0.50 mm on the anterior edge and 0.75 mm on the posterior edge should be correct.
- The suture should be applied with the globe as close to the physiological volume as possible so that the edges will be brought together as precisely as possible. If the suture is knotted with a chamber that is too deep, sealing will be abnormal when the bulb is restored to its physiological shape. If it is knotted with a shallow chamber, the sutures will be too tight and cause severe astigmatism.
- The number of sutures must be proportional to the size of the incision. Generally speaking, the larger the incision, the greater the number of sutures. Nevertheless, a few correctly placed sutures can close the wound better than a larger number of sutures that are applied incorrectly.
- The knots should always be embedded to prevent the patient from having a foreign body sensation and to avoid irritating the surrounding tissues.
- The sutures should be applied under moderate-high microscopic magnification. Perfect vision of the incision is the only route to perfect suturing. All the details, (ie, the depth the needle penetrates, the exit point, the position, the manner in which the edges are brought together during and after the knot, how the knots are closed, how the edges react once the suture has been completed, etc) can be observed better with a good level of illumination and magnification.

Once suturing has been completed, it is useful for the surgeon to control the situation by keratoscopic examination. When the surgeon has gained greater experience this examination will allow him or her to identify sutures that are too tight or whether the astigmatism is excessive. Whether it is with- or against-the-rule, oblique, etc.

## CONTINUOUS SUTURES

A continuous suture has the advantage of providing good distribution of the lines of tension while simultaneously reducing the number of knots. It can be applied in a number of ways:
- Simple—The suture begins at one end of the incision and finishes at the other.
- Return—The suture passes over the incision twice. The overcast can also be:
- Perpendicular to the incision—The needle passes obliquely through the tissue and returns to the first

edge in correspondence with the previous exit point (ie, radially to it). It passes through the tissue obliquely.
- Isosceles—The needle passes obliquely through the deeper planes and does not penetrate perpendicularly but equidistant from the exit point in relation to the entrance point.
- Oblique—The needle passes through the deep planes perpendicular to the suture line.

The ideal suture is oblique because it does not cause lateral displacement of the incision edge. It also exerts uniform compression and homogeneous sealing along the entire length of the incision.

### Rules of Continuous Sutures
- The transition of the suture must be regular; the entrance and exit points must be at uniform intervals from each other.
- The needle must catch an equal amount of tissue at the right depth on both the scleral and corneal edges.
- Every transition of the suture must have the same geometrical shape.
- Each stitch must have the correct same tension (the surgeon should avoid having parts that are tighter or looser).
- The knot should be embedded in the tissue. This will avoid any local irritation and the annoying sensation of a foreign body in the eye.

## TO SUTURE SCLERAL TUNNEL OR NOT TO SUTURE

A scleral tunnel incision with the right length, width, and shape will close spontaneously at the end of the operation. However, the surgeon should always apply one or more sutures if he or she has any doubts about its self-sealing capacity or the postoperative behavior of the astigmatism.

In these cases, the classical continuous shoelace sutures or interrupted radial sutures are not advisable because they change the relationship between the tissues inside the tunnel thus reducing the advantages this method supplies. They also induce excessive astigmatism.

In tunnel incisions, scleral in particular, the use of horizontal sutures is preferable. These involve suturing the superficial part of the incision (roof) to the deep part (floor) in a transverse manner, eliminating or reducing the radial traction. The horizontal sutures are used to bring the tissues into contact with each other without compressing the wound and avoiding or reducing the appearance of with-the-rule astigmatism, a transitory phenomenon that normally appears with radial sutures (if the incision is superior).

However, if the scleral incision (greater than 4.0 mm) is placed less than 2.0 mm from the insertion of the conjunctiva, a suture will be necessary. In this case, as the tunnel is short, radial interrupted sutures in 10-0 nylon

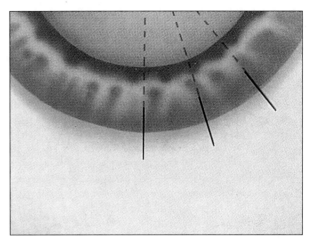

Figure 10-1. Radial placement of interrupted sutures which are also equidistant.

(Alcon CU1) are still preferable.

If the incision (greater than 4.0 mm) is placed at a distance greater than 2.0 mm behind the cornea-conjunctiva attachment point, the surgeon should check whether the aperture is self-sealing. If there are any doubts, he or she should apply a horizontal suture.

If the incision is placed 3.0 mm or more posterior to the limbus, sutures are usually not necessary and the decision of whether to apply one or not depends largely on how well the incision holds.

In order to do this, the surgeon injects balanced salt solution (BSS) through the side port incision to bring the globe to a pressure similar to physiological values or slightly higher (20 to 25 mm Hg). At this point the wound must be perfectly waterproof (ie, it must not allow even a minimal amount of liquid to escape). The control is done using a Weck-cell sponge which dries the edges of the incision and rubs repeatedly, backward and forward, on the sclera of the external incision to check whether the closure holds under external pressure.

Whether or not sutures are applied depends largely on the degree of preoperative astigmatism and the intraoperative measurement. With the eyebulb under pressure, using a qualitative keratoscope, the surgeon should evaluate the shape of the cornea. If against-the-rule astigmatism is revealed, sutures are necessary because in the postoperative period of superior tunnel incisions, there is a tendency for a certain amount of against-the-rule astigmatism to be induced.

## TO SUTURE CORNEAL TUNNELS OR NOT TO SUTURE

Corneal tunnels are performed with a different technique to scleral tunnels. They also have a different width (normally 4.1 mm or less) because in the majority of cases they are used for the insertion of foldable IOLs.

More often than not when the corneal tunnel incisions are performed correctly, sutures are not required.

However, when the tunnel is short, there are doubts about the hold, or the surgeon is worried that with-the-rule astigmatism will be induced, it is better to suture.

A corneal tunnel at least 1.5 mm long is normally sutured with a single radial suture when the width of the opening is equal to or less than 5.0 mm. For shorter tunnels (between 1.0 to 1.5 mm) or for wider incisions, the surgeon should apply a single cross stitch or three interrupted stitches.

Nevertheless, the suture must be placed following the rules mentioned previously. It must be radial and under moderate tension (to induce just a slight amount of compression on the tissues and a moderate degree of astigmatism). The surgeon should also take care to embed the knots completely.

## HORIZONTAL SUTURE TECHNIQUES FOR SCLERAL TUNNELS

There are many ways to suture a scleral tunnel. The following is a description of the more interesting techniques.

### The Rectangular Technique (Shepherd's Technique)

A horizontal suture with a single ring involves straight penetration of the needle from right to left, 1 mm inside the straight scleral incision on the floor exiting at the extreme left in the deep flap. The needle is passed through the superficial flap from the inside to the outside and through the superficial flap, this time from the outside to the inside exiting in correspondence with the initial entrance point of the needle. The thread is then knotted, with the knot remaining intrasclerally.

This suture is easy and quick. It is indicated for narrow tunnels because it allows the central portions to be brought close together if the arch is not wide. However, if the arch is wide, the flaps will tend to separate.

### Posteriorized Rectangular Suture (Singer's Technique)

At about 1.5 mm from the right lateral extremity of the tunnel, the needle enters radially on the posterior limit of the incision in the direction of the fornix. It then exits in the sclera posterior to the incision, runs through the sclera posterior to the aperture, penetrates the sclera on the left about 1.5 mm from the left lateral extremity of the tunnel, and exits on the inside of the posterior limit of the incision. It penetrates from the inside to the outside of the superficial flap. The needle then penetrates from the outside to the inside on the right hand portion of the superficial flap, exiting inside the tunnel at the initial entrance point with the knot tied inside the tunnel.

This suture is simple and easy to complete and allows the roof and floor to be brought together perfectly and the superficial portion to the deep one. It also provokes a slight radial traction.

### Infinity Suture (Fine's Technique)

The *infinity* suture devised by I. Howard Fine is the most common of these techniques. Viewed in sections, it looks like the mathematical symbol for infinity, hence its name.

The needle is passed through the superficial flap on the right side at about 1 mm from the posterior limit. It perforates the floor and then the roof again to exit onto the surface once more. The needle is passed from right to left producing a loop which takes up 40% of the tunnel width. The needle is then positioned on the left side of the tunnel and another passage is completed, from left to right, with the formation of another loop which again takes up 40% of the tunnel. The two terminals are then knotted once the threads have been sufficiently tightened. In practice the superficial part of the tunnel (roof) is fixed to the deeper part (floor) in two areas on the same transversal horizontal axis.

A variation of the infinity suture is to leave the loops larger (ie, 50%), exiting the needle after the second passage just right of the exit point of the first stitch. The knot is then brought from right to left to be embedded in the tissues.

With the infinity suture, the disadvantage is that the posterior edges of the incision tend to open considerably once the suture has been knotted. However, the thread brings the tissue very close together in the central and anterior parts of the tunnel and it is here that the wound is closed. In fact, the gaping of the posterior part of the edges is not of any great importance.

This type of closure has the advantage that the suture thread never passes radially through the incision edges, so there is no vertical stress applied to the limbus which could alter the corneal curvature. The stresses in this case are tangential to the cornea and do not change its curvature.

### Shuttle Suture (Fishkind's Technique)

In this horizontal suture method, the first step is on the floor of the tunnel. The needle is introduced at the right hand posterior extremity of the incision between the first and second quarter of the opening. After a slightly oblique passage, more or less tangential to the limbus, it exits on the floor between the third and fourth quarter of the incision. It is then passed through the superficial edge from the inside to the outside so that it will exit approximately 1 mm from the posterior extremity of the opening.

The needle is then passed through the superficial flap, approximately 1 mm from the posterior limit. It then is passed from the outside to the inside in the first and second quarter (ie, at the first entrance point of the thread). The needle is then passed through the floor again in a slightly oblique manner and exits on the posterior margin of the deep flap at the passage point between the third and fourth quarters following an oblique route from right to left.

This first arch is very important because it closes the central portion of the incision, and in view of the centralized hold on the free flap compared with the posterior hold on the deep flap, it provokes the induction of slight with-the-rule astigmatism.

The surgeon then prepares a second, wider arch. The

needle exits on the left superficial flap (from the inside to the outside). It is introduced on the right edge superficially to the deeper layers in correspondence with the initial entrance point. Then the suture thread is knotted with a suitable thread tension.

The first arch is central and small and closes the central portion of tunnel. The second, more posterior arch is used to bring the posterior part of the superficial flap to the deeper parts, also bringing the lateral extremes of the incision closer together.

However, one disadvantage is that the shuttle suture is difficult to perform. This is balanced by the excellent central and posterior closure it provides.

## Mixed Radial Horizontal Suture (Masket's Technique)

In this method, radial penetration of the needle is in the deep flap almost halfway along the incision. The needle exits from the anterior flap anteriorly, toward the cornea (halfway along the tunnel); it perforates the superficial flap on the right side. Then there is the horizontal passage through the deep flap from right to left with the first stitch which returns the needle to the initial entrance point. A second stitch takes in the left portion of the floor horizontally to reach the extreme left of the incision. The needle then enters the inside portion of the superficial flap and then another entrance point, from the outside to the inside, so that the thread ends up alongside the first stitch. The thread is knotted inside the pouch.

This is a very interesting suture. It allows the horizontal stitch in the floor to be performed under direct visual control. Moreover, it brings the floor and the roof together perfectly. It prevents the separation of the tunnel's central portion which occurs with the single arch sutures. It also avoids the anterior displacement of the external tunnel flap, consequently it avoids against-the-rule astigmatism.

## Mixed Posterior and Radial Suture (Buratto's Technique)

This method is horizontal passage from right to left in the sclera 1.0 mm posterior to the incision. Radial passage is on the tunnel floor. Exit on the superficial flap about 1 to 2 mm from the left posterior limit. Further radial penetration is toward the fornix on the superficial flap 2.0 mm more centrally. Then do a radial passage on the floor to the limit of the scleral incision, and a horizontal passage from left to right in intact sclera, horizontal to the incision. Next do radial penetration of the floor with an exit in the superficial flap 2.0 mm from the previous passage, and further lateral perforation of the superficial flap 2.0 mm from the last passage with intramural knotting of the thread.

This suture has the advantage of bringing the superficial and deep flaps together accurately and inducing a moderate radial traction through the two radial passages and the posterior scleral passages.

## Mixed Suture

This combines the rectangular suture with two interrupted sutures. It involves passing one suture transversally through the superficial flap at about half the width and then adding two interrupted radial sutures. The surgeon begins by perforating the superficial flap from the outside to the inside. The superficial flap is raised and, under direct observation, the needle is passed transversally from right to left on the posterior limit of the scleral bed. The suture begins in correspondence to the exit of the thread from the superficial flap. It is then passed from the inside to the outside through the superficial flap to return to the surface. It is then knotted with the first tail. It forms a simple horizontal rectangular suture consisting of a single arch. The surgeon then applies one radial stitch on each side, just to the side of the transversal suture. These must provide a waterproof closure with no induced astigmatism so they should be tightened just enough to bring the tissues together.

This suture has the advantage that the interrupted sutures bring the superficial flap close posteriorly to the underlying sclera and reduce the superficial flap's tendency to slide forward. The horizontal suture brings the floor close to the roof and allows good adhesion of the tissues.

In conclusion, there are many techniques for applying horizontal sutures. The method used should be chosen on the basis of the tunnel type, the degree of spontaneous self-closure of the incision, and whether a certain degree of with-the-rule astigmatism needs to be induced or not in proportion to both the preoperative astigmatism and the shape and extension of the tunnel.

# REMOVAL OF THE VISCOELASTIC SUBSTANCE

Once the implant and the suture have been completed and the surgeon has controlled the hold of the incision, he or she must remove the viscoelastic substance (VES). This is done with the irrigation/aspiration (I/A) tip with the same vacuum levels used to remove the cortex, keeping the bottle at half-mast.

First the surgeon must remove the material in the sac under the lens. This can be done by shifting the optic with a spatula or alternately pressing the optic with the distal part of the I/A tip so that the VES is expressed. All the material situated anteriorly to the IOL is then removed followed by the material in the chamber angle.

At this point, the surgeon may find it useful to introduce some drops of preservative-free 2% pilocarpine or Miochol to assist the contraction of the pupil for the following reasons:

- It reduces the postoperative pressure, freeing the corneal angle of the iris.
- It reduces postoperative photophobia associated with mydriasis.
- It increases postoperative visual acuity creating the effect of a stenopeic orifice.

However, postoperative miosis can stimulate greater uveal reactivity. It is therefore necessary to evaluate the pros and cons in every individual case.

# Chapter 11

# COMPLICATIONS
*Lucio Buratto, MD*

## INTRODUCTION

Phacoemulsification when performed by an expert, is in the vast majority of cases a simple, rapid, and safe procedure. However, for the less experienced surgeon, complications may arise in a proportion of cases. Although the causes are numerous, the effects on functional and anatomical outcome may be profound. Every phase of the operation can bring about its own set of problems. In this chapter we will examine the various parts of the surgical operation and describe all the possible complications, how to reduce them, how to avoid them, and how to treat them. To begin with, the possible complications will be listed with an overview of their treatment. A detailed discussion of these problems will take place later in the chapter.

## OVERVIEW OF COMPLICATIONS

1. Rupture of the posterior capsule and the hyaloid membrane with dislocation of nuclear material into the vitreous.

   This is the most serious complication unique to the cataract operation. Although expulsive hemorrhage is possible, this complication is common to other operations of ocular surgery; it will not be described here.

   A dropped nucleus or nuclear fragments requires a posterior approach. If the nuclear fragment stays in the anterior vitreous and if it can be easily removed, only a limited vitrectomy may be required. If there is a large volume of nuclear material dislocated deep in the vitreous, a total vitrectomy and the use of PFC are often required.

   If the surgeon does not feel confident about this procedure, he or she should refer the patient to an expert vitreo-retinal surgeon.

2. Rupture of the posterior capsule and the hyaloid membrane with vitreous prolapse (with no loss of the nuclear material in the vitreous).

   First, during emulsification of the nucleus, the incision is extended and the nucleus is extracted manually under viscoelastic. If the vitreous loss is limited, perform a mechanical anterior vitrectomy. If it is more extensive, a posterior vitrectomy is required, particularly if the cortical material is mixed with the vitreous or if it has luxated posteriorly. This complication may be aggravated if the pupil contracts and the surgeon is not properly equipped for a vitrectomy.

   Next, at the end of emulsification of the nucleus, the fragment of nucleus should be extracted with a forceps under the protection of viscoelastic substances (VES). The cortex mixed with the vitreous is removed along with the vitreous in the anterior chamber. If the number of fragments is small and they can be aspirated easily, the anterior route is appropriate; however, if the number of fragments is large, a posterior vitrectomy should be performed. This is the only way to be certain that both the anterior and posterior segments have been cleaned satisfactorily. This will reduce the risk of cystoid macular edema, inflammation, retinal detachment, and hypotony.

   Finally, during or at the end of irrigation/aspiration (I/A), proceed with an anterior vitrectomy if the opening is small and if there is little cortex remaining. When the opening is wide and the vitreous is abundant or there is a large amount of cortex present, use a posterior approach.

3. Posterior capsular rupture without vitreous loss.

   This usually occurs during I/A. If the red reflex of the fundus is clearly visible and if the microscope has been constantly focused on the posterior capsule, awareness of the probe engaging the posterior capsule should be immediate. The rupture will appear either as a straight line which crosses a portion of the pupillary area or as a broken triangular line which is clearly seen in contrast to the red reflex of the fundus. If there are any doubts about

### Table 11-1
## SUBCHOROIDAL HEMORRHAGE OR EXPULSIVE HEMORRHAGE

**Origin**

Rupture of one or two choroidal veins.

**Extension**

It can stay in the subchoroidal space (localized or widespread).
Rupture the choroid (expulsive hemorrhage).

**Predisposition**

Arteriosclerosis.
Arterial hypertension.
Glaucoma.

**Cause**

Intraoperative hypotony.

**Prevention**

Gradually reduce the IOP (side port incision).
Always maintain positive IOP.

**Diagnosis**

Sudden increase in eye pressure.
Iris prolapse.
Flattening of anterior chamber.
Appearance of a brownish color in the red reflex in the pupillary area.

**Localized treatment**

Close the incision immediately with strong silk thread 6-7/0 if the incision is limbal or scleral.
Do not pay too much attention to the quality of the work; close the incision quickly.
If there is a corneal or scleral self-sealing tunnel, immediately inject abundant Viscoat to close the tunnel from the inside (ie, make the deep flap adhere to the superficial one).
Hydrate the edges of the side port incisions.
Cut the conjuntiva in the area corresponding to the brownish shadow.
Cut right through the sclera to reach the subchoroidal space (in this situation the choroid and the retina are distant from the sclera). Channel off the blood; this will induce an immediate reduction in eye pressure and allow the surgeon to complete the sutures and/or reposition the iris if it has prolapsed.
The first sclerotomy often closes because of the formation of a clot. Reopen it or prepare a second one near an external or internal rectus (in an area of hemorrhage).
If the dark shadow proceeds rapidly and the iris prolapse increases uncontrollably, the surgeon should perform a sclerotomy, even transconjunctivally in the area corresponding to the brownish shadow.

**General treatment**

Ask the anesthetist to reduce the systemic pressure immediately.
Administer 20% Mannitol (20 cc iv).
Place the head above the feet to facilitate venous flow in trendelenburg.
Unfortunately, in the majority of cases, the expulsive hemorrhage does not give the surgeon time to perform these emergency maneuvers and the eyebulb is emptied within a matter of seconds. It is a rare occurrence with phacoemulsification. It occurs more frequently with intracapsular or extracapsular surgery or antiglaucomatous surgery.

---

whether the capsule has torn, suspend I/A, and increase the magnification and the intensity of the microscope light. Once the damage has been verified, fill the anterior chamber with an air bubble and simultaneously remove the probe. The two maneuvers must occur together; otherwise the anterior chamber will flatten, and the vitreous face may rupture with consequent vitreous loss. Inject Provisc or Healon to deepen the anterior and posterior chambers and to occlude the break in the capsule. Complete aspiration of the cortex with a *dry* technique, ie, using a one-way cannula applied to a syringe containing balanced salt solution (BSS). The surgeon should carefully and patiently peel the residual material and use as little fluid as possible. Beware; this can move the VES away from the capsular break and rupture the vitreous face (if this has not already happened).

4. Endothelial damage.

Any of the instruments which enter the anterior chamber can damage the endothelium. Phacoemulsifcation in the anterior chamber, through contact of the nucleus or fragments of the nucleus with the endothelium, probably causes the greatest amount of damage. Other reasons include flattening of the chamber, excessive turbulence, the use of an excessive quantity of irrigation liquid, injection of drugs into the chamber, etc. The use of a suitable

> Table 11-2
> ## TEARING OF DESCEMET'S MEMBRANE
>
> **Extension**
>
> The tear can be limited to just a few millimeters or be extended to involve the entire cornea.
>
> **What to do**
>
> The surgeon can proceed with phaco taking great care not to detach the membrane further.
> Reattach the membrane with air and postpone the operation.
> Fill the chamber with Viscoat opposite the detachment site to reattach the membrane and then proceed with phaco.
>
> **Cause**
>
> It always occurs close to one of the incisions and is the result of trauma in the internal incision:
>
> > Entrance to the camber with the U/S and I/A tips pushing the sleeve against the internal edge of the incision; this happens more easily with harder sleeves.
> > VES injection under the Descemet's membrane.
> > IOL is forced through an incision which is too small.
> > Use of blunt instruments.
> > Introduction of instrument with rough edges, extroversions, etc (Hirschmann spatula).
>
> **Treatment**
>
> Accurate replacement of the membrane in the tear site, followed by an injection of an air bubble is sufficient for small detachments.
> Injection of a Viscoat bubble close to the detachment site and injection of air in the more distant areas; this works well for moderately-large detachments.
> Transcorneal suture is required with large detachments.
>
> **Complications**
>
> Removal of the detached Descemet should be avoided. If the torn portion is small, it may cause the formation of transitional localized corneal edema. If the amount of membrane removed is more extensive, it may cause total edema of the cornea.

VES can significantly reduce the endothelial damage (Viscoat in some phases, Provisc or Healon in others).

5. Detachment of Descemet's membrane.

This occurs particularly during insertion of the ultrasonic probe, the cystotome, or the I/A tip. In the majority of cases it can be avoided by lifting the anterior flap of the incision with forceps. This allows better and safer access for instruments.

6. Unsatisfactory capsulotomy.

An incomplete or small capsulotomy can create a number of problems for the surgeon when fragmenting the nucleus, aspirating the cortical material, and implanting a lens. Try to correct the situation using scissors or a cystotome under viscoelastic protection.

7. Iris prolapse.

If the entry wound into the anterior chamber is too posteriorly placed, the wound is too large, or there is excessive pressure in the eye, the iris may prolapse. This is a potentially serious problem, particularly for the less experienced surgeon, as the pupil may constrict rapidly and compromise visibility.

8. Residual cortex.

The importance of residual cortex depends largely on the amount of material remaining. Small equatorial fragments will be reabsorbed rapidly within 3 to 4 weeks and therefore can be left at the end of the operation. Larger amounts may take much longer to be completely reabsorbed. They maintain a certain degree of reactivity in the anterior segment for a number of weeks. This encourages the formation of iris synechiae, opacification of the posterior capsule, and decentering of the intraocular lens (IOL). If the risk of posterior capsule rupture is small, the cortex should be removed to avoid problems of this type.

9. Zonular disinsertion.

Traction on the zonules can lead to disinsertion. This may be during capsulotomy, while emulsifying a particularly hard nucleus, or during cortical aspiration. It is more common in eyes with pseudoexfoliation. To prevent or avoid this, careful technique is required.

Less frequent complications may include:

- Epithelial damage from abrasions caused by the careless use of the instruments, incorrect application of the drapes, or through the careless application of topical anesthetics.
- Iridodialysis, which may occur during the insertion of instruments into the anterior chamber, particularly when the anterior chamber entry is too posterior. If the ultrasound (U/S) tip is forced through a small incision with a flat chamber; or whenever there is any difficulty in inserting the U/S tip.
- Rupture of the iris sphincter from incorrect use of the spatula, capture of the pupillary edge with the U/S tip, particularly during phacoemulsification with a narrow pupil. If the iris damage makes phacoemulsification difficult, the surgeon should consider converting to ECCE unless he or she feels confident to continue.
- Residual anterior capsule by incorrect or incomplete capsulotomy. It may be removed under the protection of viscoelastic.

| Table 11-3 GENERAL COMPLICATIONS WITH A TUNNEL INCISION | |
|---|---|
| Tunnel which is too long | Corneal folds. Difficulty in managing the various surgical phases. Endothelial damage. |
| Too short | Possible interference of the iris. Difficult self-sealing. |
| Too wide | Excessive BSS loss during phaco and the other phases with possible flattening of the chamber. Possible iris prolapse. |
| Too narrow | Difficult insertion of tips. Poor BSS infusion with risk of the tip overheating. Possible detachment of Descemet's membrane. |
| Too superficial | Risk of tears. Poor closure of the floor (deep flap of the tunnel). |
| Too deep | Fragile floor and risk of tearing. |
| External incision too far posterior | Difficulty in managing the tip in the chamber. Difficulty with inserting the instruments. Difficulty in using the tip correctly. |
| External incision too far anterior | The whole tunnel will be too far forward in the cornea with the possible formation of corneal folds. Difficult self-sealing. |
| Incision which is narrow externally and wide internally | Initial difficulty with inserting the tip. Good intraoperative management of the tip. |
| Incision which is wide at the entrance point and narrow internally | Facilitates the insertion of the tip. Poor intraoperative management of the tip. Formation of corneal folds. |
| Insufficient quality | Irregularity of the internal incision. Irregularity of the tunnel route. Irregularity of the internal incision, etc. |

- Insufficient cleaning of the posterior capsule caused by intraoperative miosis, vitreous pressure. This does not generally cause problems; if it does not clear spontaneously, an early capsulotomy may be required.
- Incision burn which may occur in the following situations: tight incision with inadequate BSS flow to cool the U/S tip and excessive use of high U/S power as in very hard cataracts. The latter is particularly important when low aspiration flow rates are used, and thus, there is limited tip cooling. If complete blockage of the tip or aspiration line occurs, the tip can heat up if U/S power is used to clear the block while the tip is still in the eye. Inexperienced surgeons may push the U/S tip against the edges of the wound. This flattens the silicone sleeve around the tip and allows it to heat up, causing wound burn.

## COMPLICATIONS OF THE VARIOUS PHASES OF THE OPERATION

Here is a more detailed look at the complications of phacoemulsification.

### The Incision

Phacoemulsification with a limbal incision incurs the same intraoperative and postoperative problems as with ECCE. A limbal incision can be:

- Too narrow—It will be difficult for the surgeon to introduce the probe. Even if it can be introduced, the sleeve may be compressed, making irrigation in the anterior chamber difficult. BSS cooling of the U/S tip is greatly reduced. The narrow incision also causes the formation of corneal folds which impairs visibility of the anterior chamber. The problem can be avoided by using a calibrated blade set correctly; the incision will be the right size for the tip used.
- Too wide—The anterior chamber flattens because excessive BSS escapes. The iris may prolapse or be damaged by the U/S tip. When the chamber flattens there is less room for fragmentation of the nucleus, and this may increase the damage to the endothelium. There is an increased risk of posterior capsule rupture. Iris stimulation, in association with the reduced depth of the chamber, can cause the pupil to contract and the whole operation will become more difficult. An incision which is too wide should be partially closed with one or two interrupted sutures,

or the opening can be closed and reformed in another position using calibrated instruments.
- Too far backward—If the chamber is entered too far posteriorly, the instruments may come into contact with the base of the iris along the track to the anterior chamber. There is a risk of disinsertion and trauma which will cause the pupil to constrict. A posterior incision means that the angle of the U/S tip will not be ideal for fragmenting the nucleus (this is particularly true with the inexperienced surgeon).
- Too far forward—This may cause corneal folds which will obscure good visibility and increase endothelial damage. The angle between the U/S tip and the nucleus will be too steep and the entire procedure becomes difficult and more traumatic.

Recently, cataract surgery has been become directed to small self-sealing tunnel sutureless incisions. These can be scleral, corneal, or limbal.

There are two main complications related to these techniques: scleral tunnel and corneal or limbal tunnel.

### Scleral Tunnel

Complications that can occur are:
- An incision that is too superficial—A flap which is too thin can subsequently tear. The edge of the incision can be damaged by the tip of the phacoemulsifier or other instrument. This may mean the incision is not watertight and must be sutured.
- An incision that is too deep—In myopic eyes, in elderly patients, or when the surgeon has used excessive superficial diathermy, it is possible to perforate the globe during the pre-incision. A deep incision may involve the deep blood vessels and damage the ciliary body. A very deep tunnel may not close properly and may require a suture. But if the surgeon has recognized the problem a second incision in another location should be performed. The surgeon is advised to use a blade with a rounded tip or adjustable micrometer to set the depth—normally a diamond blade—to avoid this problem.
- A wrong shaped incision—This can bring about uneven distribution of tension of the tunnel, resulting in astigmatism. A wrong shaped incision is avoidable by using one of the commercially available markers. This particularly applies to frown incisions.
- Premature entry to the anterior chamber—If the incision opens into the anterior chamber, behind Schwalbe's line and close to the angular structures, there may be damage to the trabecular meshwork or the formation of postoperative synechiae. However, it is the proximity to the base of the iris and its possible prolapse during surgery which is the main risk. The pupil may contract, leading to difficulty with the surgery and consequent iris damage. This produces greater postoperative inflammation due to breakdown of the blood aqueous barrier and release of prostaglandins. Even the introduction of the phacoemulsifier tip or frequent rubbing of the instrument sleeve during surgery can provoke tearing or disinsertion of the iris base.

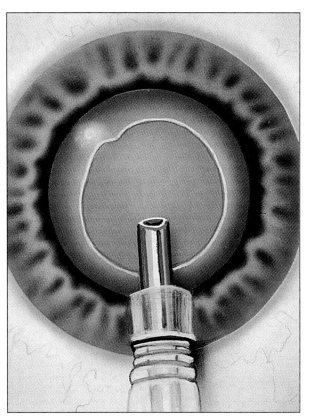

Figure 11-1. Incorrect insertion of the U/S tip can cause wrinkling of the sleeve. It happens particularly when the incision is narrow.

- A tunnel that is too short—If the tunnel is short, the corneal valve may not self-seal. A suture may be needed and astigmatism may be induced.
- A tunnel that is too long—If the tunnel has been extended too far into the clear cornea, the instruments introduced through it will be inclined upward toward the corneal endothelium. However, to work in the posterior chamber, the surgeon will have to incline the instruments downward. This will produce traction folds on the cornea which restrict visibility. All maneuvers, especially those at the incision site, will be more difficult. Phacoemulsification and the introduction of the IOL will be particularly difficult. There is an increased risk of damage to the corneal endothelium either from direct trauma from the instruments or from the large folds which have formed in the cornea. Due to the greater difficulty in aspirating cortex at 12 o'clock, there is a higher risk of capsular damage.

### Corneal or Limbal Tunnel

Although it can be made without, this incision is preceded by a vertical preincision in the majority of cases. It should be 30 to 50% of the corneal thickness.

Complications which can occur are:
- Wrong shape—Diamond blades are extremely sharp and should be used very carefully.

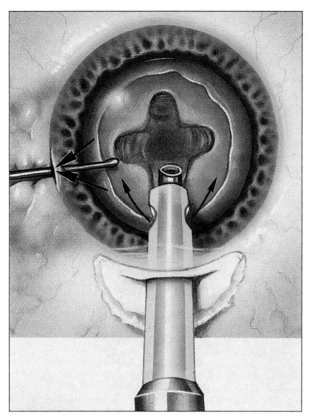

Figure 11-2. Side port incision made too posteriorly; infiltration of the perilimbal conjunctiva with BSS.

Otherwise, the surgeon may risk cutting an incision which is too long, too short, or at the wrong angle. A blocking device is useful. It is also advisable to stabilize the eye with fixation forceps. A steel blade will increase the amount of friction, causing traction folds but allowing better control of the direction of the incision.

- An incision that is too superficial—This either can be corrected immediately by deepening the incision, or it can be performed in a slightly oblique direction because of the sharpness of the diamond blade.
- An incision that is too deep—This can be avoided if the surgeon uses preset calibrated instruments for the preincision. If the eye is hypotonic, it becomes difficult to form a correct corneal tunnel so a 10-0 nylon suture can be used to close it. Another entry wound should be made. A stab incision is made with a second instrument so the anterior chamber can be filled with viscoelastic to restore the intraocular pressure (IOP), making the second tunnel easier to create.
- A tunnel that is too short—If a diamond keratome is used, the anterior chamber can be penetrated too soon. This may result in a tunnel which is too short to guarantee perfect self-sealing. One or more holding sutures should be inserted.
- A tunnel that is too long—The same problems as those for the scleral tunnel.
- Detachment of Descemet's membrane and the endothelium—If the instruments used to make the incision are blunt or if penetration in the anterior chamber is too tangential, the tip of the instrument may drag the two membranes with it. If the internal edge of the wound it is too thin, this may encourage the separation of the deep layers. Manipulation of the phacoemulsifier tip may also cause trauma. At the end of the operation, it is usually possible to re-attach the membranes using viscoelastic injected into the anterior chamber or, alternatively, an air bubble can be used.

Another frequent error in the construction of a tunnel is the dissection of multiple planes. The superficial tunnel flap will have a different thicknesses, or the dissection can be too superficial or too deep.

Excessive manipulation of the superficial flap may alter the tissues, resulting in difficult spontaneous sealing at the end of surgery. Bleeding is common when the scleral tunnel is being cut because perforating vessels are easily damaged. Hyphaema occasionally occurs in the first postoperative days as blood from the scleral vessels may enter the anterior chamber. Hyphaema can be prevented by raising the IOP by injecting BSS at the end of the operation to arrest the bleeding and prevent blood entering the tunnel.

## Side Port Incision

Two intraoperative complications may occur:
- Incisions which are placed too close to the limbus. BSS will escape from the incision and can infiltrate the conjunctiva forming a ring-shaped conjunctival swelling. This can make the operation difficult because of the poor visibility due to pooling of fluid over the cornea.
- Incisions which are too wide. Excessive loss of infusion fluid from the anterior chamber results in a disturbance of the balance between infusion and aspiration. This will cause the chamber depth to be unstable and may cause damage to the endothelium, iris trauma, and pupillary contraction.

As soon as the surgeon realizes the mistake he or she should stop the operation and open a new side port incision after closing the first one with a nylon suture.

# COMPLICATIONS DURING THE ANTERIOR CAPSULOTOMY

Capsulorhexis is one of the basic steps in phacoemulsification as it allows the surgeon to work inside the capsular bag through an elastic, strong capsular opening. This does not apply to the can opener capsulotomy because the multiple edge tears may extend through the lenticular equator. It is essential that the capsulorhexis be created with a smooth and continuous edge. The opening does not necessarily have to be round, but this is preferable. It may be oval or any other shape, but it must be continuous as any break in the edge is potentially dangerous.

The practical problems met during capsulorhexis are

Table 11-4
## COMPLICATIONS OF CAPSULORHEXIS

| | |
|---|---|
| Rhexis escape | Inject more VES to reduce the vitreal thrust and/or deepen the chamber to counterbalance the tendency of the nucleus to move toward the anterior chamber.<br>Use rhexis forceps to return the opening toward the center.<br>Cut the anterior capsule with scissors on the opposite side and restart the rhexis and try to close it to correspond with the previous escape point (in this case the rhexis will be correct), or internal to the previous (and it will still be a potential escape point).<br>Cut the capsule with very curved scissors at the escape site to return the opening toward the center.<br>Use the cystotome to cut the zonular fibers which are responsible for the poor progression of the rhexis and continue (only if there is a good red reflex and if the surgeon can see the zonular fibers).<br>Convert to a can opener. |
| If the rhexis is small | The surgeon should extend it:<br>Prior to phaco. This procedure is not easy because of the poor visibility (mobilization of the cortex) and for the nuclear thrust upward (tendency to rhexis escape).<br>After I/A prior to the implant. It should be done only if the rhexis is really very small. It is difficult because the capsule is not under tension.<br>Following the IOL implant. This is the ideal moment; the tension induced in the bag by the IOL and the abundant VES in the anterior chamber and in the bag enormously facilitate the extension. |
| Technique for extending a small rhexis | The anterior chamber and the capsular bag are filled with a high molecular weight VES (Healon GV, Healon, Provisc).<br>Using scissors, the limit of the rhexis is cut for 1.0-1.5 mm; the surgeon should remain quite tangential (angle of 30-35°).<br>The opening should be made to the right and the left of the rhexis. The surgeon should choose the sector with a greater amount of residual anterior capsule (in comparison to the pupil or the optical disc).<br>Using the rhexis forceps, the surgeon clasps the apex of the cut flap and guides it. |
| Large rhexis | Risk of luxation of the nucleus in the anterior chamber and of having to perform phaco in the anterior chamber.<br>Difficulty with correct insertion of the lens in the bag. Place the loops where there is sufficient capsule. |

visibility, control of the size, and loss of direction and escape peripherally.

## Visibility

Inadequate visibility can be due to poor corneal transparency, a very thin capsule, an incision which is too far forward in the cornea, or the lack of a good red reflex from the fundus. There are various ways of dealing with these problems.

In the event of poor corneal transparency, the surgeon must use a completely transparent viscoelastic such as Healon or Provisc. Obtain the best possible retroillumination reflex by adjusting the microscope and orientating the light correctly. The capsulotomy should be of a deliberately small diameter; it is easier to extend it at a later stage.

If the capsule is very thin and has a tendency to escape, it is better to adopt a *peeling* technique. Make the opening parallel to the pupillary edge, keeping the flap folded and close to the intact anterior capsule so that the incision is more controllable.

In the case of an overlong corneal or sclero-corneal tunnel, keep the lower edge of the capsulotomy quite central, as recovery of the flap below the incision is extremely difficult and poor visibility around the incision can result in a loss of control with the risk of capsulorhexis escape.

For advice on dealing with eyes with poor red reflex, refer to the section on capsulorhexis in special cases.

## Control of Size

The optimal diameter of the capsulorhexis is about 5.5 mm. In practice however, at the end of the capsulotomy, the diameter may be smaller or larger than this.

- Too small capsulorhexis—If the capsulorhexis is too small, movement of the phacoemulsifier will be difficult and the edge of the rhexis itself risks damage. However, it is worse to have a rhexis which goes out of control than to have one which is smaller than the desired size.

The diameter of the capsulorhexis can be extended at the end of the capsulotomy. It is easier and safer to do this after insertion of the IOL in the capsular bag. On the other hand, if the rhexis is very small and the lens cannot pass through it, the extension should be done prior to the implant with the chamber and capsular bag formed with Healon or Provisc. The viscoelastic must be injected into the capsular bag without expanding it too much, and then the anterior chamber should be filled. In this way, the anterior chamber is only moderately taut. As a result, the extension procedure is relatively simple.

The rim of the capsulorhexis is cut obliquely with

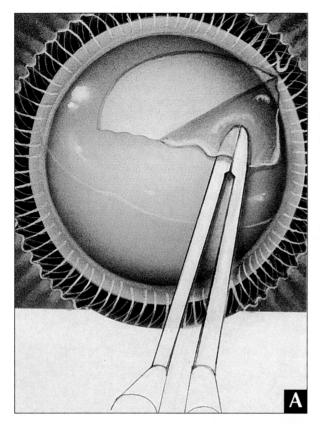
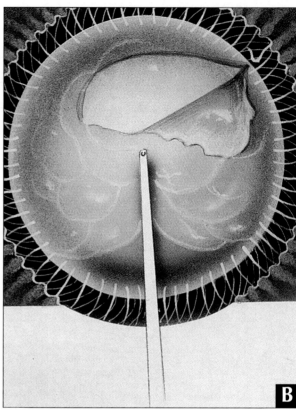
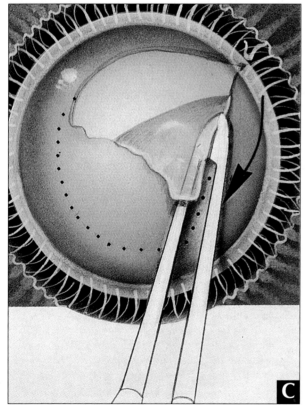

Figures 11-3A, 11-3B, 11-3C. Tendency toward rhexis escape. In the event of excessive widening of the rhexis with a tendency to escape toward the equator, the injection of additional Healon GV, Healon, or Provisc will allow the surgeon both to widen the pupil, deepen the chamber, and counterbalance any upward thrust. In this way, by catching the capsule flap with forceps (even if in the initial phase a cystotome was used) and exerting suitable traction force in the right direction (centripetal), in the majority of cases the surgeon will be able to recover the escaping rhexis.

Vannas microscissors (straight or curved) at the 4 or 8 o'clock positions, and the flap is clasped by rhexis forceps. The flap is torn with a wider diameter until the circle is completed from the opposite side. Cohesive viscoelastic is important to maintain anterior chamber depth during this maneuver.

- Wide diameter capsulorhexis—If the capsulorhexis is too large it may complicate the operation because it is unlikely that the edge of the capsule will be able to contain the nucleus during hydrodissection or phacoemulsification. In the case of a very wide capsulorhexis, it is advisable to limit the hydrodissection to a minimum without mobilizing the nucleus (which otherwise could luxate in to the anterior chamber) and resort to techniques of in situ phacoemulsification, given that a portion of the anterior capsule which holds the nucleus is too small for any of the other methods.

Viscoat is very useful in these cases, both during hydrodissection and during the phase of nucleus mobilization and phacoemulsification as it remains

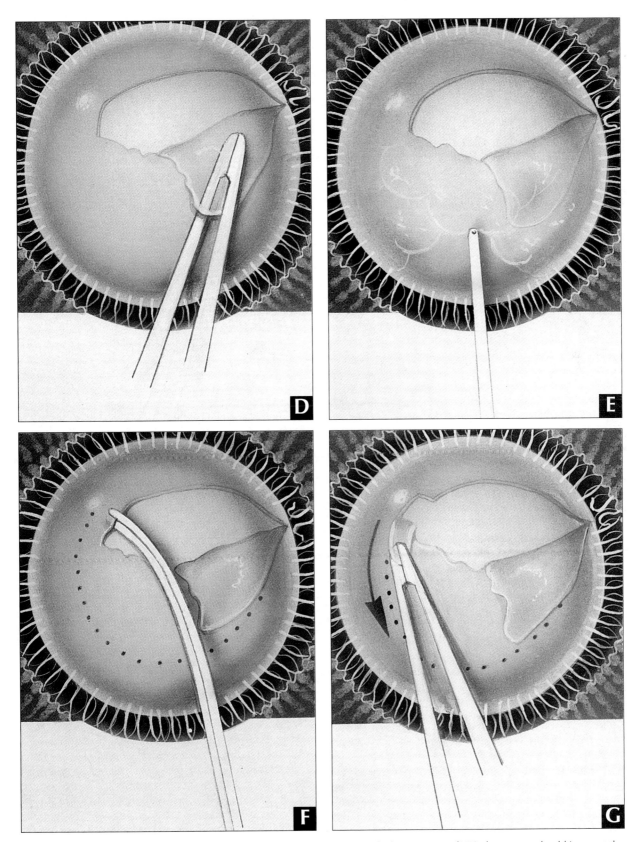

Figures 11-3D, 11-3E, 11-3F, 11-3G. If the rhexis still tends to escape despite a further injection of VES, the surgeon should interrupt the operation and change the technique. One alternative is to enter with a curved scissors to perform a small capsular incision which should be the start of a new capsulorhexis in a direction opposite to the previous one. The closure of this should then coincide with previous point of maximum opening (not always an easy procedure) or just inside it. In the latter case, the surgeon should remember that the rhexis is not intact for the successive phases of the operation.

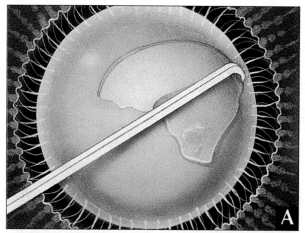

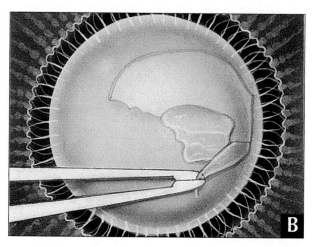

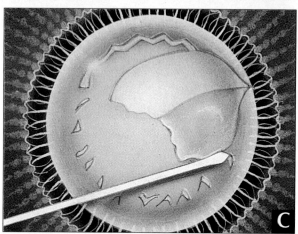

Figures 11-4A, 11-4B, 11-4C. What to do if the rhexis escapes. If the zonular fibers are visible, the surgeon can use the cystotome to break the few fibers that are responsible for preventing the progression of the rhexis, and then he or she should proceed with the forceps. Alternately, the surgeon can convert to a can opener.

in place even if BSS is injected. The nucleus is kept in place during hydrodissection and mobilization. Even during phacoemulsification, if the surgeon manages to keep a suitable volume of viscoelastic in the anterior chamber, the nucleus will remain inside the capsular bag. If the nucleus escapes from the capsulorhexis during hydrodissection, the surgeon can try to reposition it with a spatula.

The phacoemulsification should be by cruciate sculpting and fracture even though further luxation of the nucleus into the anterior chamber may easily occur. If repositioning is difficult, phacoemulsification can be done using the Kratz-Maloney technique or a procedure in the anterior chamber.

Other possible complications during capsulorhexis are:
1. Incomplete capsulorhexis (ie, a capsulorhexis which is not 360°).

The surgeon must proceed carefully. If the capsular bridge is very narrow, he or she should inject Provisc or Healon. Use rhexis forceps to grasp the capsule; the rhexis should then be completed. If the bridge is too wide and/or peripheral, the remaining flap should be cut. When this is close to the incision, it is sufficient to penetrate the incision with the tip of one arm of the scissors and cut. But if the bridge is in the inferior sector, the maneuver may be more complex. A high molecular weight VES must be used. In these cases, Sutherland's scissors can prove very useful.

During each of these maneuvers it is very important to avoid pulling on the fragments of the capsule attached to the remainder of the capsular bag. This may detach the zonules and cause equatorial escape of the rhexis, posterior capsular rupture, and other problems.

2. Escape of the capsulorhexis.

The tension of the capsule, its convex shape, and the action exerted by the zonular fibers provoke tension radially toward the equator. This tends to induce a centrifugal tearing of the capsular rim. The counter-pressure exerted by a high molecular weight VES is important as it reduces the zonular tension, pushing the nucleus downward and countering the vitreal thrust and the tendency to escape. Loss of control in the direction of the capsulorhexis can occur during this procedure and cause a widening of the capsulorhexis toward the periphery.

Awareness of what is happening may allow the rim of the capsulotomy to remain inside the zonular insertion. A choice of methods are then available to help regain control of the procedure:

- The chamber can be reformed with a high molecular weight cohesive VES (Healon GV, Healon, Provisc), creating a space for the maneuvers and opposing the vitreous pressure which contributes to the extension of the escape. The flap is caught again very carefully using the peeling technique with the cystotome. The flap is fixed near to the free edge, depressed slightly, and brought gently toward the center of the pupil. A tearing movement will tend to enlarge the capsulorhexis, particularly if the capsule is thin or if the operation is being performed in an area close to the zonular attachment area.
- The flap can be recovered using Buratto or Utrata's capsulorhexis forceps. After filling the anterior chamber with a high molecular weight VES (which

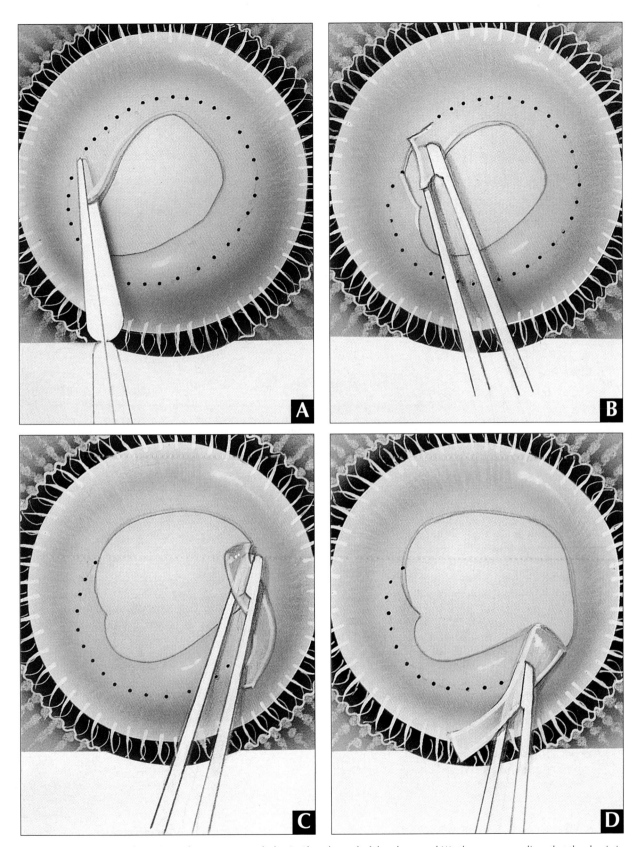

Figures 11-5A, 11-5B. Enlargement of a narrow capsulorhexis. If, at the end of the phaco and I/A, the surgeon realizes that the rhexis is too small for the IOL implantation, or if after having implanted the IOL, he or she sees that there is too much capsule overlapping the lens optic, the surgeon will have to widen the rhexis. The surgeon deepens the anterior chamber and the bag with Healon GV, Healon, or Provisc and with straight scissors (though curved scissors are preferable) then performs a cut tangential to start the rhexis external to the previous one. Figures 11-5C, 11-5D. This will be wider than the previous one—though not excessively so to avoid the risk of escape. If the new rhexis closes precociously, the opening will still be small, and the surgeon should consider repeating the procedure.

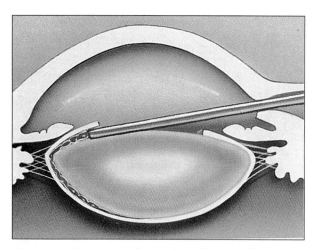

Figure 11-6. Correct procedure for hydrodissection. The cannula penetrates just below the rhexis, slightly lifts the capsule, and then BSS is gradually injected.

can also widen the pupil in that particular area) and increasing the magnification of the microscope, the forceps are introduced and the flap is caught at the most peripheral point of escape. With a gentle centripetal movement, the rhexis is brought once again toward the center.

- The free edge of the capsulorhexis is cut with curved microscissors and the flap is caught with a tearing technique in an attempt to bring the edge of the capsulotomy in a centripetal direction. In this case, to obtain a true capsulorhexis, the cut with the scissors must be curved and must correspond exactly to the opening so it can be returned to the center. Alternatively, the scissors can cut in the part of the rhexis that was done correctly. The surgeon tears in the opposite direction, attempting to close the previous escape. If this proves difficult, the closure can be done on the inside. The problems are the same as that for a capsulorhexis with an extremely wide diameter.
- If the red reflex is optimal and the mydriasis is wide enough to give a view of the zonular fibers which caused the blockage of the capsulorhexis, some of the fibers can be detached in the escape area using the cystotome. The free capsular edge may be recovered and the capsulorhexis may be completed.
- If the escape occurs at the end of the capsulorhexis, the residual portion of the capsule can be completed using the can opener technique. The edge of the anterior capsule which remains may be insufficient for standard phacoemulsification in the posterior chamber and an implantation within the capsular bag.
- In the event of a tear that extends beyond the insertion of the zonular fibers, a complete change in technique is required. Traction on the flap should be stopped immediately and the extension of the peripheral escape should be carefully evaluated. Hydrodissection should be avoided because the escape line, under the effects of the fluid pressure, can easily extend with the risk of capsule rupture or zonular dialysis during phacoemulsification.

If the patient is elderly and the nucleus hard, irrespective of when the capsulorhexis escape occurs, it is advisable to convert the technique into a can opener capsulotomy which guarantees better safety. In this case, hydrodissection should not be used, and the surgeon should resort to non-endocapsular phacoemulsification. If the nucleus is soft, the surgeon can carefully proceed with a technique of phaco aspiration.

3. Tearing of the capsulorhexis rim during the operation.

This normally happens during phacoemulsification or occasionally during the I/A phase. It usually starts from an irregularity in the capsulotomy, especially at the junction point of the capsular incision.

- In the initial phase of phacoemulsification—Accidental snagging with the U/S tip should be recognized quickly in order to avoid further problems at the same site. It is advisable to use the U/S tip as far away as possible from the break in the capsular edge and to avoid extending it further. It is also important to avoid anterior chamber collapse so the foot pedal should not be brought into the Position 0 when a considerable portion of the nucleus is still inside the capsular bag.
- During phacoemulsification—Tearing of the capsulorhexis may occur if the surgeon tries to mobilize a hard, large nucleus with the one-handed technique as the equator of the nucleus overlies the edges of the capsulorhexis. It may also occur with an overzealous nuclear fracture. If the anterior capsule opens or if there is any doubt, it is better to stop phacoemulsification, inject a VES, and carefully examine the extension of the tear. It is advisable to mobilize the remaining lens manually and to emulsify it outside the capsular bag to avoid further stress on the capsular zonules.
- Tearing of the capsulorhexis during I/A—The starting point is generally a broken anterior capsular edge and traction exerted by the cannula in order to reach the peripheral portions of the cortex especially when the capsulorhexis is small. This occurs more frequently close to the incision, particularly under a sclero-corneal tunnel, where the removal of the cortex may lead to poorly controlled maneuvers with the I/A tip. If problems arise, change technique or instruments for cortex removal below the capsulorhexis at the 12 o'clock position.

Early recognition of a broken rhexis should lead to swift removal of the I/A tip to prevent the irrigation pressure extending the escape route posteriorly. The chamber must be reshaped with a cohesive VES in order to control the size of the rhexis break more easily. If the latter does not exceed the zonular limits, automated I/A can continue. If there is any doubt, it is better to avoid irrigation and proceed with a dry manual technique.

4. Flattening of the anterior chamber.

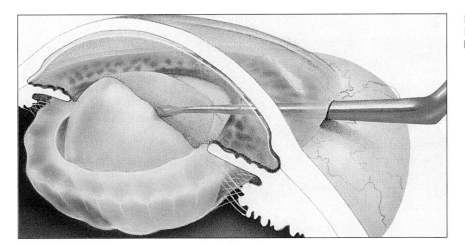

Figure 11-7. Replacement of the luxated nucleus in the capsular bag.

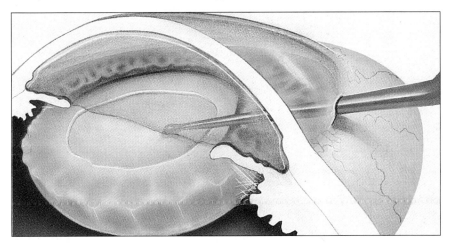

Figure 11-8. Replacement of the luxated nucleus in the capsular bag.

This is most common when BSS is used for chamber maintenance. The chamber can flatten because the saline escapes due to excessive pressure or traction exerted by the cystotome on the edges of the incision. Alternately, the corneal incision may be too wide compared to the diameter of the cystotome resulting in excessive fluid loss. Flattening of the anterior chamber should be dealt with immediately; otherwise there will be rhexis escape. Viscoelastic should be substituted for BSS as the means of deepening the anterior chamber to continue the rhexis safely.

5. Rupture of the zonules.

Zonular rupture is most common in elderly patients when the zonular fibers have already been weakened. It can also occur in cataracts where the anterior capsule is rigid or difficult to cut, or if the cataract is intumescent because the two capsules, anterior and posterior, are under a lot of tension and are very fragile. A portion of the zonule may also rupture during phacoemulsification in a morgagnian cataract. Here the capsule is often fibrotic, the zonules are weak, and the patient is elderly—all elements which encourage the disinsertion of the zonules. Cataracts associated with pseudofoliation also have weak zonules so special care and attention are necessary.

6. Vitreous in the anterior chamber.

This occurs when there is zonular rupture. If it happens before the capsule is cut or early in the capsulotomy, widen the incision and extract the whole cataract. If it happens when the capsular opening is wide, extend the corneal incision, extract the nucleus, and perform an anterior vitrectomy with removal of the anterior and posterior capsules, in addition to the cortical material.

## Hydrodissection

Hydrodissection is a very important step for successful phacoemulsification with the endocapsular technique. Hydrodissection should be performed only with an intact rhexis—never when it has escaped—because there is a high risk of it extending to the posterior capsule. The can opener capsulotomy should also be avoided.

The quantity of BSS injected at one time should not exceed 1 mL. Take care to decompress the capsular bag with every injection of fluid. Decompress by exerting pressure on the central part of the nucleus with a cannula in order to express the liquid trapped between the nucleus and the posterior capsule. An excessive quantity of BSS with inadequate decompression can rupture of the posterior capsule, cause luxation of the nucleus into the anterior chamber, or rupture of the rhexis.

- Rupture of the posterior capsule—Even though the posterior capsule has ruptured, the nucleus and the cortex remain in their original positions.

### Table 11-5
### COMPLICATIONS OF HYDRODISSECTION

| | |
|---|---|
| Rupture of the rhexis | Perforation or rupture with a sharp cannula. |
| | Excessive equatorial pressure with the cannula. |
| | Excessive injection pressure. |
| Over deepening the chamber | No VES escapes from the chamber when the BSS is injected. In order to avoid this problem, the BSS injection should be performed through the main incision, pushing gently on the deep flap of the tunnel if necessary. |
| | Injection of excess BSS. |
| Luxation of the nucleus in the anterior chamber | The rhexis is too wide. |
| | The nucleus is small. |
| | The rhexis has ruptured. |
| Rupture of the posterior capsule | Too much liquid is injected. |
| | Under excessive pressure. |
| | Too quickly. |
| Luxation of the nucleus in the vitreal chamber | Rupture of the posterior capsule. |

### Table 11-6
### COMPLICATIONS OF HYDRODISSECTION

| | |
|---|---|
| Insufficient hydrodissection | The nucleus stays attached to the cortex; as a result every technique of endocapsular phaco becomes more difficult. |
| | The surgeon would be wise not to start phaco if hydrodissection has not produced sufficient mobilization of the nucleus (if the nucleus cannot rotate sufficiently inside the bag). |
| Injection of an excessive quantity of BSS in the bag or with excessive pressure | Luxation of the nucleus in the anterior chamber. This happens if the size of the rhexis in comparison to the size of the nucleus will allow this to happen. |
| | Anterior prolapse of the nucleus with rhexis rupture. The surgeon should carefully continue the phaco in the anterior chamber. |
| | Rupture of the rhexis without nuclear prolapse. Transform the rhexis to a can opener. Continue using the technique of phacoemulsification on the pupillary plane. |
| Rupture of the posterior capsule | Due to excessive injection of BSS and high pressure: |
| | If the surgeon is not aware immediately, there is the risk of posterior luxation of the nucleus on the introduction of the U/S tip or following the initial phases of phaco. |
| | If the surgeon is aware, the nucleus should be luxated mechanically in the anterior chamber and then an anterior vitrectomy should be performed with removal of the cortical masses. |
| Possible sectorial or total dislocation of the lens | Excessive injection of BSS in the chamber without the simultaneous escape of VES. |
| | Excessive pressure from the BSS injection. |
| | Following hydrodissection with an open rhexis or after a can opener; the surgeon extends the equatorial escape. |

Subluxation or posterior luxation may occur during nuclear rotation or fragmentation. Immediately after the rupture of the posterior capsule, the nucleus displaces posteriorly. Techniques for dealing with this are described later in the chapter.

- Rupture of the rhexis—By appropriately modifying technique, an experienced surgeon can complete phacoemulsification as planned. However, the novice surgeon should change the capsulotomy into a can opener and perform the phacoemulsification in the pupillary plane, alternately converting to ECCE.
- Luxation of the nucleus into the anterior chamber—Perform a partial phacoemulsification and then, with the help of a spatula, attempt to return the nucleus to the posterior chamber. If this is not successful, proceed with a phacoemulsification in the anterior chamber, being very careful not to damage the corneal endothelium. If the corneal structures are at risk, convert and express the nucleus.
- Insufficient hydrodissection—This is the most common complication which makes all the successive maneuvers of nuclear fracture or phacoemulsification in the bag more difficult. A nucleus which does not rotate or rotates with difficulty provokes excessive traction on the zonules and the capsule. Awareness that insufficient hydrodissection has complicated the procedure requires cessation of phacoemulsification and repeat of the hydrodissection. Do not attempt to force this situation or else a number of complications—such as rupture of the capsulorhexis, disinsertion of the capsular bag, or rupture of the equatorial or posterior capsule—may arise.

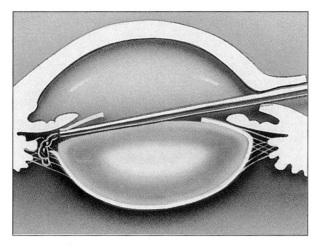

Figure 11-9. Equatorial capsular rupture through careless use of the cannula.

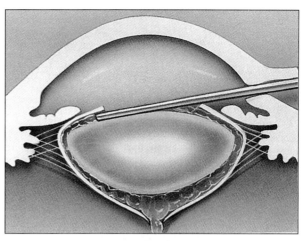

Figure 11-10. Excessive injection of liquid with high pressure and rupture of the posterior capsule.

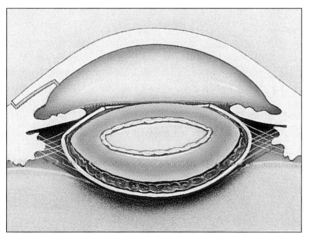

Figure 11-11. Excessive BSS injection.

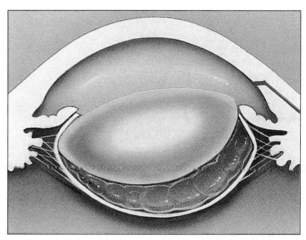

Figure 11-12. Excessive injection of BSS can cause an anterior luxation of the nucleus.

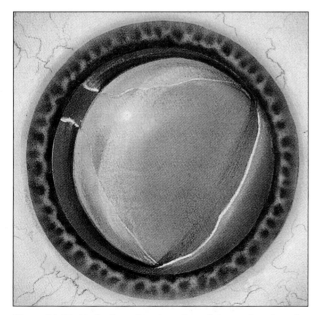

Figure 11-13. Hydrodissection. Luxation of the nucleus into the anterior chamber. Rupture of the rhexis.

## COMPLICATIONS DURING THE INTRODUCTION OF THE U/S TIP INTO THE ANTERIOR CHAMBER

The phaco tip can cause iris dialysis at the point of entry, sometimes followed by hyphaema and contraction of the pupil. As the tip enters, it may come into contact with the endothelium or detach Descemet's membrane. If this latter occurs, fill the eye at the end of the operation either with low molecular weight adhesive viscoelastic or air to encourage the two layers to adhere to each other.

## COMPLICATIONS DURING PHACOEMULSIFICATION

Many problems can occur during phacoemulsification. Some are to be anticipated because of the nature of the individual eye undergoing surgery. This may be seen in eyes with hard nuclei or where there is pseudoexfoliation. Other complications such as poor hydrodissection or difficulty in clean nuclear fracture are not expected. If

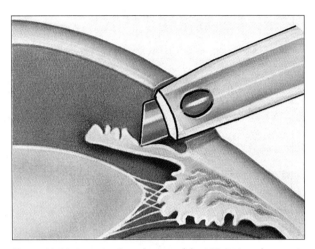

Figure 11-14. Incorrect introduction of the U/S tip into the anterior chamber with iris contact.

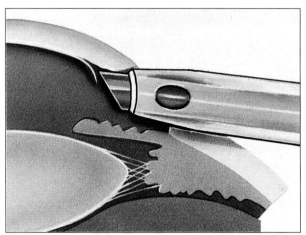

Figure 11-15. Incorrect introduction of the U/S tip. Detachment of the endothelium-Descemet's membrane.

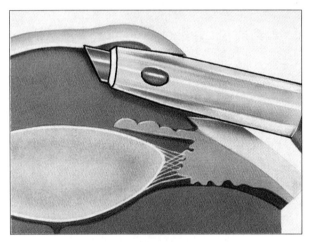

Figure 11-16. Incorrect introduction of the U/S tip. Trauma to the endothelium.

any serious problems arise, it may be better to convert from phacoemulsification of the nucleus to its manual removal. The first step in the conversion consists of extending the incision done for the phacoemulsification.

The incision which is most suitable for conversion is the limbal incision on two planes. This permits easy access to anterior chamber and is therefore particularly suitable for the beginner surgeon. Scleral tunnel or other incisions require a limbal extension of the incision which can be performed using scissors. The cut proceeds at a limbal level beside the original incision.

A corneal incision is extended more easily in its superficial component, while it is necessary to pay special attention to extending the deep parts of the corneal incision in order to avoid creating two different incision planes which would produce negative effects on the apposition and the postoperative astigmatism. More often than not, if conversion is necessary after having performed a corneal tunnel, it is better to start over again with another incision with a more suitable shape.

## Anterior Chamber Phacoemulsification

This technique is rarely performed. Such complications as those which arise with anterior chamber phacoemulsification are related to the hardness of the nucleus. As the nucleus is close to the endothelium, it is advisable to minimize U/S power in order to avoid excess vibration and cellular damage. Try to use a technique of phacoemulsification which will progressively reduce the size of the nucleus without having to use high U/S energy levels. It is also important to use an accessory spatula to control the movements of the nucleus during fragmentation.

When the residual nucleus has been significantly reduced in size, avoid damage to the adjacent structures by reducing the flow and U/S power and increasing the vacuum. This will minimize unnecessary movement of the nuclear fragment. Although operation times may be extended, it is easier to maintain contact with the residual nucleus by the U/S tip and to fragment it in the most suitable manner and position.

Viscoat is very useful during anterior chamber phacoemulsification to protect the corneal endothelium. It must be partially injected before the nucleus is positioned in the anterior chamber. Following the anterior luxation, the chamber is then completely filled; phacoemulsification can be safely begun. If the procedure is too long or when the viscoelastic close to the endothelium has been aspirated, more should be injected, particularly into the space between the nucleus and the cornea. If safe completion of phacoemulsification seems unlikely, convert to an extracapsular technique. Here the most suitable VES are those with a hyaluronic base (Provisc, Healon).

The procedure of conversion is quite simple. The nucleus is already in the anterior chamber, so the original incision for the phacoemulsification just needs to be extended to reach the dimensions suitable for extracting the remainder of the nucleus.

If the nucleus is still large and the posterior capsule is still intact, use pressure and indirect counterpressure on

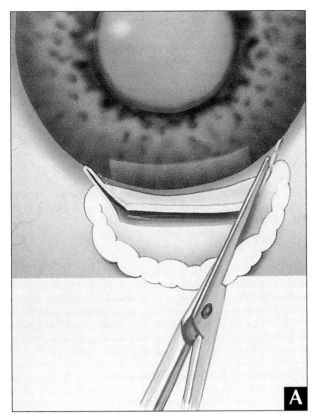 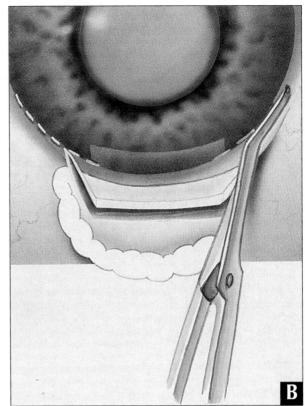

Figures 11-17A, 11-17B Technique for widening the scleral tunnel. If it is necessary to convert from a scleral tunnel, the surgeon should open the two lateral parts with straight scissors or instruments to reach the limbus and proceed in this site with curved scissors to extend the opening further. The incision will then be closed with two single sutures applied radially to the two angles where the sclera has been cut. Other sutures can be applied where necessary.

the nucleus. With a blunt instrument, press at approximately 2.0 mm from the limbus on the sclera at 12 o'clock to open the incision and expose the upper equatorial edge of the crystalline lens. At the same time, scleral counterpressure is exerted with forceps or a rectus hook at 6 o'clock and this is transmitted from the vitreous to the lower and posterior equatorial portion of the nucleus. The combination of the two forces will cause the exit of the nucleus from the anterior chamber. Use a rotation movement on the exposed pole of the nucleus to bring it out of the incision.

If the residual nucleus is small, removal can be completed using a loop. A cohesive VES such as Healon and Provisc is the most suitable for this procedure. Using a simple irrigation loop without viscoelastic is an alternative, but this will cause greater endothelial damage. The loop is introduced into the incision and inserted with irrigation between the iris and the posterior pole of the nucleus. Irrigation is then suspended, and the loop is raised slightly and pulled backward toward the incision along with the nucleus.

Reasons for abandoning anterior chamber phacoemulsification:
- Prolonged U/S times.
- A nucleus which is too hard.
- A shallow anterior chamber.
- Endothelial damage, especially in a cornea with preexisting pathology.
- Doubts about the integrity of the posterior capsule.
- Doubts about completing the procedure without significant complications.
- Narrow miosis and iris lesions due to contact with the U/S tip earlier in the operation.

Complications more likely with anterior chamber phacoemulsification are:
- Damage to the endothelium—Particularly if the viscoelastic protection is not adequate, the damage to the endothelium is directly proportional to the hardness of the nucleus, the time needed for the phacoemulsification, and the degree of trauma involved, etc. Endothelial damage also can occur when the chamber flattens with a hard nucleus that has been partially fragmented. Damage from excessive movement of a hard nuclear fragment in the chamber can be minimized by using Viscoat.
- Rupture of the posterior capsule—This may occur from excessive pressure exerted by the nucleus on the posterior capsule, involuntary perforation, or rupture of the capsule with one of the instruments introduced at the equator or under the nucleus to mobilize or extract it. This also may occur at the end of fragmentation when, due to excess U/S power, the residual nuclear fragments start moving around uncontrollably in the anterior segment.

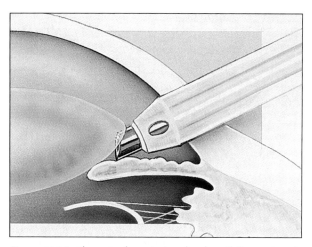

Figure 11-18. Phaco in the anterior chamber. If the nucleus is emulsified from the deep layers, the iris can be damaged.

- Luxation of the nucleus into the vitreous—More often than not, this happens when the posterior capsule has ruptured but the surgeon is unaware and continues fragmentation. The treatment is described at a later stage.

## During Phacoemulsification in the Pupillary Plane Following a Can Opener Capsulotomy

This technique of phacoemulsification is done in the iris plane following a can opener capsulotomy. Problems may be related to poor nuclear mobilization or unexpected nuclear hardness.

- Difficult mobilization of the nucleus—Ideally the nucleus is partially luxated from the capsule in the 12 o'clock position. Having been centrally sculpted, the nucleus is pushed up by the vitreous pressure as the manipulator pushes the nucleus toward 6 o'clock. The phaco tip then impales the superior pole and infusion fluid is turned on, which cleaves between the nucleus and the cortex allowing mobilization.

  However, this maneuver is technically difficult, and while it frequently allows fixation of the equator of the nucleus by the U/S tip, it is often not performed satisfactorily so as to provide sufficient mobilization.

It may be difficult to rotate the nucleus to expose new equatorial positions to the U/S tip due to the incomplete cortico-nuclear cleavage. If inadequate pressure is exerted by the spatula during the rotation of the nucleus, there is the risk of zonular dialysis. If the residual nucleus is large, a partial luxation may be sufficient to capture a portion of the equator of the nucleus with the U/S tip and continue the phacoemulsification as planned.

If, in the final phases of removal of the residual nucleus after having emulsified the equatorial crown, the posterior layers of the nucleus are extremely adherent to each other and to the cortex, use vacuum values which are suitable for mobilizing the residual nucleus and bringing it to the center of the pupillary field. This is according to the methods described in the previous chapters, without the risk of involving the posterior capsule in this maneuver. An alternative is to remove the U/S tip and inject Viscoat under the nuclear plate. This will not only raise it but will also form a protective layer of product between the capsule and the residual nucleus, which makes continuing the procedure safer.

With the chamber filled with viscoelastic, use a spatula and try to rotate the nucleus without exerting excessive traction until the cortical adhesions are free. Another method involves depressing the nucleus at 6 o'clock with a spatula to expose the equator at 12 o'clock; then inject Viscoat underneath. A viscoseparation between the nucleus and the cortex is obtained.

A more experienced surgeon can avoid this last maneuver by using the occluded phaco tip as the tool for freeing the residual nucleus. First, expose the inferior pole by pressing with the spatula at 12 o'clock and then engaging the nuclear edge that presents. Pull the nucleus away from the capsule for safe emulsification.

- Unexpected hardness of the nucleus—If the nucleus is unexpectedly large and hard and concern is felt about a successful outcome, it is better to luxate the nucleus into the anterior chamber in order to complete phacoemulsification there or to convert to a manual extracapsular technique. Problems of hard nuclei in this position have already been discussed.

If it is felt prudent to change technique due to nuclear hardness, the decision should be taken on the basis of the patient's endothelial picture, the type of anesthesia used, and general reflections regarding the length of the operation, the appearance of the anterior segment, the surgeon's expertise, the quality of the instruments, etc. In any case, the alternative choice must be adopted rapidly, in that the conversion to a manual extracapsular technique is easier if the nucleus is still large.

Other problems during phacoemulsification in the pupillary plane are:

- Difficulty luxating the nucleus superiorly—This happens more frequently with soft nuclei where the spatula is not able to exert sufficient pressure inferiorly to luxate the nucleus. Here, phacoemulsification must continue in the posterior chamber but this will make the operation more difficult.
- Rupture of the posterior capsule—This problem with or without vitreous loss will be analyzed in the following pages.
- Luxation of the nucleus or parts of it into the vitreous chamber—This will also be covered in the pages that follow.
- Iris damage on the inferior pupillary margin—This occurs when the ultrasound tip in the initial phase of sculpting the nucleus moves too close to the iris. If they come into contact, the iris can be sucked in and damaged. This can lead to other problems because the iris filaments are repeatedly aspirated toward the U/S tip which provokes further iris damage. Iris contacts can be a strong stimulus for miosis which will make the entire procedure more difficult.

### During Endocapsular Phacoemulsification

Endocapsular phacoemulsification requires good hydrodissection to avoid problems. Such difficulties that arise with this technique and its solution are determined by the fact that the procedure takes place in the posterior chamber behind the capsulorhexis which should be preserved if possible.

## COMPLICATIONS DURING ENDOCAPSULAR TECHNIQUES WITHOUT NUCLEOFRACTURE

The hardness of the nucleus causes most problems. During sculpting, the surgeon will form a clear idea as to whether the consistency of the nucleus is the right grade of hardness for the planned technique. If the nucleus is harder than expected, it is advisable to abandon this technique to avoid the risk of complications in the posterior capsule and the zonules.

The alternative choices depend on the experience of the surgeon. With suitable capsulorhexis and hydrodissection, the best choice is that of performing a nuclear fracture under the protection of Viscoat. A less experienced surgeon should resort to conversion with manual extraction of the nucleus. However, the size of the capsulorhexis may be important. If the diameter is small, there is a risk that the anterior edge will open with consequent tear toward the equator.

Try to reduce the volume of the nucleus to a minimum (remembering that a hard nucleus is almost always large) before converting to the manual extracapsular technique. Alternatively, if the rhexis is of sufficient size, do viscoexpression by injecting a VES posterior to the nucleus. If the rhexis is small, two relaxing incisions should be done on the capsulorhexis at 10 and 2 o'clock under Provisc or Healon protection, though by doing this the surgeon loses the benefits of the capsulorhexis. If mydriasis permits and if the surgeon feels confident enough to perform the operation, try to extend the capsulorhexis to allow the nucleus to exit.

Once the nucleus has been brought into the anterior chamber, remove it manually with the help of a loop. The presence of a capsulorhexis changes the distribution of the pressure and counter-pressure lines, and the expression of the nucleus by pressure and counter-pressure may be difficult.

- Good hydrodissection will ensure that there are few problems with the rotation of the nucleus for the removal of the equatorial crown. The problems differ depending on the consistency of the material.

If the nucleus is soft, it is possible that the U/S tip will sink into the equatorial tissue and put the posterior capsule under tension. On the other hand, if the nucleus is hard, the rotation with the tip can cause zonular traction. In the latter, it is advisable to repeat the hydrodissection to obtain the mobilization of the nucleus and then rotate it with the spatula.

The hydrodissection cannula is used again to inject fluid between the capsule and the residual nucleus. If this is still not successful, try viscoelastic. The anterior chamber is filled first, and then slowly and gradually the fluid is injected between the capsule and the nucleus. Using the cannula, the nucleus is then mobilized enough to be rotated with the spatula.

- Problems can also arise with the removal of the equatorial parts of the nucleus. By changing the parameters of the phaco machine, such as raising the level of vacuum, occlusion can be obtained more easily and subsequently the capture and fragmentation of the residual nucleus will occur. However, there is also an increased risk of aspirating the posterior capsule. Vice versa, by keeping the vacuum low (around 40 to 60 mm Hg), the risks for the capsule decrease but there is an increase in the difficulty of retaining occlusion of the phaco tip by the nucleus and its subsequent removal.

## COMPLICATIONS RELATING TO ENDOCAPSULAR TECHNIQUES OF NUCLEOFRACTURE

In the event of an unexpectedly hard nucleus, the surgeon must proceed as described in the previous paragraph.

To avoid complications with nuclear fracture, a perfect capsulorhexis is highly desirable. In the absence of this, the eye is exposed to the risk of complication. Therefore, it is advisable either to change the capsulotomy (and the phaco technique) or to convert. Respect the integrity of the edge of the anterior capsule during the maneuvers of aspiration and fragmentation of the peripheral nuclear material.

Satisfactory hydrodissection is extremely important; without this, the nucleus will not rotate and the entire procedure will become much more difficult. If the nucleus moves excessively during sculpting, stabilize it with a spatula and reduce the values of the U/S power, increasing vacuum. It is also useful to reinject Viscoat into the anterior chamber.

The spatula should not exert excessive traction forces during the rotation movements of the nucleus nor should it go beyond the edge of the nuclear material in order to avoid the risk of capsular tears.

When the technique involves the preparation of one or more grooves, the U/S power must be proportional to the hardness of the nucleus.

- If the nucleus is medium-hard or soft (Grade 2 or 3), the groove must extend toward the equator of the nucleus but should not be too deep, as this would cause problems in obtaining fracture.

  If a hydrodelineation was performed, impaling a fragment will normally separate the piece of nucleus from the epinucleus. In order to protect the posterior capsule, the epinucleus should remain in situ. Avoid aspirating it with the quadrant as this will normally cause the simultaneous mobilization of the other nuclear sectors still contained by the epinucleus.

Once the removal of the quadrants has been completed, the epinucleus can be aspirated in the pupillary plane,

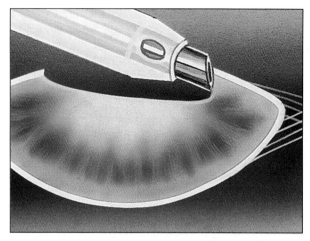

Figure 11-19. During sculpting, the surgeon should avoid bringing the U/S tip into contact with the edge of the rhexis.

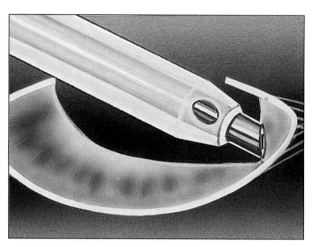

Figure 11-20. During sculpting, the surgeon should avoid going in too deep. This can happen easily distally.

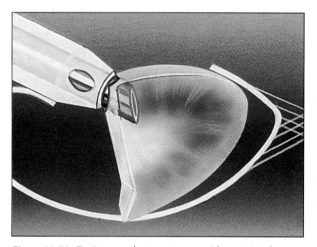

Figure 11-21. During quadrant capture, avoid rupturing the posterior capsule with the inferior edge.

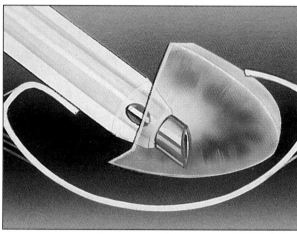

Figure 11-22. During quadrant fragmentation, avoid rupturing the posterior capsule with the U/S tip.

facilitated by the spatula which rotates the epinucleus on itself in order to bring it to the U/S tip (the *flip* maneuver).
- Vice versa, in the event of a hard nucleus, the groove must be as deep as possible until the red reflex of the posterior cortex appears. This allows the combined action of the instruments for nuclear fracture to be used to maximum advantage. The deepening may require several rotations of the nucleus with consequent increase in surgical time.
- When the nucleus is hard, there is little, if any, epinucleus. It is a single unit with the nucleus, and the peripheral cortex is reduced to a thin layer.

In hard nuclei, avoid the fractured edge tilting toward the posterior capsule by impaling nuclear quadrants at the apex, brought toward the U/S tip through the combined, coordinated action of the nucleus manipulator and the phaco tip.

If a large nuclear fragment splits into several parts which move around uncontrollably in the anterior chamber, try pulsed U/S phaco or raising the vacuum levels and lowering the flow. Viscoat is also very helpful.

## Possible Complications of Nucleofractis

1. Complications which arise during the preparation of the cross.
   - Rupture of the capsulorhexis flap—This may occur when the arms of the cross are too long and the phaco tip comes too close to the anterior capsule and ruptures it. Also, this may occur when the nucleus is fragmented close to the surface or the tip comes into contact with the capsular rim. It occurs more frequently when the rhexis is small.

Phacoemulsification can continue but proceed very carefully. The situation will become more difficult if there is more than one tear. Here the nucleus will continue to escape from the bag and enter the anterior chamber. Attempt to reposition it in the bag with the help of a dispersive viscoelastic, but this is still very dangerous. It is better to phacoemulsify the nucleus anterior to the iris plane. If the nucleus is hard, convert to an ECCE, extending the incision.

If there is even a suggestion of equatorial or posterior extension of capsular rupture, interrupt the procedure

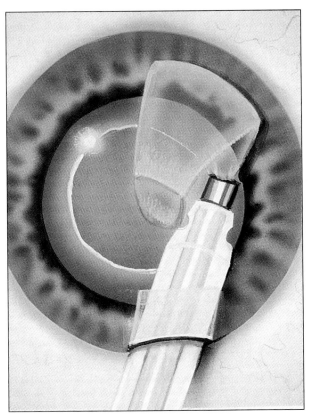

Figure 11-23. The quadrants should be approached in a comfortable position; otherwise occlusion will be difficult.

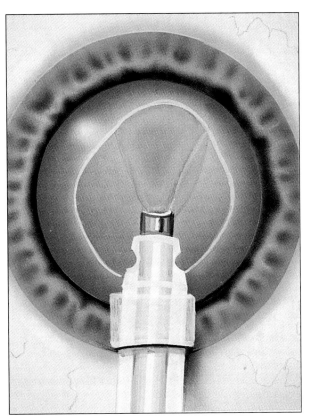

Figure 11-24. During fragmentation of the quadrants, avoid pressing on the edges of the rhexis.

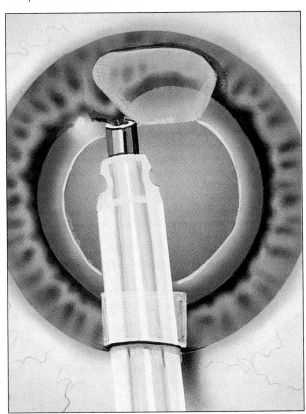

Figure 11-25. If done improperly, the capture of the free quadrants in the chamber can damage the iris.

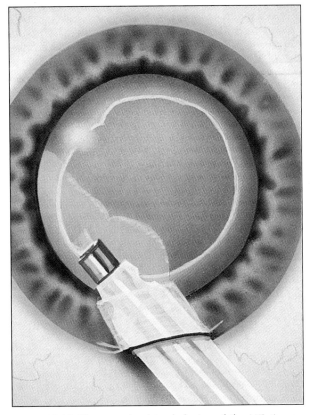

Figure 11-26. The excessive lateral sloping of the U/S tip can reduce irrigation through compression on the sleeve. Among other things, it can burn the incision if U/S is used extensively.

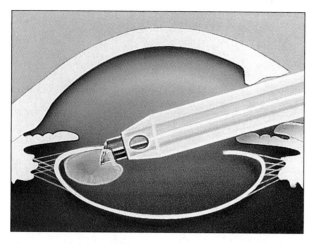

Figure 11-27. The U/S tip can rupture the rhexis during capture of one of the quadrants.

immediately, and prolapse the nucleus into the anterior chamber (possibly following some relaxing incisions in the rhexis or after having converted to a can opener). The incision is then extended and the nucleus is extracted manually.

Once the removal of the nucleus and the cortex is completed, an IOL with 5.5 to 6.0 mm optic and length of 12.0 to 12.5 mm is implanted in the bag. In order to prevent decentering of the IOL through postoperative contraction of the bag—necessarily asymmetrical—cut the rhexis directly opposite to the first tear.

- Perforation of the posterior capsule—This happens if the groove is cut too deep, through the involuntary occlusion of the tip because of excessive vacuum strength (as a result, too much material is removed at once and there is perforation of the capsule). If the cross has been extended too far toward the equator, the capsule may also be ruptured. In this situation, stop the phacoemulsification, fill the chamber with Provisc or Healon, and manually extract the nucleus once the anterior capsular opening has been extended.
- Sectoral zonular rupture with disinsertion of the capsular bag—If the phaco tip pushes too hard on the nucleus the zonules may disinsert. There may also be weak zonules, as in patients with pseudoexfoliation or following trauma. However, this usually happens during fragmentation or during rotation of the nucleus.

It can happen in a number of situations:
- Disinsertion of a partially fragmented nucleus with an intact capsule and hyaloid. Hydrodissection is repeated. If the nucleus rotates, proceed with a cross-shaped phacoemulsification under Viscoat protection in order to keep the shape of the bag. Here, prior to implanting the IOL in the bag, it is better to insert an intracapsular ring to distend uniformly the equator of the bag.
- Disinsertion with rupture of the anterior hyaloid with vitreous in the anterior chamber. The nucleus or part of the nucleus still remains in the bag. A vitrectomy is performed under Viscoat in the anterior chamber. Then the tip of the vitreous cutter is passed through the disinsertion zone into the vitreous chamber and the widest possible vitrectomy is produced. Viscoelastic is injected, even posteriorly, to replace the vitreous removed. Then the hydrodissection is repeated by slowly rotating the nucleus. The incision will be extended and the procedure should be converted to ECCE. If the disinsertion increases during these steps, the surgeon should continue with an intracapsular extraction with the cryo tip resting on the capsulorhexis.

2. Complications during the rotation of the nucleus.

The most frequent complications are zonular disinsertion and the rupture of the bag. If the epinucleus has not been adequately detached from the capsule during hydrodissection, rotation becomes much more traumatic. If it becomes apparent that the nucleus is not sufficiently mobile inside the bag, continue with more hydrodissection to mobilize it.

3. Complications which occur during nuclear fracture.

The biggest risk is the rupture of the posterior capsule. This can occur in the following circumstances: when the grooves have been sculpted incorrectly and when excessive movement of the two hemi-nuclei is needed to fracture the nucleus. It also due to a thin spatula perforating the soft nucleus and rupturing the capsule or if excessive pressure is used because the grooves are not deep enough. During nuclear fracture the rhexis may be torn particularly if it is small and the maneuvers of nuclear fracture are too great.

4. Complications during the capture and the fragmentation of four nuclear quadrants.
- Rupture of the posterior capsule—This can happen after division if the remaining quadrants are excessively mobile. They can rupture the posterior capsule. If there is a poor relationship between infusion and aspiration with continual collapse and refilling of the anterior chamber, this can damage the lens capsule, the corneal endothelium, or the zonular fibers.

This complication can also be caused by too high vacuum, particularly when the consistency of the nucleus is very soft, or when attempting to obtain occlusion in a section of the quadrant with very little material (in this case the posterior capsule is captured).

- Other complications—During the fragmentation of the nuclear quadrants, avoid emulsifying too close to the posterior surface of the cornea. This will prevent damage to the corneal endothelium. Also avoid fragmenting too close to the iris or too tightly in contact with the posterior capsule.

Frequently there are mini collapses of the anterior chamber. These happen mainly when fragmentation is done under high vacuum and strong flow rate, using phacoemulsifiers which do not have an adequate anti-surge mechanism.

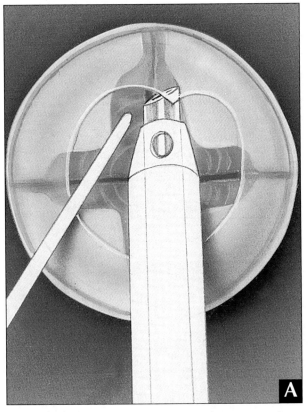 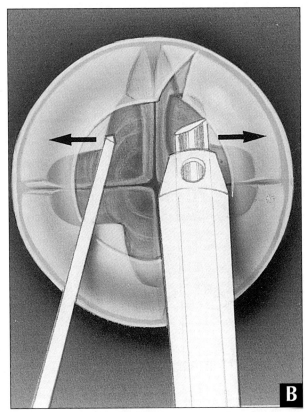

Figures 11-28A, 11-28B. Nucleofracture or other intraoperative reason may induce rupture of the rhexis.

## Complications With the Phaco Chop Technique

In the Phaco Chop technique, some problems may arise with the use of the chopper, the instrument used in combination with the U/S tip to fragment the nucleus. The greatest risk involves going in too deep, especially when the nucleus is still compact and adequate visualization of the deep planes is difficult.

In the Phaco Chop technique, it is not always easy to impale the nucleus well. High vacuum should be used. The operator should aim directly toward the center of the nucleus. Once the nucleus has been impaled and split, even the transport of the first nuclear segment to outside the capsular bag is difficult to achieve. This is due to the fact that the various segments adhere to one another inside the capsular bag. This is more likely if the surgeon is not very experienced and the various nuclear segments are not separated in an optimal manner.

Viscoat should be injected into the anterior chamber and the bag. Then repeat the maneuver made with the chopper. Alternatively use the chopper to disinsert the relevant section of nucleus. If it is not possible to remove this sector, it is best not to persist. Repeat nuclear fixation after having rotated it and then try again. And if at once you do not succeed, rotate and try again.

Alternately, one can use the variations of the Stop and Chop and the Mini Chop described in other chapters.

## POSTERIOR CAPSULE RUPTURE

The rupture of the posterior capsule, with or without rupture of the hyaloid face, with or without material falling into the vitreous, is undoubtedly the main complication in the U/S phase. This deserves more detailed description. In phacoemulsification, the rupture of the posterior capsule usually occurs for the following reasons:
- Discontinuity of the anterior capsulotomy with a tear which extends posteriorly beyond the zonules.
- Zonular disinsertion through traction linked to the manipulations on the nucleus with the residual anterior capsule intact.
- Direct action of the U/S tip on the capsule during the formation of the grooves or during other fragmentation maneuvers.
- Lacerations of the capsule during splitting into sectors or quadrants.
- Flattening of the chamber and the capsular bag allowing sharp nuclear fragments to come into contact with the posterior capsule.

The presence of nuclear material, whether or not vitreous, is in the anterior chamber. There are some unusual aspects caused by the presence of a large portion of the anterior capsule.

Capsulorhexis in a closed system creates an important barrier which helps to balance the pressure values between the vitreous and the anterior chamber. This is even more important the smaller the diameter of the cap-

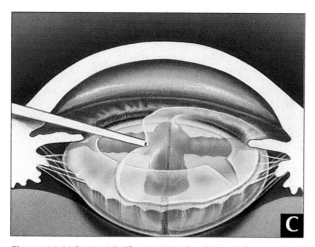
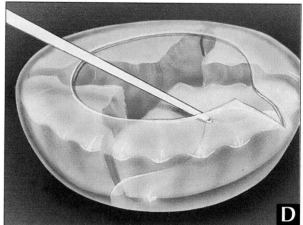

Figures 11-28C, 11-28D. The anterior chamber, not the capsular bag, is filled with viscoelastic.

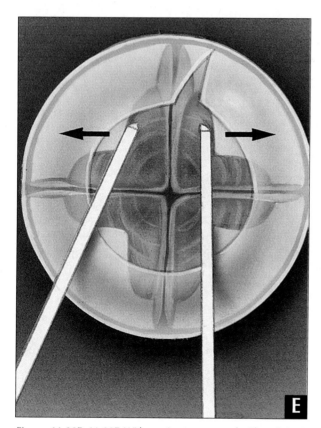
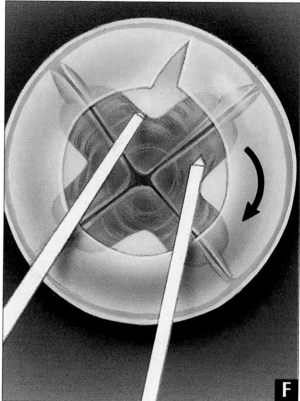

Figures 11-28E, 11-28F. With two instruments and without irrigation, nucleofracture is delicately completed. Rotation allows the nucleus to be divided into four pieces.

sulorhexis. For this reason, even in the presence of a large rupture or a large posterior zonular disinsertion (90 to 120°), it is possible to implant in the ciliary groove with a good safety margin. The rim of the anterior capsule left by the capsulorhexis acts as a support. Careful cleaning of the capsular bag of all the nuclear material and the vitreous has to be undertaken.

At the surgeon's discretion, some cortical residues in the capsular bag can be left without any great risk, as long as they are very small and are not in contact with the vitreous. In this case, an implant in the ciliary sulcus will cause the anterior and posterior flaps to stick together, trapping the residual cortex. In time, it will become fibrous and membranous but there will be no inflammation. The stage of the operation will influence the best approach.

1. In the initial phases, rupture of the posterior capsule occurs because of an extension in the edge of the rhexis. This is usually due to direct action of the U/S tip on the edge of the rhexis and it happens during sculpting or the formation of the grooves. Initially it involves the anterior capsule. It then extends to the equatorial sectors and sometimes even posteriorly.

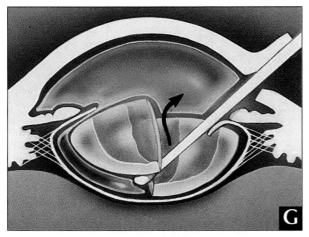 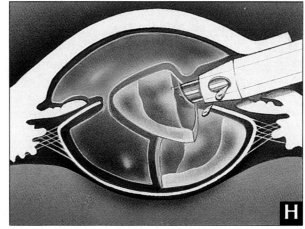

Figures 11-28G, 11-28H. Rupture of the rhexis during the techniques of nucleofracture. After having delicately divided the nucleus, manually luxate and then emulsify one quadrant.

Table 11-7A
## COMPLICATIONS OF PHACO

| Problem | Cause | Prevention/treatment |
|---|---|---|
| Capture of the iris with the U/S tip | Use of high vacuum. The tip comes too close to the iris. Mobile, flaccid iris. | In the initial phases of phaco, keep vacuum levels low. In all phases of the operation, particularly when vacuum is high, stay away from the iris. |
| Rupture of the rhexis | Use of high U/S in contact with the capsule. During the division into quadrants or the splitting (Phaco Chop). Through mechanical traction with instruments (spatulas, U/S tips). | Avoid using the U/S against the capsule of the rhexis edge. Limit gaping during the division of the nucleus. Be very careful when using the instruments in the chamber. |
| Damage to the incision | Incision which is too narrow. Use of U/S which is too strong. Insufficient flow rate. Pressure of the U/S tip against the incision (sectorial obstruction of the irrigation). | Extend the opening slightly. Reduce the U/S power. Increase the exchange rate of BSS in the chamber. Reduce the pressure exerted by the U/S tip on the incision. |
| Endothelial damage | Emulsification of the nucleus in the anterior chamber. Emulsification close to the endothelium. Emulsification without VES protection. Fragments of nucleus which are excessively mobile in the chamber. | Try to emulsify the harder portions inside the capsular bag or on the pupillary plane. During the entire procedure, avoid free fragments rotating freely inside the anterior chamber. If for any reason it is necessary to emulsify inside the anterior chamber, avoid using high U/S. It produces continual movement of the fragments and continual escape of the material from the tip. It is better to use high vacuum, low flow rate, and low U/S to work predominantly in occlusion so that the material remains in close contact with the tip. Inject Viscoat into the chamber to form a uniform layer on the entire internal surface of the cornea. In case of long phaco time, inject Viscoat many times into the chamber to give a continuous endothelial protection. Excessive mobility of the fragments at the end of phaco. To restrict the turbulence and facilitate the capture of the fragments, the surgeon should use low flow rate and high vacuum. He or she can also inject abundant Viscoat to protect the cornea and the posterior capsule. |

Table 11-7B
# COMPLICATIONS OF PHACO

| | Cause | Prevention/treatment |
|---|---|---|
| Rupture of the posterior capsule | Surgeon's ego. | The surgeon should be able to evaluate when the operation is not easily controlled and/or unsafe and be able to stop in time to modify the procedure. |
| | Sculpting of the nucleus which is too deep during the creation of the grooves with perforation of the capsule. This occurs more frequently distally. | Observe the changes in the red reflex of the fundus. Keep a check on the various layers of the nucleus and evaluate when a sector (usually the distal one) is sculpted more than the others. Always use the diameter of the U/S tip or that of the sleeve as the reference for evaluating the depth of the sculpting. |
| | Collapse of the chamber, ie, sudden occlusion break when working under high vacuum and flow rate inside the capsular bag. | This happens largely with phacoemulsifiers which are not fitted with a good anti-surge system. At the occlusion break, there is a sudden withdraw of fluid and with it anything mobile in the area. The posterior capsule may be caught and ruptured. Don't remain in occlusion for long time. Don't preset high vacuum. |
| | During the division of the nucleus into quadrants. | This happens mainly if the two retractors operate too close to the posterior capsule. When the hydrodissection has not sufficiently separated the deep layer of the nucleus from the posterior capsule. With equatorial and posterior extension of the rhexis opening. This happens particularly during nucleofracture. |
| | Excessive mobility of one quadrant with rupture of the posterior capsule. | This occurs particularly if the last quadrant consists of hard material. It can be dangerous if it has sharp edges. Under the effect of a high flow rate or through excessive mobility, it can bump into the posterior capsule and rupture it. |
| | Collapse of the chamber. | Because of bending in the irrigation tube. Because of emptying of the BSS bottle. Rupture of the capsule occurs when the tip works close to the posterior capsule. |
| Rupture of the posterior capsule (continued) | During peeling and capture of the epinucleus. | Excessive manipulation can induce capsular rupture. When the surgeon tries to luxate the epinucleus with the spatula. When the posterior epinucleus is intact and is bowl-shaped and remains attached to the posterior and equatorial capsule (particularly if there has been poor hydrodissection). The surgeon will be tempted to bring the U/S tip into close contact and use relatively high vacuum to detach it. However, the surgeon is dealing with soft material. Aspiration allows very easy capture of the underlying capsule, which can rupture. |
| | Use of unsuitable parameters. | |
| | | Lack of concentration. This can happen if the surgeon relaxes toward the end of phaco in the belief that he or she has overcome all the obstacles. |
| | Incorrect use of the accessory instrument or the use of an instrument which is too sharp. | The spatula or the chopper can rupture the posterior capsule particularly when they are used in close contact with it. |

Table 11-8
## CONVERSION

| | |
|---|---|
| When | The pupil is too narrow and it is difficult for the surgeon to see what he or she is doing. |
| | The posterior capsule has ruptured. |
| | On any occasion that the surgeon does not feel qualified to complete the phaco. |
| | The U/S device of the phaco is broken or the machine is not functioning properly. |
| How | Inject a thin layer of Provisc or Healon into the anterior chamber to protect the endothelium. |
| | Then inject a greater quantity under the nucleus to facilitate the luxation from the posterior to the anterior chamber. |
| | Extend the incision in proportion to the diameter of the nucleus. |
| | Extend the pupillary diameter (iridotomy). |
| | Extend the capsulotomy if it narrows (if there is a rhexis, perform two to three relaxing incisions). |
| Luxation of the nucleus | Perform mechanical luxation of the nucleus into the anterior chamber under the control of viscoelastic (Provisc or Healon). Please refer to the techniques of anterior luxation of the nucleus. |
| Extraction of the nucleus | Perform a viscoextraction with a rough loop. |
| | Perform a viscoextraction with Sheets' slide. |
| I/A cortex | Perform in a closed chamber after having sutured the incision carefully. |

Table 11-9
## EXTENSION OF THE INCISION FOR THE CONVERSION

| | |
|---|---|
| Limbal incision | Simply extend the incision by continuing with the same type of incision. Two pairs of scissors can be used (right and left) or a blade. It should be done under viscoelastic protection. |
| Posteriorized scleral incision | Perform two short radial incisions in the sclera to approach the limbus. |
| | Extend toward the limbus as said earlier. |
| Scleral tunnel | Using scissors or knife, perform a cut on the left or right side of the tunnel to reach the anterior limbus. The cut can be radial or, better still, angled in such a way as to reach the limbus almost tangentially. |
| | The surgeon can then proceed by extending at the limbus. |
| Corneal tunnel | If the tunnel is superior: |
| |     Cut the conjunctiva. |
| |     Perform a limbal incision posterior to the two sides of the tunnel. |
| |     Reach the tunnel with two radial incisions. |
| | If the tunnel is temporal: |
| |     Suture it with one or more 10-0 nylon sutures. If self-sealing, no suture is required. |
| |     Perform a new limbal incision superiorly. |

If rupture occurs, the entire procedure should be slowed down. Various maneuvers should be used to reduce the extension:
- Avoid pressure of the U/S tip on the nucleus.
- Avoid engaging too much material in the tip.
- Above all, avoid trying to bring this material into the anterior chamber through the rhexis.
- Keep the chamber depth stable (in particular, avoid flattening and excessive deepening).
- Avoid maneuvers of nuclear fracture particularly in the area of the rhexis opening.

2. Capsular rupture in the intermediate phases of phacoemulsification happens when the nucleus is mobilized or the surgeon tries to impale large nuclear fragments with sharp edges.

With a large nuclear remnant still in the posterior chamber, it is of the utmost importance to recognize early rupture of the posterior capsule. To continue with the procedure may result in an increase in the size of the opening because the pressure of the infusion on the inside of the capsular bag can extend the rupture and dislocate the nucleus into the vitreous with all of its consequences.

If the surgeon is aware immediately of a capsular opening in this phase, he or she has time to stop phacoemulsification and decide how to continue. This will depend once again on the residual size and hardness of the nuclear material and the presence of vitreous or not.

3. Capsular opening in the final stages of phacoemulsification (when less than a quarter of the nucleus remains).
- If the hyaloid face is intact, Viscoat is injected into the bag to try to close the opening, and the fragment is brought into the anterior chamber. Using a suitable level of vacuum the piece is emulsified.
- If the hyaloid face is broken and the vitreous has prolapsed, Viscoat is injected to push the vitreous away. Before the residual nucleus is emulsified, an anterior vitrectomy is performed which is just large enough for the removal of the vitreous from the anterior chamber. Then after having reformed the

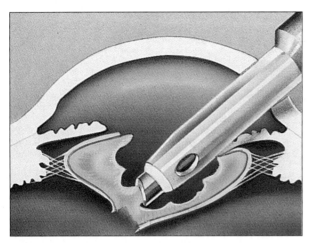

Figure 11-29. Rupture of the posterior capsule through careless phaco.

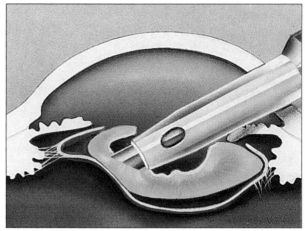

Figure 11-30. Zonular rupture during phacoemulsification. The tip of the instrument has pulled the nucleus, detaching the zonule.

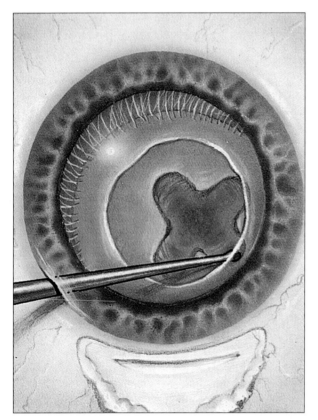

Figure 11-31. Zonular rupture during the rotation movements of the nucleus.

anterior chamber with a thick layer of Viscoat, the piece of nucleus is emulsified.
- If the hyaloid face is broken and the vitreous in the anterior chamber is abundant, it is better to do a preliminary anterior vitrectomy. Then extract the piece using a loop, widening the incision if necessary. After this, complete the anterior vitrectomy.

It cannot be over emphasized how important it is to perform the most accurate anterior vitrectomy possible to reduce postoperative complications to an absolute minimum and condition the eye for the best IOL implantation. Following anterior vitrectomy strategy depends on the quantity and the location of the residual cortex.

It is sometimes necessary to perform a posterior vitrectomy. This is decided on the basis of the amount of cortex and/or nuclear material present in the posterior chamber or in the vitreous. It also depends on the amount of vitreous remaining in the anterior segment.

There are particular problems related to posterior capsular rupture which will now be considered.

### Rupture of the Posterior Capsule Without Hyaloid Face Rupture

There are three alternatives:
1. If the nucleus is still intact, make relaxing incisions on the rhexis and perform an ECCE.

   Inject viscoelastic into the anterior chamber and most importantly under the nucleus. In this case Healon GV and Viscoat are both needed. A moderate quantity of Healon GV is injected under the nucleus. Too much viscoelastic can cause an extension of the capsular opening. A thin layer of Viscoat must be injected between the Healon GV and the vitreous face.

   A relaxing incision in the anterior capsule is performed with the cystotome at 2 and 10 o'clock. The corneal or scleral incision is then extended and the nucleus is extracted with the least traumatic technique possible. Use a method which does not require pressure on the nucleus because this may induce its luxation into the vitreous chamber. A knurled loop introduced underneath the nucleus is used to extract it.

   The corneo-scleral incision must be wide for nucleus removal to reduce the traction to a minimum.
2. Another alternative for expert surgeons especially if the nucleus is soft is to inject Viscoat under the nucleus and then proceed with emulsification under low power U/S and flow rate, and high vacuum, proceeding slowly with the bottle lowered.

   Viscoat is fundamental for this procedure. It adheres well to the tissues and stays in the position it was injected. This means that it forms a useful barrier between the nucle-

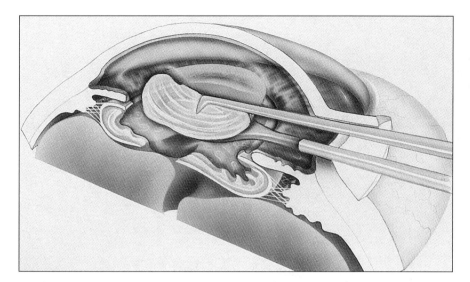

Figure 11-32. In the event of capsular rupture without vitreous loss, if the nuclear material is still large, the surgeon should extend the incision and perform a manual extraction under VES protection.

Table 11-10
## SIGNS OF POSTERIOR CAPSULE RUPTURE

| | |
|---|---|
| The first most common sign is a slight deepening of the anterior chamber | This happens because the posterior capsule behaves like a hammock which supports the lens. If the capsule opens, the nucleus will penetrate (initially only partially, then completely), thus deepening the anterior chamber. |
| Rupture of the rhexis outside visible limits | In this situation, the surgeon should always suspect progression toward the posterior capsule and he or she should react accordingly. In fact, the zonule is a barrier which provides sufficient resistance to the extension of the rhexis. |
| Reduction of the aspiration | This may mean that the vitreous has obstructed the tip's orifice. |
| A piece of nucleus appears smaller | If a piece of nucleus of known dimensions becomes smaller or appears to decrease in size, it means that part of it has inserted into the opening. |
| Loss of a piece of nucleus | It may have disappeared into the vitreous through a zonular opening or through a capsular opening. |

Table 11-11
## IF THERE IS A DOUBT ABOUT THE RUPTURE OF THE POSTERIOR CAPSULE

| | |
|---|---|
| Stop phaco immediately | If the surgeon continues, it means that pieces of the nucleus will be lost in the vitreous. Moreover, the vitreous is aspirated through the orifice. Remember that the U/S tip and/or the I/A tip cannot perform a vitrectomy or remove the vitreous. |
| Reduce the pressure and the external traction | This can force the vitreous out through the opening. |
| Lower the bottle | Excessive pressure of the infusion liquid can extend the opening and/or push the vitreous out through the opening. |
| Display the opening well by adjusting the focus, the degree of magnification, etc of the microscope | Site, size, shape, etc of the opening. |
| Check if there is vitreous in the anterior chamber | It can be seen by careful observation. Alternately, use a spatula to check. Rubbing a swab sponge along the incision can help the diagnosis. |

us and the vitreous and allows the surgeon to finish the operation with limited damage to the surrounding tissues.
3. If the portion of the nucleus is hard or medium-hard and moderate in size, it is possible to complete the phacoemulsification. The vitreous pressure must be counterbalanced by a viscoelastic which can remain in place even with an irrigation flow with relative turbulence (Viscoat). It is injected under the residual nucleus and must create a uniform layer deposited in the capsular break.

Remember that maintenance of positive pressure by BSS flow opposes the vitreal thrust but this pressure, at a

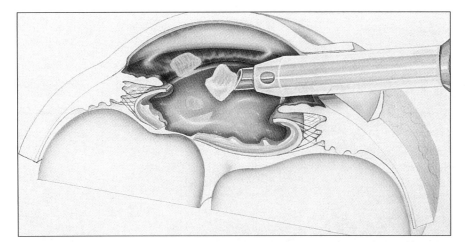

Figure 11-33. When the capsular rupture is limited and there is only a small amount of nuclear material left, under certain conditions, phacoemulsification can be continued. The use of Viscoat to close the rupture is mandatory.

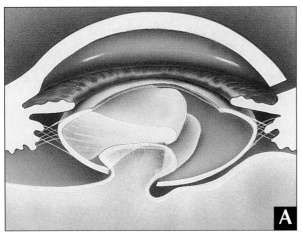
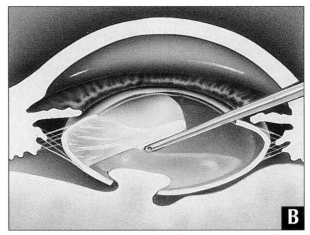

Figures 11-34A, 11-34B. Behavior in the event of posterior capsular rupture with intact hyaloid during phacoemulsification. In the event of a capsular opening with an intact hyaloid, the surgeon should inject Viscoat inside the capsular bag and close the opening, pushing the vitreous behind the pupillary plane.

later stage, can increase the size of the capsular aperture. Here, an adequate layer of Viscoat will reduce the negative effect that the irrigation flow and the increase in depth of the anterior chamber may have on the capsular opening. In addition, it counters the tendency of vitreous loss, preventing the irrigation liquid or the fragment of nucleus from rupturing the hyaloid membrane.

In this way it is possible to complete phacoemulsification without luxation, reducing the values of flow and bottle height and increasing the values of vacuum. The surgeon must remember to replace the VES periodically as it is gradually aspirated so that the layer always provides sufficient protection of the posterior chamber and the vitreous.

Once the piece of nucleus has been removed, the anterior chamber is filled with a non-adhesive VES (Provisc or Healon). Using a syringe, manually remove all the cortex (dry technique).

The injection of VES will be repeated several times so that the anterior chamber is always the right size and the cleaning is complete. Then proceed to implant the IOL in the posterior chamber in the sulcus in front of the rhexis.

### Rupture of the Posterior Capsule With Hyaloid Rupture Without Luxation of Nuclear Material into the Vitreous

When the hyaloid face is ruptured and the vitreous prolapses into the anterior chamber, it is necessary to proceed with an anterior vitrectomy. The procedure used depends on the quantity of material present.

- If the portion of nucleus is very large, it is advisable to convert.

Viscoat is injected into the capsular bag under the nuclear material to limit the progression of the vitreous and to avoid posterior luxation of the nucleus. Then Provisc or Healon is injected between the Viscoat and the nuclear material, and between the latter and the endothelium.

The incision is extended to allow for the size of the nucleus so that it will exit easily with the loop. The incision should be sutured and then a vitrectomy done via an anterior route with cleaning of the residual cortex.

- If the residual nuclear material is small in volume proceed as follows. Viscoat is injected under the residual nucleus in order to avoid its luxation into

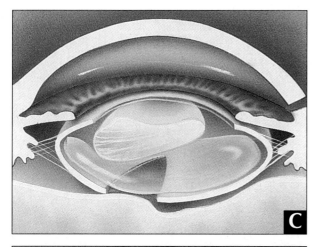
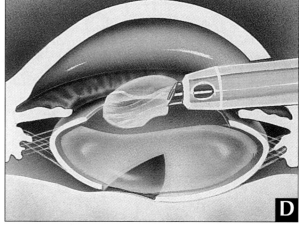

Figures 11-34C, 11-34D. Behavior in the event of posterior capsular rupture with intact hyaloid during phacoemulsification. The residual nucleus can then be positioned with the spatula or the VES cannula in a suitable position for the phacoemulsification. This should be performed under high vacuum, low flow rate, low bottle, and low U/S working always or mainly in occlusion.
Figure 11-34E. Alternately, the material can be extracted with a loop after extending the incision.

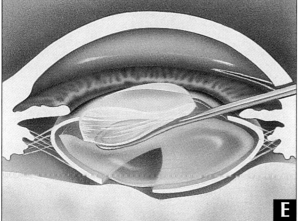

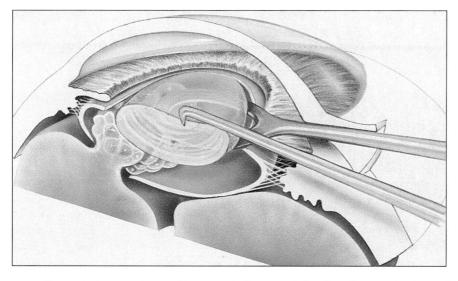

Figure 11-35. In the event of capsular rupture and vitreous loss, the surgeon should remove the nuclear material manually particularly when the pieces are large. VES protection is mandatory.

the posterior chamber and to separate the material itself from the vitreous. The remaining bag and chamber are filled with more Viscoat (care must be taken not to inject too much and risk extending the capsular opening).

A dry anterior vitrectomy is performed through the incision opened for the phaco beginning in the anterior chamber. When the cornea begins to collapse, more Viscoat is injected into the anterior chamber. The injection first coats the entire endothelial surface and then moves downward to fill the space left by the aspirated vitreous.

Continue the vitrectomy until the entire anterior segment has been cleaned. When the vitreous has been separated from the nuclear residue, carefully emulsify the residual nucleus. If some Viscoat is aspirated, more can be injected if necessary.

Phaco in this situation is done using high vacuum (150

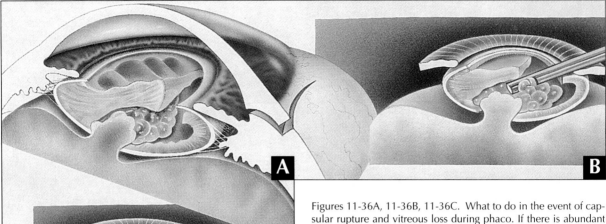

Figures 11-36A, 11-36B, 11-36C. What to do in the event of capsular rupture and vitreous loss during phaco. If there is abundant nuclear material mixed with the vitreous, the surgeon should inject VES under the residual nucleus to partially occlude the capsular orifice, to push part of the vitreous back, and to create spaces. Then, using the vitrectomy cutter, the surgeon removes part of the vitreous mixed with the material. In this way, the nuclear material is freed from its vitreal adhesions. If possible, the surgeon should also separate the vitreous which escapes from the incision from that surrounding the nuclear material.

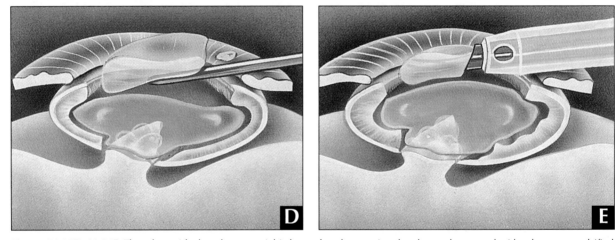

Figures 11-36D, 11-36E. Then the residual nuclear material is luxated to the anterior chamber and extracted with a loop or emulsified after more Viscoat has blocked the capsular opening.

to 200 mm Hg) but low flow (10 to 15 cc/min) U/S should be at 30 to 50%. The vacuum exerts a holding force on the nucleus and the low flow allows the surgeon to proceed slowly, reducing the BSS exchange and keeping the Viscoat in place for a longer period of time. The reduction of turbulence in the anterior segment can reduce mobilization of the free vitreous.

If the vitreous tends to block the aspiration orifice, after positioning the residual nucleus in a safe place, well coated in Viscoat, continue with a moderate dry vitrectomy. Viscoat is injected once again and phacoemulsification is performed.

Alternatively, the incision is extended, and the nuclear fragment is extracted with forceps. The wound is closed, and a dry, anterior vitrectomy is performed.

Once the vitrectomy in the anterior chamber has been completed, the surgeon introduces the tip of the vitrectomy cutter into the vitreous chamber through the anterior capsulorhexis and tries to remove the retrocapsular vitreous mass to a depth of 4 to 5 mm.

The cortical residues are normally removed during the vitrectomy. If some remain in the capsular fornix, they will be removed by aspirating with a cannula mounted on a syringe (dry technique).

Be very careful during the operation that nuclear and cortical materials do not fall into the vitreous or fragments descend to the posterior pole. If this happens, apply a vitrectomy lens to the cornea and proceed with a posterior vitrectomy (see later sections in this chapter). The fragments are identified by the coaxial illumination

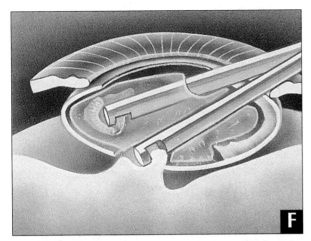

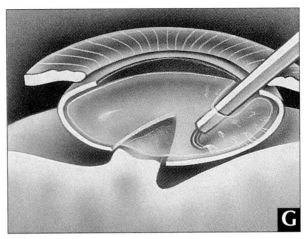

Figures 11-36F, 11-36G, 11-36H. Once the nuclear material has been removed, the remaining vitreous is removed from the capsular opening. Then the cortical material is removed from the capsular bag, partly with the dry technique. An IOL is then inserted in the sulcus.

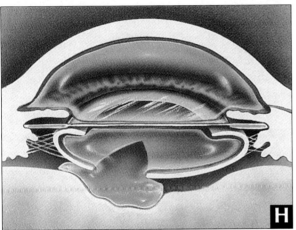

of the microscope, and the vitrectomy cutter is moved close with the tip open. When the port and the fragment are in contact, the instrument is activated—cut and aspirated—stopping as soon as the debris has been removed.

The same technique applies to fragments floating freely in the vitreous cavity as for fragments resting on the retinal plane.

Having completed this, inspect the anterior capsule and the capsulorhexis. If it is intact, this plane will be ideal for an implant in the sulcus. If it is torn, decide whether the peripheral capsular remnants will provide adequate support to implant the IOL. However, if there are any doubts, the surgeon can either postpone the implant for a few months, or he or she can implant a lens with scleral fixation. Implantation in the anterior chamber has a higher incidence of some complications (bullous keratopathy—secondary glaucoma).

### Rupture of the Posterior Capsule and Hyaloid Face With Total or Partial Luxation of the Nucleus into the Vitreous

This may occur during hydrodissection, rotation of the nucleus, creation of the cross, and emulsification of the quadrants. A posterior vitrectomy is necessary.

The instruments are removed from the anterior chamber; the tunnel is normally not sutured. A scleral incision is made about 3.5 mm behind the limbus in the inferior temporal zone using a disposable 0.9 mm blade for the endovitreal infusion route.

At 10 and 2 o'clock, again with a disposable 0.9 mm blade, make two perforating sclerotomies 3.5 mm from the limbus in order to insert the vitrectotomy cutter (right hand) and the fiber optic wand (left hand). A contact lens is then applied to the cornea and the microscope light turned off. The fiber optic light is turned on and the vitreous is completely removed. Then PFCL (liquid perfluocarbonate) is injected into the vitreous cavity using a syringe.

PFCL is a heavy liquid used in vitreo-retinal surgery which is heavier than BSS and therefore does not mix with the infusion liquid (BSS). It is used to push to the surface the smaller, lighter pieces of nuclear material.

Six mL of PFCL are drawn up in a normal syringe which is then used to mount the blunt cannula fitted with a luer-lock device. The cannula is placed in the vitreous cavity through the same scleral incision used to insert the vitrectotomy cutter and is brought close to the optic disc under fiber optic illumination.

By slowly pushing the piston of the syringe, the PFCL is expressed, and it coats the posterior part of the retina, slowly filling the entire vitreous cavity. This will bring the nucleus or its residues to the PFCL-BSS interface. If the injection of heavy liquid is continued, the debris may be brought into the pupillary field immediately under the iris.

The removal of the nucleus is always done with a phacoemulsifier, either in the posterior chamber or vitreous cavity. If the nucleus is particularly hard, there is also a third alternative.

1. In the posterior chamber.

As was mentioned earlier, the nucleus floats on the anterior surface of the PFCL. On further injection, it can be brought to its natural position behind the iris. Initially, the upward movement is followed with the fiber optic light. Once the nucleus is in an anterior position, the fiber

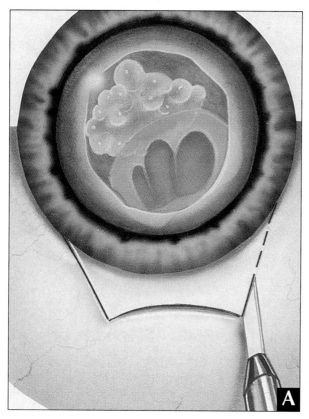

Figure 11-37A. What to do in the event of large capsular rupture and vitreous loss during phaco. If there is abundant escape of vitreous with a large piece of nucleus, the surgeon should inject some Viscoat under the material to prevent it dislocating into the posterior chamber. Then widen the tunnel incision.

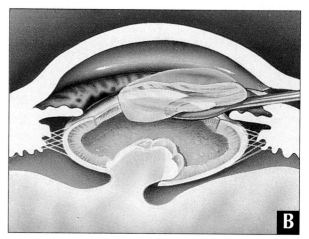

Figure 11-37B. Extract the material with a loop.

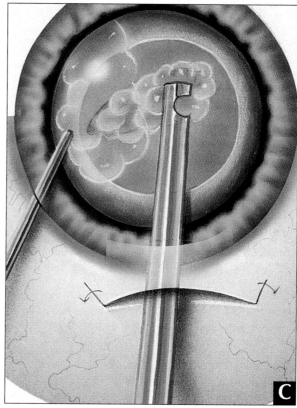

Figure 11-37C. Partially close the incision and perform a dry vitrectomy or use non-coaxial irrigation in the vitrectomy probe.

optic wand is removed and the coaxial light of the operating microscope is turned on to allow the further upward movement of the nucleus to be watched until it is behind the iris.

At this point, stop the PFCL infusion and lower the infusion bottle to rest just above the patient's head. Seal the two sclerotomies at 10 and 2 o'clock in the pars plana using special clips. The handle of the phacoemulsifier is brought into the anterior chamber through the previous corneal or sclero-corneal opening and the nucleus or its residues are emulsified. All the small fragments which remain will float on the PFCL surface with no danger of falling to the posterior pole. Any cortical residues positioned at the fornix of the bag are then aspirated using the I/A handpiece.

Once aspiration of the cataract has been completed, the surgeon removes the two clips which closed the scleral incisions, the infusion bottle is raised to the height of the surgeon's head, and a cannula (open both proximally and distally) is introduced to the vitreous cavity. The distal portion is brought to the level of the optic disc under fiber optic light control. The PFCL will exit from the eye under the pressure of the infusion liquid.

Separation between the two liquids is always obvious so the surgeon can observe the PFCL volume reducing to a small bubble at the posterior pole which is then completely aspirated by the cannula. Small fragments of nucleus which may have become detached during fragmentation and which float on the anterior surface of the heavy liquid are aspirated through the cannula used to aspirate the PFCL.

Once the globe has been filled with the infusion liquid, the sclerotomies are closed with PDS (8-0) (polydioxanone), a synthetic absorbable suture. The bottle of the infusion liquid is lowered bringing the ocular pressure to approximately 18 mm Hg.

Table 11-12

## HOW THE SURGEON SHOULD BEHAVE IF THE POSTERIOR CAPSULE RUPTURES WITH THE HYALOID INTACT AND NUCLEAR MATERIAL IS PRESENT

1. Small nuclear material
   - Inject Viscoat into the opening of the capsular bag to close the opening itself; do not fill excessively.
   - Move the nuclear material to the anterior chamber with a spatula or with the Viscoat cannula.
   - Emulsify the material with short bursts, working mainly in occlusion. Use the spatula to keep the material in contact with the U/S tip.
   - Alternately, after having injected Viscoat, enter the bag with the U/S tip. Look for occlusion with the nuclear fragment immediately. Transport the piece to the anterior chamber and fragment it.
   - Operate with suitable parameters: bottle very low, 20-30-40 cm above the patient's head. Flow rate low: 10-15 cc/min; vacuum high: 120-200 mm Hg in proportion to the hardness of the piece; U/S low: 20-40%—pulsed if necessary.
   - Replace the viscoelastic that is aspirated.

2. Large nuclear material
   - Inject Viscoat to plug the hole, then Healon or Provisc above and below the nuclear material.
   - Extend the incision so that it is larger than the fragment.
   - Introduce Sheets' glide into the posterior chamber and occlude the orifice.
   - Use a spatula or other instrument to place the nucleus in a good position, preferably in the anterior chamber.
   - Enter with the loop and extract the material.
   - Suture incision.

3. Removal of the cortex
   - Remove the cortex with the dry I/A technique as described previously. If irrigation is used through the accessory incision, keep the bottle very low.

Various options for implantation in the posterior chamber and the sulcus include:

- In front of the anterior capsule if the capsulorhexis is still intact.
- On the remainder of the anterior capsule in the event that the capsulorhexis has ruptured but there is sufficient peripheral capsular support.
- With scleral fixation when the capsular residues around the sulcus leave some doubts about the reliability of the IOL anchorage.

The corneal or sclero-corneal opening is extended. Prior to implanting the IOL, inject Viscoat into the anterior chamber. The high viscosity of this product offers many advantages over the other viscoelastics. It remains in the anterior chamber even if there is a modest endovitreal infusion required to keep the IOP within normal limits. It also provides considerable endothelial protection and once the operation has been completed, it can be left in the anterior and vitreous cavity because it does not cause a significant postoperative increase in the ocular pressure. Use lenses for the sulcus with an optic of diameter 6.5 mm. The incision may be self-sealing (ie, sutureless). However, it may be necessary to suture the wound for incisions of this size, in which case use a horizontal suture which will normally not induce any deformation of the cornea.

Once the implant has been completed, remove the endovitreal infusion, taking care to leave the pressure inside the globe within normal limits.

Extreme care is needed when the cannula used for endovitreal infusion is removed. Quickly tighten the sutures around the scleral incision to prevent the escape of liquid and avoid hypotony. If liquid escapes, correct the situation immediately by introducing fresh BSS into the vitreous cavity through a 20 G cannula mounted on a syringe.

2. In the vitreous cavity.

Using the technique described previously, the nucleus or its residues are brought to about two-thirds of the depth of the vitreous cavity using the PFCL. The sleeve of the phaco tip enters the vitreous cavity through the scleral incision at 10 o'clock.

Under fiber optic light, perform the emulsification and aspiration of the nucleus inside the vitreous cavity. Following this, the procedure is the same as that described for limbal removal of the nucleus.

3. If the nucleus is particularly hard, fragmentation may be an excessively lengthy process. As the nucleus will not float on top of the PFCL, another technique is used.

Perform a complete vitrectomy and position a Flieringa ring. The infusion bottle is raised slightly above the patient's head and the anterior chamber is opened with a limbal incision of 180 to 200°. Endovitreal infusion is stopped while the assistant keeps the cornea raised with a forceps. All the infusion liquid contained in the vitreous chamber is aspirated through a cannula mounted on a syringe. The fact that the vitreous cavity is empty makes the subsequent maneuvers easier because the visibility from the light of the microscope alone is, in these conditions, very good with accurate control.

An endocryoprobe (diameter of 0.9 mm) is introduced into the vitreous cavity and is brought slowly into contact with the nucleus positioned at the posterior pole. As soon as there is contact, the surgeon freezes the probe and raises it to detach the nucleus from the retinal plane. A few seconds later, when the *hold by freezing* is good enough, the surgeon slowly withdraws the probe and in this way the nucleus is removed.

The absence of liquid makes this easier as it is almost impossible for the iris to become frozen. This means that the probe does not have to be thawed which would involve the risk of losing the hold on the nucleus. If this happens,

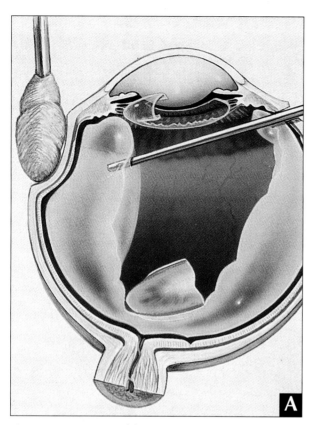

Figure 11-38A. Rupture of the posterior capsule and hyaloid face with total or partial luxation of the nucleus into the vitreous.

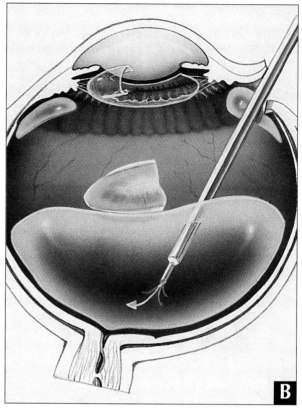

Figure 11-38B. PFCL is injected to raise the piece of nucleus.

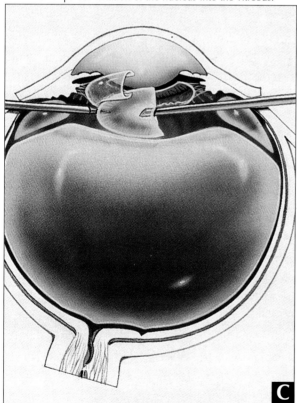

Figure 11-38C. When the fragment is in the posterior or anterior chamber, it can be easily emulsified. Alternately, it can be fragmented in the vitreous chamber.

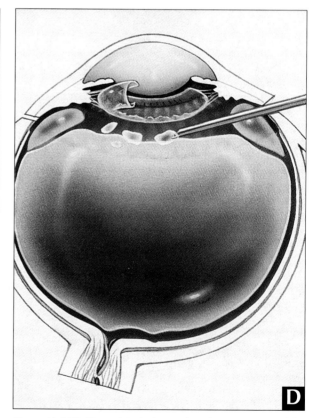

Figure 11-38D. The residual pieces of nucleus are removed by fragmentation or aspiration.

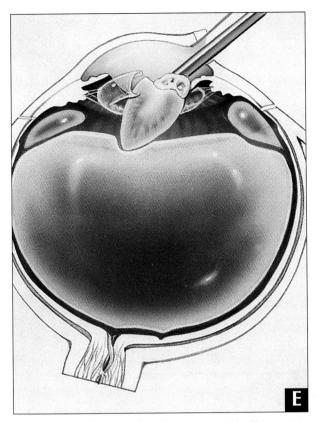

Figure 11-38E. If the piece of nucleus is very hard and large, it can be removed by cryoextraction.

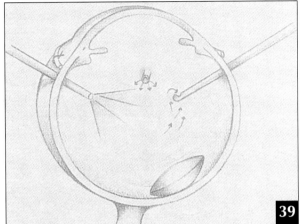

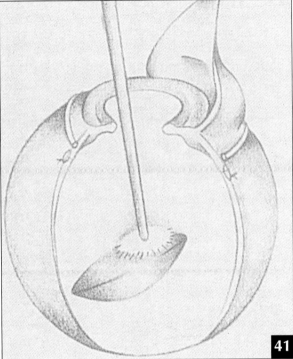

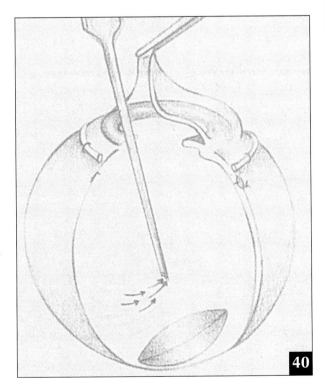

Figures 11-39, 11-40, 11-41. With posterior luxation of the nucleus, the surgeon must perform a complete posterior vitrectomy. Then he or she performs the limbal incision and aspirates the BSS. With a vitreous cryoprobe, the operator removes the nucleus.

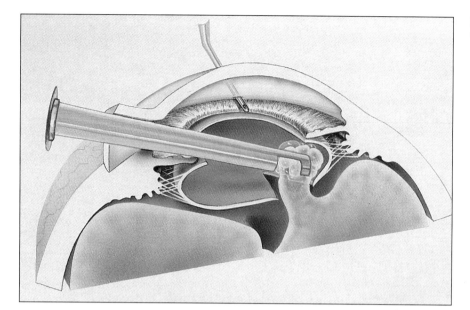

Figure 11-42. Anterior vitrectomy with closed anterior chamber.

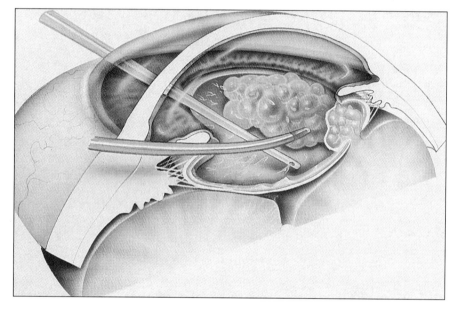

Figure 11-43. In the anterior vitrectomy, it is necessary that the irrigation occurs through an incision different to the one with the vitrectomy cutter.

the nucleus can fall toward the retina at the posterior pole.

With the bottle just slightly above the patient's head, infusion is opened immediately to fill the vitreous cavity slowly.

Having sutured the sclero-corneal wound, the bottle is raised very slowly to bring the endocular pressure to 20 mm Hg gradually. The implant can be placed in the posterior chamber or on the capsular residues, or fixed to the sclera either immediately or 6 months later.

## Anterior Vitrectomy for the Anterior Segment Surgeon

The surgical response to rupture of the posterior capsule depends on a number of factors:
- The extension of the capsular opening.
- Whether vitreous is present in the anterior chamber.
- The type of material present (cortex and/or nucleus).
- Location of the material (anterior chamber, posterior chamber, or vitreous cavity).
- The type of anterior capsulotomy performed.
- What stage the operation was at when the posterior capsule ruptured.

If anterior vitrectomy becomes necessary, proceed as follows. To reduce the likelihood of extending the capsular break and minimize the amount of the vitreous prolapse, use either dry vitrectomy or only minimal BSS through a side port incision (don't use coaxial irrigation during vitrectomy).

It is advisable to begin the vitrectomy dry and then infuse BSS gently if the chamber tends to collapse (always through a side port incision).

For the vitreous, the cutting speed must be 250 to 350 cuts per minute (mean values) with aspiration at 100 to 300 mm Hg, increasing if necessary to 350 with flow 10 cc/min. These values avoid unnecessary traction on the vitreous.

Table 11-13
## DRY I/A TECHNIQUE WITH THE POSTERIOR CAPSULE OPEN AND THE HYALOID RUPTURED

### If the opening is limited

Inject Viscoat in correspondence to the opening. Inject the product slowly and carefully. Avoid injecting it with excessive pressure; otherwise the opening can extend.

Injection of Provisc or Healon in the remainder of the capsular bag and in the anterior chamber.

Perform a dry vitrectomy firstly in the area anterior of the opening and then in the area which involves the capsular opening. If necessary, enter the opening and remove more vitreous for 1-2 mm. Proceed carefully so the opening is not extended.

Inject more Viscoat into the opening.

Using the spatula, check that the opening is free from vitreous. Perform a posterior capsulorhexis and complete the vitrectomy if necessary.

Prior to removing the cortex, proceed as described previously.

### If the opening is wide

Possibility 1:

Perform a dry vitrectomy in the anterior chamber and in the capsular bag. Then enter the opening. If necessary, use the accessory cannula or the irrigation cannula of Buratto's two-handed I/A system to irrigate the chamber distally.

Avoid pulling or pushing inside the capsular opening.

Penetration of air into the chamber may indicate an adequate vitrectomy.

Occlude the opening with Viscoat and reshape the anterior chamber and the bag with Provisc or Healon. Proceed with a posterior capsulorhexis and then with the dry technique.

Possibility 2:

Inject Viscoat into the anterior chamber and under the iris.

Perform the anterior vitrectomy dry, ie, with no irrigation.

Remove the equatorial cortex using the vitrectomy cutter working with aspiration just sufficient to capture the cortex. Cut and remove the vitreous which has entered the opening of the vitrectome.

The anterior vitreous and particularly the central and equatorial cortex must be completely removed from the opening.

Possibility 3:

The vitrectomy cutter can be inserted through a service incision (suitably enlarged) to remove the vitreous and the subincisional cortex.

The amount of viscoelastic in the chamber should be gradually increased as the vitreous is removed. The VES must replace the vitreous removed. This to avoid that more vitreous moves from the posterior segment to the anterior.

Use the right setting; otherwise the VES can also partially obstruct the orifice of the vitrectomy cutter. Vacuum of 200-300 and a flow rate of 10-18 cc/min are suitable to avoid this sort of problem.

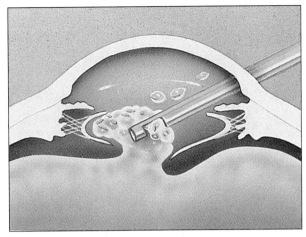

Figure 11-44. First the surgeon removes the cortical material which has not been mixed with vitreous by dry aspiration, then the cortex-vitreous mixture.

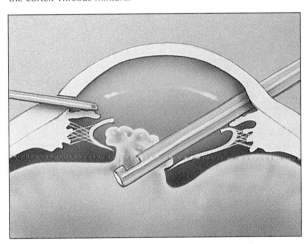

Figure 11-45. The vitreous should also be removed from just inside the capsular opening.

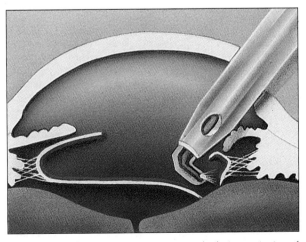

Figure 11-46. Rupture of the posterior capsule during aspiration of the cortex at 12 o'clock.

| Table 11-14 | |
|---|---|
| **DRY TECHNIQUE OF I/A WITH POSTERIOR CAPSULE OPEN AND INTACT HYALOID** | |
| *Procedure with a syringe and a cannula* | |
| When | If the posterior capsule has ruptured but the hyaloid is intact. |
| Preparation | Close the capsular opening by injecting Viscoat at the rupture site and the surrounding area. The injection serves to plug the hole and to keep the vitreous back. Because of its adhesion properties, Viscoat will stay where is injected and will not move under irrigation (as long as the levels are moderate). Inject Provisc or Healon in the remainder of the capsular bag and in the anterior chamber, ie, an injection of a pseudoplastic substance. Using this substance the surgeon can also separate the anterior capsule from the posterior one to open the capsular bag well. |
| Instruments | Three cc BSS syringe, smooth running and free from air. Fitted with a blunt 25-27 G cannula. |
| Aspiration | Bring the orifice of the cannula close to a cortical mass. Aspirate until the tip is occluded. Pull the mass toward the center of the chamber detaching it from the capsule. Free the mass by pushing gently on the piston thus injecting a few drops of BSS. Repeat the maneuver with another fragment close to the one which has just been removed. Always keep the chamber well-formed with Provisc/Healon, and ensure that Viscoat always occludes the capsular opening. If the opposite is true, inject one or the other. Avoid aspiration of the material in contact with or mixed with Viscoat. Too must exertion on the syringe is necessary. As the cannula is thin, the Viscoat will tend to occlude it so very little cortex will be aspirated. When an adequate quantity of material has been freed in the anterior chamber, push gently on the deep part of the incision to remove some Provisc or Healon along with the cortex it contains. Inject more viscoelastic and repeat the procedure until complete or almost complete removal of the cortex has been obtained. This entire procedure should be performed very carefully. The hyaloid is extremely fragile. |
| Comment | This technique requires time and patience. The surgeon must operate with due care and precision. Haste will inevitably cause rupture of the hyaloid. |

The vitrectotomy cutter must be used to prevent the fragments moving to the posterior vitreous. In order to reduce this risk, the cutting speed should be reduced to about 100 cuts/min and the vacuum increased to 200 to 250 mm Hg.

Following satisfactory vitrectomy, a high adhesion viscoelastic is injected into the capsular opening (Viscoat), the anterior chamber is reshaped with Provisc or Healon, and the residual cortical material can be removed with a dry manual technique.

Once cleaning has been completed, inject air and use a spatula to check that the anterior chamber is free from vitreous. If all is well, implantation in the ciliary sulcus of the posterior chamber can take place.

If the nucleus or part of it is luxated into the posterior segment, a posterior vitrectomy must be done. A surgeon with appropriate posterior segment experience or a vitreoretinal colleague can perform an immediate vitrectomy.

## COMPLICATIONS DURING I/A

### Rupture of the Posterior Capsule

This is the most frequent complication during the aspiration of the cortical material. Although the posterior capsule is stronger than one would imagine, it usually ruptures because the capsule is aspirated into the port of the I/A tip and traction is then applied by the surgeon.

Factors likely to increase the frequency of such complications are:
- Excessive vacuum.
- Aspiration with the port close to the posterior capsule.
- Aspiration with a shallow chamber.
- Reduced resistance of the capsule.
- A sharp, rough edge around the port.
- Venting which is not working properly.

The rupture can be small or large, a variety of shapes, and it can occur centrally or peripherally. It is often associated with the rupture of the anterior hyaloid with vitreous loss.

If the capsule is thought to have torn, stop I/A immediately, and increase the magnification and illumination of the microscope to check whether the suspected complication has really occurred. Once the damage has been assessed, fill the anterior chamber with an air bubble, removing the probe at the same time. These two operations must occur simultaneously or else the anterior chamber will flatten and the hyaloid face may rupture with vitreous loss.

Then inject Provisc or Healon to reform the anterior and posterior chambers and to block the orifice created in

> **Table 11-15**
>
> ## BEHAVIOR IN THE EVENT OF POSTERIOR CAPSULE RUPTURE WITH VITREOUS MIXED WITH NUCLEAR MATERIAL NOT DISLOCATED INTO THE VITREOUS
>
> **Case A: Small fragment of nuclear material in the capsular bag mixed with vitreous and cortex**
>
> **Case 1:** The vitreous is separated from the nuclear material.
> - Viscoat is injected under the residual nucleus and into the rest of the bag. Always inject the product from below or in such a way as to push the nuclear material toward the surface. Then inject the product into the capsular opening.
> - Introduce the U/S tip (bottle low, flow rate low, vacuum high) and try to occlude immediately with the piece of nucleus. If the Viscoat injection has been performed correctly, no vitreous will adhere to the nuclear material.
> - Bring the piece to a safe position, preferably in the anterior chamber, and emulsify with low U/S, always maintaining contact with the material. A slide or a spatula can be placed underneath the nucleus to maintain its contact with the U/S tip and to prevent fragments falling into it. Viscoat prevents fragments from falling back the vitreous.
>
> **Case 2:** The piece of nucleus is enveloped in vitreous.
> - Inject Viscoat under the nuclear material, in the capsular bag, in the capsular opening, and in the anterior chamber. Bring the nuclear material to a safe position.
> - Proceed with the dry vitrectomy of the vitreous which has escaped from the opening. Try to remove all the vitreous present in the anterior segment. If that is not not possible, remove the material manually. It is sufficient to free the material from all the vitreal connections.
> - As soon as the nuclear material is free from the vitreous, proceed as for case 1.
>
> **Case B: Large nuclear pieces**
> - Inject Provisc or Healon under the nucleus and into the capsular opening.
> - Extend the incision.
> - Enter with the loop and extract the nucleus.
> - Reshape the anterior chamber with Provisc or Healon, but without exaggerating (ie, without widening the posterior capsular opening).
> - Close the incision.
> - Perform the anterior vitrectomy under the following parameters. Cut rate: 300-400 cuts/min; flow rate 10-12; aspiration 80-120°. If the surgeon uses a two-handed technique with irrigation through an accessory cannula, the bottle must be low (30-40 cm). However, it is preferable without irrigation (ie, dry). If the chamber tends to collapse, inject more VES or BSS through the side port incision.
> - Perform a vitrectomy to remove all the vitreous anterior to the capsular opening and that contained inside the opening.
> - Plug the capsular hole with Viscoat, fill the capsular bag with Provisc or Healon, and remove the cortex with a dry technique.

the capsule. Complete the aspiration of the cortex with a *dry* technique using a one-way cannula mounted on a syringe containing BSS. Be careful and patient when detaching the residual material and use the smallest amount of fluid possible as this can shift the viscoelastic from the rupture zone and cause the rupture of the hyaloid face (if this has not happened already).

## Vitreous Loss

This is found in association with or following capsular rupture or when there is zonular detachment; it requires an anterior vitrectomy. The amount of vitreous removed varies from case to case, the size of the break, the amount and type of vitreous which prolapses from the capsular opening, and from the quantity of residual cortical material.

If the vitreous face is broken and mixed with the cortex, perform an anterior vitrectomy. Try to remove all the cortical material present in the bag and all the vitreous which has prolapsed from the break. All this should be completed while trying to keep the rhexis intact so that the IOL can be implanted in the sulcus in front of it.

## Rupture of the Anterior Capsule

When the rhexis is small, attempts to reach the cortex situated at the equator can lead to anterior capsular breaks. This is not a serious problem and the surgeon can still implant in the bag with only a small risk of the optic decentration due to postoperative capsular retraction. Alternatively, implant in the sulcus.

## Equatorial Disinsertion of the Capsule

This can occur through inherent weakness of the zonular fibers, through damage caused during the capsulotomy and nuclear fragmentation, or through traction exerted by the I/A tip.

This last situation occurs during the aspiration of cortex which is strongly adherent to the peripheral posterior capsule.

The zonules can also tear when a very large amount of cortex is aspirated. Because of a large area of contact with the posterior capsule, the strong power exerted during aspiration may lead to a localized rupture of the corresponding zonular fibers. In the majority of cases, rupture of the zonules occurs because a fragment of anterior capsule is unwittingly trapped inside the aspiration port as

| Table 11-16 |||
|---|---|---|
| **BEHAVIOR IF THE POSTERIOR CAPSULE IS RUPTURED WITH VITREOUS MIXED WITH CORTICAL MATERIAL AND/OR THE NUCLEUS DISLOCATED INTO THE POSTERIOR SEGMENT** |||
| Case A: small nuclear fragment dislocated in the vitreous | Perform the anterior vitrectomy and try to recover the piece through the posterior capsule opening. Perform anterior and posterior vitrectomy to remove the piece. Perform the anterior vitrectomy, clean the anterior segment from the cortex, implant the IOL, close, and refer the patient to a surgeon expert in vitro-retinal surgery within 2-3 days for a posterior vitrectomy. ||
| Case B: Large piece or entire nucleus dislocated in the vitreous | 1. Once the vitrectomy has been performed via pars plana, raise the nucleus from the retinal plane with PFCL and proceed with phacoemulsification in the vitreal chamber. PFCL protects the retina during this phase (bringing the nucleus into the anterior chamber, particularly if we are dealing with a whole nucleus or a large piece of nucleus, as this would compromise the capsulo-zonular support which is usually sufficient for an implant in the posterior chamber). 2. Perform a total posterior vitrectomy via pars plana. Using PFC bring the nuclear material to the anterior chamber. Phacoemulsify (PFC prevents the fragments falling into the posterior segment). Implant the IOL in the sulcus if the conditions of the capsular residue permit. Alternately, fix the IOL sclerally, or the surgeon can postpone in favor of a secondary implant. 3. Perform the best anterior vitrectomy possible and the best cortex removal. Do not implant an IOL. Refer the patient to a vitro-retinal surgeon within 2-3 days. Perform the anterior vitrectomy. Carefully removing all the cortical material. Implant the IOL in the sulcus, close, and refer the patient to an expert surgeon in vitro-retinal surgery within 3 days. An IOL correctly positioned in the posterior chamber, even if there is capsular rupture, will not affect the cleaning procedures via pars plana (vitrectomy and phacoemulsification in the vitreal chamber). ||
| Case C: Only cortical material | A good anterior vitrectomy which also extends to the vitreal chamber in the area of the opening is normally sufficient to remove the cortical material in the anterior portion of the vitreous. This is because the cortex will tend to float on the vitreous, particularly if it is dense. If the material is not accessible from the main entrance, use a second or third entrance, extending the existing ones or performing a new side port incision. If the material cannot be removed, perform a posterior vitrectomy. ||

Table 11-17

## BEHAVIOR WHEN THERE IS A NUCLEAR FRAGMENT PARTIALLY DISLOCATED INTO THE VITREOUS

At a certain point during the operation, the surgeon may realize that the posterior capsule has ruptured and that a quadrant or a hemi-nucleus has moved into the opening and is about to fall into the vitreal chamber. In this situation, continuing with irrigation extends the opening and causes the piece to fall into the vitreous. The surgeon should therefore move the pedal to Position 0 and remove the tip, leaving the bulb in a hypotonic state. Injecting VES into the chamber would cause the material to fall further, so it should be avoided.

### Case A

If the vitreous provides sufficient support for the nuclear material, enter with the spatula and gently insert it in the opening, trying to raise the material and transport it to a safer position. Without removing the spatula from the opening, use the other hand to inject Viscoat into the opening itself and around the material. Then continue as described before.

### Case B

If the surgeon believe that the vitreous is not providing sufficient support:
Cut the conjuntiva in a convenient site (the most comfortable working position for the surgeon).
Use a caliper to measure the entrance point for pars plana: 3.5-4.0 mm from the limbus.
Cut the sclera with a vitreal knife, producing a full-thickness perpendicular incision, 1.5 mm wide.
Insert the nucleus spatula through the pars plana incision, reach the capsular opening. From below, raise the nuclear residue to the anterior chamber.
With the other hand, VES is injected under the piece of nucleus and in the capsular orifice. The spatula is removed and the surgeon injects a thin layer of VES between the nucleus and the endothelium.
Extend the phaco incision enough to allow a loop to be inserted and to allow the extraction of the piece of nucleus.
Carefully suture the incision in the pars plana, and ensure that all vitreal filaments are cut.
Proceed as for capsular rupture with vitreal escape.

the tip is moved from the periphery to the center of the posterior chamber dragging the capsule with it.

## Incomplete Removal of the Cortical Masses

This may be associated with poor mydriasis and therefore insufficient exposure of the cortex. A few drops of adrenaline for intracardiac use in the bottle of irrigating solution may help. Otherwise, hold back the iris with a Hirshman spatula.

A second reason is positive vitreous pressure with difficulty in forming the posterior chamber and particular difficulty in obtaining sufficient separation of the iris from the posterior capsule. Use some interrupted sutures to seal the chamber. The bottle should also be raised in order to increase the irrigation flow rate.

If the cortex adheres tightly to the posterior capsule and will not detach despite the strong aspirating power at the tip, rather than rupturing the capsule, detach it gradually with the irrigating cannula. An insufficient or poorly shaped capsulotomy may be difficult to correct during surgery so the aspiration of the cortex is blocked.

Finally, another reason is aspiration performed with an incision which is too large. Here the excess leakage of fluid prevents the anterior chamber from allowing easy access to the I/A tip and an adequate exposure of the cortex.

# COMPLICATIONS DURING CLEANING OF THE POSTERIOR CAPSULE

The capsule may tear because of excessive pressure with the cleaning instrument, use of an unsuitable instrument, aspiration of a capsule which is too thin, violent maneuvers with a capsule under tension, and cleaning with a flattened anterior chamber. If a vacuum technique is used, tearing will almost certainly be due to an incorrect selection of the aspiration parameters (excessive vacuum and/or flow rate). Rupture of the capsule can also be associated with rupture of the hyaloid face with vitreous loss.

# COMPLICATIONS DURING THE INSERTION OF THE IOL

The insertion of the IOL into the anterior and then the posterior chamber can:
- Disinsert Descemet's membrane—When the lens insertion is done through an incision which is too narrow and excessive pressure is exerted.
- Damage the endothelium—If the anterior chamber flattens, particularly if the lens is inserted without protection of a viscoelastic, the endothelium is damaged when it comes into contact with the optic of the IOL. Use of viscoelastic will avoid this damage.
- Damage the iris—This occurs through excessive contact between the lens and the iris. The contact can be avoided with a small quantity of Provisc or Healon between the two surfaces.
- Rupture the posterior capsule—This may occur when there is excessive pressure of the distal loop, particularly if the lens is inserted at an incorrect angle. Pressure on the distal portion of the IOL optic or careless positioning of the insertion instruments may also induce a rupture. Viscoelastic acts in this situation as an excellent buffer.
- Disinsertion of the zonules—When the lens is inserted into the bag under excessive pressure using lenses with less flexible loops, it is possible to disinsert the zonules. Provisc and Healon are useful again for the same reasons as described above. This complication occurs mainly when trying to force a large lens through small rhexis.
- Rupture the rhexis—This is a relatively rare complication. It is more likely to happen through careless use of the hooks or spatulas rather than be caused by the lens itself.

# COMPLICATIONS FROM THE INSTRUMENTS USED IN THE ANTERIOR CHAMBER

During phacoemulsification, the instruments which can or must enter the anterior chamber are, in order:
- Cystotome and rhexis forceps.
- Forceps for removing the anterior capsule.
- Devices to mobilize and remove the nucleus: cannulas, spatulas, ultrasound tips, etc.
- I/A probe.
- Scrapers for the cleaning of the posterior chamber.
- IOL.
- Hooks used to position the lens or to retract the iris.

Each one of these instruments can cause damage or complications.

Cystotome—This is a sharp, cutting instrument and its penetration in the anterior chamber can cause damage if not used carefully. If the instrument is inserted through a tunnel incision and withdrawn slowly and gradually, it is unlikely to cause any damage. However, it can sometimes provoke small iris tears and restricted disinsertions at the base of the iris. They can also cause localized damage to the endothelium or detachment of Descemet's membrane.

Cystotomes which enter the anterior chamber directly with no preliminary incision (a cystotome made by bending an insulin needle) require a certain amount of pressure to perforate the cornea. If the penetration site has not been calculated exactly, the needle may be introduced at the base of the iris and this will provoke the disinsertion, tears, or the rupture of a blood vessel with hemorrhage. If the instrument penetrates in the center of the cornea, it may cause the formation of an uneven localized opacity. However, this normally will not have postoperative consequences.

## Instruments for Mobilizing or Luxating the Nucleus

There are a number of different types of instruments:
- Instruments which are used in the anterior cham-

Table 11-18

## THE RULES OF AN ANTERIOR VITRECTOMY

| | |
|---|---|
| Do not pull the vitreous, do not put it under tension, do not lengthen it, and do not damage it: | With the tip. <br> With the spatula. <br> With the sponge swab. |
| Do not wet it. | Do not use irrigation; hydration of the vitreous involves further swelling and further prolapse of the vitreous. <br> If irrigation is necessary, it must not be coaxial with the vitrectomy tip. |
| If you need to use irrigation, do that through a lateral incision and direct the fluid in the anterior chamber toward the iris plane (not toward the capsular opening). | This will limit the stimulus of the vitreous and the fluid will only partially hydrolyze the vitreous. |
| Touch the vitreous as little as possible. | Reduce the use of instruments in the chamber to a minimum. |
| Remove only the amount of vitreous necessary. | Just the vitreous that protrudes from the capsular opening or just slightly more. |
| Free the corneal or scleral incision from any vitreal filaments. | They can induce significant postoperative complications. |
| Remove the vitreous completely from the anterior chamber and the capsular bag. | Clean the orifice and remove a small amount of vitreous inside the opening. |
| In the event of miosis: | Be aware if there are mechanical retractors for access to the subiris masses or the vitreous. |
| If it is difficult to remove/cut the trapped filaments: | Remember that with a lateralized incision, the use of microspatulas can resolve the problem. |
| Suggested parameters: <br> Vacuum—200-350. <br> Aspiration flow rate—10-18. <br> Cut rate—200-300. | Optimize the procedure. <br> The main concept is that the vitrectomy must be performed under the constant control of the operator. So aspiration must progress in a linear fashion until indirect signals (progression of the pigment particles, or small pieces of cortex, small movements transmitted by capsular rupture or the pupillary edges) indicate that the vitreous is inside the orifice of the vitrectome. At this point the surgeon should keep aspiration constant. <br> By increasing the cut rate (interrupting the mass aspirated with greater frequency), there is less danger of capturing the edges of the capsule of the pupil with the vitrectome, making the whole operation safer and allowing the surgeon to increase aspiration. |
| At the end, using a sponge swab, and check that there is no vitreous in the incision. | Identify the vitreal filaments and cut them with scissors without placing them under tension. |
| Check the pupil with a spatula. | Remove any filaments with vitrectomy. <br> A round pupil is a good indicator that vitreous is not trapped in the incision. |
| Check the pupil by instilling a miotic. | If the pupil contracts rapidly and uniformly, it means that there are not vitreal filaments. |
| Check using an air bubble. | If the anterior chamber and the iris-capsular diaphragm balloon well and are a good convex shape, it means that vitreous is absent. |

ber in front of the nucleus (cystotomes, hooks, etc). These can tear the zonular fibers and provoke peripheral disinsertion; alternatively they may rupture the posterior capsule if used with excessive, inappropriate pressure.

- Instruments which are used underneath the nucleus (cannulas for irrigating or other) can rupture the posterior or anterior capsule.
- Irrigating instruments, particularly the hydrodissection cannulas—These can rupture the posterior or equatorial capsule either through the injection of an excessive quantity of BSS or through direct mechanical trauma.
- U/S tip—Complications with this instrument are undoubtedly more frequent. As it enters the chamber it can disinsert Descemet's membrane, the root of the iris, or damage a portion of the endothelium. During emulsification the iris near the pupil rim or the intermediate part can be damaged by rubbing. The rhexis can be ruptured either mechanically or because of the U/S vibration. The posterior capsule in particular can rupture, occasionally through the excessive pressure exerted through the nucleus but more frequently through direct perforation. Finally,

### Table 11-19
### ANTERIOR VITRECTOMY AND IRRIGATION

| | |
|---|---|
| It is not correct to perform a vitrectomy with an irrigating coaxial probe | The flow of the infusion will be directed in the same direction as the tip (ie, toward the internal part of the eye), toward the vitreous which will be hydrated. This will cause an increase in volume of the vitreous. If the vitreous expands, it can only go toward the anterior chamber through the opening. Coaxial irrigation therefore induces further prolapse of the vitreous. The forward movement of the vitreous puts the vitreous itself under tension with the added risk of traction-complications of the retina. |
| Infusion | Through the opening of the posterior capsule, it hits the edges of the capsular opening and will tend to separate them, extending the opening. This will cause greater prolapse of the vitreous and it will be put under tension. |
| Infusion | It pushes the vitreous and moves it forcefully in all directions. This will involve movement toward the anterior segment and involves an increase in the amount of vitreous which has to be removed. |
| It is possible and correct to have infusion separate from the vitrectomy tip | The surgeon must limit the infusion to a minimum. It should not be directed toward the capsular opening. Ideally it should be directed toward the irido-corneal angle or between the cornea and iris to avoid obstructing the visibility during the vitrectomy. |

### Table 11-20
### CAUSE OF ABSENT OR REDUCED IRRIGATION DURING PHACO

| Possible cause | Treatment |
|---|---|
| Irrigation line pinched (pinch valve closed). | Remove the pinching by moving the pedal to Position 1, 2, or 3. |
| Irrigation tube completely opened. | Remove the obstacle to the drainage. |
| Irrigation bottle too low. | Raise the bottle. |
| Irrigation tube bent. | Ask the assistant to hold the tube. |
| Fluid loss along the irrigation line (broken tube). | Replace the tube. |
| Irrigation tube not connected properly to the handpiece. | Correct the tube connection. |
| Aspiration pump of the phaco positioned above eye level. | Align the patient's eye with the machine's pump (ie, place them on the same level). |
| Incision too narrow compared to the irrigation sleeve. | Widen the incision to suit. |
| Bottle still under vacuum, particularly in the event of intraoperative replacement of the bottle. | Ventilate the bottle with a 20-23 G needle. |

### Table 11-21
### SURGICAL CAUSE OF INTRAOPERATIVE FLATTENING OF THE CHAMBER

| Cause | Treatment |
|---|---|
| Incision is too wide and there is excessive fluid escape (the most common cause). | Suture the incision to make it suitable for the tip used. |
| Rupture of the posterior capsule and the zonules with irrigation of the vitreous and its hydration. This causes the iris and the anterior capsule to move forward. | Interrupt the operation immediately and proceed as described in the chapter on anterior vitrectomy. |
| Penetration of air behind the iris. | Remove the air with a suitable syringe and cannula. |
| Vitreal Thrust. | If things are extremely difficult, close and wait for 1 or 2 hours. Change the anesthesia and continue the operation (perform an ecography to exclude choroidal hematomas). |
| Choroidal Hemorrhage. | See the specific table. |
| Insufficient anesthesia/local akinesia and consequent contraction of the eyelids. | Improve akinesia using O'Brien's infiltration technique. |
| Retrobulbar Hematoma. | Do not start the operation. If it has already started, stop immediately, suture, and postpone for a day or two. |

### Table 11-22
### CAUSE OF ABSENT OR POOR ASPIRATION DURING PHACO OR I/A

| | Cause | Treatment |
|---|---|---|
| Problem at the tip and/or the aspiration tube of the handle | Obstruction by part of the dense nuclear material or by the material that has not been completely fragmented. | Remove the tip from the eye. Insert the tip in the test chamber (an artificial anterior chamber in silicone), and select maximum flow rate and vacuum. Move the pedal to its limit and push alternately with a certain degree of power on the test chamber. This maneuver will free the line. Remove the tip from the eye and inject BSS quite forcefully using a syringe through the connector. |
| | Preoperative obstruction because the sleeve was not perfectly clean. | Replace the sleeve and the tip. |
| | Sterilization causes solidification of the lens material which was not removed after the operation. This can partially obstruct the tube. If this material is freed inside the eye, it can cause violent inflammatory reactions. | After the operation rinse the U/S or I/A tip under twice distilled hot water. Clean only the U/S I/A tip and not the piezoelectrical one. Dry carefully. |
| | Damage to the 0 ring (circular washer). | Replace the 0 ring. |
| Problems with the aspiration tube | Obstruction by dense or large pieces of material. | Use a syringe to wash the tube or replace it. |
| | Manufacturing flaws in the tube. | Replace the tube. |
| | Obstruction because of damage to the tube through prolonged sterilization (in those machines with reusable tubes). | Replace the tube. |
| | Air in the tube (never activate the aspiration in air). | Remove the air from the tube. |
| | Bending of the tube (very dangerous, particularly when the surgeon is working under high vacuum). | Ask the assistant to hold the tube. |
| | A hole in the tube. | Replace the tube. |
| | Incorrect locking-in of the aspiration to the sleeve. | Lock the tube in better. |
| Problems with the machine | Wrong settings of vacuum or flow rate (too low). | Set the machine values correctly. |
| | Blockage or fault of the pump. Incorrect function of the pump. | Ask for a technical control. |
| | Incorrect insertion of the tubes on the pump rollers. | Position the tube correctly. |
| | Detachment of the tube from the rollers. | Reposition the tube. |
| | Incorrect insertion of the cassette in the slot on the pump. | Extract the cassette and replace it correctly. |
| | Complete filling of the discharge cassette and the liquid bag (relative to those machines that | Empty the cassette or replace it. |

the endothelium can be severely damaged if emulsification takes place in the anterior chamber in the dome of the cornea.

- I/A tip—The metal tip is usually smoothly rounded and blunt so it will unlikely cause any damage. The iris can be slightly damaged (enough to create an area of atrophy postoperatively) through the backward and forward movement of the sleeve and the anterior portion, the edge of the port. If the instrument has entered the incision with the chamber well-shaped and irrigation open, there should not be any contact with the iris or the endothelium. On the other hand, if the chamber flattens, the iris can be damaged quite easily. Careless introduction of the I/A tip can cause disinsertion of

### Table 11-23
### COMPLICATIONS WITH I/A

| | |
|---|---|
| Insufficient cortex removal can occur: | Because of intraoperative miosis.<br>Because of a rhexis which is too small.<br>Because of an increase in IOP.<br>Because of iris prolapse and problems. |
| Rupture of the rhexis or the can opener. | This may occur for excessive pressure by the I/A tip on the edge of the capsulotomy. What should be done:<br>  Avoid traction or maneuvers in that area.<br>  Avoid excessive widening of the chamber and/or the capsular bag.<br>  Use the two-handed technique.<br>  Use the *dry* technique.<br>  If difficulties arise, leave the remaining cortex in situ. |
| Rupture of the posterior capsule with the hyaloid intact and part of the cortex still in position. | Inject Viscoat into the opening and close to it to push the vitreous backward. The product remains in position. Completely fill the chamber and the bag with Healon or Provisc<br>If there is a lot of cortical material, proceed with a *dry* technique.<br>If there is only little material, it can be removed with a two-handed technique or left in position. In the latter case, the lens should be implanted in the sulcus. |
| Rupture of the posterior capsule with a ruptured hyaloid and the vitreous mixed with cortex. | The surgeon should perform as complete an anterior vitrectomy as possible using the dry technique or alternately with irrigation through a side port incision (never use coaxial irrigation with the vitrectotome).<br>Once the vitrectomy has been completed, inject Provisc or Healon and insert the IOL with a method to be decided. Alternately, the incision can be closed and the surgeon performs a secondary implant. |

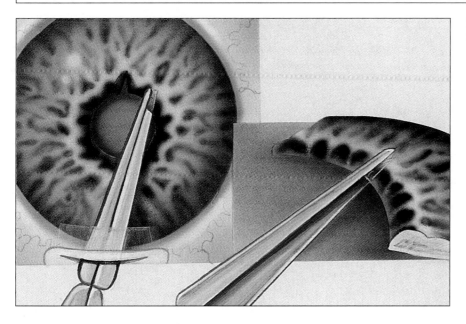

Figure 11-47. Multiple sphincterotomies with scissors.

Descemet's membrane (normally a triangular shape with the base toward the incision).

When Descemet's membrane is free in the anterior chamber, it strongly resembles a fragment of the anterior capsule. It is an instinctive reaction to remove it. However, there are three factors which should prevent this mistake which can jeopardize the transparency of the cornea:
- The certainty that the capsule has been removed in the previous phases of the operation.
- The knowledge that this floating membrane appeared following the introduction of the I/A tip into the anterior chamber.
- After careful examination of the cornea, particularly its posterior portion, one or more straight lines in the depth of the cornea which start from the edge are seen.

Spatula—This can damage the iris sphincter or detach the posterior layer of the iris with pigment loss into the anterior segment. Occasionally it can perforate the iris. When used roughly to retract the iris to the root, it may rupture some small blood vessel in the iris or in the angle. The spatula may also tear the posterior capsule and cause vitreous to escape to the anterior chamber.

Scrapers and polishers—These rough instruments are used to remove the capsular opacities. If used without care or with the capsule under inappropriate tension, they can cause rupture.

Hooks—Iris or lens hooks can damage the endotheli-

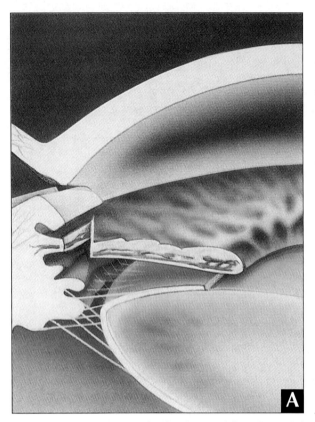 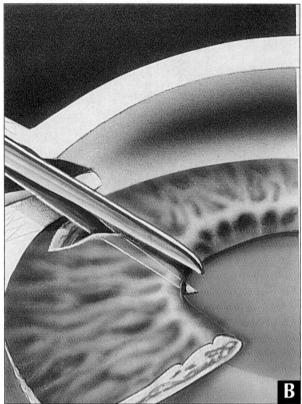

Figures 11-48A, 11-48B. Peripheral iridectomy followed by radial iridotomy.

um or the iris locally. Usually, the damage is not of any great importance. Sometimes the pupillary sphincter can be torn.

IOL—The complications of the implantation of the IOLs have been described previously.

## MIOSIS

### Preoperative Miosis

It is not uncommon to have to operate on a cataract in patients with a small pupil that will not dilate. Planning how to handle these cases is crucial in phacoemulsification. Therefore, the surgeon must be able to offer a patient with a narrow pupil all the benefits of phacoemulsification without changing the appearance or the function of the pupil. When planning this type of surgery, preoperative and postoperative factors must be taken into account.

#### Preoperative Factors

Obtain and note maximum possible mydriasis and establish what factors can influence it. If the narrow pupil remains immobile after application of mydriatics used in the normal preoperative routine, the iris is abnormal.

The removal of any posterior synechiae will increase mydriasis by 1 or 2 mm.

When planning the operation, the patient's age, his personal needs, and the hardness of the nucleus should be taken into consideration. Hard nuclei and small pupils can prove a daunting prospect even for the expert.

#### Intraoperative Factors

In phacoemulsification, the choice of technique will be based on the mydriasis obtained after manipulating in the anterior chamber to increase the dilatation.

Mydriasis can be increased by:
- Synechiolysis.
- Iridotomy.
- Multiple sphincterotomy/sphincterectomy.
- Instrumental mechanical dilatation.

Synechiolysis—After having completed the main 2.8 to 3.2 mm incision and one or two accessory incisions, a high molecular weight VES (Healon GV) is injected. A button-tipped spatula is inserted under the pupillary plane and moved around the entire circumference, trying to reach the peripheral zones, to liberate as much of the posterior surface of the iris as possible.

If synechiae are the only cause of miosis, sufficient mydriasis (4 to 6 mm) can be obtained in order to perform capsulorhexis under direct visual control.

The use of the high molecular weight VES is an important tool for increasing and maintaining the mydriasis during the capsulotomy. Capsulorhexis can then be completed. With an enlargement to 4.5 to 5 mm, any of the endocapsular techniques can be used, depending on the hardness of the nucleus and the surgeon's normal operating routine.

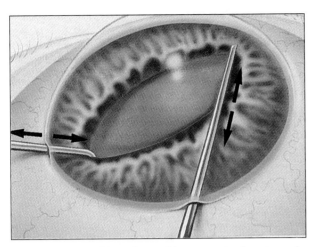
Figure 11-49. Stretching using an iris retractor hook and a push-pull.

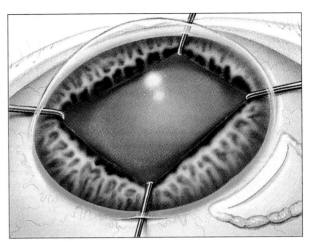
Figure 11-50. Mechanical dilatation of the pupil with four hooks.

If the mydriasis remains limited (2 to 3 mm) or reduced (3 to 4 mm) a surgeon with little or moderate experience must resort to using one of the pupillary extension techniques which will be dealt with later in this chapter. On the other hand, an experienced surgeon can proceed with capsulorhexis and then decide how to proceed on the basis of the hardness of the nucleus.

Iridotomy—Radial iridotomy is the simplest procedure for making the nucleus accessible in the event of a non-reversible closed miosis.

If not already present, a baseline iridectomy is performed at 12 o'clock. Starting from this point, the iris is cut to the pupil with microscissors presuming that the incision is performed superiorly. This technique is particularly suitable if a can opener capsulotomy is planned with a phacoemulsification technique in the pupillary plane, as the upper sector is more accessible. If the surgeon wishes to use an endocapsular technique, particularly with nuclear-fracture, it is preferable to perform an iridotomy distally (ie, at 6 o'clock) as the action zone is largely in this sector. In this case, the iridotomy is centrifugal and does not require an iridectomy.

For the best postoperative appearance and functional result, use a prolene 10-0 suture to reconstruct the pupil at the end of the operation.

Pupil reconstruction can be avoided in an elderly, extremely sedentary patient. In other cases (where phenomena of glare and reflection could reduce the quality of sight after the operation) pupil reconstruction is essential.

Multiple sphincterotomies—These will provide adequate mydriasis for phacoemulsification with satisfactory postoperative appearance and some pupillary function.

With 6 to 8 mini-sphincterotomies (each of length 0.5 to 0.7 mm) it is usually possible to create mydriasis sufficient for any technique of phacoemulsification under completely safe conditions. The outcome depends on the residual elasticity of the iris tissue.

The sphincterotomies are performed after the injection of Provisc or Healon to maintain the anterior chamber and once any posterior synechiae have been removed with a spatula. It is also useful to inject a small quantity of VES under the iris to raise the pupillary margin. In addition to the above functions, the VES has an important role in limiting iris bleeding which may occur during the operation.

The sphincterotomies can be performed with a variety of instruments (there are also special scissors—Rappasso Scissors), but normally long-armed Vannas microscissors are sufficient. Ideally these should be angled in order to reach the pupillary margin under the incision.

Sphincterectomy—This involves the complete removal of an entire sector of the pupillary sphincter.

A VES is injected into the anterior chamber and between the iris and the anterior capsule. With a curved Vannas scissors, a curved incision of the iris is performed to extend the pupillary field. The incision can also be performed with straight scissors after the iris tissue has been placed under tension with a hook or a fine forceps.

Instrumental mechanical dilatation—There are two methods which are the easiest to use in those cases where the iris tissue will not dilate with the methods described previously.
1. Stretching of the iris using mobile hooks.
    Two iris hooks can be used inserted through two counterpositioned side port incisions. Each hook, having fixed the iris near to the pupil, is pulled toward its insertion incision in the opposite direction of the other hook. The maneuver is performed from the 3 o'clock position to 9 o'clock and then at the 6 and 12 o'clock positions.
    The result depends largely on the residual elasticity of the iris. If the iris constricts again following this stretching, resort to another procedure (eg, a multiple sphincterotomy).
2. Stretching of the iris with fixed hooks.
    Four nylon hooks (Grieshaber) are inserted through 0.5 mm limbal incisions. They are adjustable thanks to a silicone button which prevents them sliding along the incision. By this means, the desired mydriasis can be obtained to allow for the technique planned for the individual case.

> **Table 11-24**
>
> **PREVENTION AND TREATMENT OF INTRAOPERATIVE MIOSIS**
>
> Preoperatively
> - Check the maximum mydriasis possible.
> - Evaluate the presence of synechiae.
> - Suspend the miotizing treatment.
> - Avoid dilating the patient during the 2 days prior to the operation.
> - Administer inhibitors of prostaglandin release (Ocufen, Voltaren, etc).
>
> Intraoperatively
> - Synechiolysis.
> - Iridotomy.
> - Multiple sphincterotomy.
> - Sphinterectomy.
> - Mechanical instrumental dilatation.
> - Using mobile hooks.
> - Using fixed hooks
> - Using a pupillary ring.
> - Using suture threads.

> **Table 11-25**
>
> **WHEN IRIDECTOMY SHOULD BE PERFORMED IN PHACOEMULSIFICATION**
>
> On any occasion that there is the risk that during the postoperative there may be a pupillary block:
>
> - When the incision may not have a perfect hold or closure.
> - When there is residual cortical material.
> - When the operation has been long and traumatic.
> - When the IOL is implanted in the ciliary sulcus.
> - When there is cortical material mixed with the vitreous.
> - In the event there is an anterior incomplete vitrectomy.
> - When there is uveitis or inflammation in the past (chronic uveitis).
> - In juvenile cataract and children.

## Intraoperative Miosis

The pupil may contract during surgery due to a variety of factors:

- Unsuitable preoperative preparation due to insufficient instillation of the mydriatic eyedrops.
- Poor individual sensitivity to the pharmacological products used, which can be tested a few days prior to the operation.
- Intraoperative manipulation of the iris.
- Repeated instability of the anterior chamber.
- Excessive duration of the operation.

Use pure, preservative-free adrenaline diluted in the infusion liquid (0.25 to 0.50 cc in 500 cc). If for local or general reasons the use of adrenaline is not advisable, it is necessary to adopt suitable measures to be able to proceed safely with the operation.

Let us consider what happens if intraoperative miosis occurs during the various phases of the operation.

Capsulotomy—The likelihood of miosis at such an early stage is not high. However, if it does occur, what happens next depends on the type of capsulotomy being performed.

A can opener incision generally does not cause problems as it can also be done blind, under the iris. Try not to move too peripherally with the cystotome.

If a capsulorhexis was being performed (or a capsulorhexis was planned), use a further injection of high molecular weight VES to dilate the pupil and then try to complete it. Another option is to convert it to a can opener in order to avoid completing the capsulorhexis without direct visual control, which may be dangerous.

Hydrodissection—It is a rare occurrence for miosis to occur during hydrodissection. However, if the chamber is lost once or twice or if the cannula touches the iris or numerous maneuvers are necessary to complete the operation, the pupil may constrict.

If the miosis permits the surgeon to see the edge of the capsulorhexis, the hydrodissection can be completed without difficulty:

If this is not the case, one of two things can be done, depending on the surgeon's experience and the anatomical and clinical characteristics of the individual case.

1. Continue with the hydrodissection. The hydrodissection cannula must pass without visual control peripherally to obtain good separation. The success of this maneuver depends mainly on the hardness and the extension of the nucleus. By observing the behavior of the cortex-nucleus material in the pupillary field, one can evaluate the effect of the BSS injection.

   After every injection, slight decompression will allow any liquid trapped in the capsular bag to escape and to overrule the effect of the BSS injection.

2. It is safer to stop the hydrodissection or abandon it completely, reenter with the cystotome, and perform can opener incisions of the anterior capsule, blind if necessary. Use a phacoemulsification technique which involves the total mobilization of the nucleus (technique in the anterior chamber or on the pupillary plane). Alternatively it would be better to perform a planned extracapsular extraction.

Phacoemulsification—Miosis is more common in this part of the operation. It can also be rather frustrating. If the surgeon lacks experience, the wisest choice is to bring the nucleus into the anterior chamber with one of the maneuvers described in the initial chapters. The size of the pupil is not so important since an anterior chamber technique will now be used. Nevertheless, luxating the nucleus into the anterior chamber is still not an easy process. Occasionally it is necessary to resort to the radial incision of the iris.

The best technique for completing phacoemulsification in a narrowing pupil is nuclear fracture with a cross-technique on the condition the capsulorhexis is intact and the hydrodissection can be completed. This is because all the maneuvers of this technique take place in the central or paracentral zone where direct vision is still sufficient even when the pupil narrows.

With other techniques in the posterior chamber, especially if the nucleus is not sufficiently mobilized (and this is the determinant factor), proceed with extreme caution. Plan every step of the phacoemulsification and be ready

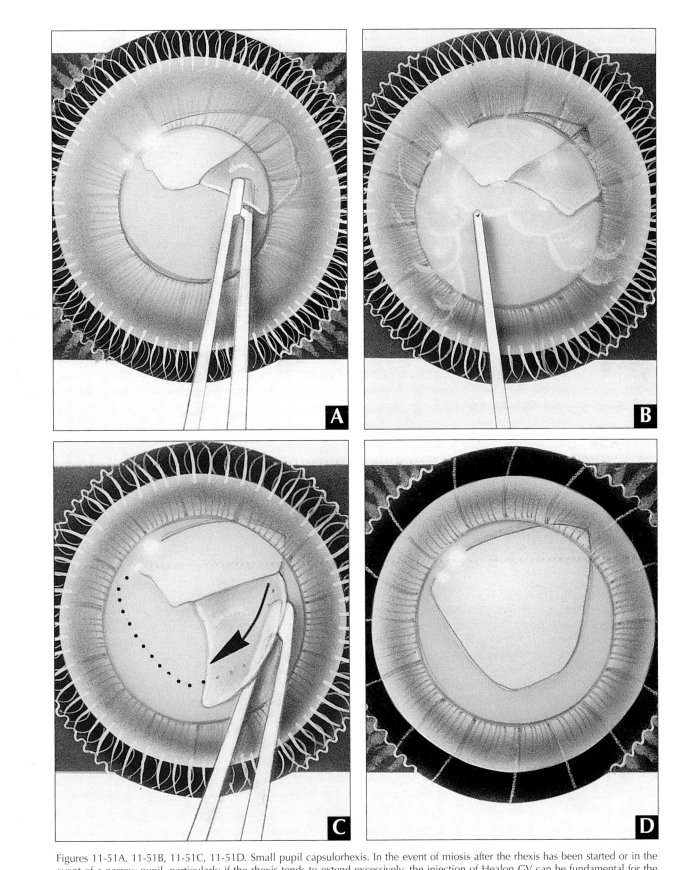

Figures 11-51A, 11-51B, 11-51C, 11-51D. Small pupil capsulorhexis. In the event of miosis after the rhexis has been started or in the event of a narrow pupil, particularly if the rhexis tends to extend excessively, the injection of Healon GV can be fundamental for the progression of the procedure. This widens the pupil, flattens the capsule, and counterbalances any vitreal thrust. In practice, in the majority of cases, it allows the surgeon to complete the rhexis even if it is not likely to be perfectly circular.

for extremely long operation times.

It is very important to be patient and take your time, as complications are always waiting round the corner.

If two phases for each step are used the whole procedure will be much easier.
1. Stop the phacoemulsification, create space with viscoelastic, and mobilize the nuclear material with a spatula.
2. Further phacoemulsification of the material made accessible to visual control and in a more favorable position for access by the U/S tip.

The safety of the operation is also increased through separation and protection provided by viscoelastic of the posterior capsule. In this case, Viscoat plays a very important role. It can actually form a cushion between the remaining nucleus and the posterior capsule and can maintain the integrity of the posterior capsule even in difficult situations.

Under critical conditions, it is advisable to resort to an intraoperative iridotomy.

## Aspiration of the Cortex and IOL Implant

Miosis in these phases normally does not create any great difficulty. Regarding aspiration of the cortex, it is advisable to expose the material to be captured with the help of a spatula and a suitable hook.

The Buratto two-handed technique using two separate cannulas is extremely useful. With this system it is possible to aspirate all the cortex satisfactorily even with marked miosis. Even for the implantation of the IOL, the use of a high molecular weight VES and high cohesion (Healon, Provisc) has proved extremely beneficial.

The use of both products is expensive but the former creates the spaces better while the latter maintains them better. This is the current trend in other steps of phacoemulsification.

## CONCLUSION

Phacoemulsification is undoubtedly the technique which gives the best results in cataract surgery. The skills need to be acquired but with adequate training this should not result in adverse results for the patient.

Phacoemulsification, because of the small incision, allows the surgeon to perform self-sealing incisions with excellent anatomical healing. More importantly, its rapid functional recovery allows the patient to return quickly to his or her normal daily routine with innumerable personal, social, and economic benefits. It also permits a marked drop in the number of postoperative visits and cuts down expenditure by eliminating provisional spectacles. The patient (and the doctor) are spared irritating suture removal.

Phacoemulsification induces little astigmatism. The resulting wound is also resistant to postoperative trauma in both the short- and long-term.

Phacoemulsification also allows the surgeon to remove the nucleus and the cortex through a continuous capsulotomy which can be even smaller than the size of the nucleus itself. This is a great help when the IOL is positioned, but particularly advantageous in the postoperative period.

During surgery, the improved visibility of the capsular rim allows safe insertion of the IOL into the capsular bag. This isolates the surrounding structures, gives excellent centering, makes the IOL optic adhere well to the posterior capsule, and limits the frequency and speed of posterior capsule opacification.

In the postoperative period there is superb tolerance of the artificial lens because of its placement in the capsular bag. It does not alter or modify the nearby structures, and it does not undergo any alteration of material. This is particularly true if a one-piece PMMA IOL is implanted.

Phacoemulsification allows the insertion of lenses with small optics and the insertion of foldable IOLs, thus considerably reducing the size of the surgical wound. This has the advantage of keeping anatomical damage to a minimum and accelerating the healing process.

In conclusion, phacoemulsification offers these and many other advantages over ICCE and ECCE. They are now a fundamental part of current basic training and therefore must be learned. In order to reduce the risks to a minimum, the surgeon must have a good theoretical foundation, appropriate familiarity with the machine, adequate experience in surgery, but also a clear concept of the surgical mistakes which can cause complications and how best to avoid them.

# Chapter 12

# VISCOELASTIC SUBSTANCES AND CATARACT SURGERY

*Lucio Buratto, MD*

## GENERAL CONCEPTS

In recent years, numerous articles have described the characteristics of viscoelastic substances (VES) and their ability to facilitate cataract surgery and help the surgeon operate in conditions of greater safety. All surgeons performing this type of surgery are well aware of the advantages provided by these products during the various surgical steps. However, the perfect VES does not exist, at least not yet. While some products are excellent auxiliaries in some situations, their inherent chemical and physical characteristics make them totally unsuitable in others.

They all must have at least one basic feature—high viscosity with a zero shear rate to stabilize and maneuver tissues and structures inside the eye, while guaranteeing adequate space necessary for the procedures.

Naturally, all the other physical characteristics (cohesiveness, elasticity, pseudoplasticity, etc) will influence the degree and ease with which the product can be injected and removed, and the length of time it will remain in the eye during surgical maneuvers. These are important features that should not be underestimated by the surgeon.

According to Steve Arshinoff, MD, VES can be divided into two main groups based on certain characteristics they are:
1. Substances with very high viscosity and cohesive substances with high viscosity with zero shear rate and high molecular weight.
2. Substances with a lower viscosity at zero shear rate with a low molecular weight which will tend to disperse inside the eye.

If we take a closer look at viscosity with zero shear rate and the cohesiveness, the surgical objectives will be obvious.

The very cohesive VES with high viscosity—such as Healon GV, Healon, Provisc, Amvisc Plus, Amvisc, and Biolon—are very useful in creating space and stabilizing the tissues, increasing the mydriasis, stabilizing the nucleus during capsulorhexis, deepening the anterior chamber, separating the synechiae, opening the capsular bag, and maintaining this space during implantation of the IOL, creating counterpressure on the vitreous in the event of capsular rupture, etc.

The dispersive VES (ie, those with lower viscosity and lower cohesiveness) may break up easily when injected into the eye and therefore *disperse* in small fragments. This group includes Viscoat, Vitrax, and the methylcellulose products. These products form a layer that will adhere and coat the posterior surface of the cornea to protect the endothelium during phacoemulsification, allow selective mobilization and isolation, and capture nuclear fragments. They are also used if the phacoemulsification tip accidentally catches the iris, in the event of zonular disinsertion, rupture of the posterior capsule, etc. In addition, they can be used to allow phacoemulsification to be performed on eyes with a low number of endothelial cells.

Healon GV is the reference substance in the first group of VES. Viscoat is the reference substance in the second group.

The choice of VES varies with the surgical requirements of that particular case. Each surgeon must be trained sufficiently to choose the most appropriate substance for the individual patient and the specific technique. The ideal situation would be to have more than one VES available during the operation. This will provide the patient with all the intraoperative and postoperative advantages of the substance without being subjected to any of the drawbacks.

The question of endothelial protection continues to present problems. Some surgeons feel that the dispersive VES provide better protection. Others feel that the cohesive VES protect the endothelium better by forming chemical bonds with the cornea and protecting it from

| Table 12-1 |
|---|
| **WHEN A VES IS REQUIRED** |
| Filling the anterior chamber |
| During capsulorhexis |
| During hydrodissection |
| During phacoemulsification |
| With I/A |
| When filling the capsular bag |
| To maintain good capsular opening during insertion, unfolding, and positioning of the IOL |

the release of free radicals during phacoemulsification. This bonding will provide even better protection for the endothelium, compared with the adhesive substances that coat the posterior face of the cornea, providing mechanical protection.

I will now analyze the substances which are appropriate for the various steps of cataract surgery.

## FILLING THE ANTERIOR CHAMBER

Filling the anterior chamber with an appropriate VES is fundamental for the optimal performance of phacoemulsification. If the pupil is narrow, the chamber is shallow, or the surgeon is performing the capsulorhexis with forceps, the substance used must be transparent and also maintain the spaces within the anterior chamber to allow the surgical steps to be completed in a satisfactory manner.

There are three basic characteristics for the VES:
1. Maintain the space—High viscosity with zero shear rate is indicated.
2. Ensure good visibility of the structures in the anterior chamber—A very transparent substance is indicated.
3. Be easy to inject—A substance with high pseudoplasticity is indicated.

## CAPSULORHEXIS

For the surgeon to perform continuous curvilinear capsulorhexis (CCC) four basic requirements of the appropriate VES must be satisfied:
1. A deep anterior chamber. A substance with high molecular weight and high viscosity with zero shear rate is required.
2. Excellent visibility. The substance must be very transparent.
3. Stabilize the capsular flap to keep it immobile and pushed downward. The substance must have the same properties as a soft permanent spatula.
4. Allow the surgical instruments to be maneuvered. A substance with high pseudoplasticity and high elasticity is indicated.

I feel that Healon GV is undoubtedly the ideal substance for both routine capsulorhexis and for more complicated cases. This will be followed by the products containing high molecular weight hyaluronic acid such as Healon and Provisc.

## CLEAVAGE OF THE LENS STRUCTURES

One basic requirement of a substance that will have to resist all the maneuvers which take place during hydrodissection and hydrodelamination is that the injected fluid wave be able to circulate freely. It must flow between the separated tissues and then escape toward the anterior chamber.

The ideal VES must:
- Maintain the shape of the anterior chamber during the injection of balanced salt solution (BSS). It must have high viscosity with low shear rate.
- Avoid a strong pressure increase in the event an excessive quantity of BSS is injected, so it must be highly cohesive and have high pseudoplasticity. The substance must be able to leave the eye easily if an excess quantity of BSS is introduced.

The surgeon would thus be advised to choose a cohesive, pseudoplastic product with high viscosity with zero shear rate. Both Provisc and Healon appear to satisfy these requisites.

Healon GV may be too heavy in some cases and make the BSS flow from the bag more difficult.

It may also be difficult for adhesive materials such as Viscoat to leave the anterior chamber if excess BSS is injected. Moreover, the fluid flow injected can create cleavage lines in the product, making it more difficult to see the structures lying behind.

In addition to the use of the appropriate pseudoplastic, cohesive VES, the surgeon must exert a small degree of pressure on the posterior edge of the surgical incision prior to hydrocleavage. This will allow a small quantity of VES to escape and permit easier circulation of the fluid injected and it will escape more easily from the bag.

## PHACOEMULSIFICATION

During the phase of nuclear fragmentation using ultrasound (U/S), the surgeon has the following needs:
1. A product that can resist the applied forces and which will remain in the eye to protect the endothelium because phacoemulsification is a turbulent procedure with elevated fluid flow during irrigation and aspiration (I/A). This continuous flow will tend to remove the viscoelastic.
2. A product that will protect the surfaces, the corneal endothelium in particular.

In fact, emulsification of the nucleus produces:
- Nuclear fragments that float in the anterior chamber.
- Air bubbles through cavitation which can damage the endothelium.
- A high degree of fluid turbulence.
- A high degree of fluid exchange during which the VES will tend to be removed.

Table 12-2
## THE BEST VES IN THE PRELIMINARY PHASES OF A PHACOEMULSIFICATION OPERATION

| Operating phase and surgeon's requirements | Required characteristics and recommended product |
|---|---|
| **For filling the chamber** | |
| Easy to inject. | High pseudoplasticity. |
| For filling the spaces. | Low viscosity with high shear rate (when the viscoelastic is moving). |
| | High viscosity with zero shear rate. |
| The best VES for this operating phase are (in order of preference): | Healon GV. |
| | Healon. |
| | Provisc. |
| | Viscoat. |
| **The capsulorhexis must** | |
| Maintain the depth of the anterior chamber. | High viscosity. |
| Allow good visibility. | High elasticity. |
| Avoid the flap moving uncontrollably. | Transparency. |
| Keep the capsular flap pushed downward. | *Permanent spatula* to keep a firm hold on the capsule |
| Allow instruments to be moved easily in the capsule. | Transparent to allow good visibility. |
| | *Permanent spatula* to prevent cortical material entering the anterior chamber. |
| | *Soft spatula* to remove the capsular flap. |
| The best VES for this operating phase are (in order of preference): | Healon GV. |
| | Healon. |
| | Provisc. |
| | Viscoat. |
| For maintaining the chamber during the injection of BSS. | Pseudoplasticity. |
| **Hydrodissection** | |
| It must be able to leave the eye if an excessive volume of BSS is injected. | |
| The best VES for this operating phase are (in order preference): | Healon GV. |
| | Healon. |
| | Provisc. |
| | Viscoat. |

3. A product that protects the eye structures from the mechanical vibrations produced by the phacoemulsification tip.
4. Assurance that there is no massive or uncontrolled escape of VES. The surgeon must ensure that the product leaves the chamber slowly and is under his or her complete control throughout the entire phacoemulsification procedure. It must be completely removed at the end of the procedure.
5. The product must maintain the spaces, despite the various movements of the phacoemulsification tip, the spatula, and the nucleus.

I will discuss those five points in detail and explain which VES is most suitable for each one.

1. The property of low cohesion is required in order to remain in the anterior chamber despite the significant flow of irrigation.

    As previously mentioned, the irrigation solution used during phacoemulsification will tend to remove viscoelastic from the anterior chamber. Substances are not very cohesive with short-chain molecules and low molecular weight and will persist. In this case Viscoat is particularly indicated.

2. Good adhesion is needed for protection of the corneal endothelium.

    Adhesive substances such as Viscoat will tend to adhere to the cells of the corneal endothelium, protecting it. The high degree of coatability is a fundamental requirement for good adhesiveness. Adhesive substances such as Viscoat are preferable from this point of view.

3. Protection from mechanical vibrations requires a substance with a high degree of elasticity.

    During the procedure, the phacoemulsification tip vibrates in a closed system. These vibrations are transmitted to the internal structures of the eye, where VES should act as a sort of shock absorber.

    If the surgeon has to choose between a product that is not very elastic but will remain in the anterior chamber, and a product that is very elastic but will escape quickly, he or she should opt for the former.

    Again Viscoat is a preferred VES under these conditions and the most suitable VES product for phacoemulsification.

4. The ability to remain in the anterior chamber during the introduction of the instruments requires a product with low cohesion.

    During insertion of the phacoemulsification tip or the

Table 12-3A

# THE BEST VISCOELASTIC DURING THE PHASE OF U/S IN THE PHACOEMULSIFICATION TECHNIQUE

| Surgeon's requirements during phaco | Quality required and product recommended |
|---|---|
| A substance which will preserve the spaces even when the phaco tip, the spatula, and the nucleus are moving and when irrigation is active. | Low pseudoplasticity. The CDS in Viscoat is a low pseudoplastic Newtonian substance. |
| Phaco is a turbulent process with high liquid flow during irrigation and aspiration. The continual flow will tend to remove the viscoelastic. The surgeon requires a product which will resist the applied forces and which will remain in the eye to protect the endothelium. | This short-chain substance with low molecular weight is less cohesive. Viscoat has low cohesion properties so it will persist longer in the eye. |
| Remain in the chamber even with the introduction of instruments or alternately. | The viscosity drops slightly with the movements, so with BSS-phaco movement, for example, the spaces are maintained longer. |
| Escape gradually and/or controllably and/or partially. | Escape of Viscoat from the chamber during the procedure will therefore be slow. Provisc, Healon, and Healon GV are products with high cohesion thanks to the long molecular chains with high molecular weight. These will tend to escape in a single drop as the phaco tip is inserted. |
| Protect all the surfaces but particularly that of the endothelium. | A highly wettable product is required. With its high wettability, Viscoat provides excellent coating of the epithelium and the tissue surfaces. The low wettability of Provisc, Healon, and Healon GV has a poor coating ability. Products (Healon, Healon GV, Provisc) which bind chemically with the endothelial receptors are also valid (binding sites and scavenger effect). |
| During the phase of U/S the best VES are, in order: | Viscoat, Healon GV, Healon, Provisc. |

Table 12-3B

# VES AND THE PRODUCTION OF NUCLEAR PARTICLES

| Emulsification of the nucleus produces: | The surgeon requires: |
|---|---|
| Particles of nucleus. Air bubbles which may damage the endothelium. High liquid turbulence. High liquid exchange which tends to induce the escape of VES. The introduction of the phaco tip, the spatula, and other instruments also contribute. | High protection of the endothelium, obtained by coating the surfaces adequately to protect the epithelium from trauma. Trauma is induced by rapidly moving nuclear particles or the air bubbles and from the current of irrigation liquid. A highly adhesive product, one which provides long-lasting coverage of the corneal endothelium and the tissues. A highly wettable product. A viscoelastic product which persists in the anterior chamber and in contact with the endothelium. The optimal choice would be a low viscosity product (Viscoat) as opposed to a high viscosity product (Healon GV). |
| Mechanical vibrations of the phaco. | In order to protect the tissues, the elasticity of the product is extremely important (the elasticity depends on the viscosity and the molecular length). |
| During phaco, the best VES are (in order): | Viscoat. Healon GV. Healon. Provisc. |

| Table 12-4 |
|---|
| **THE IDEAL VISCOELASTIC DURING I/A OF THE CORTEX** |

| The surgeon needs to have: | Characteristics of the VES: |
|---|---|
| A substance which resists high flow rates of BSS in the chamber and protects the endothelium. | High adhesion. |
| A substance which stays where it is placed (on the endothelial surface) and which does not mix and alter the cortex or modify its removal. | Poor cohesion. |
| A substance which does not leave the anterior chamber in a single bubble with introduction of the tip it is gradually removed. | Poor removability. |
| A substance which will not obstruct the aspiration of the cortex. | |
| As with phaco, in I/A the VES which are more adhesive to the internal surfaces of the cornea are: | Viscoat. Healon GV. Provisc. Healon. |

spatula, Viscoat with its low cohesiveness is the VES that maintains the space best without escaping. If Viscoat does escape, it will do so slowly and in a controllable manner.

On the other hand, products such as Healon GV, Healon, and Provisc will tend to escape in a single bubble from the anterior chamber because of their long molecular chains and high molecular weight.

5. Maintenance of the space.

Once the phacoemulsification tip has been introduced into the anterior chamber, the elements responsible for the constant maintenance of a deep anterior chamber are determined by the machine settings (bottle height, level of the flow rate, values of the vacuum, the type of pump, and the presence of continuous irrigation). These elements, and not the presence of VES, will provide the surgeon with the deep chamber.

If the product has a low degree of pseudoplasticity, it is more likely to persist in the anterior chamber without escaping, so Viscoat is preferable.

## IRRIGATION/ASPIRATION

During I/A of the cortex the main needs of the surgeon regarding the ideal VES are:

1. A substance that will remain in the anterior chamber under the high flow rate of BSS to maintain the protection of the endothelium. The description provided for endothelial protection during phacoemulsification is also valid here. A substance such as Viscoat is preferred as it will adhere to the endothelium and persist in the anterior chamber despite the high BSS flow.
2. A substance that will remain on the endothelial surface and will not mix with the cortex, altering or modifying its removal. A substance with low cohesiveness is preferable in this case.
3. A substance that will not leave the anterior chamber in a single bubble when the tip is introduced, but can be removed gradually. In this case, the surgeon should choose a substance that will disperse; the optimal choice would be a product which is not very cohesive,

| Table 12-5 |
|---|
| **VES TO FILL THE BAG AND IMPLANT THE IOL** |

| The surgeon needs: | Qualities required of the VES: |
|---|---|
| Substances that are easily injected. | High pseudoplasticity. |
| Substances that occupy spaces (which stay in place). | High molecular weight. Spreads smoothly. |
| The best VES to fill the capsular bag are (in progressive order): Viscoat. | Healon GV. Healon. Provisc. |

with short-chain molecules.

One could argue that the complete removal of the VES at the end of surgery will also be more difficult. Many authors report that the time needed to perform I/A is increased, causing damage to the corneal endothelium. However, in my opinion, the products that are adhesive and have low cohesiveness are still preferable. Once again, the choice is Viscoat.

## FILLING THE CAPSULAR BAG

After completing phacoemulsification and aspirating the residual cortex, the surgeon must expand the capsular bag with VES in preparation for the intraocular lens (IOL) implant.

The basic requirements of an ideal VES to fill the capsular bag are:
- The viscoelastic should be easy to inject and therefore highly pseudoplastic.
- The product must occupy the space, but remain immobile, thus acting as a permanent spatula.
- It must allow good visibility; it should be transparent.
- It must be easily removed from the bag following IOL implantation and be highly cohesive.

Table 12-6

# MAINTENANCE OF A GOOD CAPSULAR OPENING DURING INSERTION OF THE IOL

| The surgeon's needs | Characteristics required of the product |
|---|---|
| Maintenance of the space. | High molecular weight. High viscosity. |
| | Sodium hyaluronate provides: High viscosity and thus a high capacity for maintaining the spaces (bag and chamber). CDS, which is not very good at maintaining spaces because of its low viscosity. |
| If the IOL comes into contact with the delicate structures the best VES to maintain the chamber and the bag prior to the insertion of the IOL are: | Healon GV. Healon. Provisc. Viscoat. |
| During insertion the IOL and its positioning: The VES must not resist the entrance of the IOL. The VES must allow easy manipulation of the IOL. | High pseudoplasticity. |
| As the lens is unfolded: The VES must provide resistance against rapid unfolding of the lens (if it is a foldable IOL). | Low pseudoplasticity. |
| Depending on the type of IOL and the clinical situation, the chosen VES must have a high or a low pseudoplasticity The best VES are: | Healon GV. Healon. Provisc. Viscoat. |
| Cover the IOL with a uniform layer of substance (high *wettability* of the IOL). | The *wettability* of Viscoat is superior to that of the other substances. |
| Removal of the VES, the possibility of easy aspiration of the substance from the capsular bag and the anterior chamber. | Low viscosity with high shear rate. Good cohesion. |
| The best substances, in terms of removability, are: | Healon GV. Healon. Provisc. Viscoat. |

For an optimal filling of the bag, my choice would be Healon GV, Healon, and Provisc, because of their easy injectability (pseudoplasticity) and excellent permanent, soft spatula effect (high molecular weight, high viscosity with a low shear rate). Moreover, these substances are very transparent and extremely cohesive, which means that they will be easily aspirated from the bag.

## MAINTENANCE OF A GOOD CAPSULAR OPENING DURING IOL IMPLANTATION

Recently, the popularity of foldable IOLs has increased dramatically and thus acquired a strong market position.

Implantation in the capsular bag of a hard lens does not involve any significant dynamic problems. The VES plays an important role in maintaining the spaces within the chamber. For the foldable lenses introduced when folded and which open once inside the eye, there are many notable problems concerning dynamics. The VES chosen by the surgeon must allow him or her to implant the lenses while:

- Maintaining the spaces in the anterior chamber (and avoiding traumatic contact of the IOL with the cornea and the iris). The ideal VES will maintain good aperture of the capsular bag during all the implantation maneuvers. In addition, it will have high viscosity with zero shear rate and high molecular weight.
- Ensuring good visibility.
- Enabling easy entrance of the IOL and not obstructing its passage in any way. The VES should have high pseudoplasticity.
- Opposing the rapid unfolding of the lens and avoiding abrupt whipping by the distal loop of the IOL when it is released in the bag. The VES should have high elasticity and low pseudoplasticity.
- Not oppose the IOL's movements in the bag when centering the IOL. It should have high pseudoelasticity and high viscosity.

Table 12-7
## ASPIRATION OF THE VISCOELASTIC

Enter the chamber with the probe and press down on the posterior edge of the flap to allow some of the product to escape (some escaped already when the IOL was implanted); the pedal has been moved to Position 0.

Move the foot pedal to Position 2 and aspirate in the anterior chamber.

Starting distally, remove the material present at the circumference of the rhexis.

Push down on the lens to allow the material trapped between the lens and the posterior capsule to escape and aspirate it.

If possible, enter just under the rhexis with irrigation alone open and then activate the aspiration.

Aspirate the product at the camerular angle passing the I/A tip over the accessible angular portion.

When it looks as though all the material has been aspirated, repeat the control procedure of the capsular bag.

Table 12-8
## I/A PARAMETERS FOR REMOVING VES FROM THE ANTERIOR CHAMBER

| VES | Vacuum | Flow Rate | Tip |
|---|---|---|---|
| Healon GV | 400 mm Hg | 20 mL/min | 0.3 mm |
| Healon | 300 mm Hg | 15 cc/min | 0.3 mm |
| Viscoat | 500 mm Hg | 30 cc/min | 0.3 mm |
| Provisc | 250 mm Hg | 15 cc/min | 0.3 mm |

Table 12-9
## THE USE OF VES DURING PHACOEMULSIFICATION

In conclusion, in order to take full advantage of the clinical and physical characteristics of the VES during the phacoemulsification operation, at least two VES must be used.

| | |
|---|---|
| To maintain the anterior chamber | Use Provisc. Healon. |
| Capsulorhexis Hydrodissection | Healon GV. |
| For phacoemulsification I/A | Use Viscoat. |
| To fill the bag To maintain the opening of the bag To insert, unfold, and position the IOL | Use Provisc. Healon. |
| To remove the VES | Healon GV. |

In view of all these considerations, we can conclude that for IOL implantation, a VES with high molecular weight, high viscosity, high elasticity, and high pseudoplasticity is preferable with Healon GV, Healon, and Provisc at the top of the list.

## REMOVAL OF VES

It is well-known that VES facilitates surgical maneuvers, protects the tissues, and aids in the surgeon's manipulation of the tissues. However, the postoperative complications of increased intraocular pressure (IOP) caused by any remaining VES in the eye are just as well-known and have been extensively documented.

When choosing a VES, the surgeon should consider the ease of removal after surgery, both in terms of time required to complete this procedure and the ease of completion of the procedure. Substances that are highly cohesive and have low viscosity with a high shear rate (such as Provisc, Healon, and Healon GV) are aspirated very quickly and the aspiration times coincide for partial or complete aspiration. Thus the product will be removed completely and immediately from the eye. On the other hand, less-cohesive VES (Viscoat) have partial aspiration times which can mean taking between three and six to eight times longer for complete removal from the eye.

## USING TWO VISCOELASTICS

As demonstrated so far, in every phase of the operation, there are characteristics that enhance the physiochemical features of the VES and reject others. When the surgeon chooses a particular VES, some steps of the operation will benefit from the substance while others will not. The idea of using two viscoelastics was developed, thus gaining the advantages of each product and reducing the drawbacks.

### Capsulorhexis

In this case it is possible to position a VES (Healon GV, Healon, or Provisc) below in contact with the anterior capsule. These particular products have:
- Excellent transparency.
- High pseudoplasticity.
- High molecular weight.

This will allow the surgeon to have a better view of the flap even in conditions of poor visibility. The surgeon will also be able to perform capsulorhexis more easily to block the capsular flap or to move it as desired. The escape of the endolenticular milky liquid from intumescent cataracts can also be controlled.

The surgeon can then position an adhesive substance such as Viscoat which:
- Is highly adhesive.
- Has low pseudoplasticity.
- Has low molecular weight.

The product placed superiorly will remain in contact with the endothelium and will protect it during phacoemulsification. During phacoemulsification and hydrodissection, the lower product can leave its position and allow a wave of BSS to leave the capsular bag (eg, during the maneuvers of hydrodissection). Also, without the presence of the VES in contact with the material, the maneuvers of phaco fracture are performed easily.

Table 12-10
## PRECAUTIONS WHEN USING VISCOAT DURING PHACOEMULSIFICATION

| | |
|---|---|
| Enclosure of air bubbles due to the poor cohesion of the product. | The bubbles injected with the syringe which are already inside the chamber tend to remain trapped in the product. The bubbles which are produced during phaco because of cavitation of the tip will remain trapped inside the product and will reduce the visibility. |
| Transparency: The intrinsic characteristics of the product make it less transparent than sodium hyaluronate. During surgery, irregular cleavage lines form, which produce irregular surfaces at the interface of the irrigation liquid Viscoat | This causes visibility problems. At the beginning of phaco, it is advisable to remove the layer of product which is more in contact with the nuclear material. |
| Resistance to removability: The poor cohesion of Viscoat makes the product resistant to high flow rates and is therefore difficult to remove at the end of the operation. | The long maneuvers necessary and the high flow rates required for the complete removal of the product can damage the corneal endothelium. |
| Tendency to occlude the U/S tip. | This may happen with the techniques that require zero vacuum and low flow rate. To avoid this problem, at the beginning of the procedure, remove the layer of VES in contact with the nuclear material. |

Table 12-11
## SIMULTANEOUS USE OF TWO PRODUCTS IN THE SAME OPERATION

| | |
|---|---|
| For capsulorhexis, hydrodissection, phacoemulsification: The product on top must be the more adhesive one with a lower molecular weight. In this way, the product will stay in position for the entire operation. This provides cellular protection. | Viscoat on top, ie, the product which: Is more adhesive. Is less pseudoplastic. Has lower molecular weight. |
| The lower product must be heavier: This improves the visibility during the rhexis. This improves the ease of management of the instruments. This can be removed easily during the initial stages of phaco. | Provisc, Healon, or Healon GV underneath, the product which: Is more transparent. Is more pseudoplastic. Has greater molecular weight. |
| During the implant of the IOL: To form the bag properly. To coat the IOL. To facilitate the penetration of the lens in the capsular bag and to facilitate its rotation and manipulation. | Underneath: use Provisc, Healon and Healon GV again, the product which: Is more pseudoplastic. Has a greater molecular weight. Still less cohesive. More adherent to the tissues. On top: use Viscoat. |
| Removal of the VES. | Provisc is removed more easily so it is better to place it in the bag. Viscoat is more difficult to remove; it is placed outside the bag and in the anterior chamber. |

## IOL Implantation

The capsular bag is filled with cohesive, high molecular weight, pseudoplastic VES (Healon, Provisc, etc). On top of this, the surgeon can place another more adhesive product, such as Viscoat, between the iris and the corneal endothelium. This solution has a number of advantages.

A cohesive, high molecular weight VES with high viscosity and low shear rate placed in the bag greatly facilitates the bag distention, the insertion of the IOL, and its unfolding. It absorbs any negative shock waves as it enters the bag. At the same time, because of the cohesive characteristics, the substance will be aspirated more easily.

A mechanical protective barrier for the corneal endothelium and the iris will be created by the injection of an adhesive VES in the anterior chamber, in contact with the cornea (eg, Viscoat). The passage of the IOL and any contact with the ocular tissues will aid in the protection. In addition, the VES will not tend to escape from the anterior chamber as a result of pressure on the tunnel entrance caused by the surgeon as the IOL is inserted through a very small incision. Moreover, it will keep the anterior chamber deep and should always be present during the unfolding maneuvers of the IOL.

## Ease of Removal at the End of the Operation

Using these injection methods of VES, removal is encouraged because the cohesive substance underneath can be easily removed from the capsular bag, even from behind the IOL. The substance positioned above (such as Viscoat) which previously seemed more difficult to remove, is now clearly visible because of its positioning in the highest portion of the anterior chamber. It can be clearly identified and removed.

I advise using two different complementary viscoelastics in order to satisfy the different requirements during surgery.

# Section II

# PHACOEMULSIFICATION TECHNIQUES

# Chapter 13

# SURGICAL PHARMACOLOGY: INTRAOCULAR SOLUTIONS AND DRUGS USED FOR CATARACT SURGERY

*Henry F. Edelhauser, PhD*
*David B. Glasser, MD*

*Supported in part by NIH grants P30 EY06360 and EY00933 and Research to Prevent Blindness, Inc. Dr. Edelhauser is a Research to Prevent Blindness Senior Scientific Investigator Awardee.*

## INTRODUCTION

The cataract surgeon uses an impressive array of pharmacologic agents before, during, and after cataract surgery. These include sedatives and analgesics, local anesthetics, preoperative antiseptics, irrigating solutions, viscoelastics, mydriatics and miotics, antibiotics, anti-inflammatory agents, and a growing number of other products designed to enhance intraocular surgery and its outcome. Sedatives and local anesthetics have the potential for causing serious systemic reactions. All surgical solutions and additives have the potential for injuring the tissues they contact: the cornea, lens, trabecular meshwork, uvea, vitreous, and retina. The potential for injury is much greater when a solution is used inside the eye rather than when it is applied externally, because the concentrations to which the sensitive intraocular tissues are exposed are much higher. Due to the potential for toxicity, there should always be a specific indication for the use of an intraocular solution of medication. It should never be used *routinely*. In this chapter, we will discuss the use of solutions and drugs employed in ocular surgery and the means of avoiding and managing toxic reactions associated with these agents.

## ANTISEPTIC SOLUTIONS

Cleansing of the periocular skin with an antiseptic scrub solution is a routine step in preparing the eye for surgery, and is designed to reduce the risk of bacterial contamination. Toxicity of these solutions is related to inherent toxicity of the antiseptic itself, concentration, presence of a detergent, and contact time. Recent reports of keratitis resulting from accidental exposure to Hibiclens highlight the potential for toxicity if the scrub solution is allowed to enter the conjunctival sac.[1-4]

Phinney and associates[2] reported five patients accidentally exposed to Hibiclens who presented symptoms of pain and decreased vision. A large corneal epithelial defect was usually present, although punctate keratitis was described in one patient. Stromal edema and vascularization developed and progressed over a period of 2 to 10 weeks. Intrastromal hemorrhages occurred in areas of stromal neovascularization in one patient. Two patients developed irreversible bullous keratopathy and required penetrating keratoplasty. The edema cleared within 6 to 7 months in the remaining three patients, leaving reduced endothelial cell density and mild stromal scarring. Two of five patients had a decreased corneal sensation. Hamed and associates[1] reported stromal thinning and ectasia in

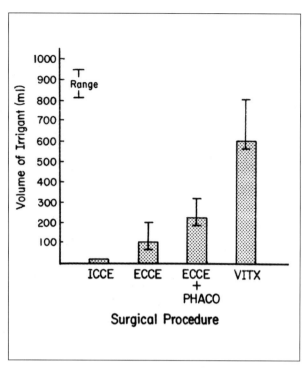

Figure 13-1. Comparative volumes of irrigating solutions used for various surgical procedures. (Reprint with permission *Ophthalmic Surgery*.[9])

two cases with persistent epithelial defects treated with steroids. Dense irreversible corneal scarring occurred in both cases.

In contrast, Shore[4] reported two cases of accidental Hibiclens exposure which were limited to epithelial involvement and which recovered without sequelae within 5 days. The benign course was attributed to routine irrigation of the conjunctival sac with balanced salt solution after the skin prep. It is noteworthy that eight of the nine reported cases of severe keratitis[1-3] occurred in association with non-ocular surgery performed by non-ophthalmologists. The paucity of cases related to ophthalmic procedures may be related to the tendency of many ophthalmologists to irrigate the conjunctival sac at the end of the prep.[5] Irrigation reduces contact time and the potential for toxicity.

Hibiclens contains chlorhexidine gluconate 4% in a detergent vehicle and has bactericidal activity against a wide range of gram-positive and gram-negative bacteria. Chlorhexidine itself is toxic to corneal epithelium and endothelium, and penetration may be enhanced by the detergent present in Hibiclens.[1,6] Chlorhexidine also binds to stromal proteins and is slowly released,[6] which may explain the progressive course of stromal edema and vascularization noted in the clinical reports.

MacRae and associates[7] studied the ocular toxicity of several antiseptics and found marked corneal de-epithelialization, conjunctival chemosis, and anterior stromal edema in rabbits treated with Hibiclens, tincture of iodine, 3% hexachlorophene with detergent (pHisoHex), 70% ethanol (Lavacol), and 7.5% povidone-iodine with detergent (Betadine Surgical Scrub). Only 10% povidone-iodine without detergent (Betadine Solution) prevented the severe toxic reactions seen with the other antiseptics in this study.

Corneal toxicity from antiseptic solutions is a potentially blinding complication. Since the potential for corneal exposure to the scrub solution cannot be completely simulated, we recommend the use of a non-toxic antiseptic: 10% povidone-iodine without detergent (Betadine Solution). This solution is germicidal against a broad range of gram-positive and gram-negative bacteria, fungi, yeasts, viruses, and protozoa. Apt et al[8] placed half strength (5%) Providine-iodine without detergent (Betadine Solution) directly into the conjunctival sac prior to ocular surgery in 30 patients. They found no significant toxicity and a 91% reduction in colonies cultured. In addition, we recommend irrigation of the conjunctival sac after completion of the skin prep, especially if the antiseptic used is toxic or contains a detergent.

## IRRIGATING SOLUTIONS

An essential component in most intraocular surgical procedures is a safe irrigating solution. The irrigant keeps the globe inflated and maintains normal pressure-volume relationships during surgery. The rapid increase in the number of surgical procedures being performed over the last decade has been paralleled by an increase in the number of commercially available irrigating solutions.[9]

The potential for damage to the corneal endothelium and other tissues is related to the chemical composition, pH, and osmolality of the solution which bathes those tissues. As intraocular manipulations have become more complex, the duration and volume of irrigation have increased.[1] Despite a lack of controlled clinical studies, longer irrigation times, higher flow rates, and larger volumes are probably more traumatic to the corneal endothelium.[10]

### Evolution of Modern Irrigants

A review of the development of modern intraocular irrigants will set the stage for an understanding of their toxicity. This subject was last reviewed by McDermott[9] and Edelhauser.[11] Normal saline was the predominant irrigant until Merrill, Fleming, and Girard[12] showed that its acidic pH of 6.8 and incomplete electrolyte balance are toxic to intraocular tissues. The balanced salt solution (BSS) developed by Merrill and associates has a stable but non-physiologic citrate-acetate buffer, a pH of 7.5 to 8.2, and contains sodium, potassium, calcium, magnesium, and chloride. This composition began to approximate that of aqueous humor. When BSS was introduced, the short surgical procedures of the 1960s demanded only small volumes of irrigating solution, and 15 mL squeeze bottles met these needs. In the 1970s, greater volumes of irrigating solutions were needed to support procedures such as lensectomy, vitrectomy, phacoemulsification, and extracapsular cataract extraction (ECCE). Many prospective irrigants were evaluated in laboratories and operating rooms. In 1972, Dikstein and Maurice[13] used in vitro

Table 13-1
## CHEMICAL COMPOSITION[1] OF HUMAN AQUEOUS HUMOR, BSS PLUS[2], AND SMA-2[3] AND HARTMANN'S LACTATED RINGERS SOLUTION[4]

|  | Human aqueous humor | BSS Plus | BSS | Hartmann's SMA-2 | Lactated Ringers |
|---|---|---|---|---|---|
| Sodium | 162.9 | 160.0 | 155.7 | 145.7 | 131 |
| Potassium | 2.2-3.9 | 5.0 | 10.1 | 4.8 | 5 |
| Calcium | 1.8 | 1.0 | 3.3 | 1.2 | 2 |
| Magnesium | 1.1 | 1.0 | 1.5 | — | — |
| Chloride | 131.6 | 130.0 | 128.9 | 120.1 | 111 |
| Bicarbonate | 20.15 | 25.0 | — | 25.0 | — |
| Phosphate | 0.62 | 3.0 | — | — | — |
| Lactate | 2.5 | — | — | — | 29 |
| Glucose | 2.7-3.7 | 5.0 | — | 8.3 | — |
| Ascorbate | 1.06 | — | — | — | — |
| Glutathione | 0.0019 | 0.3 | — | — | — |
| Citrate | 0.12 | — | 5.8 | 3.4 | — |
| Acetate | — | — | 28.6 | 4.4 | — |
| pH | 7.38 | 7.4 | 7.6 | 7.3 | 6.4 |
| Osmolality (mOsm) | 304 | 305 | 298 | 290 | 258 |

[1]All concentrations are in millimoles or milliquivalents/liter.
[2]BSS Plus, BSS manufactured by Alcon Laboratories, Inc, Fort Worth, TX.
[3]SMA-2 manufactured by Senju Pharmaceutical, Osaka, Japan.
[4]Baxter Healthcare, Ltd, Thetford, Norfolk, England.

corneal endothelial perfusion technique to show that a modified bicarbonate Ringer's solution containing glutathione, glucose, and adenosine (GBR) could preserve corneal endothelial function and ultrastructure. Edelhauser and associates,[14,15] using the same in vitro perfusion techniques, compared GBR to four other commonly used irrigants (normal saline, Plasma-lyte 148, lactated Ringer's, and BSS). In each case, GBR was superior at maintaining corneal endothelial function (as measured by corneal swelling rates) and ultrastructure.

These studies further emphasized the importance of supplying organic and inorganic constituents similar to those of aqueous humor during intraocular irrigation. However, commercial formulation of a stable GBR solution was difficult because of the instability of reduced glutathione, adenosine, and bicarbonate. To circumvent these problems, BSS Plus (Alcon Laboratories) was formulated to be as similar to GBR and aqueous humor as possible while maintaining pharmacologic sterility, stability, and shelf-life. BSS Plus is a two-component bicarbonate-buffered electrolyte solution containing oxidized glutathione and glucose but no adenosine. Once reconstituted, the solution will maintain a physiologic pH for 6 to 24 hours.[9,10]

## Laboratory Studies

Laboratory studies of isolated perfused human corneas indicate that BSS Plus maintains normal corneal thickness. It will cause human eye bank corneas stored at 4°C to deturgese as the temperature is increased to 37°C. The endothelial metabolic pumps become functional and endothelial ultrastructure is maintained, while lactated Ringer's, BSS, SMA-2, and Hartmann's lactated Ringer's (HLR) do not.[16,17,18] Araie has shown that endothelial permeability is substantially increased after perfusion with SMA-2, an intraocular irrigating solution produced in Japan.[19] This suggests that the corneal swelling seen in SMA-2 perfused corneas is due in part to compromised endothelial barrier function. Increased permeability is consistent with the disruption of intracellular junctions observed in scanning and transmission electron micrographs of corneal endothelium after perfusion with SMA-2 and BSS. The large surface area paucity of lateral cell membrane area (where the $Na^+/K^+$ ATPase pump are located) and the presence of abnormal mitochondria in these corneas suggest a decrease in endothelial pumping capacity as well.

In vivo anterior chamber irrigations in cats and monkeys[10,17] confirm that BSS and SMA-2 can reversibly stress the endothelium, inducing corneal swelling after 1 hour and abnormal cell morphology after as little as 15 minutes of irrigation. BSS Plus prevented changes in cell morphology and corneal swelling after irrigation lasting 2 hours. In a more recent study by Nuyts et al[18] to evaluate HLR, it was shown that HLR caused corneal swelling and endothelial cell ultrastructural changes (endothelial cell edema and cytoplasmic vacuolization). The results of this study suggest that the clinically observed corneal clouding during irrigation with HLR is due to endothelial cell edema and decreased endothelial pump function. BSS Plus can reverse the corneal swelling induced by HLR.[18]

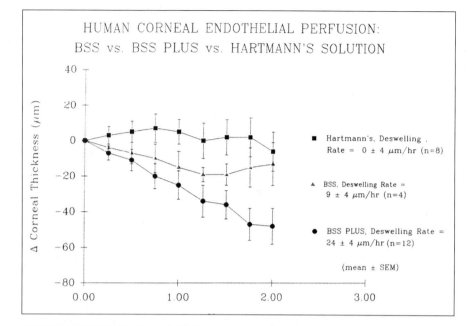

Figure 13-2. A comparison of corneal swelling rates following 120 minutes of endothelial perfusion with HLR solution, BSS, and BSS Plus. (Reprint with permission Graefes Arch Clin Exp Ophthalmol.[18])

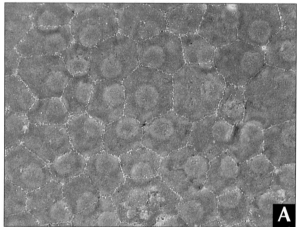

Figure 13-3A. Human corneal endothelium following 3 hours of in-vitro perfusion with BSS Plus SEM sowing hexagonal cells (x 1000).

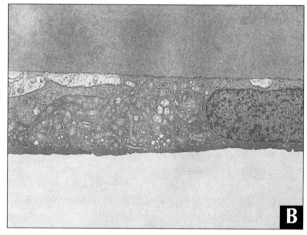

Figure 13-3B. TEM electron micrograph. The endothelial cell junctions are tight and the cytoplasmic organelles are normal (x 5220).

In a recent study of the electroretinographic effects of intravitreal irrigation, BSS Plus was able to maintain normal retinal function while BSS did not.[20] Post-vitrectomy retinal vascular permeability and retinal edema in rabbits was also reduced with the use of BSS Plus compared with BSS.[21]

## Clinical Studies

There are fewer clinical studies comparing BSS with BSS Plus. Kline and associates[22] found significantly less endothelial cell loss with BSS Plus (15.4%) than with BSS (22.7%) in 100 patients after ECCE and posterior chamber lens implantation performed without viscoelastic. However, the use of narrow-field specular microscopy (with its high inherent sampling error) to calculate cell density and the relatively high mean cell loss compared to other reports (8% after similar surgical procedures)[23] make it difficult to generalize these results.

Benson,[24] in a well-designed prospective study, found significantly less corneal edema on the first day after vitrectomy with BSS Plus than with lactated Ringer's. This concurs with the report by Matsuda[25] of significantly less cell loss after vitrectomy with BSS Plus than with lactated Ringer's. However, Rosenfeld[26] was unable to demonstrate any difference in cell loss between BSS and BSS Plus use during vitrectomy.

## Clinical Correlates

Many studies have been published evaluating the effects of irrigating solutions on rabbit corneal endothelium, which may be less susceptible to injury than human tissue. The rabbit eye is young, presumed free of disease, has the capacity for endothelial cell regeneration, and can withstand great metabolic stresses.[7] Conclusions about rabbit tissue may not reflect the behavior of human tissue 60 to 70 years old. Therefore, use of drugs or solutions shown to be safe for rabbit endothelium may still result in damage to some human patients.

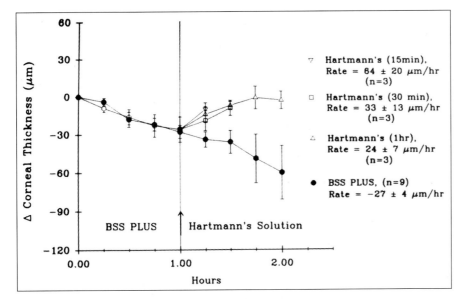

Figure 13-4. Human corneal in vitro endothelial perfusion (1 hour) followed by endothelial perfusion of HLR for 15 minutes, 30 minutes, and 1 hour. Note the increased corneal swelling with HLR solution. (Reprint with permission *Graefes Arch Clin Exp Ophthalmol*.[18])

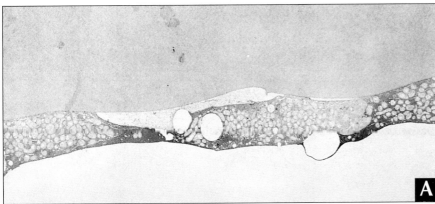

Figure 13-5A. TEM of a human cornea following a 30 minute endothelial perfusion with HLR solution. Note the marked vacuolation of cytoplasm, swelling of mitochondria, and endothelial edema (x 3420).

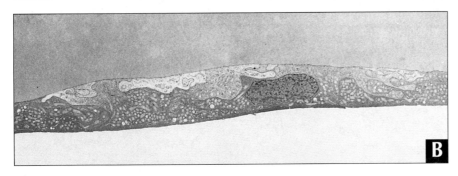

Figure 13-5B. TEM of the paired human cornea following a 30 minute endothelial perfusion with BSS Plus. The outer plasma membrane is smooth and the intracellular organelles are normal (x 3420). (Reprint with permission *Graefes Arch Clin Exp Ophthalmol*.[18])

Nevertheless, it has been difficult to demonstrate significant differences in cell loss in clinical studies comparing BSS and BSS Plus. However, lack of a significant decrease in endothelial cell density (ECD) does not necessarily mean that the endothelium is undamaged. ECD measurements are not that accurate. Sampling errors based on the size of the patient sample and the number of cells counted may be significant.[27,28] Wide-field specular microscopy with analysis of cell morphology and density is a more sensitive and reliable indicator of endothelial cell change or stress.[10]

In addition, follow-up times for most clinical studies are too short to detect significant changes in ECD. Cell loss associated with the mechanical trauma of surgery is probably too great to allow more subtle changes associated with an irrigating solution to be detected in the early postoperative period. We know that cell loss continues throughout life and that the cornea remains clear by virtue of the tremendous cell reserve with which we are born. Any surgical or nonsurgical insult shifts the cell loss curve toward decompensation.[29] Even a slight increase in the rate of cell loss can significantly reduce the useful life span of the corneal endothelium. The meaning of abnormal morphology many years after surgery remains unknown, but it is unlikely that these changes are associated with a slowing of endothelial cell loss.[30]

Patients with low cell densities or morphologic abnormalities of the endothelium (diabetics for example) are known to be more susceptible to surgical trauma[31-34] and

**IRRIGATION SOLUTION IN POSTOP EYE**

**Aqueous Replacement vs Time**

*Fluid Capacity*

| | |
|---|---|
| Anterior Chamber | 0.250ml |
| Posterior Chamber | 0.060ml |
| Space Left by Extracted Crystalline Lens | 0.250ml |
| Subtotal Fluid Capacity | 0.560ml |
| Posterior Chamber IOL (Average) | -0.035ml |
| Total Capacity | 0.525ml |

*Aqueous Flow Rate*

Normal Non-Geriatric Eye (Average) .002ml/min

*Aqueous Replacement*

Minimum Time $\dfrac{0.525\text{ml}}{0.002\text{ml/min}}$ = 262.5 mins (4 hours, 23 minutes)

*Flow Rate Following Surgery*

Aqueous flow is nearly always reduced by surgery. A 50% reduction is not uncommon. Thus, irrigation solution often remains in the postop eye for up to 8-3/4 hours.

Figure 13-6. A theoretical calculation of fluid volumes and replacement in the eye following cataract surgery. Note the prolonged turnover time for the solution present in the anterior chamber at the completion of surgery. (Reprint with permission *Ophthalmic Surg.*[9])

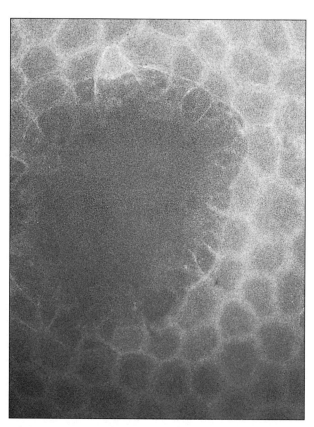

Figure 13-7. Corneal endothelial damage following air bubble touch to the endothelium during phacoemulsification. The dark area is where the air bubble touches the endothelial cells. The endothelial cell f-actin has been stained with phallacidin (x 480).

Table 13-2
**CORNEAL LONGEVITY**

| % Cell loss/year | Longevity (years) |
|---|---|
| 0.5 (normal) | 200 |
| 1.0 | 100 |
| 2.0 | 50 |
| 3.0 | 33 |

other stresses, such as contact lens wear,[35] which might result in corneal decompensation. Diabetics are also more likely than others to require cataract surgery or vitrectomy. Many young patients with diabetic retinopathy or who have suffered ocular trauma are undergoing vitrectomy with encouraging results. In some instances, the nature of their disease dictates repeated procedures. In these cases where the endothelium is already compromised, it is especially important to be as gentle as possible to the endothelium by using the most physiologic irrigating solution possible.[36]

## Biochemical Basis for Toxicity

The ability of BSS Plus to maintain structural and functional integrity of intraocular tissues better than BSS, SMA-2, or HLR is probably related to differences in their buffers.[37] Bicarbonate (in BSS Plus) is the major buffer present in aqueous and is effective in the physiologic pH range of 6.0 to 8.0. Bicarbonate is also important for normal retinal function.[20,27,38] Citrate-acetate (in BSS and SMA-2) buffers are effective at non-physiologic pHs from 3.6 to 6.2. Citrate may also chelate calcium, thereby disrupting cell junctions and barrier function.[39,40] HLR lacks a buffer all together.

Other chemical differences between the solutions may play a role. Glutathione is needed for maintenance of cell junctions and barrier function, and it also plays a role in endothelial fluid transport.[41,42] Glucose is an essential energy source[43] for maintenance of aerobic metabolism, ATP production for the $Na^+/K^+$ pump, and NADPH production to reduce glutathione and prevent oxidative damage to endothelial cells. McDermott and Edelhauser summarized the requirements for a state-of-the-art irrigating solution in 1988 as follows: pH of 7.4, osmolality between 300 and 310 mOsm, bicarbonate buffer, glucose, glutathione, and pertinent electrolytes.[9]

Another factor, often underestimated, is that of contact time. An irrigating solution may be in use for less than 30 minutes during cataract surgery. However, given the aqueous volume after cataract surgery with lens implantation and assuming normal aqueous flow, McDermott et al[9] calculated that it takes over 4 hours for the aqueous to replace the fluid left in the anterior chamber at the end of the case. If surgery reduces aqueous flow by 50%, it may take over 8 hours for the aqueous to turn over.

Another area of concern is the proper temperature of the irrigating solution. Although 37°C is physiologic, the risk of overheating the irrigant might present a real danger to intraocular tissues. Accelerated metabolic activity with increased glucose and oxygen consumption and even denaturation of some proteins might occur at temperatures just a few degrees above 37°C.[9] Cooling irrigating solutions by running the tubing through an ice bath has also been suggested by a number of surgeons. Reduced temperature theoretically reduces the rate of biochemical reactions and might reduce inflammation. There may also be a reduced risk of a scleral burn from an overheated phacoemulsification tip. However, there have been no published reports demonstrating the efficacy of cooled irrigating solutions.

Irrigating solutions that are in polypropylene bottles or bags when used for phacoemulsification cause bubbles in the anterior chamber which can obscure the view of the surgeon and cause endothelial cell damage.[44,45] Irrigating solutions in bottles have less dissolved gas than the irrigating solutions in polypropylene bottles and bags; therefore, fewer bubbles are produced during phacoemulsification.[44]

## Formulation Problems and Contamination

There have been scattered reports of toxicity throughout the 1980s, most of which are related to microbial contamination, inadequate packaging, or improper formulation of an irrigating solution.

In 1980, Pettit[46] reported 13 cases of fungal endophthalmitis after cataract surgery. The organism responsible, *Paecilomyces lilacinus*, was traced to a contaminated lot of sodium bicarbonate used to neutralize intraocular lens (IOL) sterilizing solutions. These methods are no longer used. The filamentous fungi *Cladosporium*[47] and *Ulocladium*[48] were isolated in 1984 from separate lots of 15 mL BSS in plastic squeeze bottles. No clinical adverse reactions were reported. A *Penicillium* fungus was isolated from 500 mL bottles of irrigating solution after a fluffy white precipitate was noted in the bottles.[49] Container failure was implicated as a possible source of contamination. No clinical infections were reported.

The largest epidemic of postoperative fungal endophthalmitis was caused by *Candida parapsilosis*.[50,51] At least 19 culture-proven cases resulted from one lot of contaminated 250 mL bottles of GBR solution in use in 1983. The cases were identified in three states in the United States. Time from onset of symptoms to initiation of antifungal treatment ranged from 1 week to over 4 months and final visual outcome was count fingers or less in one quarter of the patients.[51]

These reports suggest that saprophytic fungi are ubiquitous and extremely hardy. A single lot of contaminated irrigating solution may result in widely dispersed cases of postoperative endophthalmitis, many of which may be delayed in onset or difficult to diagnose. It is, therefore,

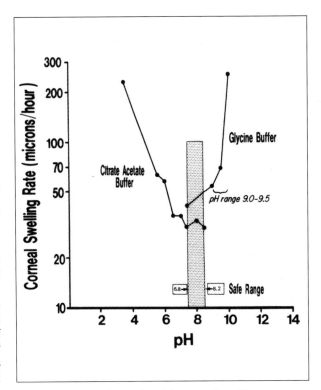

Figure 13-8. Logarithmic plot of the corneal swelling rate versus pH of the endothelial irrigating solution. Minimal swelling occurred in the pH range 6.8-8.1. (Reprint with permission *Invest Ophthalmol Vis Sci.*[53])

advisable to visually inspect the irrigating solution to assure clarity and container integrity prior to surgery.

Poor packaging led to the recall in 1983 of 500 mL bottles of BSS after reports of corneal decompensation linked to its use. Analysis of the solution revealed a pH of 9.1.[52] The glass used to package the solution reacted with the irrigant, resulting in an alkaline pH shift during storage. Gonnering and associates have demonstrated irreversible damage to rabbit and human donor corneas exposed in vitro to pHs outside the range of 6.5 to 8.5.[53] Improper formulation and variations in quality control resulted in intraoperative endothelial cell edema and temporary corneal clouding during use of another brand of BSS in 1988. The osmolality of this solution ranged from 217 to 402 mOsm/L, and the pH ranged from 6.3 to 7.2.[9,54] Balanced salt solutions with osmolalities of 200 and 240 mOsm/L were shown to induce reversible endothelial cell edema in rabbit and human donor corneas in the laboratory.[9,55]

Another source of concern is non-microbial particulate contamination of solutions, which appears to be widespread.[56-58] We are unaware of reports of clinical adverse reactions attributed to particles in solutions. Accounts of print flaking off of 15 mL plastic bottles of BSS suggest that the package itself may be a source of contamination. All of these reports emphasize the importance of packaging and maintenance of proper pH and osmolality in an irrigating solution.

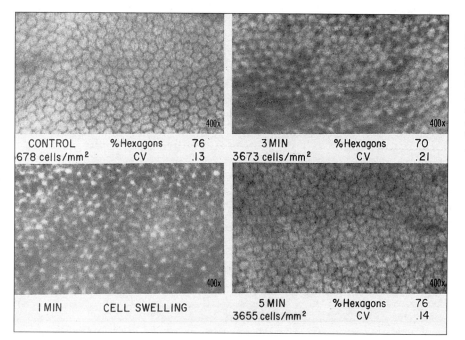

Figure 13-9. Sequential specular photomicrographs of rabbit corneal endothelium following perfusion with a 240 mOsm BSS intraocular irrigating solution. Below each photograph are the morphometric parameters: cell count, percent hexagons, and coefficient of variation. (Reprint with permission *Ophthalmic Surg.*[9])

Table 13-3
## COMPOSITION AND PROPERTIES OF VISCOELASTICS

|  | Healon | Amvisc | Occucoat | Viscoat |
|---|---|---|---|---|
| Hyaluronate Na (mg/mL) | 10.0 | 16.0 | — | 30.0 |
| Molecular Weight (kD) | 3800 | 1700 | — | >500 |
| Chondroitin SO4 (mg/mL) | — | — | — | 40.0 |
| Molecular Weight (kD) | — | — | — | 22.5 |
| HP Methylcellulose (mg/mL) | — | — | 20.0 | — |
| Molecular Weight (kD) | — | — | >80 | — |
| Sodium, mmol/L | 149.5 | 154.0 | 129.8 | 112.9 |
| Potassium, mmol/L | — | — | 10.1 | — |
| Calcium, mmol/L | — | — | 3.3 | — |
| Magnesium, mmol/L | — | — | 1.5 | — |
| Chloride, mmol/L | 145.5 | 154.0 | 103.3 | 73.6 |
| Phosphate, mmol/L | 2.2 | — | — | 19.7 |
| Citrate, mmol/L | — | — | 5.9 | — |
| Acetate, mmol/L | — | — | 28.7 | — |
| pH | 7.2+.2 | 7.6+.2 | 7.2+.4 | 7.2+.2 |
| Osmolality, mOsm/L | 308 | 340 | 285 | 325 |
| Viscosity, St @ 25°C | 2000 | 550 | 40 | 400 |

## Reuse

We strongly recommend against reuse of irrigating solutions because of the increased risk of contamination. Irrigating solutions contain no preservatives and are designed to be used once after opening. Reuse contradicts all standard infection control principles and increases the chance for error in the operating room. The reliability, safety, and resistance to breakage of devices designed to allow the use of a single bottle of solution on several patients are unknown. Their use should be avoided.

## VISCOELASTIC SUBSTANCES

Viscoelastic substances (VES) are used primarily to protect the corneal endothelium during cataract surgery and IOL implantation. The principal causes of cell loss during cataract surgery are endothelial contact with surgical instruments, the lens nucleus, lens fragments, air bubbles, and the IOL.[59-66] Viscoelastics are also used for manipulation of tissues during anterior segment surgery. They were initially developed as vitreous substitutes, but have been supplanted by the use of intraocular gases and silicone oil in vitrectomy surgery. Wide clinical experience with these solutions suggests that they are effective and well tolerated in anterior segment surgery.

## Clinical Behavior

Sodium hyaluronate (Healon, Amvisc), chondroitin sulfate/sodium hyaluronate (Viscoat), and hydroxypropylmethylcellulose (HPMC) (Occucoat) based viscous solutions are non-toxic to cat endothelial cells under conditions analogous to cataract surgery in humans.[67] They effectively protect the endothelium from trauma compared to controls in standardized models of trauma.[67-71]

However, there are marked differences between solutions with respect to their tendency to remain in the anterior chamber during surgery and their ability to maintain space or prevent shallowing of the anterior chamber. Ability to maintain space and thereby manipulate tissues is dependent upon viscosity, which is greatest with Healon.

The ability to remain in the anterior chamber in large quantities during irrigation is greatest with Viscoat and Occucoat, and is more important during phacoemulsification than during extracapsular surgery.[71] This is because flying fragments of lens nucleus and air bubbles can damage the endothelium throughout the entire period of nuclear phacoemulsification, while the endothelium during extracapsular surgery is at greatest risk only during nuclear expression. Cell damage in controlled animal trials is significantly reduced when grossly visible quantities of viscoelastics are retained.

The properties which allow a viscoelastic to remain in the anterior chamber throughout surgery have not been well defined. Studies[72] have shown that retained viscoelastic in the anterior chamber has the following rank order: Viscoat, Occucoat, Amvisc Plus, and Healon.[71] A number of hypotheses based on viscoelastic coating, adherence to, or binding to the endothelium have been suggested to explain the protective effects of viscoelastics. These include binding site, electrostatic, and surface tension theories. However, unless a viscoelastic which is adhering to the endothelium has high cohesive forces within itself, most of it will be washed out of the eye or aspirated with the irrigating solution, leaving behind a thin coating. Hammer and Burch[69] have shown that a thin coating of a high viscosity substance such as hyaluronate sodium does not protect the endothelium from the shear forces encountered during cataract removal and lens implantation. A thick layer must be maintained to prevent damage from compressive (perpendicular) and shear (lateral) forces.

Molecular weight appears to be a more important determinant of viscoelastic retention than the ability to bind to or coat the endothelium. Lower molecular weight viscoelastics tend to be retained to a greater degree.[71] Longer chain molecules may be more intertwined with adjacent molecules, making the entire mass of viscoelastic more likely to be aspirated or washed out.

Ability to maintain high viscosity in the face of increasing flow or shear rates during irrigation (Newtonian behavior) could also contribute to improved retention. Loss of viscosity with increasing flow (pseudoplastic behavior) is likely to result in loss of the viscoelastic from the anterior chamber. HPMC and hyaluronate sodium are pseudoplastic fluids; chondroitin sulfate is Newtonian.[69] Therefore, the relatively low molecular weight and Newtonian characteristics of the chondroitin sulfate in Viscoat result in excellent retention characteristics. The high molecular weight and pseudoplasticity of the hyaluronate sodium in Healon and Amvisc Plus result in loss of the viscoelastic during surgery. The HPMC in Occucoat is low in molecular weight, but it is pseudoplastic, resulting in an intermediate degree of retention.

Viscoelastics, which mix slowly with irrigants, might also be expected to remain in the anterior chamber longer than those which are highly soluble in irrigating solutions, provided the cohesive forces within the viscoelastic are low. If the cohesive forces are high, the viscoelastic may be rinsed out in a bolus. This behavior is commonly seen with hyaluronate sodium. Further work is needed to determine the precise role played by each of these factors in viscoelastic retention during surgery.

There are also disadvantages to viscoelastic retention. Retained viscoelastics may trap air bubbles and lens fragments with the potential for reduced visibility, and they require more thorough aspiration for removal. However, in difficult cases or when greater trauma is encountered, it is advantageous to have a viscoelastic that will be retained throughout surgery. The extra protection may reduce the risk of later corneal decompensation.

Viscoelastic solutions do not significantly bind drugs commonly used in the perioperative period.[72] Clinical problems associated with these substances have been related to increased intraocular pressure (IOP), formulation problems, and intraocular inflammation.

## Intraocular Pressure

All viscoelastics have the potential to raise IOP to dangerous levels.[73-78] The peak pressure usually occurs within 6 to 8 hours after surgery, so studies using measurements 24 hours after surgery may miss the pressure rise.[68,77-80] The mechanism responsible for the increase in pressure is probably related to a decrease in outflow facility. Sodium hyaluronate (and probably other viscous solutions) are eliminated from the anterior chamber primarily through the trabecular meshwork.[81,82] Berson and associates found a 65% decrease in aqueous outflow facility after anterior chamber injection of 1% sodium hyaluronate into enucleated human eyes.[81] Anterior chamber washout does not eliminate the decrease in outflow facility,[81] but it does decrease the level and duration of the postoperative pressure rise.[67]

Therefore, we recommend washout or aspiration of viscous solutions at the end of surgery in all cases. Viscoat requires more meticulous aspiration (in all quadrants of the anterior chamber) than other viscous solutions. This is because Viscoat contains chondroitin sulfate, which retains its viscosity during irrigation/aspiration (I/A). This allows Viscoat to remain in place during the surgical procedure, but also prevents it from completely flowing out of the eye during removal unless it is specifically aspirated. Removal of the viscous solution

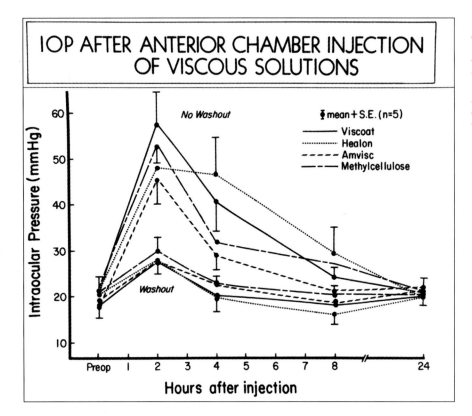

Figure 13-10. IOP after anterior chamber injection of viscoelastics in the cat. Upper four curves, no washout of viscoelastics; lower four curves, viscoelastic washout. Note that the pressure rise is less and of shorter duration if the viscoelastic is washed out. (Reprint with permission Arch Ophthalmol.[67])

will not prevent the pressure rise in all cases,[78] therefore, we also recommend the use of intraocular carbachol (Miostat), topical apraclonidine (Iopidine), or a systemic carbonic anhydrase inhibitor (CAI) for pressure control during the first 24 hours after surgery. West and associates[83] found that topical levobunolol may be more effective than timolol 0.5% or betaxolol given immediately after surgery.

## Formulation Problems

McCulley and associates have shown that the ionic composition of the vehicle used to formulate a viscous solution is an important determinant of endothelial toxicity.[84] Their conclusions are reminiscent of the work on irrigating solutions discussed above. Currently available viscous solutions are formulated in phosphate-buffered saline (Healon), physiologic saline (Amvisc), and phosphate-buffered water (Viscoat). Although none are formulated in a BSS, they are non-toxic to the endothelium in vivo.[67]

An early formulation of Viscoat did result in several cases of calcific deposits in the corneal stroma and Bowman's membrane after cataract surgery.[85,86] Calcium precipitation was attributed to excessive phosphate concentration (93 mM) in the Viscoat vehicle. Reformulated Viscoat contains less phosphate (18 mM), and there have been no further reports of calcium deposition.

## Intraocular Inflammation

Commercially available highly purified viscoelastics are non-antigenic according to the manufacturers and studies by Richter.[87,88] However, intrastromal injection of Healon, Amvisc, or Viscoat induces a mild acute inflammatory reaction in rabbit corneas.[89,90] Clinical inflammatory reactions related to the use of viscous solutions are uncommon. They can occur because of impurities or deficiencies in formulation. As early as 1959, Fleming, Merrill, and Girard[91] reported that a 0.5% solution of methylcellulose in BSS produces no inflammatory or foreign-body reaction after injection into the anterior chamber of rabbit eyes, while 0.5% methylcellulose in physiologic saline produces iridocyclitis.

Kim,[92] Breebaart, and associates[93] have reported on severe inflammation and endothelial cell destruction after the use of VES. Further investigation revealed that toxicity was due to residual detergent present in the cannulas used to inject the viscoelastics.[93,94] Residual viscoelastic in the cannula may have made it difficult to rinse out the detergent after cleaning. This highlights the importance of thoroughly rinsing reusable cannulas and reemphasizes the potential toxicity of detergents. Only disposable cannulas should be used with viscoelastics.

## MYDRIATICS AND MIOTICS

Control of the pupil during intraocular surgery can be accomplished via a variety of mydriatics and miotics. Intraocular use of drugs originally intended for extraocular use should be avoided whenever possible. Almost all drugs formulated for topical, intravenous, intracardiac, or intratracheal use contain preservatives and other chemicals which are toxic to the endothelium or may adversely affect the physiological balance of the ocular irrigant.

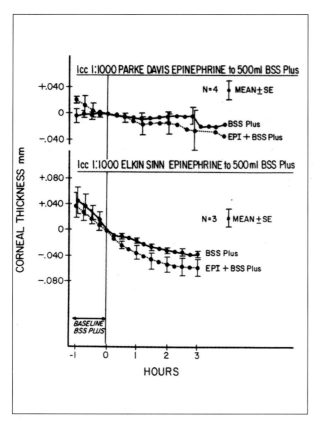

Figure 13-11. Effect of two commercially available epinephrine products on the thickness of the in vitro endothelial perfused cornea. There was a 1 hour baseline BSS Plus perfusion followed by one cornea of the pair perfused with 1 cc epinephrine added to 500 mL of BSS Plus. There was no significant difference between the two solutions. (Reprint with permission *Ophthalmic Surg*.[9])

Table 13-4
**INTRAOCULAR MIOTICS**

|  | Miochol | Miostat |
|---|---|---|
| Miotic | 1.0% Acetylcholine | 0.01% Carbachol |
| Vehicle | 3.0% Mannitol/water | BSS |
| pH/Osmolality | Physiologic | Physiologic |
| Onset of miosis | Under 1 minute | 2 minutes |
| Duration of miosis | 10-20 minutes | 2-24 hours |
| Pressure lowering | 1-6 hours | 1-3 days |

## Mydriatics

Preoperative pupillary dilation is usually accomplished with a combination of topical anticholinergic agents (tropicamide 1%, cyclopentolate 1%, homatropine 5%, or scopolamine 0.25%) and sympathetic agonists (phenylephrine 2.5% or 10%). Three or four doses 1 hour before surgery are usually sufficient. Systemic absorption of topical phenylephrine resulting in hypertension is less likely with the 2.5% than the 10% solution. Pupils will not dilate to the same degree at the time of surgery if they were dilated the day before with either tropicamide or cyclopentolate.[95] Therefore, dilated preoperative examinations should be done several days or more before surgery.

A number of authors report that preoperative topical non-steroidal anti-inflammatory drugs (NSAIDs) such as indomethacin 1%, flurbiprofen 0.03%, and suprofen 1% help to maintain mydriasis during cataract surgery.[96-100] Presumably, this is a result of prostaglandin synthesis inhibition. However, Gimbel[99] notes that intraocular epinephrine is a more potent mydriatic than NSAIDs. Bito[101] points out that no known prostaglandin is a sufficiently effective miotic in humans to account for surgical miosis.

Intraoperative mydriatic agents used in the early 1970s included repeated intraoperative application of topical phenylephrine during lengthy procedures. This was abandoned because of corneal epithelial sloughing, drug-induced stromal edema, and endothelial toxicity of commercial preparations containing a non-physiologic buffered vehicle and benzalkonium chloride.[102-104]

Intraocular epinephrine has been the intraoperative mydriatic of choice for most ophthalmologists for over a decade. In 1972 and 1982, reports of corneal edema after its use led to studies of the effects of commercially available epinephrine preparations on the corneal endothelium.[105-107] Toxicity of 1:1,000 and 1:10,000 solutions formulated for intravascular or intracardiac use was determined to be due to the presence of sodium bisulfite (a preservative/antioxidant), acidic pH 3 to 4, and a non-physiologic buffer (citrate) with high buffering capacity. The addition of 1 mL of 1:1,000 (not 1:10,000) epinephrine to at least 5 to 15 mL of BSS or BSS Plus was recommended in order to dilute the preservative and buffer. Buffer capacity, and therefore resistance to neutralization of pH, varied considerably from one manufacturer's preparation to the next.

McDermott demonstrated that the addition of 1 mL of 1:1,000 preservative-free epinephrine from certain manufacturers (Parke-Davis and Elkins-Sinn) to 500 mL of BSS Plus is nontoxic and maintains adequate endothelial function during 3 hour perfusions of isolated human corneas.[9] Slack and associates found that a preservative-free and sulfite free 1:1,000 epinephrine (American Regent) was even better at maintaining corneal endothelial function and microstructure during perfusion.[108] We recommended 0.5 mL of 1:1,000 epinephrine added to 500 mL of BSS Plus. This resulting concentration of epinephrine (1:1,000,000) will readily dilate the pupil within 1 minute during surgery. In rare instances when a more concentrated solution is necessary, 1 mL of 1:1,000 epinephrine is added to 30 mL of BSS Plus, and 0.2 mL of this mixture is injected into the anterior chamber.

## Miotics

A miotic pupil facilitates corneal trephine centration, peripheral iridectomy, anterior chamber lens insertion, and a variety of other intraocular manipulations. Most surgeons prefer a miotic pupil at the end of cataract surgery to ensure lens centration and to protect the endothelium from the lens implant. Coles has shown that

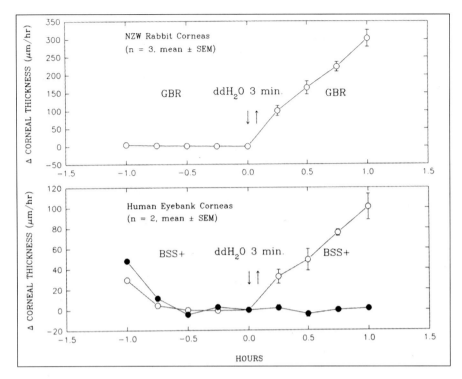

Figure 13-12. Change in corneal thickness after 3 minutes of perfusion with distilled water to rabbit corneal endothelium and human corneal endothelium. The rabbit corneas swelled at 274± 21 µm/hr and the human corneas swelled at 98 ± 12 µm/hr. The human control corneal tissue (solid circles) remained at a constant thickness with continued perfusion. NZW indicates New Zealand White and ddH$_2$O indicates double distilled water. (Reprint with permission Am J Ophthalmol.[18])

pilocarpine is toxic to the endothelium and its intraocular use should be avoided.[109] Sympatholytic agents such as thymoxamine and dapiprazole have been recommended for intracameral use in selected cases[110,111] However, they are not commercially available and have not yet undergone the type of rigorous toxicity testing used to evaluate other intraocular solutions. Currently available intraocular miotics include Miochol (Ciba Vision) and Miostat (Alcon Laboratories). Their major clinical and chemical characteristics are listed in Table 4.[112-115] In their current formulations, Miochol is a 1% solution of acetylcholine in mannitol and water, and Miostat is a 0.01% solution of carbachol in BSS. Yee and associates found corneal swelling and ultrastructural endothelial changes during perfusion of human corneas with Miochol, while Miostat prevented corneal swelling and endothelial toxicity.[116] They attributed this difference to the more physiologic vehicle used to formulate Miostat.

In contrast, Birnbaum and associates did find reversible corneal swelling without ultrastructural changes during perfusion with Miostat.[117] However, this study used rabbit rather than human tissue, and no comparison with the current formulation of Miochol was made. Ocular toxicity has occurred when the Miochol (two compartment) product was not mixed. In this case, distilled water was injected into the anterior chamber, and the patient lost 1,000 endothelial cells per mm$^2$.[118] Laboratory studies have shown marked corneal swelling and swollen endothelial cells with large vacuoles within the cytoplasm and junctional breakdown between cells.[118] Miochol has recently been reformulated in the United States (Miochol E) and contains a vehicle with ions more compatible to aqueous humor. A significant clinical advantage of miostat is IOP reduction for at least 24 hours compared to 6 hours with Miochol.[113-115] Systemic hypotension and bradycardia have been reported as idiosyncratic reactions following intraocular injection of acetylcholine.[119-121] Carbachol could cause a similar reaction in a susceptible individual. If endothelial toxicity is of particular concern, the formulation and laboratory evidence suggest that Miostat is more physiologic with the beneficial effect of lowering IOP.

## ANTIBIOTICS

Prophylactic antibiotic usage in cataract surgery is based on the determination that the risks of endophthalmitis and its consequences are greater than the risks of antibiotic toxicity, development of resistant organisms, and alteration of the microflora. The risk of infection increases with contamination of solutions, instruments, the operative site, operating room environment, prolonged surgery, and the presence of active infection of the eye or periocular structures (blepharitis, conjunctivitis, dacryocystitis, lid abscess). The risk of complications from prophylactic antibiotics is minimized by using local rather than systemic agents and by limiting usage to the short period during which the susceptibility to infection is increased.[122]

In the United States, the incidence of endophthalmitis after cataract surgery has been reported to be between 0.71% and 3.05% in various studies without preoperative antibiotics. In separate studies, the incidence of postoperative endophthalmitis was 0.056% to 0.11% when preoperative antibiotics were employed.[123,124] These studies were retrospective, lacked control groups, and failed to account for variations in surgical techniques, antibiotics used, and cleanliness of the environment. Nevertheless, the data suggest that preoperative antibiotics do play a role in the prevention of endophthalmitis following cataract surgery.

Timing and route of administration are two important considerations in the use of prophylactic antibiotics. Topical antibiotics should be administered for at least 24 hours before surgery to most effectively decrease bacterial counts in the conjunctival sac. No regimen will completely sterilize the conjunctiva and lids. Topical therapy beyond 1 week postoperatively is not effective or necessary since the wound is sealed with an epithelial plug by 3 to 5 days. Prolonged therapy may contribute to epithelial toxicity and promotes the development of resistant strains. A one-time subconjunctival injection of antibiotics at the end of surgery is a popular mode of prophylaxis and is effective in animal models.[125,126] Bacteria responsible for endophthalmitis following cataract surgery usually gain access to the eye via the anterior chamber. Subconjunctival antibiotics produce therapeutic levels in the aqueous shortly after their administration. Even higher levels would be expected when the injection immediately follows suturing of a cataract incision. The ability to delivery high levels of antibiotics to the site of a potential infection at the time of inoculation is theoretically appealing and accounts for the popularity of intraoperative subconjunctival prophylaxis. Antibiotics added to irrigating solutions or otherwise given intraocularly are not recommended. The rise of endothelial toxicity from intraocular antibiotics is greater than the risk of endophthalmitis when topical and subconjunctival prophylaxis are used.

Gritz et al[127] recently evaluated the antibiotic supplementation of intraocular irrigating solutions. They found that exposure to antibiotics for a short period of time, such as during intraocular surgery, has no effect on the organisms commonly responsible for endophthalmitis.

The particular antibiotics chosen for prophylaxis vary immensely among authors. Broad spectrum coverage is popular. Subconjunctival aminoglycosides (gentamicin or tobramycin 20 mg) and cephalosporins (cefazolin 50 mg) are commonly used for intraoperative prophylaxis. Some surgeons use subconjunctival vancomycin to reduce the risk of chronic Propionibacteria endophthalmitis. Given the high concentrations achieved with topical antibiotics at the ocular surface, almost any topical antibiotic should decrease bacterial counts preoperatively. Consider, however, that no antibiotic completely sterilizes the ocular surface. The most effective means of preventing postoperative infection include proper surgical preparation, good surgical technique, and maintenance of sterile conditions.

## ANTI-INFLAMMATORY AGENTS

Topical anti-inflammatory agents are typically used to control postoperative inflammation. Corticosteroids are the mainstay of therapy. Prednisolone phosphate or acetate 1%, dexamethasone sodium phosphate 0.1%, or fluorometholone 0.25% drops are commonly administered four to eight times a day initially, with tapering as

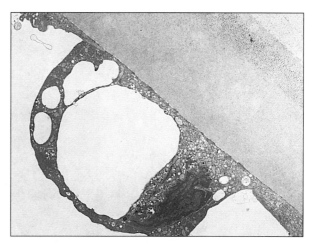

Figure 13-13. TEM of human corneal endothelial cell after 3 minutes of perfusion with distilled water. Marked corneal endothelial swelling occurs with large vacuoles present within the cytoplasm and junctional breakdown is evident (x 5220). (Reprint with permission Am J Ophthalmol.[118])

indicated by the degree of inflammation. Dexamethasone sodium phosphate 0.05% ointment can be administered at bedtime for overnight control of inflammation when necessary. Steroids have the potential for increasing IOP, and they reduce wound healing and local immune competence. These effects do not usually result in clinically significant complications. Patients with elevated IOP often respond to topical beta blockers or CAIs. Fluorometholone is less likely to increase IOP than the other topical corticosteroids.

Topical NSAIDs have also been shown to reduce inflammation after cataract surgery.[128-131] While there is not as much experience with these agents as with corticosteroids, they do hold promise for the future. They may be particularly useful in patients who can not tolerate steroids because of IOP elevation.

It has also been suggested that topical anti-inflammatory medications decrease the risk of cystoid macular edema (CME) after cataract surgery. Much of the data for corticosteroids is anecdotal, as there are no properly controlled studies of the effects of steroids on post-cataract CME. Topical NSAIDs alone and in combination with corticosteroids have been shown to reduce the risk of CME if the nonsteroidal agent is begun prior to surgery.[132-137]

## OTHER AGENTS

Glucose, tissue plasminogen activator, thrombin, antibiotics, steroids, and a host of other drugs have been suggested as useful intraocular agents or as additives to irrigating solutions. It must be emphasized that almost all drugs which are formulated for extraocular use contain vehicles, preservatives, antioxidants, and solubilizers which are not intended for intraocular use. The potential, therefore, exists for direct toxicity from the drug itself, its vehicle, preservatives, or any number of interactions which might alter the electrolyte balance, pH, or osmolality of the irrigating solution. The surgeon must be aware that such additives render the solution formulation, stability, and toxicity unknown, and that use of such a solution constitutes an in vivo human experiment.[9] Accordingly, additives should only be used for specific indications, never *routinely*.

## Preservative

Sodium bisulfite, a preservative/antioxidant, was the endothelial toxin responsible for cases of corneal edema associated with epinephrine use discussed above.[106-107] Other preservatives present in drugs include propyl- and methyl-parabens, benzalkonium chloride, cetylpiridium chloride, benzyl alcohol, chlorhexidine, and thimerosal. All have been shown to adversely affect endothelial structure and function, particularly benzalkonium chloride.[63,138-143] Preserved solutions should not be used within the eye.

Another potential source of preservative toxicity is reuse of instruments and irrigation tubing. Human corneal endothelium can withstand exposure to levels of ethylene oxide and the reaction products ethylene glycol and ethylene chlorohydrin 25 times higher than those recommended for ophthalmics by the US Food and Drug Administration. However, ethylene oxide gas sterilization of plastic irrigation tubing may cause release of complex compounds (plasticizers, clarifiers, monomers, polymers) which can combine with sterilant residues, resulting in toxicity[144] or inflammation.[145] Kim reported three cases of iritis and corneal decompensation after cataract surgery due to toxicity from thimerosal residues in reused viscoelastic cannulas.[92] Breebaart and Nuyts have reported 18 cases of severe postoperative corneal edema caused by a non-ionic ethoxylated fatty acid detergent residue inside irrigating cannulas.[93,94]

## Glucose

In diabetic patients, intraoperative posterior subcapsular opacification can be prevented by adding glucose to the BSS Plus during vitrectomy.[146,147] Diabetics have polyols trapped within the lens, which causes the lens itself to become hyperosmotic.[148] Osmotic equilibrium with the aqueous is maintained under normal circumstances in diabetic patients. During vitrectomy, osmotic stress leads to posterior subcapsular opacification during irrigation with solutions of normal osmolality (305 mOsm). The addition of 3 mL of 50% dextrose (in sterile water with no preservatives) to a 500 mL bottle of BSS Plus increases its osmolality to 330 mOsm, restoring osmotic equilibrium. This modification of BSS Plus appears to be non-toxic.[147]

## Thrombin

Commercial preparations of bovine thrombin designed for topical application have been added to irrigating solutions and used during vitrectomy for diabetic retinopathy and retinopathy of prematurity, trabeculectomy for neovascular glaucoma, and keratoplasty in a vascularized recipient bed.[149-151] Although thrombin (100 U/mL) is effective in reducing intraoperative and postoperative bleeding, it is associated with a 20% incidence of severe postoperative inflammation with sterile hypopyon formation and fibrin deposition.[149]

McDermott, Edelhauser, and Mannis[58] investigated the toxicity of two commercially available thrombin preparations: Thrombinar (Armour Pharmaceutical) and Thrombostat (Parke-Davis). Gel electrophoresis exhibited multiple peaks suggestive of proteins other than thrombin in Thrombostat which might be immunogenic. Particulate analysis demonstrated up to 700, 5-20 μm particles in the Thrombinar and up to 21,000 particles in the Thrombostat. In addition, 100 U/mL solutions of Thrombostat contain 70 mg/dl of glycine. Serum glycine levels in excess of only 30 mg/dl have been associated with temporary graying of vision and electroretinographic changes in patients undergoing bladder irrigation after prostate surgery.[152] Therefore, Thrombostat should not be used inside the eye.

In two studies, sheep and rabbit corneas exposed to 100 U/mL and 1,000 U/mL concentrations of thrombin showed no damage with vital-dye staining.[151] However, thrombin solutions containing 1,000 U/mL are hyperosmotic and perfusion of the human donor corneas with this concentration causes intracellular vacuolization and disruption of junctions between endothelial cells. The pH and osmolality of a 100 U/mL solution of Thrombinar in BSS Plus is physiologic. Perfusion of the human donor cornea with this solution significantly inhibited corneal deswelling but did not cause ultrastructural damage to endothelial cells.[58] These findings highlight the importance of testing toxicity by evaluating endothelial function in human donor tissue.

In eight patients, human thrombin (80 U/mL) was infused continuously during vitrectomy without a marked increase in inflammation or development of sterile hypopyon after surgery.[153,154] While this solution was free of non-human proteins, it was not tested for presence of non-thrombin proteins, particulate contamination, or endothelial toxicity. There is also the need to insure against transmission of infectious diseases when thrombin derived from human blood is used.

Concern for the purity, immunogenicity, and toxicity of currently available thrombin preparations has led Aaberg to comment that intraocular thrombin must be used prudently as an adjunct during uncontrolled hemorrhage or as prophylaxis to prevent hemorrhage.[155] Injection of limited quantities of thrombin followed by thorough washout may reduce but will not eliminate the potential for adverse reactions. Thus, conventional techniques for control of bleeding, such as tamponade, are preferred.

## REFERENCES

1. Hamed LM, Ellis FD, Boudreault G, et al. Hibiclens keratitis. *Am J Ophthalmol*. 1987;104:50-56.
2. Phinney RB, Mondino BJ, Hofbauer JD, et al. Corneal edema related to accidental Hibiclens exposure. *Am J Ophthalmol*. 1988;106:210-215.
3. Apt L, Isenberg SJ. Hibiclens keratitis, correspondence. *Am J Ophthalmol*. 1987;104:670.
4. Shore JW. Hibiclens keratitis, correspondence. *Am J Ophthalmol*. 1987;104:670-671.

5. Apt L, Isenberg SJ. Chemical preparation of skin and eye in ophthalmic surgery: An international survey. *Ophthalmic Surg.* 1982;13:1026-1029.

6. Green K, Livingston V, Bowman K, Hull DS. Chlorhexidine effects on corneal epithelium and endothelium. *Arch Ophthalmol.* 1980;98:1273-1281.

7. MacRae SM, Brown B, Edelhauser HF. The corneal toxicity of presurgical skin antiseptics. *Am J Ophthalmol.* 1984;97:221-232.

8. Apt L, Isenberg S, Yoshimori R, Paez JH. Chemical preparation of the eye in ophthalmic surgery. III. Effect of povidone-iodine on the conjunctiva. *Arch Ophthalmol.* 1984;102:728-729.

9. McDermott ML, Edelhauser HF, Hack HM, Langston RHS. Ophthalmic irrigants: A current review and update. *Ophthalmic Surg.* 1988;19:724-733.

10. Glasser DB, Matsuda M, Ellis JG, Edelhauser HF. Effects of intraocular irrigating solutions on the corneal endothelium after in vivo anterior chamber irrigation. *Am J Ophthalmol.* 1985;99:321-328.

11. Edelhauser HF. Intraocular irrigating solutions. In: Lamberts DW, Potter DE, eds. *Clinical Ophthalmic Pharmacology.* Boston: Little, Brown and Company; 1987:431-444.

12. Merrill DL, Fleming TC, Girard LJ. The effects of physiologic balanced salt solutions and normal saline on intraocular and extraocular tissues. *Am J Ophthalmol.* 1960;49:895-898.

13. Dikstein S, Maurice DM. The metabolic basis to the fluid pump in the cornea. *J Physiol.* 1972;221:29-41.

14. Edelhauser HF, Van Horn DL, Hyndiuk RA, Schultz RO. Intraocular irrigating solutions: Their effect on the corneal endothelium. *Arch Ophthalmol.* 1975;93:648-657.

15. Edelhauser HF, Van Horn DL, Schultz RO, Hyndiuk RA. Comparative toxicity of intraocular irrigating solutions on the corneal endothelium. *Am J Ophthalmol.* 1976;81:473-481.

16. Edelhauser HF, Gonnering R, Van Horn DL. Intraocular irrigating solutions: A comparative study of BSS Plus and lactated Ringer's solution. *Arch Ophthalmol.* 1978;96:516-520.

17. Glasser DB, Matsuda M, Edelhauser HF. Comparison of corneal endothelial structural and functional integrity after irrigation with bicarbonate-buffered and acetate-citrate-buffered solutions. In: Cavanagh HD, ed. *The Cornea: Transactions of the World Congress on the Cornea.* III. New York: Raven Press; 1988:101-106.

18. Nuyts RMMA, Edelhauser HF, Holley GP. Intraocular irrigating Solutions: A comparison of Hartmann's Lactated Ringer's solution, BSS and BSS Plus. *Graefes Arch Clin Exp Ophthalmol.* 1995;233:655-611.

19. Araie M. Barrier function of corneal endothelium and the intraocular irrigating solutions. *Arch Ophthalmol* 1986;104:435-438.

20. Moorhead LC, Redburn DA, Merritt J, Garcia C. The effects of intravitreal irrigation during vitrectomy on the electroretinogram. *Am J Ophthalmol* 1979;88:239-245.

21. Saornil Alvarez MA, Pastor Jimeno JC. Role of the intraocular irrigating solutions in the pathogenesis of the postvitrectomy retinal edema. *Curr Eye Res* 1987;6:1369-1379.

22. Kline OR, Symes DJ, Lorenzetti OJ, deFaller JM. Effect of BSS Plus on the corneal endothelium with intraocular lens implantation. *J of Toxicol: Cutaneous and Ocular Toxicology.* 1983;2:243-247.

23. Bourne WM, Liesegang TJ, Waller RR, Ilstrup DM. The effect of sodium hyaluronate on endothelial cell damage during extracapsular cataract extraction and posterior chamber lens implantation. *Am J Ophthalmol.* 1984;98:759-762.

24. Benson WE, Diamond JG, Tasman W. Intraocular irrigating solutions for pars plana vitrectomy. *Arch Ophthalmol.* 1981;99:1013-1015.

25. Matsuda M, Tano Y, Edelhauser HF. Comparison of intraocular irrigating solutions used for pars plana vitrectomy and prevention of endothelial cell loss. *Jpn J Ophthalmol.* 1984;28:230-238.

26. Rosenfeld SI, Waltman SR, Olk RJ, Gordon M. Comparison of intraocular irrigating solutions in pars plana vitrectomy. *Ophthalmology.* 1986;93:109-114.

27. Bourne WM. Morphologic and functional evaluation of the endothelium of transplanted human corneas. *Trans Am Ophthalmol Soc.* 1983;81:403-450.

28. Hirst LW, Auer C, Abbey H, et al. Quantitative analysis of wide-field endothelial specular photomicrographs. *Am J Ophthalmol.* 1984;97:488-495.

29. Mishima S. Clinical investigations on the corneal endothelium. XXXVIII Edward Jackson Memorial Lecture. *Am J Ophthalmol.* 1982;93:1-29.

30. Edelhauser HF. Discussion of: Rosenfeld SI, Waltman SR, Olk RJ, Gordon M. Comparison of intraocular irrigating solutions in pars plana vitrectomy. *Ophthalmology.* 1986;93:114-115.

31. Rao GN, Shaw EL, Arthur EJ, Aquavella JV. Endothelial cell morphology and corneal deturgescence. *Ann Ophthalmol.* 1979;11:885-899.

32. Rao GN, Aquavella JV, Goldberg SH, Berk SL. Pseudophakic bullous keratopathy. Relationship to preoperative corneal endothelial status. *Ophthalmology.* 1984;91:1135-1140.

33. Foulks GN, Thoft RA, Perry HD, Tolentino FI. Factors related to corneal epithelial complications after closed vitrectomy in diabetics. *Arch Ophthalmol.* 1979;97:1076-1078.

34. Schultz RO, Matsuda M, Yee RW, et al. Corneal endothelial changes in type I and type II diabetes mellitus. *Am J Ophthalmol.* 1984;98:401-410.

35. Nirankari VS, Baer JC. Persistent corneal edema in aphakic eyes from daily-wear and extended-wear contact lenses. *Am J Ophthalmol.* 1984;98:329-335.

36. Chung H, Tolentino FI, Cajita VN, et al. Reevaluation of corneal complications after closed vitrectomy. *Arch Ophthalmol.* 1988;106:916-919.

37. Winkler BS, Simson V, Benner J. Importance of bicarbonate in retinal function. *Invest Ophthalmol Vis Sci.* 1977;16:766-768.

38. Negi A, Honda Y, Kawano S. Effects of intraocular irrigating solutions on the electroretinographic b-wave. *Am J Ophthalmol.* 1981;92:28-37.

39. Stern ME, Edelhauser HF, Pederson HJ, Staatz WD. Effects of ionophores X537A and A23187 and calcium-free medium on corneal endothelial morphology. *Invest Ophthalmol Vis Sci.* 1981;20:497-507.

40. Kaye GI, Mishima S, Cole JD, Kaye NW. Studies on the cornea. VII. Effects of perfusion with a $Ca^{++}$-free medium on the corneal endothelium. *Invest Ophthalmol Vis Sci.* 1968;7:53-66.

41. Whikehart DR, Edelhauser HF. Glutathione in rabbit corneal endothelia: The effects of selected perfusion fluids. *Invest Ophthalmol Vis Sci.* 1978;17:455-464.

42. Ng MC, Riley MV. Relation of intracellular levels and redox state of glutathione to endothelial function in the rabbit cornea. *Exp Eye Res.* 1980;30:511-517.

43. Mishima S, Kudo T. In vitro incubation of rabbit cornea. *Invest Ophthalmol.* 1967;6:329-339.

44. Watsky MD, Edelhauser HF. Intraocular irrigating solutions: The importance of $Ca^{++}$ and glass versus polypropylene bottles. *Internat Ophthalmol Clinics.* 1993;33:109-125.

45. Kim EK, Cristol SM, Geroski DH, McCarey BE, Edelhauser. Corneal endothelial damage by air bubbles during phacoemulsification. *Arch Ophthalmol.* 1997;115:81-88.

46. Pettit TH, Olson RJ, Foos RY, Martin WJ. Fungal endophthalmitis following intraocular implantation: A surgical epidemic. *Arch Ophthalmol.* 1980;98:1025-1039.

47. O'Day DM, Sommer A. Clinical Alert 1/1. American Academy of Ophthalmology, October 18, 1984.

48. Isenberg RA, Weiss RL, Apple DJ, et al. Fungal contamination of balanced salt solution. *J Am Intraocul Implant Soc.* 1985;11:485-486.

49. Samples JR, Binder PS. Contamination of irrigating solution used for cataract surgery. *Ophthalmic Surg.* 1984;15:66.

50. O'Day DM. Special note. *Am J Ophthalmol.* 1984;97:128.

51. Stern WH, Tamura E, Jacobs RA, et al. Epidemic postsurgical Candida parapsilosis endophthalmitis. Clinical findings and management of 15 consecutive cases. *Ophthalmology.* 1985;92:1701-1709.

52. Googe JM, Mamalis N, Apple DJ, Olson RJ. BSS Warning. *J Am Intraocul Implant Soc.* 1984; 10:202.

53. Gonnering R, Edelhauser HF, Van Horn DL, Durant W. The pH tolerance of rabbit and human corneal endothelium. *Invest Ophthalmol Vis Sci.* 1979;18:373-390.

54. Briggs RB, McCartney DL. Balanced salt solution infusion alert. *Arch Ophthalmol.* 1988;106:718.

55. Edelhauser HF, Hanneken AM, Pederson HJ, Van Horn DL. Osmotic tolerance of rabbit and human corneal endothelium. *Arch Ophthalmol.* 1981;99:1281-1287.

56. Winding O, Gregerson E. Particulate contamination in eye surgery. *Acta Ophthalmol.* 1985;63:629-633.

57. Neumann AC. Particulate and microbial contamination of intraocular irrigating solutions. *J Cataract Refract Surg.* 1986;12:485-488.

58. McDermott ML, Edelhauser HF, Mannis MJ. Intracameral thrombin and the corneal endothelium. *Am J Ophthalmol.* 1988;106:414-422.

59. McCarey BE, Polack FM, Marshall W. The phacoemulsification procedure. I. The effect of intraocular irrigating solutions on the corneal endothelium. *Invest Ophthalmol Vis Sci.* 1976;15:449-457.

60. Polack FM, Sugar A. The phacoemulsification procedure, II: corneal endothelial changes. *Invest Ophthalmol Vis Sci.* 1976;15:458-469.

61. Kaufman H, Katz J. Endothelial damage from intraocular lens insertion. *Invest Ophthalmol Vis Sci.* 1976;15:996-1000.

62. Binder PS, Sternberg H, Wickham MG, Worthen DM. Corneal endothelial damage associated with phacoemulsification. *Am J Ophthalmol.* 1976;82:48-54.

63. Irvine AR, Kratz RP, O'Donnell JJ. Endothelial damage with phacoemulsification and intraocular lens implantation. *Arch Ophthalmol.* 1978;96:1023-1026.

64. Waltman SR, Cozean CH. The effect of phacoemulsification on the corneal endothelium. *Ophthalmic Surg.* 1979;10:31-33.

65. Holmberg AS, Philipson BT. Sodium hyaluronate in cataract surgery. II: Report on the use of Healon in extracapsular surgery using phacoemulsification. *Ophthalmology.* 1984;91:53-59.

66. Beesly RD, Olson RJ, Brady SE. The effects of prolonged phacoemulsification time on the corneal endothelium. *Ann Ophthalmol.* 1986;18:216-222.

67. Glasser DB, Matsuda M, Edelhauser HF. A comparison of the efficacy and toxicity of and intraocular pressure response to viscous solutions in the anterior chamber. *Arch Ophthalmol.* 1986;104:1819-1824.

68. Glasser DB, Katz HR, Boyd JE, Langdon JD, Shobe SL, Peiffer RL. Protective effects of viscous solutions in phacoemulsification and traumatic lens implantation. *Arch Ophthalmol.* 1989;107:1047-1051.

69. Hammer ME, Burch TG. Viscous corneal protection by sodium hyaluronate, chondroitin sulfate, and methylcellulose. *Invest Ophthalmol Vis Sci.* 1984;25:1329-1332.

70. Craig MT, Olson RJ, Mamalis N, Olson RJ. Air bubble endothelial damage during phacoemulsification in human eye bank eyes: The protective effects of Healon and Viscoat. *J Cataract Refract Surg.* 1990;16:597-602.

71. Glasser DB, Osborn DC, Nordeen JF, Min YI. Endothelial protection and viscoelastic retention during phacoemulsification and intraocular lens implantation. *Arch Ophthalmol.* 1991;109,1438-1440.

72. McDermott ML, Edelhauser HF. Drug, binding of ophthalmic viscoelastic agents. *Arch Ophthalmol.* 1989;107:261-263.

73. Binkhorst CD. Inflammation and intraocular pressure after the use of Healon in intraocular lens surgery. *J Intraocul Implant Soc.* 1980;6:340-341.

74. Pape LG. Intracapsular and extracapsular technique of lens implantation with Healon. *J Am Intraocul Implant Soc.* 1980;6:342-343.

75. Percival P. Protective role of Healon during lens implantation. *Trans Ophthalmol Soc UK.* 1981;101:77-78.

76. Lazenby GW, Broocker G. The use of sodium hyaluronate (Healon) in intracapsular cataract extraction with insertion of anterior chamber intraocular lenses. *Ophthalmic Surg.* 1981;12:646-649.

77. Cherfan GM, Rich WJ, Wright G. Raised intraocular pressure and other problems with sodium hyaluronate and cataract surgery. *Trans Ophthalmol Soc UK.* 1983;103:227-232.

78. Barron BA, Busin M, Page C, et al. Comparison of the effects of Viscoat and Healon on postoperative intraocular pressure. *Am J Ophthalmol.* 1985;100:377-384.

79. MacRae SM, Edelhauser HF, Hyndiuk RA, et al. The effects of sodium hyaluronate, chondroitin sulfate, and methylcellulose on the corneal endothelium and intraocular pressure. *Am J Ophthalmol.* 1983;95:332-341.

80. Rich WJ, Radtke ND, Cohan BE. Early ocular hypertension after cataract extraction. *Br J Ophthalmol.* 1974;58:725-731.

81. Berson FG, Patterson MM, Epstein DL. Obstruction of aqueous outflow by sodium hyaluronate in enucleated human eyes. *Am J Ophthalmol.* 1983;95:668-672.

82. Iwata S, Miyauchi S. Biochemical studies on the use of sodium hyaluronate in the anterior eye segment. III. Histological studies on distribution and efflux process of 5-amino fluorescein-labeled hyaluronate. *Jpn J Ophthalmol.* 1985;29:187-197.

83. West DR, Lischwe TD, Thompson VM, Ide CH. Comparative efficacy of the b-blockers for the prevention of increased intraocular pressure after cataract extraction. *Am J Ophthalmol.* 1988;106:168-173.

84. McCulley JP, Stern ME, Meyer DR. In vitro assessment of the comparative toxicity of viscoelastic substances. *Invest Ophthalmol Vis Sci.* 1985;26(suppl):239.

85. Nevyas AS, Raber IM, Eagle RC, et al. Acute band keratopathy following intracameral Viscoat. *Arch Ophthalmol.* 1987;105:958-964.

86. Binder PS, Deg JK, Kohl FS. Calcific band keratopathy after intraocular chondroitin sulfate. *Arch Ophthalmol.* 1987;105:1243-1247.

87. Richter W. Non-immunogenicity of purified hyaluronic acid preparations tested by passive cutaneous anaphylaxis. *Int Arch Allergy Appl Immunol.* 1974;47:211-217.

88. Richter W, Ryde M, Zetterstrom O. Non-immunogenicity of purified sodium hyaluronate preparation in man. *Int Arch Allergy Appl Immunol.* 1979;59:45-48.

89. Hoover DL, Giangiacomo J, Benson RL. Descemet's membrane detachment by sodium hyaluronate. *Arch Ophthalmol.* 1985;103:805-808.

90. McKnight SJ, Giangiacomo J, Adelstein E. Inflammatory response to viscoelastic materials. *Ophthalmic Surg.* 1987;18:804-806.

91. Fleming TC, Merrill DL, Girard LJ. Studies of the irritating action of methylcellulose. *Arch Ophthalmol.* 1959;61:565-567.

92. Kim JH. Intraocular inflammation of denatured viscoelastic substance in cases of cataract extraction and lens implantation. *J Cataract Refract Surg.* 1987;13:537-542.

93. Breebaart AC, Nuyts RMMA, Pels E, Edelhauser HF, Verbraak FD. Toxic endothelial cell destruction of the cornea after routine extracapsular cataract surgery. *Arch Ophthalmol.* 1990;108:1121-1125.

94. Nuyts RMMA, Edelhauser HF, Pels E, Breebaart AC. Toxic effects of detergents on the corneal endothelium. *Arch Ophthalmol.* 1990;108:1158-1162.

95. McCormack DL. Reduced mydriasis from repeated doses of tropicamide and cyclopentolate. *Ophthalmic Surg.* 1990;21:508-512.

96. Keates RH, McGowan KA. The effect of topical indomethacin ophthalmic solution in maintaining mydriasis during cataract surgery. *Ann Ophthalmol.* 1984;16:1116-1121.

97. Keates RH, McGowan KA. Clinical trial of flurbiprofen to maintain pupillary dilation during cataract surgery. *Ann Ophthalmol.* 1984;16:919-921.

98. Stark WJ, Fagadau WR, Stewart RH, Crandall AS, deFaller JM, Reaves TA, Klein PE. Reduction of pupillary constriction during cataract surgery using suprofen. *Arch Ophthalmol.* 1986;104:364-366.

99. Gimbel HV. The effect of treatment with topical nonsteroidal anti-inflammatory drugs with and without intraoperative epinephrine on the maintenance of mydriasis during cataract surgery. *Ophthalmology.* 1989;96:585-588.

100. Sachdev MS, Mehta MR, Dada VK, Jain AK, Garg SP, Gupta SK. Pupillary dilatation during cataract surgery - relative efficacy of indomethacin and flurbiprofen. *Ophthalmic Surg.* 1990;21:557-559.

101. Bito LZ. Surgical miosis: Have we been misled by a bunch of rabbits? *Ophthalmology.* 1990;97:1-2.

102. Machemer R. *Vitrectomy: A Pars Plana Approach.* New York: Grune and Stratton; 1975:51.

103. Edelhauser HF, Hine JE, Pederson H, et al. The effect of phenylephrine on the cornea. *Arch Ophthalmol.* 1979;97:937-947.

104. Cohen KL, Van Horn DL, Edelhauser HF, Schultz RO. Effect of phenylephrine on normal and regenerated endothelial cells in cat cornea. *Invest Ophthalmol Vis Sci.* 1979;18:242-249.

105. Dohlman CH, Hyndiuk RA. Subclinical and manifest corneal edema after cataract extraction. In: *Symposium on the Cornea: Transactions of the New Orleans Academy of Ophthalmology,* St Louis, MO: CV Mosby; 1972: 221.

106. Hull DS, Chemotti MT, Edelhauser HF, et al. Effect of epinephrine on the corneal endothelium. *Am J Ophthalmol.* 1975;79:245-250.

107. Edelhauser HF, Hyndiuk RA, Zeeb A, Schultz RO. Corneal edema and the intraocular use of epinephrine. *Am J Ophthalmol.* 1982;93:327-333.

108. Slack JW, Edelhauser HF, Helenek MJ. A bisulfite-free intraocular epinephrine solution. *Am J Ophthalmol.* 1990;110:77-82.

109. Coles WH. Pilocarpine toxicity. *Arch Ophthalmol* 1975;93:36-41.

110. Grehn F. Intraocular thymoxamine for miosis during surgery. *Am J Ophthalmol.* 1987;103:709-711.

111. Prosdocimo G, De Marco D. Intraocular dapiprazole to reverse mydriasis during extracapsular cataract extraction. *Am J Ophthalmol.* 1988;105:321-322.

112. Walsh JB, Gold A (eds). *Physicians' Desk Reference for Ophthalmology.* Oradell, NJ: Medical Economics, 1989.

113. Hollands RH, Drance SM, Schulzer M. The effect of acetylcholine on early postoperative intraocular pressure. *Am J Ophthalmol.* 1987;103:749-753.

114. Hollands RH, Drance SM, Schulzer M. The effect of intracameral carbachol on intraocular pressure after cataract extraction. *Am J Ophthalmol.* 1987;104:225-228.

115. Ruiz RS, Rhem MN, Prager TC. Effects of carbachol and acetylcholine on intraocular pressure after cataract extraction. *Am J Ophthalmol.* 1989;107:7-10.

116. Yee RW, Edelhauser HF. Comparison of intraocular acetylcholine and carbachol. *J Cataract Refract Surg.* 1986;12:18-22.

117. Birnbaum DR, Hull DS, Green K, Frey NP. Effect of carbachol on rabbit corneal endothelium. *Arch Ophthalmol.* 1987;105:253-255.

118. Grimmett MR, Williams KK, Broocker G, Edelhauser HF. Corneal edema after Miochol. *Am J Ophthalmol.* 1993;116:236-238.

119. Babinski M, Smith B, Wickerham EP. Hypotension and bradycardia following intraocular acetylcholine injection. Report of a case. *Arch Ophthalmol.* 1976;94:675-676.

120. Gombos GM. Systemic reactions following intraocular acetylcholine instillation. *Ann Ophthalmol.* 1982;14:529-530.

121. Brinkley JR, Henrick A. Vascular hypotension and bradycardia following intraocular injection of acetylcholine during cataract surgery. *Am J Ophthalmol.* 1984;97:40-42.

122. Glasser DB, Hyndiuk RA. Antibacterial agents. In: Tabbara KF and Hyndiuk RA (eds.). *Infections of the Eye.* Boston, MA: Little, Brown; 1986: 211-233.

123. Starr MB. Prophylactic antibiotics for ophthalmic surgery. *Surv Ophthalmol.* 1983;27:353-373.

124. Kattan HM, Flynn HW, Pflugfelder SC, Robertson C, Forster RK. Nosocomial endophthalmitis survey. Current incidence of infection after intraocular surgery. *Ophthalmology.* 1991;98:227-238.

125. Yannis RA, Rissing JP, Buxton TB, Shockley RK. Multistrain comparison of three antimicrobial prophylaxis regimens in experimental postoperative Pseudomonas endophthalmitis. *Am J Ophthalmol.* 1985;100:404-407.

126. Elliott RD, Katz HR. Inhibition of pseudophakic endophthalmitis in a rabbit model. *Ophthalmic Surg.* 1987;18:538-541.

127. Gritz DC, Cevallas AV, Smolin G, Whitcher JP. Antibiotic supplementation of intraocular irrigating solutions: An in vitro model of antibacterial action. *Ophthalmology.* 1996;103:1204-1209.

128. Sanders DR, Kraff M. Steroidal and nonsteroidal antiinflammatory agents. *Arch Ophthalmol.* 1984;102:1453-1456.

129. Flach AJ, Kraff MC, Sanders DR, Tanenbaum L. The quantitative effect of 0.5% ketorolac tromethamine and 0.1% dexaraethasone sodium phosphate solution on postsurgical blood-aqueous barrier. *Arch Ophthalmol.* 1988;106:480-483.

130. Kraff MC, Sanders DR, McGuigan L, Raanan MG. Inhibition of blood-aqueous humor barrier breakdown with diclofenac. A fluourophotometric study. *Arch Ophthalmol.* 1990;108:380-383.

131. Drews RC. Management of postoperative inflammation: dexamethasone versus flurbiprofen, aquantitative study using the new flare cell meter. *Ophthalmic Surg.* 1990;21:560-562.

132. Miyake K, Sakamura S, Miura H. Long-term follow-up study on prevention of aphakic cystoid macular oedema by topical indomethacin. *Br J Ophthalmol.* 1980;64:324-328.

133. Yanuzzi LA, Landau AN, Turtz AL. Incidence of aphakic cystoid macular edema with the use of topical indomethacin. *Ophthalmology.* 1981;88:947-954.

134. Kraff MC, Sanders DR, Jampol LM, Peyman GA, Lieberman HL. Prophylaxis of pseudophakic cystoid macular edema with topical indomethacin. *Ophthalmology.* 1982;89:885-890.

135. Jampol LM. Pharmacologic therapy of aphakic cystoid macular edema: a review. *Ophthalmology.* 1982;89:891-897.

136. Jampol LM. Pharmacologic therapy of aphakic and pseudophakic cystoid macular edema: 1985 update. *Ophthalmology.* 1985;92:807-810.

137. Flach AJ, Stegman RC, Graham J, Kruger LP. Prophylaxis of aphakic cystoid macular edema without corticosteroids. A paired-comparison, placebo-controlled double-masked study. *Ophthalmology.* 1990;97:1253-1258.

138. Gasset AR, Ishii Y, Kaufman HE, Miller T. Cytotoxicity of ophthalmic preservatives. *Am J Ophthalmol.* 1974;78:98-105.

139. Coles WH. Effects of antibiotics on the in vitro rabbit corneal endothelium. *Invest Ophthalmol.* 1975;14:246-250.

140. Van Horn DL, Edelhauser HF, Prodanovich G, et al. Effect of the ophthalmic preservative thimerosal on the rabbit and human corneal endothelium. *Invest Ophthalmol Vis Sci.* 1977;16:273-280.

141. Green K, Hull DS, Vaughn ED, et al. Rabbit endothelial response to ophthalmic preservatives. *Arch Ophthalmol.* 1977;95:2218-2221.

142. Weinreb RN, Wood I, Tomazzoli L, Alvarado J.

Subconjunctival injections. Preservative-related changes in the corneal endothelium. *Invest Ophthalmol Vis Sci.* 1986;27:525-531.

143. Lemp MA, Zimmerman LE. Toxic endothelial degeneration in ocular surface disease treated with topical medications containing benzalkonium chloride. *Am J Ophthalmol.* 1988;105:670-673.

144. Edelhauser HF, Antoine ME, Pederson HJ, et al. Intraocular safety evaluation of ethylene oxide and sterilant residues. *Journal of Toxicology: Cutaneous and Ocular Toxicology.* 1983;2:7-39.

145. Stark WJ, Rosenblum P, Maumenee AE, Cowan CL. Postoperative inflammatory reactions to intraocular lenses sterilized with ethylene oxide. *Ophthalmology.* 1980;87:385-389.

146. Haimann MH, Abrams GW, Edelhauser HF, Hatchell DL. The effect of intraocular irrigating solutions on lens clarity in normal and diabetic rabbits. *Am J Ophthalmol.* 1982;94:594-605.

147. Haimann MH, Abrams GW. Prevention of lens opacification during diabetic vitrectomy. *Ophthalmology.* 1984;91:116-121.

148. Kinoshita JH. Aldose reductase in the diabetic eye. XLIII Edward Jackson Memorial Lecture. *Am J Ophthalmol.* 1986;102:685-692.

149. Thompson JT, Glaser BM, Michels RG, de Bustros S. The use of intravitreal thrombin to control hemorrhage during vitrectomy. *Ophthalmology.* 1986;93:279-282.

150. Blacharski PA, Charles ST. Thrombin infusion to control bleeding during vitrectomy for stage V retinopathy of prematurity. *Arch Ophthalmol.* 1987;105:203-205.

151. Mannis MJ, Sweet E, Landers MB, Lewis RA. Uses of thrombin in ocular surgery. Effect on the corneal endothelium. *Arch Ophthalmol.* 1988;106:251-253.

152. Creel DJ, Wang JM, Wong KC. Transient blindness associated with transurethral resection of the prostate. *Arch Ophthalmol.* 1987;105:1537-1539.

153. de Bustros S, Glaser BM, Johnson MA. Thrombin infusion for the control of intraocular bleeding during vitreous surgery. *Arch Ophthalmol.* 1985;103:837-839.

154. Verdoorn C, Hendrikse F. Intraocular human thrombin infusion in diabetic vitrectomies. *Ophthalmic Surg.* 1989;20:278-279.

155. Aaberg TA. Balancing the benefits and risks of intracameral thrombin. *Am J Ophthalmol.* 1988;106:485-486.

# Chapter 14

# TOPICAL ANESTHESIA

*Matteo Piovella, MD*
*Ilvo Gratton, MD*

## INTRODUCTION

Anesthesia serves two purposes: first of all, to achieve full analgesic effect on the patient and, second, to allow the surgeon to operate in the best possible conditions and with minimal problems. Furthermore, anesthesiologic techniques and anesthetic drugs should combine the lowest possible risks with the fewest collateral effects.

In the history of cataract surgery, the second goal has long prevailed. In fact, although local anesthesia (retrobulbar or peribulbar anesthesia, orbicular block) is not a new development, until recently general anesthesia has been generally preferred as both the complete lack of movement and reaction on the part of the patient as well as the precious vitreous hypotony that comes with it were considered fundamental. All of us probably can recall the great confusion in the operating room and the hasty cries for anesthesiologic assistance whenever a patient would begin to wake a little too early from narcosis.

The risks and the problems connected with general anesthesia in the old and often sick cataract patient and the need to organize surgical activity on an outpatient basis have finally convinced an increasing number of ocular surgeons to switch to local anesthesia. Surgeons have consequently been forced to get used to head and body movements, vocal comments, sometimes outbursts of coughing. One great advantage has been a significant decrease of anesthesiologic risks and collateral effects and the possibility of a more agile organization of surgical activity.

Topical anesthesia is a further and maybe final step in the same direction. The risks and the problems connected to retrobulbar and peribulbar anesthesia are eliminated, and a quicker resumption of normal visual function is ensured if the surgeon is able to adapt to operating on an eye that is not still and therefore less under control. This situation certainly represents a disadvantage for the surgeon, as lack of immobility goes against one of the most radicated principles of ophthalmic surgery. However, we are convinced that with a change of mentality and the adoption of adequate surgical techniques, this method can be applied safely and successfully to most cataract patients.

## ADVANTAGES

Local anesthesia complications are rare but are well documented in ophthalmic literature.

As far as retrobulbar anesthesia is concerned, both local and general complications are described. General complications include bradycardia and cardiac arrest, respiratory depression and arrest, intradural injection with CNS depression, convulsions or coma. Among local complications, apart from retrobulbar hemorrhagia, which is a relatively frequent cause of postponement of operation, are optical nerve or bulbar lesions and perforation, extra and intraocular muscle paresis with ptosis, diplopia, persistent mydriasis, and lagophthalmos.

With peribulbar anesthesia, injections are limited to the extraconical space, so that anesthesiologic risks are certainly lower. However, nine cases of permanent vertical rectus paresis following peribulbar anesthesia have recently been signaled.[1] A complete list has been made by Zahl and Meltzer.[2]

Another risk factor is connected with the use of an oculopressor. With an injection of anesthesia, preoperative decompression is essential in order to favor retrobulbar diffusion of anesthetic solution and to induce a hypotonic effect on the vitreous body. Unfortunately, many cases of retinal complications have been described, especially in high myopia, such as retinal detachment and both venous and arterial occlusion, even after a correctly performed compression maneuver, which of course requires short pauses every 7 to 8 minutes.

Compression is not necessary in topical anesthesia as the bulb has a lower tone than in peribulbar, probably because no extra volume of fluid has been injected into the retrobulbar space. Of course, by adding a beta-blocker during preparation for surgery, there follows a more distinct hypotonic effect.

Local anesthesia sometimes causes persistent paresthesia, nausea, and headache. Because of long-lasting corneal anesthesia and lack of blinking reflex, many cases of keratopathy and corneal abrasions are observed.

In cases of allergic reaction to the anesthetic solution, reaction may easily be systemic with injective anesthesia, while it remains local with topical anesthesia.

A more practical advantage involves operating room organization. Topical anesthesia, in fact, consists of a single, fairly straightforward action: the repeated instillation of anesthetic eyedrops, which is familiar to ophthalmologic personnel and substantially devoid of risk. It may, therefore, be administered by paramedics, thus simplifying preoperative patient preparation and reducing operating room time.

On the contrary, local anesthesia consists of a series of maneuvers that ophthalmologists usually prefer performing personally. As an alternative, anesthesia is performed by a fellow ophthalmologist or by an anesthesiologist, but if it so happens that intraoperative anesthesia is incomplete, the surgeon will always wonder if the injections have been correctly executed. This might lead to unpleasant altercations among colleagues.

Topical anesthesia patients experience rapid physical recovery with no nausea and lethargy.[3,4] Patients report optimal analgesic effect and overall intra- and postoperative comfort. In our experience, only 3.2% reported intraoperative discomfort.[5] Most patients who have experienced peribulbar anesthesia for one eye and topical for the other prefer the latter.[6]

Both visual and motor functions promptly return close to normal early in the postoperative period,[7] as they are actually never really interrupted. Since we started using topical anesthesia for cataract surgery, we have performed automatic refraction and visual acuity tests 20 minutes to 2 hours after surgery (our operating schedule is interrupted by pauses every 2 to 3 hours for patient discharge). Elaboration of this data demonstrates that 22.2% have a visual acuity without correction of at least 20/30 and 82.5% of at least 20/80 (unpublished data). The realization that vision is fair or even good makes both patient and surgeon happy.

Patients wear an eyepatch only a few minutes and are discharged with just a pair of normal eyeglasses for protection. They feel and appear to others as people who have not been operated on, and that is gratifying or even quite useful in some cases (monocular patients, psychologically unstable subjects). The recent addition of highly hydrophilic corneal lenses (Protek, Ciba Vision), which is applied to our patients during the first 24 postoperative hours, adds to patients' sensation of well-being while preserving the psychological boost of the unpatched eye.

A faster closure of the lateral corneal wound due to the immediate recovery of normal blinking has been suggested by I. Howard Fine, while a normal lacrimal function represents a good prophylaxis against postoperative infections.

## DISADVANTAGES

It is certainly more difficult to operate on a mobile eye. A new category of complications directly connected to lack of akinesia now exists. The most frequent complication is irregular incision, which tends to cause an increase of wound suturing during the learning curve of topical anesthesia.

Probably even more important is the reduced control over ocular pressure. Although baseline pressure is usually rather low, unexpected orbicular muscle contractions may cause sudden variation of IOP and anterior chamber depth.

Potential epithelial toxicity[8] does not appear to be a problem. Many different anesthetic agents have been used.[3,4,9] We think it is important to protect the corneal surface by instilling a few artificial tear eyedrops in case of a prolonged waiting period before surgery.

No cases of untoward effects connected with the instillation of preoperative topical anesthetic agents have been reported.

Depth and length of anesthetic effect is somewhat lower than local anesthesia. Patients can feel pressure, and pressure may suddenly be transformed into a troublesome or even painful sensation after abrupt or rough maneuvers that cause traction on zonular fibers or ciliary body. Suture and scleral cautery[6] often induce discomfort or mild pain. The management of surgical complications is, of course, more difficult. However, if the surgeon remains in control, he or she can brilliantly mend very difficult situations, as a good anesthetic effect actually persists longer than 30 minutes.

All ophthalmologists should keep in mind that the pain threshold differs from one individual human being to another, depending on drug sensitivity as well as many other physical and psychological factors and that the barrier between tactile and pain sensation is very thin. As a matter of fact, the same principles apply to injective anesthesia, which some patients remember as an unpleasant or even painful experience (similar to the tension anyone feels in the dentist's chair, fearing that the drill vibratory sensation may turn into pain).

The psychological role of both surgeon and staff to avoid this transition is a nodal point in the management of topical anesthesia. With this in mind, topical anesthesia has been called *vocal anesthesia*. If one does not understand this point, topical anesthesia becomes pure surgical exercise, both dangerous and morally wrong.

As far as surgical technique is concerned, topical anesthesia is not equally applicable to all.

Even extracapsular cataract extraction can be performed, as it actually was as far back as 1988, with the sole addition of some infiltration in the superior rectus area.[10] However, the rough maneuvers of this technique

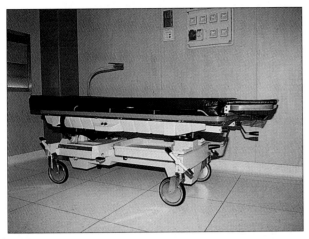

Figure 14-1. A mobile operating table is very convenient for outpatient surgery, as it allows for every possible patient position. 62-cm width provides enough room for both correct arm position and comfortable accommodation of obese patients.

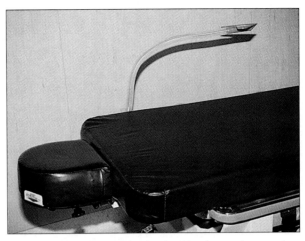

Figure 14-2. Operating table: details of headrest and oxygen bar. Foam rubber mattress is more than 10 cm thick. In fact, patient comfort is very important with topical anesthesia.

(nuclear expression, sutures) will easily stimulate pain reactions, and the lesser control over IOP and chamber depth in topical anesthesia greatly increases risks in a widely open bulb. We do not have any experience of planned extracapsular extraction, but have only performed a few conversions.

Topical anesthesia is ideal with phacoemulsification and lateral clear corneal incision, as this is a fast, atraumatic technique with the easiest approach for the surgeon and a position of the bulb that is easy to maintain for the patient by simply fixating the microscope light. It is probably not by chance that topical anesthesia was first applied in its actual form in 1992 by Fichman,[11] only 1 year after the introduction of self-sealing lateral clear corneal incision.[12]

Scleral tunnel is longer, the surgical approach at 12 is somewhat more laborious, and the patient may find it a little more difficult to find and keep the required position. Topical anesthesia is certainly possible, but patient selection should be more attentive and sedation or adjunctive anesthesia is more often required.[13]

## TRANSITION TO TOPICAL ANESTHESIA

Transition to topical anesthesia is a long and delicate process, in many ways comparable to transition from extracapsular extraction (ECCE) to phacoemulsification. Several ophthalmologists who approached phacoemulsification without adequate training had so many problems, and of such a serious nature, that they had to hastily turn back to ECCE.

So it is with topical anesthesia; even well-trained and mentally prepared surgeons have to pay a tribute in the form of a slight increase in the complication rate during their learning curve. A more superficial approach may bring about disaster, as any slight complication will become difficult to handle. After a few negative experiences, many ophthalmologists will simply give up.

The first rule for an atraumatic approach is perfect knowledge and control of phacoemulsification and one's surgical technique (eg, lateral clear corneal incision). Lack of akinesia will amplify any technical imperfection, making complications more frequent. It is advisable, therefore, to test any major technical change with peribulbar anesthesia.

Crossing the psychological barrier that a free-moving eye represents is certainly more difficult. Perfect absence of motion and of reaction has been one of the cornerstones of classical ophthalmic surgery, so much so that even rather recent treatises state that complete extraocular muscle akinesia is not only preferable but even necessary. On the contrary, topical anesthesia is applicable not only to a few ideal cases, but to the majority of uncomplicated cataract cases. The entire surgical team should be convinced of it as any negative attitude or skeptical remark makes patients insecure and difficult to control.

It may be very useful to assist during several surgical sessions in which topical anesthesia is routinely applied and observe the management of anxious patients, complicated cataracts, and intraoperative complications.

It is advisable to adopt a gradual approach. There are several possibilities.

First of all, the volume of anesthetic solution injected during peribulbar anesthesia can be gradually diminished causing a parallel increase in ocular mobility.

A second possibility is to maintain orbicular block for some time in order to exclude the problems created by orbicular muscle contraction (IOP and anterior chamber depth variability).

A third possibility may be to associate a subconjunctival injection at the incision site or to use the modified perilimbal approach (sub-Tenon's anesthesia using a blunt cannula through a small peritomy made 2 to 3 mm from the limbus).[14] The first ophthalmologist who used subconjunctival anesthesia for phacoemulsification was, to our knowledge, W. Petersen. Donald N. Serafano has proposed associating topical and subconjunctival anesthesia for scleral tunnel.

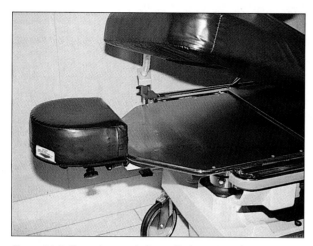

Figure 14-3. Operating angled metallic base gives the surgeon an advantage when using a lateral approach.

Due to its greater complexity, scleral tunnel construction may stimulate pain reaction more frequently than corneal incision. Serafano uses scleral tunnel when implanting 5 mm optic polymethylmethacrylate (PMMA) lenses, because he believes it to be safer due to the square shape of the tunnel. He prepares it temporally starting 1.5 mm from the limbus on the scleral side, associating 1 cc of 2% lidocaine locally to 4% Xylocaine eyedrops every 10 minutes three times before surgery. When implanting silicone lenses through a 4 mm wound, Serafano chooses lateral clear corneal incision with topical anesthesia only.

In conclusion, if one understands that the patient assumes a new role during surgery by becoming a more active agent to the point of being directly responsible for an entirely new kind of complication, it naturally follows that the doctor-patient relationship must change. Patients should be given adequate information before and during the surgery. Ideally, understanding and trust between doctor and patient should be fully established both on a professional and human level. If the ophthalmologist is not able to reach this goal, he or she probably will do better to renounce topical anesthesia.

## PATIENT SELECTION

During the learning curve of topical anesthesia, patients should be carefully selected.[15] Uncomplicated cataracts with soft nuclei, well-dilated pupils, and fully cooperative patients are ideal. Selection should eventually become less strict, as experience and confidence builds up in the surgeon.

Exclusion criteria can be divided into two groups. The first group is made of cataract cases presenting aspects of particular difficulty and being therefore at high risk of intraoperative complications. For the expert surgeon, they progressively come to coincide with cases in which phacoemulsification itself is not recommended.

The second group consists of patients who, for different reasons, are not able to collaborate: deaf people, children, uncollaborating elderly people, mentally handicapped, and usually foreigners. Overanxious patients are to be evaluated case by case, and the number of people excluded greatly decreases as the personal capability of the surgeon rises.

To our knowledge, there are no medical contraindications to topical anesthesia. On the contrary, there is at least one case that represents a strong indication for its use: hemorrhagic diseases.

High myopia is possibly a relative indication, as the reduced scleral resistance and large bulbar size may represent a risk for retrobulbar and peribulbar injections and ocular compression. Glaucoma may be another, as anesthesia may impair optic nerve blood flow and therefore damage visual field.

In order to fully exploit its advantages, topical anesthesia should become one of the favorite choices in cases of uncomplicated cataract surgery. We used topical anesthesia in 75% of our uncomplicated cataract cases in 1993, and 99% in 1996.

## DOCTOR-PATIENT RELATIONSHIP (VOCAL ANESTHESIA)

### Preoperative Examination

We advise doctors to speak to their patients about topical anesthesia right from the preoperative examination, because most people may have never heard of that possibility. Even patients who may have consulted us for the very reason that they want *no-needle* anesthesia usually do not know what it entails.

We believe that topical anesthesia should be clearly indicated in the written informed consent to surgery after advantages and disadvantages of the different anesthesiologic techniques have been explained.

We think, however, that the patient should not just be given a completely free choice between the two techniques (or between ECCE and phacoemulsification). The patient should clearly know what the doctor's preference is, because the patient will expect the doctor to suggest those solutions that are more advantageous to his or her case.

Most patients understand the concept of anesthesiologic risk; they are happy to avoid periocular injections and postoperative eye-patch and eagerly anticipate the promised faster visual recovery. However, some will have doubts about the effectiveness of eyedrops or fear they will not be able to cooperate adequately. A few even claim they want general anesthesia.

Observing patient behavior and reactions is important in identifying patients unfit for topical anesthesia.

### Preparation for Surgery

We advise doctors to spend a little time with the patient just before surgery.

The ophthalmologist should first remind the patient of the different sensations he or she will feel during surgery (microscope light, oxygen blow, dampness from fluid flowing down to the ear, tactile and pressure sensations from instruments), reassuring the patient that the sensa-

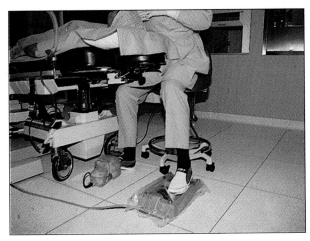

Figures 14-4, 14-5, 14-6. A demonstration of lateral surgical approach. Antitrendelemburg position is supported by the large central pneumatic cylinder.

tions are not a prelude to pain. A practical demonstration of the permanence of some eye sensitivity should be given.

While briefly reviewing the few simple positions and maneuvers the patient may be asked to take, the surgeon should stress the ease of the surgery. The patient should not be worried that loss of fixation, body movement, or a cough will compromise surgical outcome. On the contrary, the patient should know that he or she is free to express any worries, fatigue, or pain sensations so that problems may promptly find adequate solutions.

Operating room personnel should help make the patient relax by treating him or her with kindness and solicitude. The anesthesiologist should be introduced and should assure the patient that he or she will look after the patient throughout surgery.

It may help to invite the patient to think back to happy memories.

If a patient remains overanxious, some sedation may be administered, or it may be decided to switch to peribulbar anesthesia.

## Management of the Patient During Surgery

Before incision, patient reaction to corneal wetting should be controlled. If it is excessive, corneal wetting should be limited and should be done only in conditions of full safety (still and protected instruments). Ability and speed in responding to orders should be controlled. In any case, these should be limited in number and clearly stated: for example, it is wrong to say, "Look at the light" if the patient is fixating correctly already. In fact, the patient would probably think he or she is in the wrong position, and, therefore, would move in order to find the nonexistent correct aim, soon going back to microscope light. If a command is given, the surgeon should wait a few seconds to give the patient time to understand it and move to the new position. By adapting this technique to limited movements and small deviations from the ideal position, the ophthalmologist should avoid bothering the patient with excessive requests, which would confuse and finally wear him or her out.

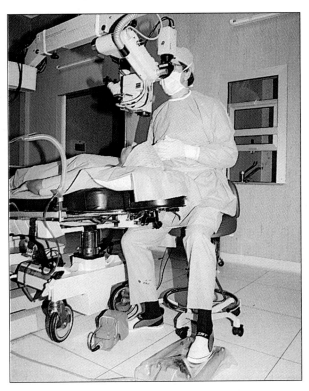

Figure 14-5.

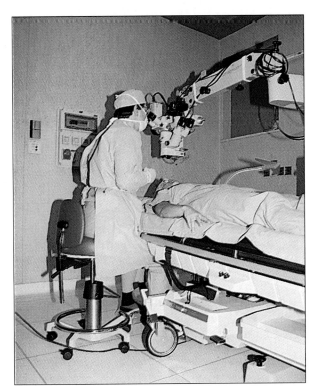

Figure 14-6.

From time to time, patients should be encouraged and in some way informed about the good progress of the operation. Any pause or unusual maneuver that might cause sudden alarm reactions should be announced and

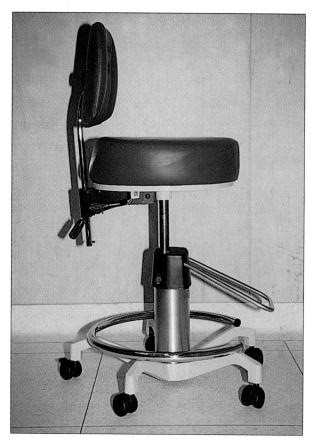

Figure 14-7. Operating chair should be stable, easy to adjust, and sufficiently compact in order to favor lateral approach. It must also be easy to move, as position has to be changed quite often with topical anesthesia.

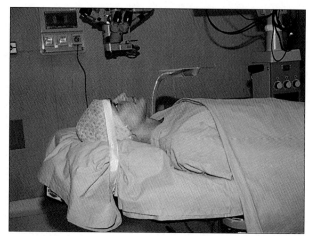

Figure 14-8. Correct head position. Head may rest more comfortably with a soft pillow. Notice horizontal oxygen bar.

explained. In any case, the surgeon and operating room staff should always appear to be in command of the situation. If the patient hears unfavorable remarks, perceives a negative attitude, uncertainty, or nervousness, he or she may suddenly lose control.

This is particularly the case when dealing with complications. Because the patient will probably notice that something is wrong, common sense would suggest giving him or her a simple, reassuring explanation, such as, "Your cataract is a little harder than expected and it will take longer to clean everything up." Long, silent pauses or altered voices should be avoided.

### Postoperative Management

Operated eyes are kept patched for about half an hour. At discharge, patients wear sunglasses for protection.

Particular attention should be given to making sure patients correctly understand postoperative prescriptions and recommendations. In day surgery, the duties of cleaning and medicating operated eyes are entrusted to people who are not experts. Therefore, it is important that patients and relatives (or neighbors or nurses) who assist learn how to properly instill eyedrops and judge the importance of symptoms that may emerge between two control examinations.

Instructions should be repeated several times, and written directions should be given for home consultation.

It should be kept in mind that lack of paresthesia and significant pain, as well as a perfectly normal exterior look, may induce patients to be excessively confident and forgo prescribed recommendations.

## PATIENT PREPARATION: MYDRIASIS AND ANESTHESIA

Our schedule of patient preparation in case of uncomplicated cataract begins the day before surgery with home instillation of sodium diclofenac (Voltaren Ofta, Ciba Vision) three times a day, completed by a single instillation of 0.5% tropicamide with phenylephrine (Visumidriatic fenilefrina, MSD).

On the morning of the day of surgery, patients are invited to arrive at the Operating Center about 1 hour before scheduled surgery time in order to complete the following preparation:

- 0.5% tropicamide phenylephrine five times every 10 minutes.
- 1% Cyclopentolate (Ciclolux, Lux ), one time.
- 1% atropine (Atropina 1%, Lux ), one time.

This schedule may seem a little complex. However, maximal and long-lasting mydriasis is of the utmost importance in topical anesthesia in order to perform a rapid phacoemulsification without iris manipulation. According to Grabow,[4] adequate cycloplegia may minimize discomfort induced by stretching of zonules and ciliary muscle.

We find that atropine does not keep the pupil from readily responding to intracameral miotics when necessary (actually we seldom use miotics). Besides, when patients are examined 12 to 24 hours after surgery, pupils are usually miotic already.

As for the anesthesiologic preparation, at the moment, each surgeon who is familiar with topical anesthesia uses a number of different anesthetic agents with personal protocols.[3,4,9] We use the following scheme:

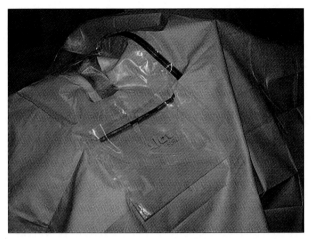

Figure 14-9. A disposable surgical drape is kept high over the patient's chest by the horizontal oxygen bar, thus creating an ample breathing space, which usually prevents claustrophobic patient reaction.

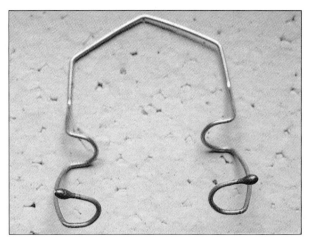

Figure 14-10. Lid speculum—Surgeon's lateral view.

- 2% lidocaine hydrochloride, five times every 10 minutes.
- 0.4% benoxinate, five times every 10 minutes.

Benoxinate is produced in Italy as monodose eyedrops by Alfa Intes, while lidocaine has to be drawn from vials (Lidrian, Bieffe Medital), using a syringe with no needle. The same syringe serves as a personal eyedropper for each patient.

In case of delay, artificial tears and occlusion are used to protect corneal epithelium.

No premedication is given. In many patients, atropine apparently causes a systemic effect vaguely resembling preoperative sedation.

A vein should be incannulated for possible intraoperative needs or emergencies. If some sedation is necessary, we use propofol (Diprivan) injecting a volume that depends on patient weight. This helps keep restless patients under control without putting them to sleep. Contrary to North American authors, we seldom recur to intravenous sedation (1.7% of cases in our first year of experience with topical anesthesia [1993], 0.61% in 1996).

The role of the anesthesiologist may seem marginal. On the contrary, we deem his or her presence necessary both before and throughout surgery. Remember that the anesthesiologist's intervention, when needed, is usually urgent.

## Operating Room—Patient Draping and Preparation for Surgery

Eye position is more difficult to control with topical anesthesia, as any kind of mechanical fixation is lacking. The eye must be horizontal and corneal limbus possibly visible at 12 o'clock. Head tilt is the fundamental factor. Having microscope light as a reference mark, neck extension tends to uncover limbus at 12. However, excessive extension may be fatiguing.

Head position should, of course, be harmonized with antitrendelemburg body position.

Patient comfort is quite important. Common operating tables are narrow, rigid, and, therefore, certainly unfit for topical anesthesia. The ideal table should be large enough to accommodate even obese patients; it should be provided with a soft, 10 cm thick mattress that may alleviate the not-uncommon back problems of the elderly. The headrest should also be comfortable and easy to regulate in any direction. Additional ring-shaped head holders should be avoided. Ideal head restraining systems must prevent sudden movements while not bothering patients. Sticking plaster should be anallergic and easy to remove.

Lid speculum cannot be too rigid as that would cause an occlusive reaction with synergic bulbar elevation. Younger patients may manage to actually expel an inadequate instrument during surgery. We suggest using a speculum with branches connected on the nasal side (which makes lateral clear corneal approach quite easy) and curved in such a way as to keep lids a little lifted from the bulb.

Care should be taken when draping the patient. A well-positioned horizontal oxygen bar sustaining the surgical drape high over the patient's chest will give him or her ample breathing space. Nasal cannulas are not suitable because they can induce patient reaction due to mechanical stimulation or chemical irritation of nasal mucosa by oxygen flow.

Microscope settings must be carefully checked before every case. Both focus and XY should not be at the end of scale, as the surgeon will need to change focus and centration quite often due to continuous eye movements.

## SURGICAL TECHNIQUE

General guidelines are rapidity, essentiality, and lightness (no touch surgery).

### Lateral Clear Corneal Incision

Incision is a very delicate step, set as it is at the beginning of the surgical act, with the patient having had no experience yet and sudden movement being possible at any time.

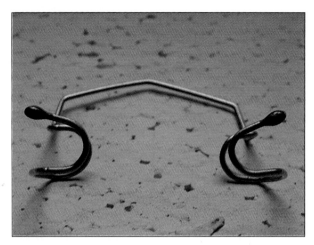

Figure 14-11. Lid speculum—Actual view in lateral surgical approach.

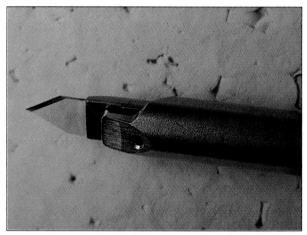

Figure 14-12. 3.2 mm diamond blade with upper cutting edge only gives optimal control over incision. The blade can be calibrated down to 250 µm during preincision.

We usually adopt a three-step, clear corneal incision in the temporal quadrant. We only employ diamond blades. The cornea should be adequately wetted before incision as a dry epithelium may be irregularly damaged. During the maneuver itself, wetting should be avoided, because possible reactive movements may end up in an irregular, not waterproof wound and greater induced astigmatism. Some surgeons use forceps to fixate the bulb. We believe that holding instruments may cause an unpleasant tactile sensation and some fear of later pain, impairing patient collaboration. Besides, if a diamond is used, the cornea does not usually offer much resistance to penetration. Once the blade has entered the stroma, control becomes much better.

## Viscoelastics and Capsulorhexis

Before capsulorhexis, the anterior chamber is filled with a viscoelastic substance (VES).

As is well known, viscoelastics will oppose the tendency of some light nuclei to readily come into the anterior chamber as the anterior capsule is being opened.

Viscoelastics are of the utmost importance in modern cataract surgery as they give protection to the endothelium and other ocular tissues throughout the entire operative act. Many products with different physical and chemical properties are available[16], and every surgeon has a preferred substance that best suits personal technique and habits. We have been routinely using a VES since 1985 (Healon [Pharmacia]); we switched to Viscoat (Alcon) in 1992. We have always removed the viscoelastic at the end of surgery.

The importance of VES increases with topical anesthesia. Risks to the endothelium are higher as a result of unanticipated ocular saccades and anterior chamber variations following sudden orbicular muscle contraction, which may cause direct trauma and make leakage of viscoelastic from incision easier. It is therefore important to choose a substance that gives the greatest possible protection and rarely leaves the anterior chamber throughout phacoemulsification. This is why we prefer viscoelastics with low cohesiveness. Within this group, Viscoat is by far the best. Its imperfect transparency makes continuous control on its protective presence possible so that timely additions can be made if viscoelastic is unintentionally removed, as is often the case during emulsification of hard nuclei.

It is certainly true that low cohesiveness makes aspiration at the end of surgery difficult. Viscoat has to be carefully removed from each quadrant. With the advances in surgical technique within the past few years, this is hardly a problem; on the contrary, it can be considered another warranty of particularly good protective qualities. Moreover, in our experience, incomplete removal does not cause significant increases of IOP.

Viscoelastic is also quite useful in isolating and selectively moving pieces of tissue: eg, blocking small capsular ruptures, protecting iris tissue damaged by phaco tip, repositioning an iris that has prolapsed into the incision. On these occasions, it serves as a precious auxiliary instrument.

Among cohesive viscoelastics, we prefer high molecular weight products such as Healon GV (Pharmacia), which works well in creating and maintaining spaces. We sometimes use one of these before lens implantation to reform the capsular bag.

We perform capsulorhexis with needle and forceps. Forceps seem to us to provide more precise control of rhexis as well as more effectiveness when it is necessary to modify direction in case of peripheral extension. It is sufficient to grasp the capsule at its very implant base and operate a perpendicular traction.

## Hydrodelineation/Hydrodissection

A complete mobilization of the cataract nucleus is quite important in topical anesthesia. If the nucleus is free from adhesions to cortex, it will be easy to rotate it without exerting any traction on zonular fibers and ciliary body, which may otherwise elicit pain reactions. In addition, separation from the epinucleus provides a cushion protecting the posterior capsule from variations in vitreous pressure.

Hydrodelineation is certainly more successful if a flat cannula is used in place of the normal round air cannula.

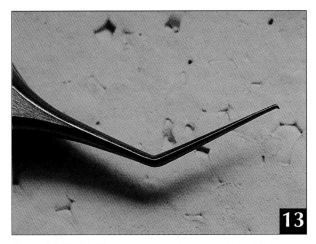
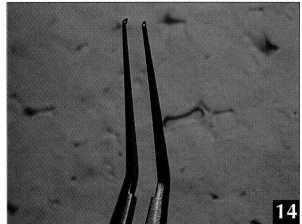

Figures 14-13, 14-14. Capsulorhexis is a particularly delicate maneuver in topical anesthesia. We recommend using forceps with pointed teeth and a perfect hold, controlled by a spacer.

The distinctive golden ring will tell the surgeon the maneuver has been completed.

Because adherence to posterior capsule is often considerable, hydrodissection of the epinucleus is also important.

## Phacoemulsification

We commonly adopt Chip and Flip phacoemulsification.

Our experience has been that the use of a second instrument may more easily generate compression sensations and, therefore, induce reaction while not enhancing eye control, confirming the philosophy that the simpler the surgical technique, the better (no touch technique).

If hydrodissection and hydrodelineation are complete, monomanual manipulation and emulsification present no problem.

## Aspiration of Epinucleus and Cortex

Usually, the epinucleus is well mobilized and can therefore easily be flipped and aspirated with the phaco tip. If there is residual adherence, it is safer to use the I/A tip with patient and delicate maneuvers.

Posterior capsule scraping is tricky, as a central rupture is always possible, especially in topical anesthesia.

## Lens implantation

We enlarge the incision to 5.25 mm or to 3.5 to 4.1 mm when implanting respectively 5 mm optic PMMA lenses or foldable lenses. Excess VES should be injected to fully reform capsular sac, repeating the injection after enlarging the incision, if needed. An incompletely filled capsule may cause posterior capsule folding or rupturing during lens implantation and rotation.

Implantation should be simple and gentle. Until 1994, we found that PMMA lenses were superior to available foldable lenses in spite of the larger incision needed.[17] With careful technique, sutures were not usually needed (9.5% in our experience). In our opinion, the main problem with foldables was the lack of well-working insertion forceps or injectors. Lenses opened inside the eye in a rather rough and abrupt, and sometimes explosive, way. Instrumentation and lens materials have since improved, and, therefore, we have switched to routine implantation of foldable lenses and 3.5 to 4.1 mm incisions since January 1995. At the moment, we prefer to use thermoplastic lenses (Memorylens [ORC]), which are provided ready for implantation and slowly unfold within the eye in a completely atraumatic way. As an alternative, we implant acrylic lenses (5.5 mm optic AcrySof [Alcon]), which have a high refractive index and are particularly thin, even for higher powers. In our opinion, they are also easy to fold with appropriate forceps and gentle in unfolding.

We now use 5 mm optic PMMA lenses primarily for low power implants.

## Concluding Surgery

After implantation, the VES is aspirated as completely as possible, and the anterior chamber is reformed, testing the incision for good self-sealing properties. With a 4.1 mm incision, suture incidence has fallen to 2.4% ( unpublished data ). If necessary, a single central suture is sufficient to make the incision perfectly watertight and has little influence on corneal curvature. In any case, the suture can be removed after a few days. Remember that most patients will feel some discomfort when the sclera is being punctured.

Time should not be wasted with unimportant details, as many patients may be at the end of their tolerance and collaboration capabilities.

Care should be taken in removing lid speculum as rough maneuvers may bring about anterior chamber loss even in the presence of a perfect incision.

## COMPLICATIONS AND COMPLICATED CASES

Among the most delicate problems one can face during topical anesthesia are a miotic pupil, a capsular rupture, an irregular incision, and a conversion to ECCE.

It is perfectly possible to manage complications in topical anesthesia if the surgeon keeps control of the situation. On the contrary, if the patient becomes restless, the surgeon should stop briefly to let the anesthesiologist give some intravenous sedation. Propofol usually calms down agitated patients while maintaining some collaboration capability. In a few cases, some kind of infiltrative anesthesia may be added. Resorting to general anesthesia should be the exception.

We have never had to switch either to general or to any infiltrative anesthesia. In case of mild pain, we have recently begun to use intracameral anesthesia[18] (injection of 0.2 cc of preservative-free 1% Lidocaine [Astra]).

We would like to highlight one point: rather than pain, the wider concept of surgical stress should be considered. Patients naturally feel the strain of undergoing an operation and also of the unusual situation of having to provide some kind of collaboration. This strain is quite different from person to person and varies with many factors, such as comprehension, mental elasticity, and the quality of the patient-doctor relationship. Strain may be high at the beginning of surgery, followed by a decrease and a subsequent increase again in the last phases of surgery. In our experience, the ophthalmologist can reasonably expect about 15 minutes of maximal collaboration. Although this begins to decrease, it is generally possible to go on with topical anesthesia for about 30 minutes. Afterward, many patients may become quite difficult to control, although very cooperative patients may feel perfectly fine for as long as 1 hour, as other ophthalmologists have confirmed.

In order to have an adequate safety margin, average surgical time for an uncomplicated cataract should be 15 minutes or less, so that there will be plenty of time to face any possible complications. Necessary instrumentation should be ready at hand, and operating room personnel should be trained in setting it up swiftly. All this implies that faster surgical techniques (eg, lateral clear corneal incisions) are ideal for topical anesthesia.

An occasional iris touch with phaco and I/A tips is not usually painful. However, repeated touch or iris manipulation is bothersome. Therefore, spatula and hooks should be used gently. VES can be ideal in repositioning iris prolapsed into the corneal tunnel and may help in slightly enlarging miotic pupils or detaching synechiae.

Capsular rupture significantly prolongs surgical time, especially if vitrectomy is needed. However, if operating room staff is efficient, it is perfectly possible to conclude surgery with topical anesthesia.

Conversion is more complex, and strategy should be decided from case to case. Intravenous sedation may be necessary, and some kind of injective sedation can be chosen as appropriate. We do not have much practical experience in this field, and we think that the cautious surgeon will seldom face that situation if he or she wisely chooses peribulbar anesthesia in cases that, according to personal experience, are to be considered at high risk.

In our opinion, suture is to be considered a complication, although minor, because it depends on an incorrect wound construction and always induces some kind of pain reaction from the patient.

New and sometimes peculiar kinds of complications are patient-related complications. They are due to orbicular muscle contraction or ocular saccades. Orbicular muscle contraction and its potentially serious effects should be prevented by careful use of viscoelastics, regulation of bottle height, accurate hydrodissection, and no-touch surgical techniques.

Complications following bulbar movements should be minimized by adequate preparation of the surgeon. The surgeon should learn to get the best possible cooperation from each patient while adapting his or her technique to small movements and positions that may not always be ideal.

## REFERENCES

1. Esswein MB, von Noorden GK. Paresis of a vertical rectus muscle after cataract extraction. *Am J Ophthalmol*. 1993;116:424.
2. Zahl K, Meltzer MA. The complications of regional anesthesia. *Ophthalmology Clinics of North America*. 1990; March: 111.
3. Kershner RM. Topical anesthesia for small-incision self-sealing cataract surgery: a prospective evaluation of the first 100 patients. *J Cataract Refract Surg.* ,1993;19:290.
4. Grabow HB. Topical anesthesia for cataract surgery. *Eur J Implant Refract Surg*. 1993;5:20.
5. Piovella M, Camesasca F, Gratton I, Scaltrini G. Topical anesthesia with lidocaine 2% for phacoemulsification. AAO 1995, *Scientific Poster*. 162.
6. Novak KD, Koch DD. Topical anesthesia for phacoemulsification: initial 20 case series with one month follow-up. *J Cataract Refract Surg*. 1995;21: 672.
7. Nielsen PJ. Immediate visual capability after cataract surgery: topical versus retrobulbar anesthesia. *J Cataract Refract Surg*. 1995;21:302.
8. Marr WG, Wood R, Senterfit L. Effect of topical anesthesia on regeneration of corneal epithelium. *Am J Ophthalmol*. 1957;43:606.
9. Gills JP, Williams DL. Advantage of marcaine for topical anesthesia (letter). *J Cataract Refract Surg*. 1993;19:819.
10. Smith R. Cataract extraction without retrobulbar injection. *Brit J Ophthalmol*. 1990;April:205.
11. Fichman RA. Topical drops replace injection for cataract anesthesia. *Ocular Surgery News*. 1992;3(4):1.
12. Fine IH. Architecture and construction of a self-sealing incision for cataract surgery. *J Cataract Refract Surg*. 1991;7(suppl):672.
13. Dinsmore SC. Drop, then decide approach to topical anesthesia. *J Cataract Refract Surg*. 1995;21:666.
14. Pallan LA, Kondrot EC, Stout RR. Sutureless scleral tunnel cataract surgery using topical and low dose perilimbal anesthesia. *J Cataract Refract Surg*. 1995;21:504.
15. Fine IH, Fichman RA, Grabow HB, eds. *Clear Corneal Cataract Surg and Topical Anesthesia*. Thorofare, NJ: SLACK Inc; 1993.
16. Arshinoff S. Comparative physical properties of ophthalmic viscoelastics. *Ophthalmic Practice*. 1989;7:16.
17. Piovella M, Gratton I, Barca M, Scaltrini G. Lateral clear corneal incision and 5 mm optic PMMA implantation with topical anesthesia. *Ocular Surg News*. 1993;4(10):58.
18. Gills JP, Cherchio M, Raahan MG. Unpreserved lidocaine to control discomfort during cataract surgery using topical anesthesia. *J Cataract Refract Surg*. 1997;23:545.

# Chapter 15

# INCISIONS
*Antonello Rapisarda, MD*

## INTRODUCTION

One of the objectives of modern cataract surgery is to rapidly improve visual performance, which will be stable in time. In order to reach this situation, techniques have been improved continually and with them the development of tools necessary for this sophisticated type of surgery—machinery, lenses, surgical instruments, and viscoelastic substances (VES)—have all been developed to suit the changing situation.

For rapid, long-lasting visual recovery, the surgeon aims to maintain corneal curvature as close to the preoperative as possible.

Phacoemulsification is a technique that allows the surgeon to remove the cataract through a very small incision. As it alters the corneal curvature less than the others, it can produce final results that are closer to the predefined objectives than other techniques.

The incisions required for this technique are sophisticated; they are small in size and allow the insertion of foldable intraocuolar lenses (IOLs).

## INCISION

An incision is an opening that allows the surgeon to gain access to an organism; the width and the depth differ in relation to the site and the type of operation planned.

In the planning phase of a phaco operation, the surgeon must examine the type of incision required and how it will be closed at the end of the operation.

The surgeon should be aware of the following:
- The width of the incision will influence the degree of movement of the instruments inside the anterior chamber, the hold of the anterior chamber during the maneuvers of phaco, and the type of lens that can be implanted.
- The length and the direction of the incision will influence its behavior in relation to the tangential and perpendicular forces, which come into play particularly in the postoperative period (endocular pressure, external forces).

A perpendicular incision will also open the wound through small displacement of the edges.

A correctly sized oblique incision will create a valve opening that will remain closed because of displacement (sliding) of the edges.

In the first case, an increase in endocular pressure intra- or postoperatively will cause the formation of a tunnel, which is opened externally; in the second case, there will be greater adhesion between the two edges of the wound.

To achieve this, when the surgeon is planning the incision, he or she should ensure that the hypothetical hinge of the wound flap is inside the wound itself and therefore distant from the edges of the incision. If this is not the case, sutures will be required.

While respecting the above *hinge rule*, the incision must have a number of well-defined features, irrespective of the site. These include the following:
- The size of the opening must be proportional to the size of the phaco tip, both to allow its introduction in the bulb, without compressing the silicone sleeve around the probe, and to allow the balanced salt solution (BSS) that flows inside the opening to reach the anterior chamber easily and continually. At the same time, it prevents the liquid introduced to the chamber from escaping through the space between the incision walls and the phaco tip. It allows it to escape almost exclusively through the phaco tip and keeps the depth of the chamber itself constant even with the modern techniques of Phaco Chop.

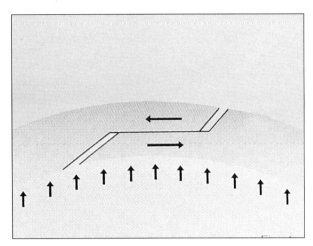

Figure 15-1. Tangential and perpendicular forces come into play, particularly in the postoperative period.

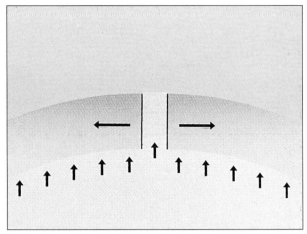

Figure 15-2. A perpendicular incision will open the wound through small displacement of the edges.

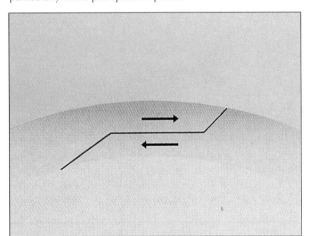

Figure 15-3. An oblique incision will create a valve opening, remaining closed during the sliding of the edges.

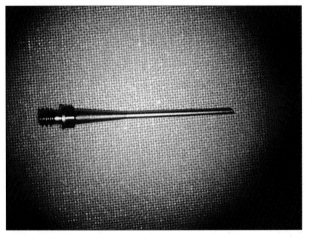

Figure 15-4. The size of the opening must be prepositioned to the size of the phaco tip.

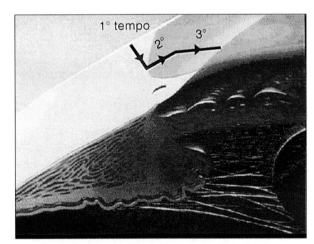

Figure 15-5. Limbo corneal tunnel.

- The surgeon must avoid damaging the corneal endothelium.
- The surgeon must avoid iris prolapse.
- The incision must either be easy to suture or not require sutures at all (sutureless).

The optimal sites for the incision include the following:
- Limbal.
- Scleral.
- Corneal.

## LIMBO-CORNEAL TUNNEL

This is certainly the easiest technique. For this reason, it is ideal for surgeons approaching phacoemulsification for the first time.

Materials recommended include the following:
- Disposable 30° blade, 9230-01 Alcon Surgical.
- Disposable rounded blade, 9400-02 Alcon Surgical.
- Disposable, preset 3.2 mm blade with a sharp tip, 9232-61 Alcon Surgical, if we have a traditional phaco tip.
- Sharp disposable 2.75 mm blade, 9927-61 Alcon Surgical, if we have a 2.8 mm phaco MicroTip.
- Disposable blunted 3.55 mm blade 9935-61 Alcon Surgical, for the implantation of a foldable acrylic IOL with a 5.5 mm optic or a silicone IOL with a 6 mm optic.
- Preset disposable, blunted 5.2 mm blade, 9656-61

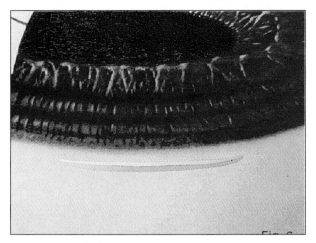

Figure 15-6. Limbal site incision.

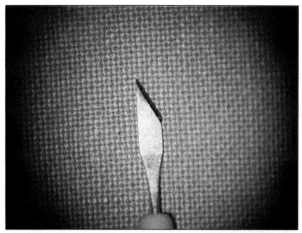

Figure 15-7. Disposable 30° blade, 9230-01 Alcon Surgical.

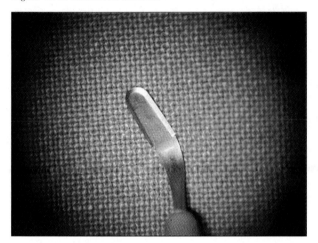

Figure 15-8. Disposable rounded blade, 9600-02 Alcon Surgical.

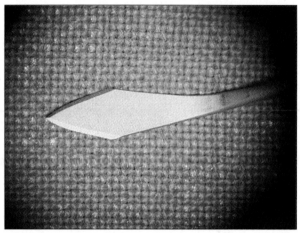

Figure 15-9. Sharp disposable 2.75 to 3.2 mm blade, 9921-61 Alcon Surgical.

Alcon Surgical, if an IOL in polymethylmethacrylate (PMMA) has to be implanted.

## Technique

The incision is cut in a limbal site perpendicular to the ocular surface, for a depth of 50% of the tissue thickness and width just slightly greater than the diameter of the lens to be implanted. A 30° blade should be used.

Prepare of a small limbo-corneal tunnel (about 2 mm in length), with a width equal to the size of the linear incision, which has already been performed. An angled bevel-up blade with a rounded tip should be used.

Enter the anterior chamber (width between 2.75 and 3.2 mm) at the end of the tunnel.

The surgeon should use a sharp preset blade between 2.75 and 3.2 mm wide.

The incision is extended when aspiration of the residual cortical masses has been completed, to allow the passage of the bulk of the lens disc for implantation. Here we will use a preset blunted 3.5 to 4.0 mm blade if a foldable IOL is to be implanted; alternately, a preset blunted 5.2 mm blade should be used if a rigid lens with a 5 mm optic disc is to be implanted. If the optic disc of the lens is larger, the incision

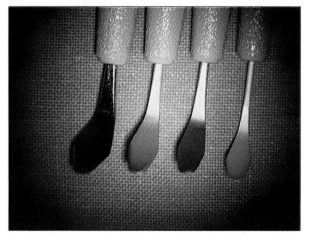

Figure 15-10. Preset disposable, blunted 5.2 mm blade, 9656-61, Alcon Surgical.

is widened using the cutting edges of the blade itself.

Advantages include the following:
- Ease of access to the anterior chamber.
- Ease of movement with the phaco and aspiration tips.

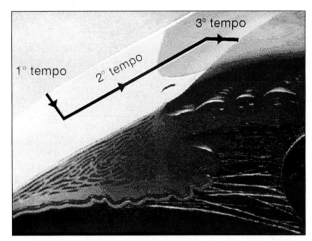

Figure 15-11. Sclero-corneal tunnel.

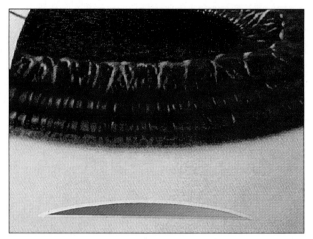

Figures 15-12, 15-13. Conjunctival flap.

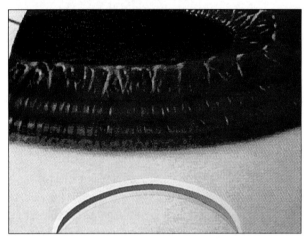

Figure 15-13.

- Ease of IOL implantation.

Disadvantages include the following:
- Moderately difficult access to the anterior chamber.
- Moderately difficult to maneuver both the phaco and aspiration tips.
- Moderately difficult to implant the IOL.

## SCLERO-CORNEAL TUNNEL

This technique has undoubtedly been used more frequently and is the most difficult of the techniques.

The materials recommended are the same as those for the limbal incision so please refer to the above section.

### Technique

The surgeon prepares a conjunctival flap measuring 5 x 3 mm.

Using a 30° blade, a first incision is made in the sclera perpendicular to the plane at least 2 mm from the limbus; the depth of the incision should be approximately 350 to 400 µm (50% of the scleral thickness). The incision can be straight, curved either limbal convex or concave, triangular with a limbal apex, or transversal radial. Irrespective of its shape, the incision must be at least 2 mm from the limbus itself.

With the rounded blade, a 3.5 mm sclero-corneal tunnel is made for a soft IOL. A tunnel of 5.0 mm is made for a rigid IOL, so that the blade enters the corneal stroma where the tissue is perfectly transparent. Irrespective of the shape of the incision, the progression of the blade in transparent tissue must be controlled very carefully.

With a preset, 3.2 mm blade, the surgeon proceeds through the sclero-corneal tunnel, and, at the end, the tip penetrates the anterior chamber.

At the end of phacoemulsification and aspiration of the residual cortical masses, the incision is extended with a blunted preset blade, to allow the passage of the optic disc of the lens to be implanted.

Advantages include the following:
- Better hold of the valve incision.
- Low degree of astigmatism in the initial postoperative period.

Disadvantages include the following:
- Difficult access to the anterior chamber.
- Difficult maneuvers with the phaco and aspiration tip.
- Difficult implantation of both rigid and soft/foldable IOLs.

## CORNEAL TUNNEL

The incision in the cornea has become the elective approach for many surgeons performing cataract extraction with phacoemulsification.

Preferably, it should be performed in a temporal site: as the corneal tunnel is short only in this sector, the pressure exerted by the eyelid favors the impermeability of the incision.

This incision is indicated for the following patients:
- Patients with coagulation disorders, because there is no blood loss because the conjunctiva is not disinserted and the sclera is not cut.
- Patients with an antiglaucomatous fistula on the 12 o'clock radius.

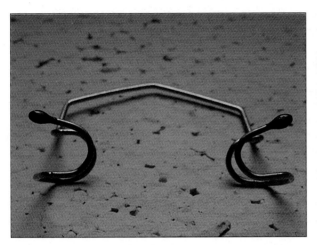

Figure 15-14. Blepharostat (retractor).

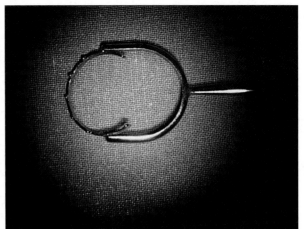

Figure 15-15. Fixing ring.

- Patients with a soft or moderately hard nucleus.
- Patients suitable for implantation of a foldable IOL.
- Patients operated under topical anesthesia.

## OPERATING ROOM CHANGES

The evolution of the surgical technique, from the sclero-corneal and limbal tunnels to the pure corneal tunnel, requires some changes to the classical organization of the operating room.

### Operating Table

The traditional table cannot be used because the surgeon must be able to sit in a comfortable position lateral to the patient and have full control over the foot pedals for the phacoemulsificator and the microscope.

For this reason, the base of the operating table must be small, leaving the space below the top half of the bed free for movement.

### Blepharostat (Retractor)

The surgeon should use a blepharostat that has been suitably modified for the temporal surgical approach. This will allow the surgeon to move more freely.

### Fixing Ring

In order to fix the bulb (under topical anesthesia) during the construction of the tunnel, a ring for bulbar fixation, such as Fine-Thornton's, can be used.

The same material used for the limbal and scleral incision can be used. Alternately, the surgeon can use diamond instruments with a preset, 3.2 mm blade fitted with micrometric screws to calibrate the protrusion of the blade. Only the tip of the blade must be sharp, not the sides (instruments by Asico Instruments); this instrument was not mentioned previously because stainless steel blades have reached such a high level of perfection, its use is superfluous in the creation of a tunnel in a sclero-corneal or limbal site. On the other hand, it is a useful tool when the surgeon has to create a tunnel in pure corneal tissue. The surgeon must remember that there is no margin for error permitted with diamond blades; stainless steel blades are more flexible from this point of view. So only surgeons with considerable experience should attempt these operations with diamond blades.

### Technique

A corneal tunnel always means the implantation of a soft IOL, and it often requires the operation to be performed under topical anesthesia. This will not completely immobilize the eyebulb, a fundamental element for the good creation of a corneal tunnel.

So, when the surgeon is performing the incision, he or she should use either a bulb-fixing ring (although the pressure it exerts may irritate the patient) or, better still, he or she should prepare a corneal wedge in a perilimbal position (using the same instruments used to create the side port incision) to allow the bulb to be steadied with a corneal forceps.

The patient is also asked to stare at the microscope's light, which will provide the most suitable position of the bulb. It will also be more comfortable for the surgeon and safer for the patient.

When the surgeon has decided on the method to use to fix the bulb, he or she can create the corneal tunnel using the technique that is more appropriate for the surgical requirements.

The corneal tunnel can be created on one plane in a single surgical step, on two planes in three surgical steps, or on two planes in three-dimensions in four steps.

#### *Incision on One Plane in One Surgical Step*

With a preset, acute 2.75 to 3.2 mm blade (the size depends on the dimensions of the phaco tip used), the corneal stroma is penetrated obliquely at the surface to half the thickness. By varying the inclination of the blade, it progresses for about 2 mm in the stroma, parallel to the corneal surface, and then enters the anterior chamber after a further variation in the inclination of the blade.

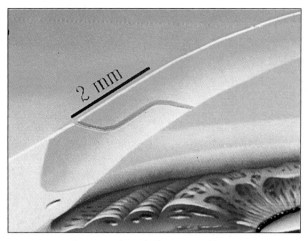

Figure 15-16. Creation of a one-plane corneal incision in one surgical step.

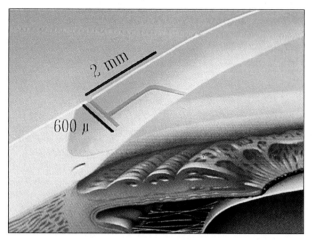

Figure 15-17. Incision on two planes in three surgical steps.

Table 15-1

## CORNEAL TUNNEL: EQUIPMENT AND TECHNIQUE BY BURATTO

| Technique | Instruments |
| --- | --- |
| Vertical preincision | Microknife with 30° blade (Alcon 5481). |
| Performance of intra-corneal delamination | Disk microknife (Alcon 6816). |
| Cutting lateral incisions | Microknife with 30° blade (Alcon 5481). |
| Entrance in the anterior chamber and incision for phaco (inside incision). | Angled 3.2 mm lancet microknife (Alcon 5485) or glazed (Alcon 93261). |
| Widening the incision to implant an AcrySof | Angled, glazed precalibrated 4.1 microknife (Alcon 64061). |
| Vertical incision | Half thickness (250-350 µm) for 4.0-4.2mm anteriorly to the vascular arcades temporal position (outer incision). |
| Formation of the tunnel | With the disc microknife the corneal tissue is cut—delaminated parallel to the epithelium in the depth of the preincision. |
| Lateral incision | Incision of the one or two lateral openings parallel to the iris plane Incision of about 1.2 mm inside and 1.7 mm outside lateral incisions are 70°-80° separate from the main opening one is on left and the other on the right of the main incision. |
| Viscoelastic | Injection of Provisc in anterior chamber. |
| Internal main incision | The 3.2 mm blade is introduced into the tunnel, the tip directed toward the lens anterior pole while the back is lifted (indentation). Penetration in the chamber is performed for the whole width of the blade. |

### Incision on Two Planes in Three Surgical Steps

#### Step 1

With a 30° blade, an incision is cut perpendicular to the corneal surface in front of the limbal vascular arches at a depth of about half the corneal thickness, with a width equal to the folded width of the soft IOL to be implanted.

#### Step 2

With a blade with a rounded tip, such as the bevel-up Crescent knife, the surgeon creates a tunnel of 2.0 to 2.5 mm in the corneal stroma.

#### Step 3

The surgeon uses a blade with an acute tip (of size variable between 2.75 and 3.2 mm) to enter the anterior chamber at the end of the newly formed tunnel with the blade inclined downward.

Once the cortical masses have been removed and the capsular bag and anterior chamber have been filled with VES, the incision is extended further with a preset blade to allow the folded IOL to enter.

If diamond instruments with preset blades fitted with micrometric screws are used, the following technique is used:

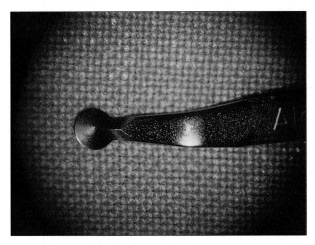

Figure 15-18. Disk knife (Alcon 968161).

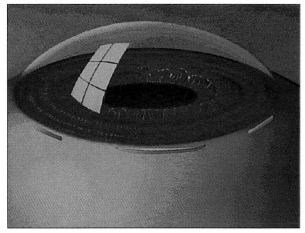

Figure 15-19. Side port incision.

### Step 1
A perpendicular incision is cut to two-thirds the thickness of the wall (about 600 µm) in clear cornea immediately in front of the limbal vascular arches for a length of between 3.5 and 4.0 mm depending on the model and the material of the foldable lens to be implanted.

### Step 2
Using the same instruments, a tunnel of about 2 mm is created in the corneal stroma (at a depth of about 300 µm). The surgeon enters the anterior chamber by changing the inclination of the blade at the end of the tunnel. The creation of the horizontal portion of the tunnel is begun prior to the end of the perpendicular incision, which gives greater flexibility in the architecture of the entire incision. It also guarantees improved impermeability of the surgical wound at the end of the operation.

### Step 3
The tunnel is widened, using a preset steel blade with a blunt tip or a diamond blade, to receive the optic disc of the soft lens, which the surgeon has decided to implant.

#### Incision on Two Planes in Three Dimensions in Four Steps
A further step is added to the previous method; the tunnel is widened using disk knife 968161 by Alcon Surgical (diameter of the blade 2.25 mm) without changing the size of the internal and external limits of the tunnel itself. This extension makes the tunnel more elastic, which facilitates the passage of the IOL.

Advantages of the corneal tunnel include the following:
- Absence of postoperative conjunctival and scleral inflammation (white eye from the first day postoperative).
- Ease of access to the anterior chamber.
- Ease of movement with the phaco tip and suction in the anterior chamber.
- Ease of implantation of the IOL particularly if the material is foldable.
- Rapid healing of the corneal epithelium.
- Low degree of induced astigmatism.
- Topical anesthesia can be used.
- Rapid visual rehabilitation.

Disadvantages include the following:
- Possible severe postoperative astigmatism in the event a suture is placed incorrectly because of a badly prepared tunnel.
- Possibility of irregular tunnel walls because of corneal edema, secondary to prolonged use of the ultrasound tip (hard nucleus).

## SIDE PORT INCISION
A side port incision is a small limbal incision about 0.5 mm wide, cut 90° from the main incision. Its natural position is to the left, but some surgeons prefer to cut a second one to the right of the main incision.

A 15 or 30° blade is recommended.

### Technique
The surgeon enters the anterior chamber in the limbal position and progresses slightly in an oblique direction through the stroma.

Advantages include the following:
- Possibility of introducing a spatula into the anterior chamber to manipulate the nucleus during the procedures of phacoemulsification.
- Possibility of manual completion of aspiration of the cortical residues at 12 o'clock, if the surgeon does not have Buratto's double handle available.
- The surgeon can fill the anterior chamber at the end of the operation, to check the satisfactory sealing of the valve-incision.
- The soft IOL can be manipulated when it is being implanted.

## REFERENCES
1. Shepherd JR. Induced astigmatism in small incision cataract surgery. *J Cataract Refract Surg*. 1989;15(1):85-88.
2. Sanders DR, Barnet RW, Brind SF, Ernest PH, Faulkner

ED, Fine H, McFarland MS. Symposium: preferred techniques for single-stitch cataract/IOL surgery. *Ocular Surg News* (suppl), Nov. 15, 1989.

3. Neumann AC, McCarty GL, Sanders DR, Raanan MR. Small incision to control astigmatism during cataract surgery. *J Cataract Refract Surg*. 1989;15:78.

4. Masket S. Astigmatic analysis of the scleral pocket incision and closure technique for cataract surgery. *CLAO Journal*. 1985;11:206-209.

5. Sanders DR, et al. Effect of incision size and suture configuration on induced astigmatism and visual rehabilitation. In: Gills JP, Sanders DR, eds. *Small Incision Cataract Surgery*. Thorofare, NJ: SLACK Inc. 1990:15-25.

6. Fine H. *Chip-and-flip phacoemulsification technique with infinity suture closure, phacoemulsification surgery and intraocular lens implantation*. Thorofare, NJ: SLACK Inc; 1992:3-22.

7. Cimberle U, Dal Fiume E. *Tipi di incisione: imparare la faco*. Milano: Fogliazza Ed. 1992:29-48.

8. Buratto L. *Iridectomia e sutura: chirurgia extracapsulare della cataratta*. 1987:251-256.

9. Eisner G. *Chirurgia dell'occhio*. Milano: Fogliazza Ed. 1992:4-118.

# Chapter 16

# THE LIMBAL INCISION
*Paul H. Ernest, MD*

## INTRODUCTION

### Background

The invention of the intraocular lens (IOL) and the development of new surgical techniques and tools to implant them has dramatically changed the way cataracts are treated. Eye surgeons have explored various incision sites, operative approaches, suture techniques, and wound configurations in their efforts to minimize trauma while restoring the best possible vision.

The advent of the foldable IOL and advances in device technologies have led to significant refinements in small incision surgery and wound closure that are revolutionizing the practice of cataract surgery. These clinical advances are leading to reductions in iatrogenic ocular trauma and postoperative astigmatism, decreased risk of hyphema, delayed filtering blebs and iris prolapse, increased wound stability, and faster recovery and vision restoration.[1-3]

### Historical Perspective

Cataract surgery techniques have evolved substantially over the years. The two-step (two-plane) limbal incision, with its perpendicular incision into the sclera and subsequent beveled incision into the anterior chamber, was used for many years. In the mid 1970s, Dr. Richard Kratz was credited with inaugurating the modern era of wound construction with his development of the scleral tunnel incision (ie, the scleral pocket incision) as an alternative to the conventional limbal incision. In January 1990, Dr. Michael McFarland contributed the next evolution—a sutureless closure.[4] He suggested that if the incision started sufficiently behind the surgical limbus and the scleral tunnel was kept very narrow, vertical cuts made in the floor to give the tunnel a spreading effect would return together following the insertion of an implant.

In February 1990, Dr. Ernest determined that the presence of an internal corneal lip was more important than having a long scleral tunnel with vertical cuts, because it could prevent hyphemas and delayed filtering blebs, as well as avoid fluid loss from the anterior chamber. Hence, Dr. Ernest modified the scleral tunnel technique into a three-step procedure with the addition of the internal corneal lip (also known as the corneal valve incision).[1,5]

The parameters and advantages of this incision were determined in a cadaver eye model in which scleral corneal incisions that have a square configuration and incorporate a 1.5 mm internal corneal lip were shown to be more stable then either rectangular scleral corneal wounds or square scleral corneal wounds where the internal lip was smaller than 1.5 mm.

The greater wound stability was attributed to the square wound configuration.[6] Ernest's three-step procedure consists of a perpendicular incision through the sclera, a horizontal incision into clear cornea, and an angled, beveled incision into the anterior chamber. The 4.0 mm wide wound incision starts approximately 2.0 mm behind the surgical limbus.

Because the three-step approach leaves an internal lip of endothelium, Descemet's membrane, and corneal stroma that self-seals once intraocular pressure (IOP) returns to normal, this technique eliminates suture-related foreign body sensation, avoids suture needle damage to the ciliary body, prevents hyphemas and delayed filtering blebs, increases wound stability, and causes only minimal iatrogenic astigmatism.[5-10]

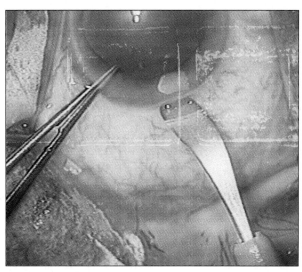

Figure 16-1. A Crescent blade is used to make an incision at the surgical limbus.

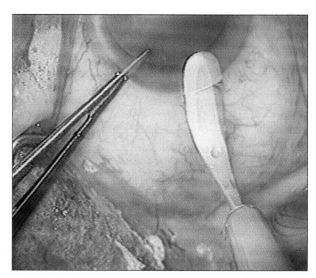

Figure 16-2. A Crescent blade is used to dissect approximately 2.0 mm of clear cornea.

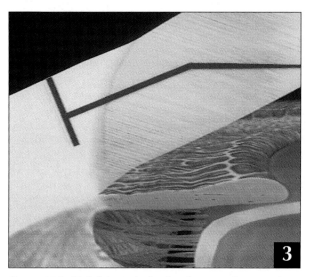

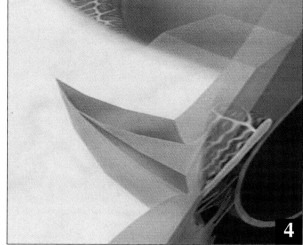

Figures 16-3, 16-4. Schematic drawing demonstrating wound construction.

## THE LIMBAL INCISION

### Anesthesia

The ability to perform modern cataract surgery with smaller, square-wound configurations has facilitated the use of the temporal approach instead of the over-the-eyebrow, superior approach. With this technique, topical anesthesia has replaced the local and periocular injections of anesthetic that would otherwise be necessary.

Prior to instillation of dilating drops, topical fl% Marcaine is instilled in the operative eye. The fl% Marcaine is again instilled prior to preparation of the eye using Betadine solution. Following completion of the paracentesis incision, 1% Xylocaine preservative-free is instilled in the anterior chamber. A waiting period of 10 seconds is taken. Viscoat (Alcon) is then instilled in the anterior chamber to give the eye the necessary firmness.

### The Limbal Incision Procedure

After instillation of Viscoat, the surgeon next inserts a closed 0.12 forceps to the paracentesis incision, gently opening it once inside to stabilize the globe. An incision is then made in the anterior limbal area, using a Crescent blade (Alcon) in the inverted position. The depth of the scleral incision should be one-half its thickness. Approximately 2.0 mm of clear cornea should be dissected with the Crescent blade.

A 3.2 mm keratome blade (Alcon) is then passed through the dissected tunnel incision, and an internal corneal lip is carefully fashioned. The surgeon should use the 0.12 forceps to draw the eye toward the tip of the keratome blade with one hand, while slowly passing the keratome blade through Descemet's membrane with the other. The resulting incision should be horizontal.

Surgeons should be particularly careful when making this cut through Descemet's membrane. Should the ante-

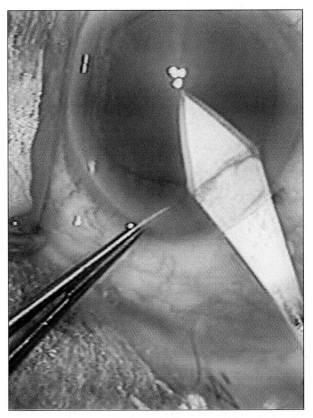

Figure 16-5. A 3.2 mm keratome blade is passed through the dissected tunnel incision and an internal corneal lip is carefully made.

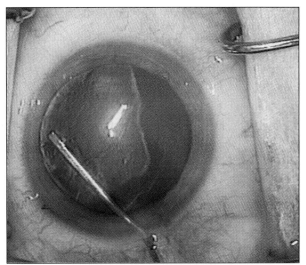

Figure 16-6. Hydrocortical cleavage is performed to separate the capsular-cortical attachments.

rior chamber be overinflated with viscoelastic—making the IOP very high—passing the keratome blade through Descemet's membrane will result in a triangular rather than horizontal cut. Making the cut too quickly or angling the keratome blade too sharply downward will also cause a triangular rather than a linear, horizontal cut through Descemet's membrane.

Following the formation of the internal corneal lip incision, the surgeon retracts both the keratome blade and the 0.12 forceps. A cystotome is then used to make a triangular flap through the central aspect of the anterior capsule. A curvilinear capsulorhexis, 5 mm in diameter, is then fashioned with Utrata forceps. The next step— hydrocortical cleavage to separate the capsular-cortical attachments and hydrocortical dissection to delineate the central nucleus from the epinucleus—is achieved using a spatula-style cannula attached to a syringe filled with balanced salt solution (BSS) (Alcon).

Using phacoemulsification, perpendicular grooves are fashioned through the central nucleus to a depth of 60%. A cyclodialysis spatula inserted through the paracentesis incision is used to steady the globe during phacoemulsification. After the procedure, the surgeon removes the spatula and inserts an Ernest nuclear cracking forceps (Katena) to crack the nucleus. The viscoelastic solution is used to protect the corneal endothelium during the cracking procedure, as well as to give adequate depth to the anterior chamber.

The Ernest forceps are removed, the phacoemulsification handpiece and cyclodialysis spatula are reinserted, and the central nucleus is removed. The epinucleus and its cortical attachments are removed using the pulsed phacoemulsification mode. Residual cortical material is removed with the irrigation/aspiration (I/A) handpiece. Viscoelastic is then used to inflate the capsular bag and to deepen the anterior chamber.

Next, a multipieced IOL (AMO SI40 style, Allergan, AcrySof MA30, Alcon) is folded longitudinally, using an Ernest-McDonald II forceps (Katena), with the leading loop tucked in upon itself. The lens is inserted through the temporal incision, while a cyclodialysis spatula inserted through the paracentesis incision is used to steady the globe. Once the lens is in the anterior chamber, the leading loop is passed under the edge of the capsulorhexis, and the lens is released.

After the trailing loop is dialed into the capsular bag, the I/A handpiece is inserted. All viscoelastic material must be removed, including any trapped behind the lens. BSS is then injected through the incision site to deepen the anterior chamber and to ensure that the inner aspect of the internal corneal lip incision has not rolled back upon itself.

The surgeon should then apply point force to the posterior aspect of the incision on high and low IOP levels to test the wound's resistance to pressure. Cauterization of the conjunctiva and closure are unnecessary. It is not necessary to cauterize the minor capillary bleeding that may occur from the limbal incision.

## Intraoperative Solutions

Antibiotics are routinely injected into the BSS used in the phacoemulsification I/A procedure, as well as in the syringes for hydrocortical cleavage, hydrodelineation, and formation of the anterior chamber at the conclusion of the operation. A commercially available, 500 mL container of BSS can be injected by the pharmacy with 20 mg of Vancomycin and 10 mg of Tobramycin. Thus, subconjunctival injection of antibiotics is unnecessary. An appropriate quantity of epinephrine is also injected into the 500 mL bottle of BSS to maintain pupil dilation and eliminate

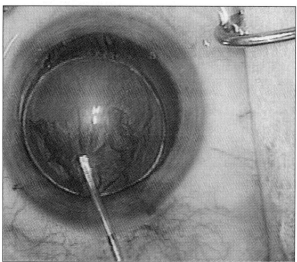

Figure 16-7. In hydrocortical dissection, a spatula-style cannula attached to a syringed filled with BSS is used to delineate the central nucleus from the epinucleus.

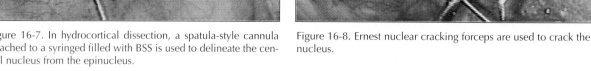

Figure 16-8. Ernest nuclear cracking forceps are used to crack the nucleus.

microbleeding from the episclera or conjunctiva incision. An eye patch is unnecessary, and the patient can see immediately.

## ADVANTAGES AND BENEFITS OF THE LIMBAL INCISION

The limbal incision has several advantages over the currently advocated clear corneal incision. Clear corneal incisions, especially those that have a vertical component, are more subject to foreign body sensation than limbal incisions. This irritation occurs because there is edema of both the anterior and posterior aspects of the incision in clear corneal incisions with vertical components, which creates a gape in the most superficial aspect of the incision. In turn, this gape forms a ridge that can irritate the patient.

The clear corneal incision is said to allow faster surgery without disturbing the conjunctiva. Experience with the limbal incision, however, shows its speed to be the same. Moreover, the minimal disturbance from limbal incisions rarely, if ever, results in subconjunctival hemorrhage. Based upon clinical experience, foreign body sensation with the limbal incision is less than that associated with clear corneal incisions.

A further concern regarding clear corneal incisions is wound stability. In cadaver eye studies, as rectangular clear corneal wounds were made more square by only 0.5 mm—from 3.2 mm x 2.0 mm to 3.2 mm x 2.5 mm—they became more resistant to pressure.[11] Once the length was increased so that the wound was square (3.2 mm x 3.2 mm) with a 1.5 mm internal corneal lip, they were capable of withstanding maximum external pressures of 525 psi. The square incision, whether scleral corneal or clear corneal, provides maximum resistance to external pressure at that level. Although square clear corneal incisions are clinically impractical either because they encroach upon the visual axis or because they are too small to be operated through, they clearly establish the incision's greater inherent stability.

In their fourth cadaver study of clear corneal incisions, Ernest et al reported that non-square clear corneal incisions have a critical width depending on wound construction.[12] Ernest et al later reported when incisions of exactly the same dimensions (width, length, and construction type) were made at the limbus and in clear cornea, the ones at the limbus demonstrated greater wound stability. The reason for this is not completely clear. It may be that the architecture of the limbus, with its circumferential fibers, allows greater resistance than the radial fibers of the cornea. The limbus also contains more elastic fibers than the cornea, which has none.[13]

## VECTOR ANALYSIS AND VISUAL RESULTS

In a recently published study of patients who had surgery with the temporal limbal incision, Ernest and associates compared the results with those of patients who had a 3.2 mm limbal incision superiorly—where peritomy incision through the conjunctiva was performed and cautery was used. Another set of reference patients had a 4.0 mm square scleral corneal wound performed with a superior approach. All of the 4.0 mm patients underwent substantial conjunctival dissection as well as cautery.

The 4.0 mm incision had significantly more diopters (D) of induced cylinder and much more axis change on Jaffe and Cravy vector analyses because of the cautery and the amount of dissection of the tissue. When the patients who underwent temporal limbal incisions were compared with those who underwent the superior limbal incisions, the results were essentially the same after 2 postoperative weeks, although the temporal limbal incision has less induced cylinder on day one.

The results achieved in 69 patients who underwent cataract surgery with the temporal approach (3.2 mm

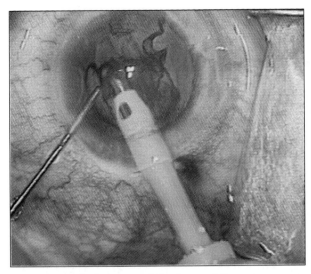

Figure 16-9. Pulsed phacoemulsification mode is used to remove the epinucleus and its cortical attachments.

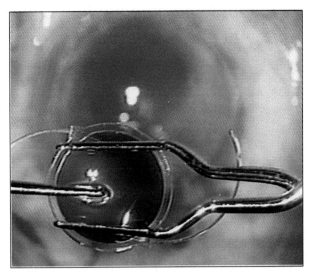

Figure 16-10. Ernest-McDonald forceps are used to longitudinally fold a multipieced silicone lens AMO SI40.

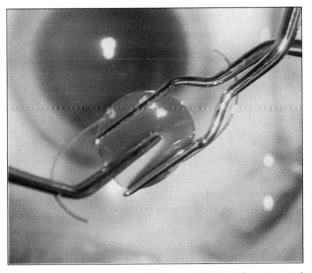

Figure 16-11. Ernest-McDonald forceps folding Alcon AcrySof MA30 lens.

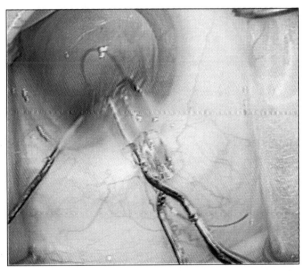

Figure 16-12. The AMO SI40 lens is inserted through the temporal incision while a cyclodialysis spatula through the paracentesis incision is used to steady the globe.

incision) versus 75 who had the conventional superior approach (3.2 mm incision) (unpublished data) suggest improvements in immediate postoperative visual acuity with greater benefit at 2 weeks post-surgery. Visual acuity was assessed on the first postoperative day and again at 14 days.

On the first postoperative day, only 24% of the patients who were operated on via the superior approach had uncorrected visual acuity of 20/40 or better, compared with 55% of the temporal surgery patients. At 14 days, 71% of the superior approach patients had achieved uncorrected visual acuity of 20/40 or better versus 81% of the temporal patients. The temporal approach results in better first postoperative day visual acuity for two reasons: less corneal folding and, consequently, less corneal edema. Any edema that is present is also further from the visual axis.

## PROCEDURAL PRECAUTIONS

Surgeons who perform the limbal incision procedures should observe several precautions. Steps should be taken to minimize fluid loss during phacoemulsification and I/A to prevent ballooning of the conjunctiva, which can obscure visualization during surgery. This can be accomplished by using one of the newer handpieces designed for safe insertion through tight wounds without cauterization of the incision site. The amount of phacoemulsification time needed for sculpting can be reduced if the surgeon uses more beveled tips in working with particularly dense nuclei. Careful hydrocortical cleavage technique can eliminate the need for I/A.

If ballooning of the conjunctiva does occur, a small peritomy through the conjunctiva posterior to the limbal incision corrects the problem. Epinephrine in the irrigating solution prevents subconjunctival hemorrhage.

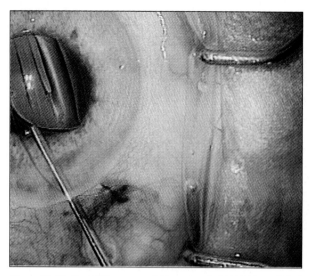

Figure 16-13. The trailing coop of Alcon AcrySof MA30 lens dialed into capsular bag.

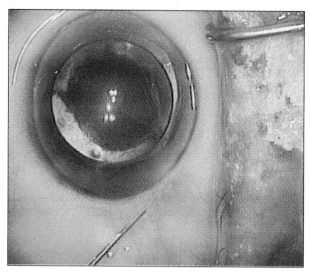

Figure 16-14. High- and low-point force is applied to the posterior aspect of the incision to test the wound's resistance to pressure.

The presence of a minimal amount of postoperative chemosis of the conjunctiva is beneficial for two reasons. The first is the presence of antibiotics within the conjunctiva to prevent infection. Second, slight chemosis causes the plane of the conjunctival incision to be at a different level than the plane of the scleral incision, thereby protecting the external aspect of the wound.

## THE THEORY OF ENDOTHELIAL PUMP

There have been numerous critics of cadaver eye models, some who claim that there is a physiologic mechanism, mainly an endothelial pump, that is a significant component in wound stability.

Dr. Carlos DeFigueiredo performed a living rabbit model comparing clear corneal incisions of three types—paracentesis, hinged, and square wound. Stromal hydration was performed in each of the incisions. He observed within 15 to 20 minutes the stromal edema had cleared in each incision type, due to the endothelial pump mechanism. Upon testing each wound with pinpoint pressure, he found the paracentesis incision was the least stable. The hinged incision was eight times more stable than the paracentesis. The square wound configuration was at least 20 times more stable than the paracentesis. His conclusion was that endothelial pump was only important in removal of stromal fluid and that wound configuration and construction were the predominant factors in early wound stability.[14]

## WILLS FELINE STUDY

Dr. Richard Tipperman, Dr. Chris Kardasis, and Dr. Ernest performed a feline study evaluating limbal versus clear corneal incisions.[15] A total of 30 cats were used. The right eye of each cat had a clear corneal incision; the left eye had a limbal incision. The incision dimensions were non-square 3.0 mm in width, 1.75 mm in length. A paracentesis type incision was made in each case. Reformation of the anterior chamber and stromal hydration were not performed.

The eyes were observed over a period of 16 days. Pinpoint pressure was applied to each eye at various time intervals. Histologic evaluation of the eyes occurred at 1 week, 1 month, and 2 month intervals.

The results showed a statistically significant difference in resistance to pinpoint deformation pressure between the limbal and paracentesis incision ($P=0.0034$). Histologic evaluations at 1 week showed no healing activity of the clear corneal incision. The limbal incision, whether it was placed anteriorly or posteriorly, showed a significant fibroblastic response causing the wound to seal. At the 2 month time interval, the clear corneal incision did heal in a manner similar to that of a corneal transplant. The degree of healing was not to the same level as the fibroblastic response in the limbal incision.

## CONCLUSION

The limbal incision is not only safe and effective, but is superior to the clear corneal incision because of its greater postoperative wound stability and lack of foreign body sensation. The ability to stretch limbal tissue compared to corneal tissue was also an advantage. Surgical time is efficient and comparable with other approaches. The limbal incision can also be formed by a temporal approach with the use of topical anesthesia. Patients are not only able to see immediately after surgery, but more likely achieve better vision than 20/40 visual acuity on the first postoperative day.

Because of the greater wound stability, patients do not require protective eyewear, either after surgery or when they sleep. Consequently, they may return to work sooner than with other techniques and enjoy recreational activities without fear of damaging or reinjuring the eye. Thus, limbal incision surgery may be considered economic and efficient as well as visually restorative and cosmetic.

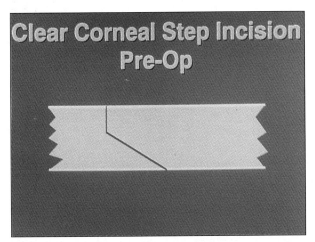

Figure 16-15. Schematic drawing of a clear corneal incision prior to phacoemulsification.

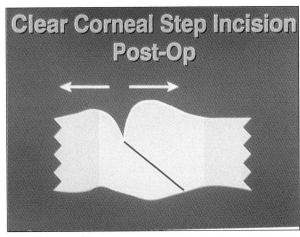

Figure 16-16. Schematic drawing of a clear corneal incision post-phacoemulsification showing cornea edema and ridge.

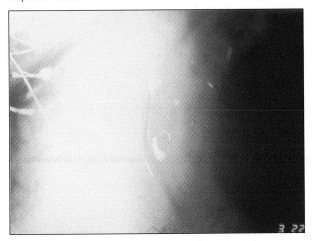

Figure 16-17. Slit lamp picture of a patient 1 day post-clear corneal incision showing corneal ridge and corneal edema.

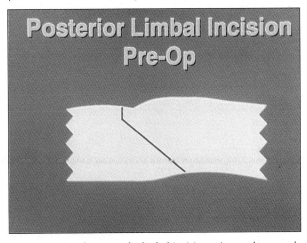

Figure 16-18. Schematic of a limbal incision prior to phacoemulsification.

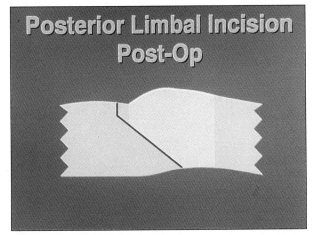

Figure 16-19. Schematic of a limbal incision post-phacoemulsification showing edema of the corneal tunnel, but no edema of the incision.

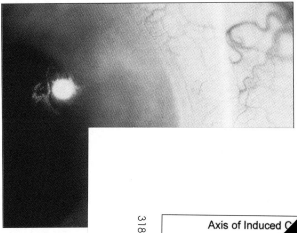

Figure 16-20. Show... sion showing no e...

## REFERENCES

1. Ernest PH, Kiessling LA, Lavery KT. Relative strength of cataract incisions in cadaver eyes. *J Cataract Refract Surg.* 1991;17(suppl):668-671.
2. Koch PS. Structural analysis of cataract incision construction. *J Cataract Refract Surg.* 1991;17(suppl):661-667.
3. Obstbaum S... improved stability... *Refrac Surg.* 1991;1...
4. McFarland... The first modern... Sanders DR, eds...

Table 16-1
## JAFFE VECTOR ANALYSIS
## MEAN DIOPTERS OF INDUCED CYLINDER (STANDARD DEVIATION)

| Exam | 3.2 mm temporal limbal | 3.2 mm superior limbal | 4 mm superior scleral corneal |
|---|---|---|---|
| 1 day | 0.66 (0.44) | 0.97 (0.68) | 1.54 (0.96) |
| 2-3 weeks | 0.65 (0.45) | 0.65 (0.49) | 1.11 (0.59) |
| 1-3 months | 0.62 (0.47) | 0.50 (0.38) | 0.98 (0.66) |
| 4-8 months | 0.58 (0.32) | 0.58 (0.52) | 0.74 (0.46) |
| 1 year | | | 0.66 (0.32) |
| 2 years | | | 0.91 (1.01) |

Table 16-2
## CRAZY VECTOR ANALYSIS
## MEAN AXIS OF INDUCED CYLINDER (STANDARD DEVIATION)

| Exam | 3.2 mm temporal limbal | 3.2 mm superior limbal | 4 mm superior scleral corneal |
|---|---|---|---|
| 1 day | 0.40 (0.66) | -0.26 (1.20) | 0.88 (1.49) |
| 2-3 weeks | 0.14 (0.82) | -0.11 (0.76) | 0.74 (1.01) |
| 1-3 months | 0.19 (0.74) | -0.15 (0.61) | 0.43 (1.17) |
| 4-8 months | 0.05 (0.60) | -0.04 (0.83) | 0.06 (0.86) |
| 1 year | | | -0.17 (0.74) |
| 2 years | | | -0.69 (0.73) |

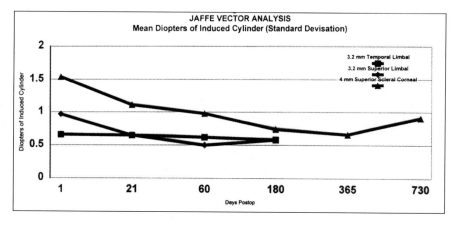

Figure 16-21. Vector analysis of induced cylinder/Jaffe.

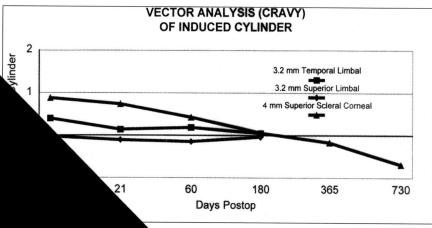

Figure 16-22. Vector analysis of induced cylinder/Cravy.

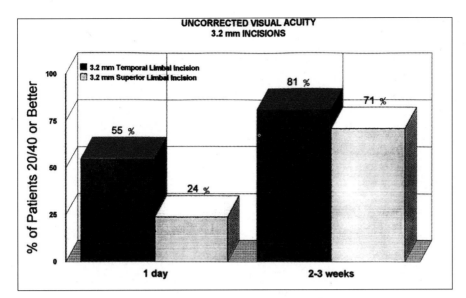

Figure 16-23. Uncorrected visual acuity/3.2 mm incisions.

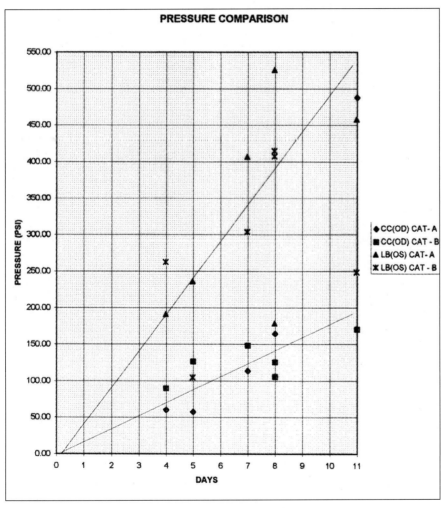

Figure 16-24. Graph comparing resistance deformation pressure for clear corneal and limbal incisions over time.

Table 16-3

## UNCORRECTED VISUAL ACUITY % OF PATIENTS WITH 20/40 OR BETTER

| Exam | 3.2 mm temporal limbal incision | 3.2 mm superior limbal incision |
| --- | --- | --- |
| 1 day | 55% | 24% |
| 2-3 weeks | 81% | 71% |

Table 16-4

## UNPAIRED T-TEST FOR PRESSURE GROUPING VARIABLE: TECHNIQUE HYPOTHESIZED DIFFERENCE

| | Mean difference | DF | T-value | P-value |
| --- | --- | --- | --- | --- |
| CC, LB | -0.319 | 22 | -3.278 | 0.0034 |

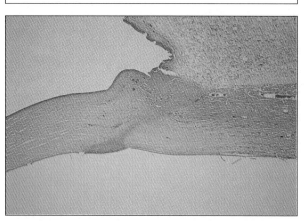

Figure 16-25. Limbal incision 1 week post-surgery demonstrating significant fibroblastic activity completely sealing the incision.

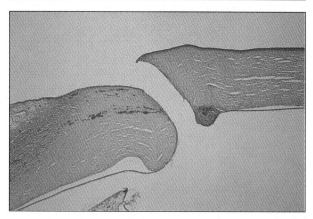

Figure 16-26. Clear corneal incision 1 week post-surgery showing no wound healing.

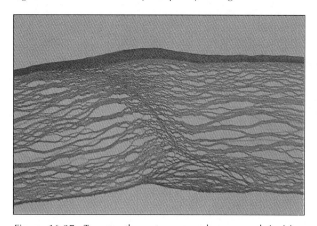

Figure 16-27. Two-month post-surgery clear corneal incision demonstrating the incision is healed through binding of the stromal keratocytes as seen in corneal transplant surgery.

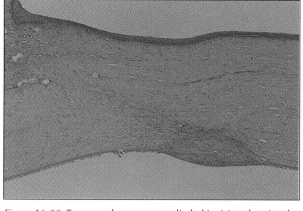

Figure 16-28. Two-month post-surgery limbal incision showing the same fibroblastic activity and the same degree of healing as 1 week post-surgery.

SLACK Inc; 1992:3-5.

5. Ernest PH. *Grand Rounds Lecture and Patient Presentation: Single Stitch Cataract Surgery.* Kresge Eye Institute, Wayne State University, Detroit, Michigan. Feb 1990.

6. Ernest PH, Lavery KT, Kiessling LA. Relative strength of scleral tunnel incisions with internal corneal lips constructed in cadaver eyes. *J Cataract Refract Surg.* 1993;19:457-461.

7. Ernest PH. The corneal lip tunnel incision. *J Cataract Refract Surg.* 1994;20:154-157.

8. Ernest PH. The self-sealing sutureless wound: Engineering aspects and experimental studies. In: Gills JP, Martin RG, Sanders DR, eds. *Sutureless Cataract Surgery.* Thorofare, NJ: SLACK Inc; 1992:23-39.

9. Fine IH. Architecture and construction of a self-sealing incision for cataract surgery. *J Cataract Refract Surg.* 1991;17(suppl):672-676.

10. Masket S. One year postoperative astigmatic comparison of sutured and unsutured 4.0 mm scleral pocket incisions. *J Cataract Refract Surg.* 1993;19:453-456.

11. Ernest PH, Lavery KT, Kiessling LA. Relative strengths of scleral corneal and clear corneal incisions constructed in cadaver eyes. *J Cataract Refract Surg.* 1994;21:39-42.

12. Ernest PH, Lavery KT, Kiessling LA. Relative strength of scleral corneal and clear corneal incisions constructed in cadaver eyes. *J Cataract Refract Surg.* 1994;20:626-629.

13. Ernest PH, Neuhann, T. Posterior limbal incision. *J Cataract Refract Surg.* 1996;22:78-84.

14. DeFigueiredo CG. Relative strength of clear corneal incision sealed by organic glue in the rabbit eye. Presented at the American Society of Cataract and Refractive Surgery annual meeting, April 1995, San Diego, CA.

15. Ernest PH, Tipperman, R, Kardassis C, Lavery, KT, Sensoli AM. The Healing Process Based on Incision Location. Presented at the American Society of Cataract and Refractive Surgery annual meeting, June 1996, Seattle, WA.

# Chapter 17

# CAPSULORHEXIS: PRINCIPLES AND TECHNIQUES

*Aldo Caporossi, MD*
*Stefano Baiocchi, MD*
*Paolo Frezzotti, MD*

## THE HISTORY

The objective of cataract surgery using an extracapsular technique is to maintain a space between the anterior segment and the vitreal chamber while maintaining the bag intact. The incision methods (can opener, Christmas tree, etc) used to open the anterior capsule allow the surgeon to reach this objective immediately, but in the long-term, the rough, asymmetrical edges condition the stability of the pseudo-phaco inside the posterior chamber, through the stress lines of non-uniform size and direction. Development of the surgical procedure (envelope), which provides a more regular incision edge, has possibly improved but not eliminated this problem; the cut is still asymmetrical, and this causes stress lines that are markedly weighted in one direction. Through the intuition of Gimbel, Neuhann, and Shimizu, a symmetrical, well-centered tear method—continuous circular capsulorhexis (CCC)—was presented. It has the great advantage of long-term stability.

## ANATOMY

The lens capsule is a basal membrane rich in carbohydrates and therefore strongly positive to PAS staining. The capsule appears to be very uniform when examined under the optical microscope. However, when observed under TEM, it shows an ultra-structure with very fine filaments, a network of Type IV collagen tetramers linked together by small globular components (NC1-domains). In the young eye, the thickness at the anterior pole is about 8 µm but only 2 µm at the posterior pole; in the equatorial region, this thickness varies between 8 µm and 12 µm. The preequatorial regions are particularly thick, reaching 15 µm anteriorly and 22 µm posteriorly.

In adulthood, the preequatorial region can thicken to a mean value of 21 µm, while the posterior thickness remains constant. The lens is supported by four bundles of zonular fibers that are inserted in the anterior, posterior, and equatorial surfaces of the capsular bag. The posterior orbicular-capsular fibers can be clearly observed; they originate more posteriorly and proceed along a curve that follows the shape of ciliary body from their origin point, close to the ora serrata to their insertion located peripherally to Wieger's capsular hyaloid ligament. In sections, these fibers run in front of the anterior vitreal surface. They are small in number and large in size.

The anterior orbicular-capsular fibers are the thickest and largest of the system; originating in the posterior part of the pars plana, they proceed in large bundles to the insertion zone situated 1.5 to 2 mm in front of the lens equator in the younger patient. In older patients, the insertion point tends to anteriorize by as much as 2 mm. The posterior cilio-capsular fibers are thin strips; they are the most numerous of the zonular component. They originate in the grooves of the ciliary processes and then proceed axially and posteriorly, crossing the anterior cilio-equatorial fibers to insert posterior to the posterior orbicular-capsular fibers.

The equatorial ciliary fibers are very numerous and thin in the young patients but are absent in patients older than 80. They originate in the anterior portion of the apex of the ciliary processes and proceed to the equatorial region of the lens. As the anterior fibers are inserted 1.5 to 2 mm from the equator in young human lenses, the anterior surfaces—free from zonular fibers—normally have a diameter of 6.5 to 7 mm, which can drop to 4 mm in very elderly patients or in patients with uveal pathologies.

Abnormal insertion of the anterior zonular fibers can sometimes be observed, and the free area may be just 2 mm in diameter. If the surgeon is familiar with all these anatomical features, it will help him or her overcome any

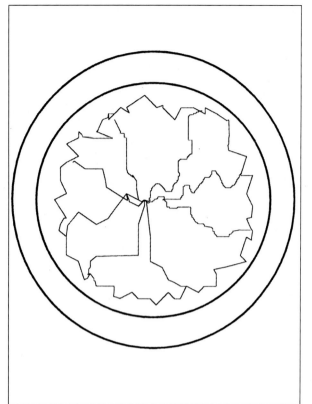

Figure 17-1. The coarctation vectors in the can opener capsulotomy.

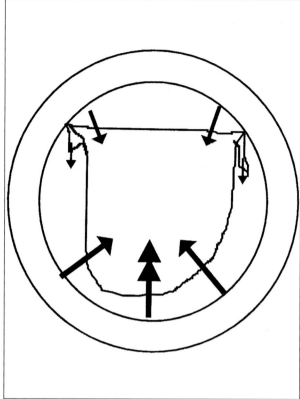

Figure 17-2. The coarctation vectors in the envelope capsulotomy.

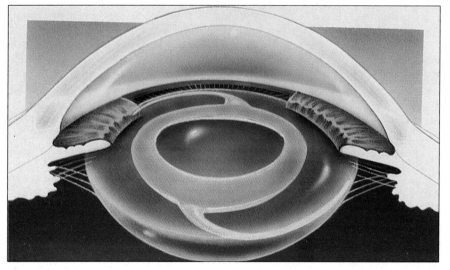

Figure 17-3. CCC with an IOL implanted in the capsular bag.

difficulties should there be an anterior capsular opening during the operation.

## TECHNIQUE

Capsulorhexis is performed on a surface that is convex and rounded anteriorly; the anterior capsule is stable and distended under the effect of the fibers (which contain the capsule) and the endocapsular thrust, and through the radial traction that the zonules exert on the bag. For these reasons, it is important that the surgeon begins to tear the CCC near the center of the surface. Once the capsule has been opened, the endocapsular pressure exerted by the contents of the bag on the anterior capsule is expressed through two vectors: one directed posterior-anteriorly, which will tend to raise the capsular flap, and one directed centrifugally (radially), which will tend to bring the edges of the opening toward the equatorial region. These radial centrifugal forces work in harmony with the tractional vector determined by the zonular fibers and facilitate the progression of the tear from the center toward the equator.

Table 17-1
**PATIENT TO BE SUBJECTED TO CAPSULORHEXIS**

A) Optimal conditions for a capsulorhexis
   1. Absence of enophthalmus
   2. Nuclear opacity of moderate hardness (high retro illumination grading)
   3. Wide, regular mydriasis
   4. Anterior chamber of normal depth
   5. Perfect transparency of the cornea
   6. Hypermature intact zonular apparatus
   7. Absence of situations which favor the vitreal thrust
   8. Efficacious anesthesia and akinesia

B) Non-optimal conditions for capsulorhexis
   1. Enophthalmic bulb or markedly reduced eyelid rim
   2. Low retroillumination grading
   3. Capsular pathologies
   4. Poor mydriasis
   5. Poor depth of the Anterior chamber
   6. Over-ripe cataract or with degenerative capsular processes
   7. Zonular pathologies
   8. Imperfect transparency of the cornea
   9. Presence of non-dissectable irido-capsular synechiae

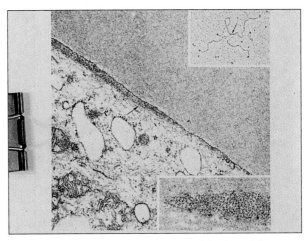

Figure 17-4. Faintly fibriller architecture of the human lens capsule. Actin filaments (arrow) at edge of lens epithelial cell (X 65,500). Upper insert—Typical tetramer of Collagen IV from bovine lens capsule. The four molecules are linked together in the center by their carboxy terminal ends (7S region—arrow) (X 108,000). Lower insert—Fibrillar inclusion from mid lens capsule (X 70,000). (From Albert and Jackobiek. *Principi e Pratica di Oftalmologia*, Vol 1 p. 608.)

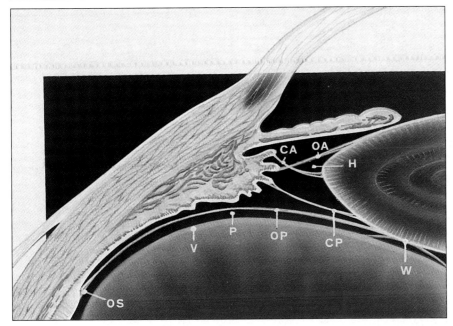

Figure 17-5. Diagrammatic representation to show the main systems of zonular fibers.
OP: Orbiculo-posterior capsular fibers.
OS: Ora Serrata.
OA: Orbiculo-anterior capsular fibers.
CP: Cilio-posterior capsular fibers.
CA: Cilio-equatorial capsular fibers.
V: Vitreous.
W: Hyaloideo-capsular ligament of Wieger.
P: Canal of Petit.
H: Canal of Hannover.
(From Duke-Elder: *System of Ophthalmology*. Vol II p. 337 modified.)

Once the tear has been started, in order to completely understand how the CCC will be completed, we feel it is useful to go over some physical principles regarding the mechanics of the tear. There are two basic theoretical principles for tearing the anterior capsule. It requires two different amounts of force applied in a conceptually different manner. However, they can produce similar effects through very different physical principles:

1. Tearing by coplanar orthogonal traction (tearing by stretching).

The traction force is applied along a traction plane that is the same as the material to be torn but which is the plane of maximum resistance to the tear. The force is applied perpendicular to the direction of the tear; to obtain the tear, the surgeon must apply a force superior to the resistance of the capsule, which as we said is at a maximum on this plane. This principle of tearing was presented by Gimbel and Neuhann, and the authors use it simply because exerting traction on the free flap of the capsulorhexis, pulling it toward the center of the lens to continue the tear in a circular direction, will mean that the tear will not escape out-of-control toward the equator. So, in order to obtain a variation of the tear direction, either toward the center or externally, the surgeon

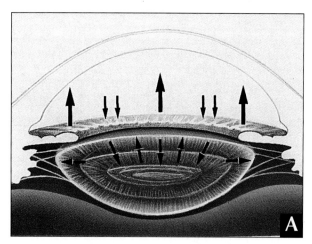

Figure 17-6A. Anterior-posterior vector raises the capsular flap.

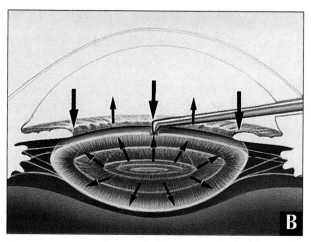

Figure 17-6B. Centrifugal (radial) vector will bring edges of the opening toward the equatorial region.

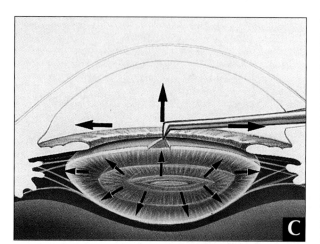

Figure 17-6C. Radial centrifugal forces work in harmony with the tractional vector determined by the zonular fibers and facilitate the progression of the tear from the center of the equator.

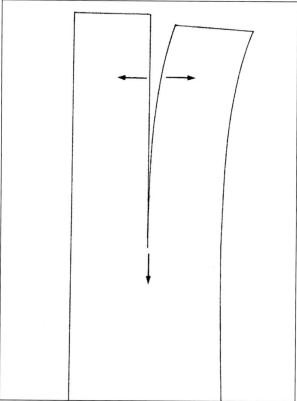

Figure 17-7. Force is applied perpendicular to the tear.

must apply further traction forward or backward respectively.

As the surgeon must apply sufficient force to overcome the maximum resistance of the capsule, once this type of tear has been started, it will tend to progress rapidly and can easily escape control. In addition, with this method, the capsule may tear in a direction different from the desired one, and the procedure will not be easy to control, even if the force applied is far less than that required to obtain the tear in the direction desired. This uncontrolled progression appears particularly when the traction applied is not perpendicular to the desired direction and explains why it is necessary to change the point of application of the force.

However, this technique has the advantage that it can absorb even very brusque changes in tear direction. This theoretical model is closer to the cystotome technique; it adds a component of anterior-posterior compression on the free flap.

If this compression is excessive, it can induce two types of complications:
- Excessive contrast of the endocapsular thrust force and zonular traction (centrifugal) with resulting predominance of the centripetal forces, which determine an excessively small diameter of CCC.
- Perforation of the flap with accidental opening of the underlying capsule and snagging of the lens cortex by the cystotome; this will slow down the tear technique. Control of tear progression will deteriorate, and there will be a marked reduction in the visibility.

2. Tearing through traction on parallel planes by pulling the flap (tearing by shearing).

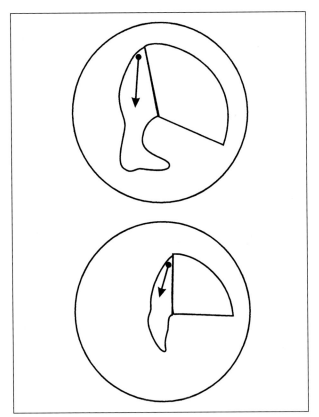

Figure 17-8. To obtain a variation of the tear direction, either toward the center or externally, the surgeon must apply further traction forward or backward respectively.

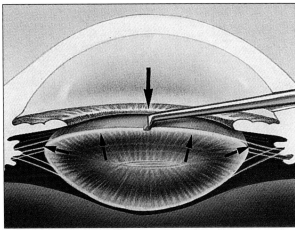

Figure 17-9. Centripetal forces caused by excessive contrast of endocapsular thrust force and zonular traction.

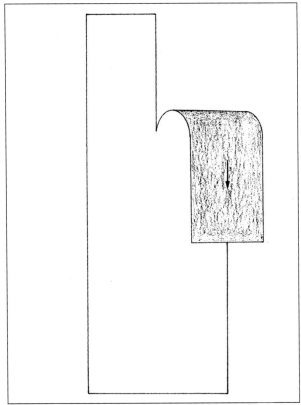

Figure 17-10. Force required to tear is minimal.

The direction of the main force vectors acts along the plane of minimal resistance (perpendicular to the plane itself) so the force required to tear the material is minimal. The traction force is applied in a direction that is parallel to the desired tear direction; the minimal force permits an extremely slow tear progression with good control of the capsular opening. Greater traction force is required only if the surgeon wishes to modify the tear direction or change the diameter of the CCC as it loses its orthogonality of the applied forces and the torn surface.

To maintain this relationship of parallelism between the traction force and the tear direction, the surgeon should frequently change the application point of the force, which must always lie close to the tear point. This theoretical model is closest to the tear method using forceps with converging or coaxial arms.

## METHODS

For a correct CCC, we must examine some parameters of the eye itself and take a look at the instruments available:
1. Characteristics of the eye.

The optimal conditions for a good CCC, from an anatomical point of view, are the good exposure of the bulb, depth of the anterior chamber (mean 3.0 to 3.5 mm), regular mydriasis, total uniformity, and total integrity of the anterior capsular surfaces and the zonular fibers, with good retroillumination grading and good visibility. Conditions to the contrary represent relative or absolute contraindications to the correct performance of a capsular opening using CCC.
2. Contents of the anterior chamber.

During capsulorhexis, the anterior chamber can be formed with balanced salt solution (BSS), air, or viscoelastic substance (VES). Apart from the operator's preference, the choice depends on the method used, the instruments, and the conditions of the bulb.

Capsulorhexis with the chamber formed with BSS requires the capsule to be opened with the cystotome; the

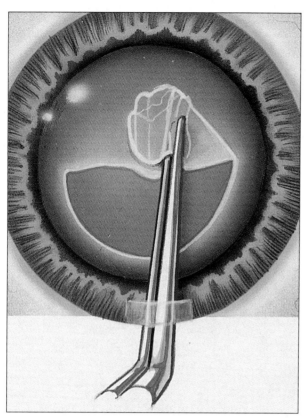

Figure 17-11. Tear method using forceps with converging or coaxial arms.

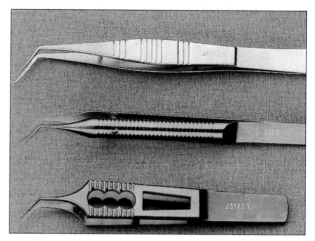

Figure 17-12. Some of the converging capsular forceps available on the market.

BSS can be introduced into the anterior chamber either directly through the discharge pipe (a fixed constant quantity that enters and depends on the height of the bottle) or through the use of an automated I/A machine (with the possibility of interruption the flow). Also, the BSS supply can reach the anterior chamber either through the irrigating cystotome or alternately through the anterior chamber maintainer.

BSS in the anterior chamber gives the surgeon excellent vision of the anterior structures; moreover, the use of an irrigating solution containing adrenaline can improve poor mydriasis. The use of an I/A machine allows fluid to enter the chamber only when necessary. This avoids the chamber deepening or flattening excessively, something that may occur with direct infusion.

However, BSS has some disadvantages; under BSS flow, the flap of the anterior chamber tends to move about and is difficult to control. Because of the low surface tension, BSS will tend to escape from the anterior chamber so it is not the ideal substance for maintaining the spaces of the bulb. It is therefore unsuitable for young eyes or bulbs with increased endovitreal pressure. As the temperature of the BSS is lower than body temperature, it can induce miosis (particularly if adrenaline has not been added to the bottle).

The fact that the cystotome must be used to perform the capsulorhexis when BSS is used to form the anterior chamber is a huge disadvantage; the same applies to the anterior chamber maintainer, which must be used if the surgeon wishes to use forceps. In our opinion, forceps require an excessively wide opening, and this carries the risk of variations in the chamber depth.

The anterior chamber can be formed with air, which provides good vision of the zonular fibers and the edges of the rhexis. It is particularly indicated if there is poor red reflex of the fundus and/or when the surgeon wants to perform a wide capsulorhexis under conditions of retroillumination, which are far from optimal. It is ideal with a capsulorhexis in over-ripe or brunescent cataracts, or when the surgeon has to operate in patients of oriental races. This high surface tension liquid allows the surgeon to perform the rhexis through the opening of the cystotome (with the cystotome or the forceps with coaxial arms, such as Caporossi forceps) without air tending to escape and with constant chamber volume.

The capsular flap is kept very stable through the presence of air, which makes it easier to capture. However, there is an interface phenomenon that makes it more difficult to see the structures clearly, partly because of the large difference in the refractive index between air and the cornea, which may cause spherical and cylindrical aberrations.

In addition, because of the high surface tension, any variation within the chamber will always be important because of the large amount and the rapid fluid escape that may occur.

Naturally, forming the chamber with air or BSS is low-cost, but this advantage is off-loaded by the fact that the surgeon cannot use openings between 3.0 and 3.5 mm, which would permit him or her to use forceps with converging arms. The formation of the anterior chamber with VES is probably the best solution for an easy capsulorhexis. Based on hyaluronic acid (with either high or low molecular weight), VES injected into the anterior chamber allows good exposure of the structures in the anterior segment. If VES containing chondroitin sulfate and hyaluronic acid is used, the anterior chamber should be filled using the single bubble technique to avoid the interface phenomenon between the various layers of VES, which could make the exposure of the structures more critical. However, if the VES used has a cellulose

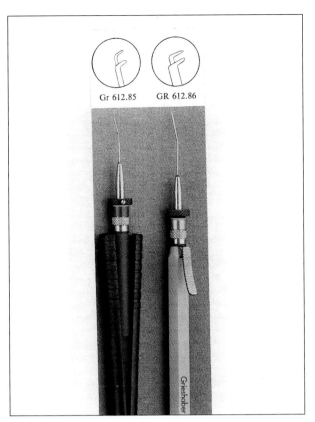

Figure 17-13. Coaxial forceps with Sutherland-Grieshaber handles. On the left the Caporossi forceps (caliber 27G, with blunt tips) and on the right Dossi Forceps (caliber 23 G with sharp tips).

Figure 17-14. Free flap of the capsule pushed toward the periphery of the lens and raised.

base, the technique used to fill the anterior chamber must permit slow, total hydration of the macro-molecule, otherwise layers with different refractive indices will be formed (layering phenomenon).

VES with high molecular weight and those with non-Newton fluid characteristics maintain the chamber very well; they also have a low tendency of escaping from the anterior chamber and allow the surgeon to perform a corneo-scleral opening of 3.0 to 3.5 mm with no appreciable variations in the chamber depth even during capsulorhexis using forceps with converging arms. Another advantage of using VES in the anterior chamber is the protection that these substances provide for the anterior chamber structures. In addition, the stabilizing action on the free capsular flap should not be underestimated.

The biggest drawback attached to shaping the anterior chamber with VES is the cost. With some types of VES, air bubbles that may become trapped in the VES may disturb the visibility and in some cases can be difficult to remove.

3. Surgical instruments.

The instruments used for CCC can be split into three basic classes:

- Cystotomes—Irrigating, non-irrigating, pre-prepared, or self-forming, with a variety of angulations, with the direction of the cutting surface equal to or opposite to that of the irrigation. The calipers used vary from 23 to 30 G depending on the surgeon's preference.

- Forceps—With converging arms, produced along the same lines as the capsular forceps with a disc-capturing tip or a blunt lock-in tip, with ergonomic or flat handles, with arms available in a variety of angle or designs. They are produced in stainless steel or titanium and have either a sharp or blunted tip. There are numerous types: Corydon, Kershner, Kraff-Utrata, McPherson, Piovella, Buratto, etc.

All the forceps operate according to the same principles and need to be handled with extreme precision inside the anterior chamber, especially if the surgeon has used a VES that cannot maintain the chamber sufficiently. However, these forceps grip firmly on the flap even when conditions are far from optimal (ie, a non-uniform capsule, insufficient mydriasis, abnormal working/operating angles) allowing the surgeon to complete the CCC, even of large dimensions.

An important parameter for evaluation is the ratio between the size of the bulb and the forceps used, which may not be optimal. An abnormal shape of the orbit may result in difficult access with this type of forceps. The cost of the high molecular weight VES and the possible supply requirements are a purely economical disadvantage.

- Forceps with coaxial arms were born from the principles of endovitreal surgery. Some models have been studied by various surgeons, the most paradigmatic are without a doubt the Caporossi and the

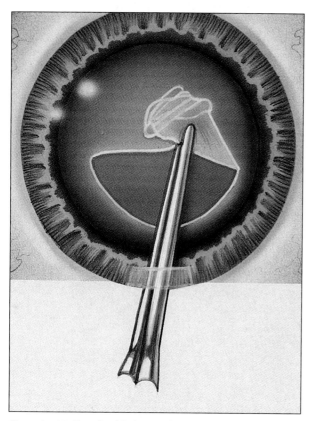
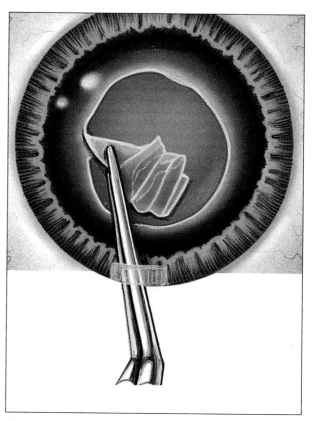

Figure 17-15. Flap should close to the edge during tearing movement.

Figure 17-16. Completion of the circumference should meet the starting point externally to avoid the formation of points of lesser resistance.

Dossi forceps. The former has a blunt tip and is built around a mandrill with a very small diameter (27 G) while the forceps created by Dossi are somewhat larger (21 G). They have sharp edges to avoid the passage with the cystotome.

The coaxial forceps are smaller than the converging forceps and provide the possibility of operating in a closed anterior chamber through an opening of 1.0 to 1.4 mm. This means that a smaller amount of VES is required, the depth of the anterior chamber is controlled, and the control of the rhexis is more or less identical to that obtained with converging forceps.

As the instrument is very thin, the Caporossi forceps are the only ones currently available that allow the surgeon to perform or complete the rhexis through a side port incision, if necessary. VES must be used to maintain the shape of the anterior chamber when the surgeon uses these forceps and there is a lower probability of replacement during surgery.

Once the capsule has been opened centrally with the cystotome or the sharp or blunt tip of the forceps, the free flap of the capsule is pushed toward the periphery of the lens and raised. Once the flap has been raised, it is folded back over the intact capsular surface. Forceps or cystotomes are used to capture the flap and pull it in the direction of the cut, either clockwise or counterclockwise. Once the first 45 to 60° have been completed, the surgeon should change the point where the traction force is applied. He or she should catch the flap close to the edge once again and repeat the tearing movement for a further 45 to 60°. This action should be repeated until the entire circumference has been treated. The completion of the circumference should meet the starting point externally to avoid the formation of points of lesser resistance within the CCC.

The optimal diameter of the CCC in phacoemulsification depends on two factors: diameter of the mydriasis and the diameter of the intraocular lense's (IOL's) optic disc. It is potentially dangerous to perform the CCC below the iris. As a result, the surgeon must have a visible surface of the anterior capsule equal to the diameter of the rhexis. The first step is to adjust the pharmacological approach in proportion to the iris response to pharmacological stimulation.

The most common mydriatic drugs used in cataract surgery are rapid-action para-sympathicolytic energics, which frequently contain the active ingredients tropicamide and cyclopentolate. These have rapid-action, and one of their most important advantages is that they can be easily counterbalanced through the direct use of cholinergics. As these drugs act on the post-synaptic muscarinic receptors, they paralyze the sphincter muscle of the iris, stimulating the dilating muscle of the iris with consequent mydriasis. This action mechanism—passive induction of mydriasis—is the system's limitation. So the second way of obtaining optimal mydriasis is direct stimulation of the adrenergic receptors of the muscle that dilates the iris.

These drugs have two important classes of side-effects:

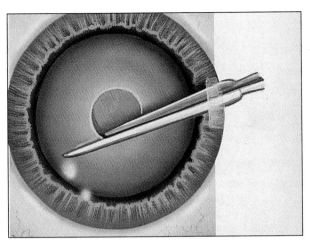

Figure 17-17. Concentric tearing by shearing with forceps.

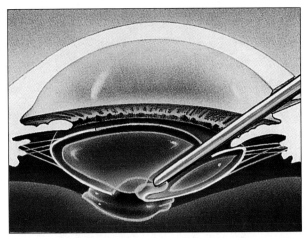

Figure 17-18. Tearing by shearing technique creating capsular opening with a diameter in the region of 3 mm.

- A topical effect is the epithelial toxicity, which can cause deterioration of the corneal transparency.
- A systemic effect linked to the positive inotropic, heart-stimulating, and hypertensive action of the adrenergic drugs; this means that the use of these drugs is not recommended in patients affected by hypertension or heart pathologies.

If the drug treatment does not produce sufficient dilatation, the surgeon must use more aggressive surgical methods:

- Posterior synechiotomy.
- Removal (if possible) of the atrophic membrane of the pupillary edge.
- Sphincterotomy. Interruption of the atrophic areas of the pupillary edge without tearing allows the surgeon to maintain good pupil kinetics even though there is a high risk of hemorrhage. Surgically, it is not a difficult maneuver, but in order to maintain the sphincter intact, the surgeon must have good surgical sensitivity.
- Stretching the pupillary edge is easier than the sphincterotomy. It requires special instruments such as Zanini's double hook or the simultaneous use of *push and pull* with an iris hook. The main disadvantage of the method is the pupillary atony that is a consequence of the multiple rupture of the sphincter produced by the stretching. There is also a high frequency of bleeding, but it is less important.
- Use of fixed dilatation systems for traction (Arpa's hook) and tension (Zenoni's ring) are the extreme solutions borrowed from vitreoretinal surgery. They leave total pupillary atony, which is frequently asymmetrical.

The choice of a CCC diameter 0.5 mm less than the optical disc of the IOL would appear to be the most logical. With this condition, we have the overlap of the anterior lens tissue on the anterior surface of the IOL for about 0.2 to 0.3 mm. This allows the bag to remain closed without a large ring of opaque capsule, which may interfere with vision of the peripheral retina.

## ADVANCED CCC TECHNIQUES

### Two-Step Capsulorhexis

This technique is often used to convert small capsular openings into rhexis with an adequate diameter. It has the advantages of the capsulorhexis when this is difficult or if the capsular opening is smaller than expected.

Small capsulorhexises are often performed in intumescent or brunescent cataracts, when the red reflex is poor or if the pupil is narrow. In these cases, after hydromanipulations of the nucleus and after removing the lens material, the capsular bag is filled with high molecular weight VES. Prior to or after having implanted the IOL, an incision is created tangentially to the edge of the capsulorhexis. Using forceps, the surgeon performs concentric tearing by shearing as for a primary capsulorhexis. During extension of the two-stage capsulorhexis, the edge of the rhexis must always be captured close to the base of the cut. So the point where the traction force is applied must be changed frequently. This technique is particularly useful in conditions of poor mydriasis. The extension capsulorhexis can be performed following mechanical dilatation or sphincterectomy of the pupil.

### Posterior Capsulorhexis

Circular continuous posterior capsulorhexis can also be considered an emergency method in the event of posterior capsule rupture or a method to prevent the opacification of the posterior capsule in high-risk patients (ie, post-uveitic, with retinitis pigmentosa, high myopias, children). The technique is performed is a similar way to the anterior capsulorhexis even though there are some slight differences that are directly linked to the inherent details of the structure to be treated.

The first is that the capsular bag is carefully filled with high molecular weight VES; it is then cut carefully (the thickness at the center of the posterior capsule is one-third that of the anterior capsule). A small quantity of low-cohesion VES is injected into the space behind the lens to distance the anterior hyaloid and put the posteri-

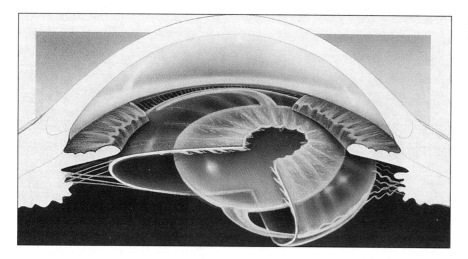

Figure 17-19. Side view of a single piece IOL in the bag

or capsule under tension. This way, it is given an anterior convex shape that is similar to the anterior capsule. Once the surgeon has turned over the flap, he or she can proceed with the tearing by shearing technique, creating a capsular opening with a diameter in the region of 3 mm.

## INTRAOPERATIVE COMPLICATIONS

### Capsulorhexis Escape

During the creation of a CCC, the cut may progress beyond the margins. The reasons for this unwanted centrifugal progression may be connected to the inherent nature of the capsule itself (non-uniform resistance to the tearing tension, in pseudoexfoliative cataracts for example), with abnormal insertion of the zonular fibers; or it may be due to insufficiently counterbalanced endovitreal or endocapsular pressure (insufficient or inadequate formation of the anterior chamber). Lastly, it may also be due to incorrect maneuvers with the instruments—referring to the precise relationship between the application of the forces and the cutting direction (the orthogonal and parallel force lines must be respected), and unexpected pressure on the scleral edges, which can cause a sudden flattening of the anterior chamber.

In all these cases, precocious diagnosis of incorrect progression of the tear is the only thing that will allow the surgeon to intervene efficaciously and successfully to complete the CCC.

However, if the technique cannot be used, the surgeon should convert the CCC to a can opener. However, for the good functional outcome of the operation, the capsular structures must remain intact.

If there is centrifugal escape of the tear edge, the surgeon should stop and reform the anterior chamber with abundant high molecular weight VES. He or she should check the stability of the chamber depth, and, catching the free flap as close as possible to the incision edge with very gentle traction, try to return the incision edge to the center of the lens, maintaining the orthogonal direction of the flap tear in respect to the intact capsule and the parallelism of the direction of the traction force in respect to the wanted tear direction.

The surgeon should eliminate any abnormal zonular insertions prior to restarting the capsulorhexis. If the escape has brought the edge of the incision to lie under the iris plane, the surgeon should first shape the chamber with VES. Then he or she should try to obtain better mydriasis using hooks or iris retractors and if possible with a targeted injection of VES so that he has a better view of the edges of the tear progression.

If this maneuver is successful, he or she should proceed as previously described. However, if the maneuver is not successful, the surgeon can use one of the following alternatives.

He or she can go back to the CCC starting point and proceed in the opposite direction; however, if the new circumference is not *ab esterno*, a point of lesser resistance will be formed.

The second alternative involves converting the opening from a CCC to a can opener, as long as the torn edges do not exceed two-thirds of the circumference. While this is unfortunate, the surgeon should not view it as a defeat.

Another possible intraoperative complication is the centrifugal escape in the event of hydromanipulations of the nucleus or during phacoemulsification. In the former, there will always be an area of lower resistance, which will be the cause of numerous complications. This is usually when the circumference closes inside the limits of the planned diameter. If this happens, the surgeon should luxate the nucleus mechanically either in the posterior chamber or in the anterior chamber, depending on the hardness of the nucleus and the condition of the endothelium, and then perform phaco.

It goes without saying that these maneuvers are only possible if the tear has not exceeded the lens equator. If it has, the surgeon should convert to a planned ECCE.

In the second case, the reasons can be traced to two different origins: rupture of the incision edges caused directly through contact with the phaco tip and rupture due to pressure of the infusion liquid. The liquid acts on the point of least resistance, which results from the *backward closure* of the capsulorhexis.

Irrespective of the reason, the subsequent behavior is conditioned by which phase of phaco the rupture occurred in and the degree of extension.

If the rupture occurs during the sculpting phase of the nucleus, the surgeon should luxate and fracture the nucleus in the posterior chamber as described previously.

If rupture occurs after nuclear cracking, the volume of infusion liquid should be reduced (and in parallel, the parameters of vacuum and flow rate), and the surgeon should complete the phaco under low flow rate and low turbulence.

A final possible complication of CCC is the disinsertion of the zonule, which will condition how the rhexis will progress. The surgeon should limit the dialysis area by creating the opening by bringing the flap toward the disinsertion area and never pulling it toward the center.

## POSTOPERATIVE COMPLICATIONS

The most frequent postoperative complication observed is undoubtedly the opacification of the anterior capsule. A more serious complication is the contraction of the capsular bag with phimosis of the rhexis.

Opacification of the anterior capsule is a very serious complication and involves the part of the anterior capsule in contact with the IOL. The opacification is caused by fibrotic metaplasia of the subcapsular anterior epithelium with the formation of collagen tissue.

This phenomenon depends on the type of material (silicone produces it to a greater extent than polymethylmethacrylate (PMMA), while acrylic and Hema would appear to induce it to a lesser degree, and certainly with greater latency).

Phimosis of the rhexis and the contraction of the capsular bag are important phenomena; though they are rare occurrences, they require surgical or para-surgical treatment. The ratio between the size of the rhexis and the size of the optical disc play an important role, as does the lens material, the loop material, the distention of the bag and the ability to keep it distended, and any concomitant pathologies (myopia, exfoliation, glaucoma, residues of retinal detachment, etc).

Following an observation period where the surgeon has observed the progression of the symptoms, surgical treatment, or treatment with YAG laser must be planned. The treatment will interrupt the phimotic fibrous ring and/or liberation of the bag from the adhesions, recenter the lens, or its replacement with a one-piece with an even larger optical disc, or use the same lens and the distention of the capsular bag with a PMMA ring.

As the residual epithelium and lens fibers are involved, Nishi suggested a very careful 360° aspiration of the residual anterior capsule. One important preventive measure is to perform a wide capsulorhexis (demonstrated particularly in the event of relaxed zonules). In any case, the problem can be resolved quite easily by surgery (radial cuts with scissors) or parasurgically (YAG laser: relaxing incision).

Another postoperative complication is over-distention of the capsular bag due to VES trapped inside the IOL. This will happen early on in proceedings and can be seen as a flattening of the anterior chamber with an increase in myopia of 3 to 4 diopters (D) because of the anteriorization of the IOL and an excessive distance between the posterior capsule and the IOL, which can be shown biomicroscopically.

This complication can be resolved by surgically removing the material trapped behind the IOL using two-handed aspiration. This maneuver has been enormously facilitated by the increased ease with which the VES can be aspirated. Due to the length of time the VES has been in the capsular bag, it will have been hydrolyzed making it easier to remove.

## CONCLUSION

The advantages of CCC can be summarized as follows:

- CCC allows better centering of the IOL in the capsular bag both in the long- and short-term.
- Capsulorhexis reduces the frequency of opacification of the posterior capsule particularly if a bi-convex or posterior convex lens has been implanted inside the capsular bag. In these cases, the posterior face of the IOL will remain in close contact with the capsule. (There is reduced opacification with an IOL implanted in the bag compared to full size; this may possible be due to a more uniform application of the tensile forces to the lens equator.)
- Resistance and elasticity of the capsulorhexis allows the surgeon to perform the endocapsular phacoemulsification through a small opening. This improves the overall safety of the procedure and allows him or her to implant an IOL with a large optical disc, with loops that have excellent extra-capsular stability in the postoperative period.
- The maintenance of a good bag shape with continuous edges allows the surgeon to perform nuclear fluid-manipulation inside the bag. This will successfully separate the various lens layers without exerting excessive zonular traction and with little risk of tearing the anterior edge of the capsule (infusion with hydrodissection, hydrodelineation, and nuclear hydrodelineation with ultrasound [U/S]).
- It allows good centering of the IOL, which has led to the development of lenses with diameters of 5.0, 5.25, and 5.5 mm suitable for phaco and small incisions. It has favored the developments in the phacoemulsification techniques through the development of the in situ techniques. Last but not least, it has helped standardize the position of the IOL in the posterior segment and improved the potential of biometric calculation.
- In the event of posterior capsule rupture, the anterior capsule can be used to support the IOL implanted in the groove (which has a continuous edge).
- The absence of free capsular flaps in CCC prevents the formation of posterior synechiae between the iris and the free capsular flaps, which may cause distortions and deformation of the pupil. In some cases, it may also lead to pupillary capture of the IOL.
- In the postoperative, capsulorhexis prevents contact between the iris and the structures in the posterior chamber or the anterior segment. The only excep-

tion is the anterior surface of the capsule, which would actually appear to be further away from the iris postoperatively than it was preoperatively. This reduced iris rubbing by the IOL inside the bag reduces uveal contact and irritation to a minimum.
- The certainty that the implant will be stable inside the capsular bag is a huge advantage for patients affected by uveitis (and patients with glaucoma). As the IOL is inserted inside the bag, uveal contact and irritation are reduced to a minimum.

## REFERENCES

Arshinoff S. Mechanism of capsulorhexis. *J Cataract Refract Surg*. 1992;18(6):623-628.

Amstrong TA. Refractive effect of capsular bag lens placement with the capsulorhexis technique. *J Cataract Refract Surg*. 1992;18(2):121-124.

Caporossi A, Baiocchi S. Original forceps for capsulorhexis. *Ocular Surg News International Ed*. 1992, May. 13.

Caporossi A, Baiocchi S, Simi C. Capsulorhexis. In: Buratto L, ed. *Facoemulsificazione tecnica e stato dell'arte*. Vol. II. Milano: Camo Ed. 1996.

*Caporossi A, Frezzotti R*. Capsulotomia: una metodica in evoluzione. Presentato al Congresso SOI 1991. Pubblicato su Viscochirurgia Vol. XI Spec. 1992.

Gimbel HV, Neuhann T. Development, advantages and methods of the continuos circular capsulorhexis technique. *J Cataract Refract Surg*. 1990;16:31-37.

Haefliger E, Neuhann T. The Neuhann capsulorhexis. A safe technique for all-in the bag implantation. *Klin Monastbl Augenheilkd*. 1988;192(5):435-438.

Komatu M, Shimizu M. Circular capsulectomy in extracapsular extraction. *Jpn J Clin Ophthalmol*. 1988;42(8):909-912.

Neuhann T. Theory and surgical technique of capsulorhexis. *Klin Monastsbl Augenheilkd*. 1987;190(6):542-545.

Shimizu K. Continuos circular capsulorhexis (CCC). *Eur J Implant Surg*. 1990;2(2):115-117.

# Chapter 18

# PHACOEMULSIFICATION TECHNIQUE

*Stephen F. Brint, MD*

## INTRODUCTION

Removal of the cataractous lens through clear corneal incisions dates back to ancient time, even more recently using the von Graffe knife, with the use of no sutures and requiring long stabilization of the head and eye for the initial repair of the wound. More recently, Dr. Kimiya Shimizu has been advocating clear corneal incisions for phacoemulsification, however using 5 to 6 mm polymethylmethacrylate (PMMA) lenses, thus requiring either a single interrupted or an x suture to close the corneal incision.

At the 1992 ASCRS meeting in San Diego, papers were presented by Dr. Richard Fichman, who demonstrated use of phacoemulsification using scleral tunnel approach, but being done under topical Tetracaine anesthesia, as well as by Dr. I. Howard Fine, who advocated using clear corneal incisions for routine cataract surgery, with the use of foldable intraocular lenses (IOLs), but under conventional peribulbar anesthesia. Subsequently, after these two excellent presentations, a number of doctors, including Dr. Fine, Dr. Harry B. Grabow, Dr. Charles Williamson, Dr. Andrew Lyle, and myself, began using the idea of the clear corneal tunnel for phacoemulsification and implantation of a small incision foldable lens under topical anesthesia. This has met with some controversy as other physicians have tried it. Each one has used his own individual technique, some operating from the normal superior position, others using various metal keratomes, and some surgeons shunning small incision IOLs in favor of one-piece PMMA lenses, which leave a rather large, questionably self-sealing corneal tunnel. Because of this, there have been problems reported, such as excessive endothelial cell loss and, worse yet, cases of endophthalmitis.

The clear corneal incision, when properly done, can be a very satisfying procedure for both the patient and the doctor. Mastering the instrumentation and techniques of the clear corneal incision follows previous confidence gained from experience with the no-stitch, self-sealing, scleral tunnel incision. It does require a commitment to excellent surgery, as once the surgeon has committed himself to a clear corneal incision, he must be able to perform state-of-the-art capsulorhexis, in situ phacoemulsification, and be comfortable with the use of the various foldable IOLs. Routine performance under conventional retrobulbar or peribulbar anesthesia provides confidence in this total technique; the surgeon can then feel comfortable adding *the icing on the cake* topical anesthesia.

Dr. Grabow was one of the first to actually analyze his results using clear corneal incision with topical anesthesia. Initially, he began using a conventional superior incision. However, using the incision in this location, he reported excessive endothelial cell loss (approximately 15%). This was reduced to 7% when the incision site was moved temporally.

Clear corneal incisions with topical anesthesia are obviously not for every patient. Communication of the concept of maintaining fixation on the operating microscope light and keeping the eye still is essential. Those patients with chronic obstructive pulmonary disease, who have heavy body movement on breathing, are difficult to do. Younger patients tend to be more anxious and less cooperative. Patients who are non-English speaking, deaf, or otherwise uncooperative are also poor candidates. For the surgeon beginning clear corneal phacoemulsification under topical anesthesia, cases that we ordinarily consider difficult should probably not be performed with this technique, such as cases of compromised cornea with guttata, pseudoexfoliation, miotic pupils, and deeply brunescent lenses that will require prolonged phaco time.

Having moved to a temporal approach for clear corneal incision, I have realized that it has many other

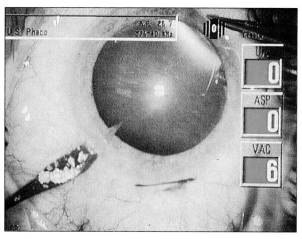

Figure 18-1. 22.5° sharp point knife used for paracentesis, 60° away from primary corneal/limbal incision.

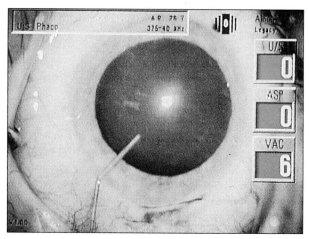

Figure 18-2. Instillation of 0.25 cc of 1% Xylocaine for intracameral addition to topical anesthesia.

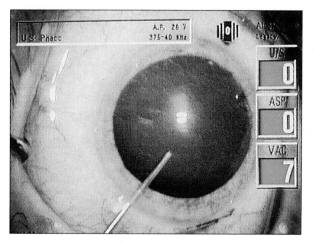

Figure 18-3. VES injected into anterior chamber to flush out aqueous and Xylocaine.

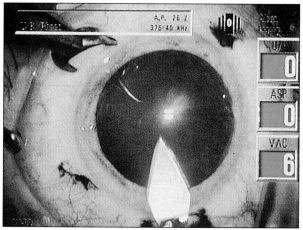

Figure 18-4. 2.65 metal keratome used to develop corneal tunnel, approximately 2 mm in length.

advantages, primarily, better visibility with an improved red reflex. As the balanced salt solution (BSS) outflow is in a more natural position, there is less pooling and therefore decreased dependence on the need for the surgical assistant to either drop the cornea or to mop up any excess fluid. The stability of the K reading is also improved, with less induced astigmatism and obviously less tendency to against the rule shift. The patient is also more comfortable postoperatively when a scleral tunnel is done laterally rather than superiorly, because the lid rubs perpendicularly along the edge of the peritomy, as opposed to parallel across the entire length of the peritomy incision.

Working from the side also has its disadvantages, in that it requires a new learning curve for the surgeon. The bed must be adjusted higher to allow more room for the knees, as well as perhaps even changing the surgical bed. The patient's head tends to drift away from the surgeon and may need to be taped or stabilized by the assistant. If the scleral tunnel approach is chosen, the conjunctiva tends to be more thin temporally than above and more friable.

## ANESTHESIA

The technique for topical anesthesia that I prefer is to begin with two drops of 0.5% Tetracaine prior to dilation, one drop of Ocufen, and then dilation with cyclopentolate 1% and NeoSynephrine 2.5%. This is begun approximately 40 minutes prior to the procedure. In the 30 to 40 minute range prior to the procedure, 4% Xylocaine, sterile nonpreserved, is drawn up into a 5 cc syringe and four drops are initially instilled. Two drops every 5 minutes are given until the time of surgery throughout the prepping and draping process. At the time the initial drops are instilled, normally 1 mg of Versed is given to afford mild sedation for the patient; however, in virtually all cases, no other sedation is necessary. Anesthesia should begin approximately 30 minutes prior to surgery. I have found the timing of the instillation of the Xylocaine to be extremely important, as it appears to reach peak effect at 30 minutes. Even though the drops are continued, if they are begun too early, their effect tends to wear off, not allowing the patient to maintain a good level of anesthesia. Therefore, it is very important for the nurses to observe where you are in each particular case

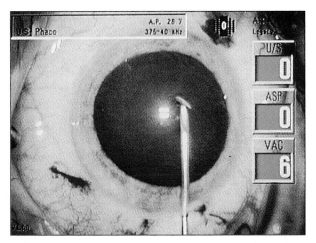

Figure 18-5. Capsulorhexis initiated in center to mid periphery with bent 26 gauge needle.

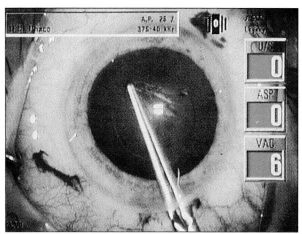

Figure 18-6. Capsulorhexis completed with Utrata forceps.

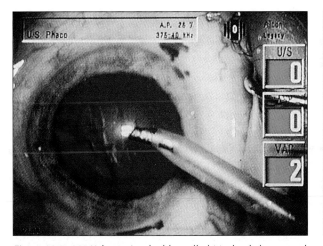

Figure 18-7. 30° Kelman tip, double-walled Mackool sleeve used for phaco.

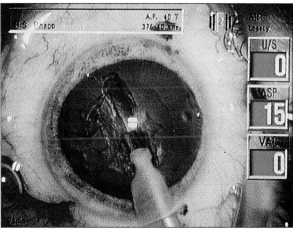

Figure 18-8. First groove made as deeply as possible, facilitated with downward curve of the 30° Kelman tip.

and to know that some cases may take longer than others so the anesthesia timing may need to be adjusted.

The obvious advantages of topical anesthesia are in avoiding all of the potential complications of injection, such as globe perforation, retrobulbar hemorrhage, optic atrophy, vascular occlusion, or allergic or toxic reactions. It affords the patient essentially instant vision, as the eye does not have to be patched because of the lack of akinesia, as well as improved vision on day 1, because of the more normal tear film pattern. It is also less expensive than injection anesthesia. The disadvantages include the learning curve, and the potential of eye movement during the procedure, especially during the capsulorhexis, which is critical to all the subsequent steps in the operation. In the rare case in which vitrectomy has been necessary, I have not found that the topical anesthesia posed any additional difficulties in management of the vitrectomy. There is increased patient anxiety, and therefore the surgeon and his staff need to constantly communicate with the patient and reassure him or her. Thus, one needs to make a great effort to educate the entire staff on the benefits of topical anesthesia for the patient. Therefore, the staff can help calm the patient as soon as the patient enters the room and assist the surgeon in maintaining a calm operating environment during the procedure.

For the last 6 months, in addition to the above description of my topical anesthesia technique, the initial groove is made just posterior to clear cornea with the diamond trifacet knife, and the paracentesis incision is made with the 22.5° metal blade knife. This occurs after 0.25 cc of Xylocaine is injected with a BSS injection cannula into the anterior chamber. This intracameral Xylocaine mixture has previously been made for the entire day's cases, consisting of 2% nonpreserved Xylocaine and BSS in equal amounts (a 50:50 mixture), thus resulting in an effective 1% Xylocaine concentration. The mixing with BSS seems to buffer the solution, however, and the subsequent injection of 0.25 cc of this mixture into the anterior chamber is more comfortable to the patient than injecting the straight 1% nonpreserved Xylocaine, which I had previously tried.

Following the injection of Xylocaine into the anterior chamber, the anterior chamber is filled with viscoelastic, usually Provisc (sodium hyaluronate), which flushes most of it out of the anterior chamber. I have found that

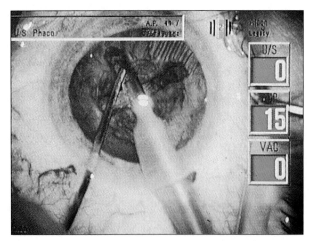

Figure 18-9. Second groove made narrow and perpendicular to first groove, with nucleus rotated in clockwise manner with 0.5 mm wide flat spatula.

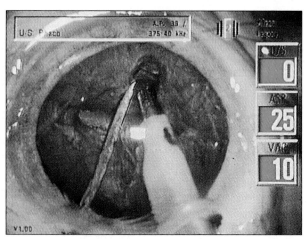

Figure 18-10. After all four grooves are made, approximately 90% deep, broad wide spatula and curve of phaco tip placed deep in the groove to initiate cracking.

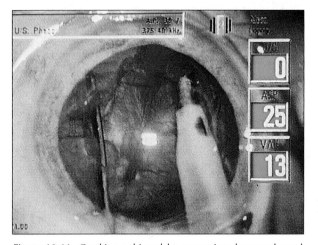

Figure 18-11. Cracking achieved by separating the spatula and phaco tip, ensuring that crack continues through posterior nuclear plate past the midline.

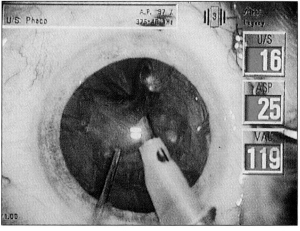

Figure 18-12. After all quadrants are cracked, the first quadrant is occluded at its side and then lollipopped to the center for emulsification.

the addition of the intracameral greatly increases patient comfort during phacoemulsification and decreases the patient's awareness of pressure changes in the eye as the insertion and removal of the phaco tip and the insertion and removal of the irrigation/aspiration (I/A) tip occur.

## INCISION

The clear corneal incision, which I prefer, has evolved over the 4 years that I have been using this technique. The creation of the corneal tunnel has been described both with the making of a corneal or clear corneal/limbal groove or going directly in without the groove, using either a diamond or metal blade keratome. I have always preferred the creation of a groove initially and have always used a nonguarded diamond trifacet knife to create the groove.

Even though the trifacet knife depth is not controlled, I feel that it should be approximately 450 to 500 μm deep, and should be very carefully made to curve exactly parallel to the limbus. The length of the groove should be approximately 3.5 mm, as this will be the width that is necessary for the most comfortable insertion of the foldable acrylic IOL.

Following the work of Paul Ernest, based on cadaver and human studies, bringing the clear corneal groove back into the limbal vascular arcade area gives a more stable wound, as well as reported faster wound healing. I have over the last 6 months adopted this technique and am now making the groove without a peritomy, but in the vascular arcade area of the limbus, so that it is common and even anticipated that there will be a small amount of bleeding when creating the groove.

The biggest advantage in moving the groove back a bit from where I previously made it is increased patient comfort. Although rare, it was troubling to have a patient continue to complain of a foreign body sensation at the corneal incision site several months following a beautiful,

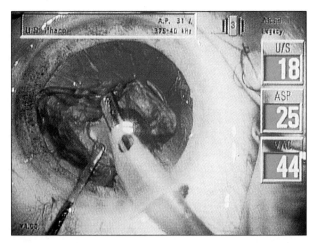

Figure 18-13. Final quadrant is emulsified, facilitated by spatula, which then is placed behind the phaco tip to protect posterior capsule.

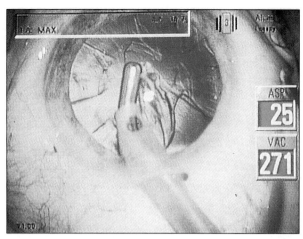

Figure 18-14. I/A of cortex using 45° curved ultraflow I/A handpiece.

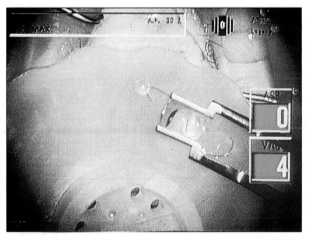

Figure 18-15. AcrySof MA30 IOL placed on plate of wagonwheel holder, folded with Alcon folding forceps.

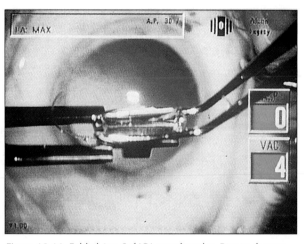

Figure 18-16. Folded AcrySof IOL transferred to Buratto forceps.

uncomplicated procedure. By moving the incision back into the vascular arcade area, the incision site is covered with conjunctiva and has eliminated this rare but troublesome patient complaint.

After the creation of the clear corneal/limbal groove, a paracentesis incision is made approximately 60º away from the primary incision, which in almost all cases has been placed temporally, and the above-mentioned intracameral Xylocaine is injected, followed by the filling of the anterior chamber with viscoelastic material, so that the anterior chamber will be very firm to allow the creation of a good corneal tunnel, with the proper keratome.

I am now in the process of decreasing my phaco incision from the 3 mm, which I have used for many years with the standard phaco tip, to 2.8 mm that we are using with the new MicroTip, and eventually anticipate a 2.6 mm incision using the Mackool system phaco tip (we are correspondingly in an evolution of keratomes). With the 3 mm incision, I prefer the 3 mm diamond keratome from HUCO.

As we are rapidly changing incision sizes, we have not continued to buy diamond keratomes of the appropriate size for these new reduced incisions, and are therefore using metal keratomes. The disadvantage that I see in the metal keratome is that one cannot control the entry into the anterior chamber as well; therefore, the length of the corneal tunnel is not as consistent. In my opinion, the length of the corneal tunnel should ideally be between 1.75 to 2.0 mm, and this is not always easily achieved using the metal keratome.

The most appropriate keratome that I have used for the 2.8 mm incision for the MicroTip has been the 3D diamond keratome, developed by I. Howard Fine (Rhein Medical). I anticipate that when we have completed our transition to the Mackool size incision, that the 2.6 mm version of this keratome will be my keratome of choice.

## CAPSULORHEXIS

Under the previously instilled viscoelastic, a 26 gauge needle, bent preoperatively to fashion a cystotome, is used to initiate the capsulorhexis. The anterior capsule is punctured centrally, then extended to the mid periphery

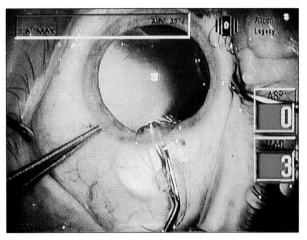

Figure 18-17. Insertion of AcrySof IOL with leading haptic engaged between the jaws of the pronated Buratto forceps through a 3.5 mm incision.

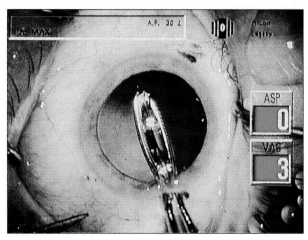

Figure 18-18. AcrySof IOL rotated so that first haptic is in the bag.

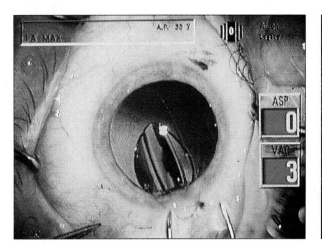

Figure 18-19. AcrySof IOL released from direct action Buratto forceps.

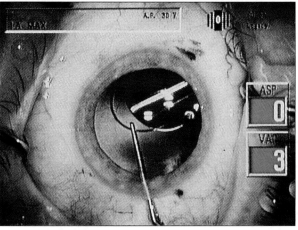

Figure 18-20. Trailing haptic placed in capsular bag with Kelman-McPherson forceps.

to the surgeon's right. Placing the cystotome under the tear for elevation, a dog ear is created which is then carried 360° using the Utrata forceps, regrasping near the edge every 90° to insure control. It is essential to complete the circle tearing from outside to in for integrity. A diameter of 5 to 5.5 mm is preferred, allowing a slight anterior capsule overlap of the IOL optic after lens insertion.

## HYDRODISSECTION

On a 3 cc syringe filled with BSS, a flat 25 gauge hydrodissection cannula is placed to the surgeon's left just under the margin of the capsulorhexis. The capsule is elevated slightly and the BSS is injected quickly to create a fluid wave which moves right watching for the nucleus to rise as if it is trying to *come out of the bag*. Usually only one injection of fluid is needed to elevate the nucleus, but additional injections at other positions along the rhexis margin may be necessary.

## PHACOEMULSIFICATION

The phacoemulsification machine that I am using presently is the Alcon Legacy, and the preferred tip is the MicroTip with the 30° bevel of Kelman design. The choice of the MicroTip for me is not so much that a 2.8 mm incision is required, rather than the traditional 3.0 mm, but because of the decreased lumen of the tip, with the proper settings on the machine, improved fluidic performance is achieved, and stability of the anterior chamber during emulsification and aspiration of the nucleus is increased.

The phaco technique of choice in over 90% of the cataract cases continues to be the four quadrant Divide and Conquer technique as originally described by John Shepherd. The curved 30° Kelman MicroTip facilitates this technique even more by creating very narrow, precise grooves, which can be made quickly and at a deeper level due to the downward curve of the Kelman tip. By creating these precise grooves, a larger amount of nuclear material can be left in place to provide more substance

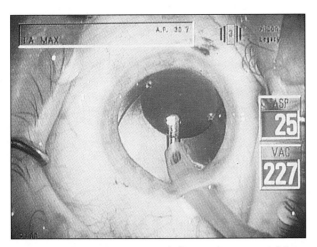

Figure 18-21. Careful aspiration of all viscoelastic material from both behind as well as in front of IOL.

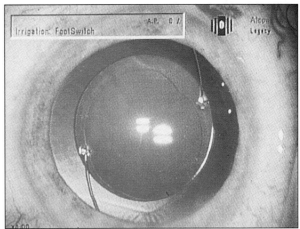

Figure 18-22. Excellent centration of acrylic IOL achieved.

against which to place the second instrument (0.5 mm Knolle spatula) and the smaller phaco tip, to facilitate a complete crack in both average, as well as softer nuclei.

The nucleus is rotated in a clockwise manner, as the four grooves are made to approximately 80% depth, extending just underneath the edge of the capsulorhexis. Then the cracking of the nucleus is accomplished using the bimanual technique with the infusion on (the continuous irrigation setting on the Alcon Legacy is useful in preventing inadvertent loss of infusion during the cracking phase).

After all four sections are completely cracked and free from each other, the port of the 30° downward bevel is then occluded directly into each quadrant, which is brought to the center. With the port either turned to the side or turned downward toward the posterior capsule, the quadrant is emulsified. With the port of the 30° tip turned downward and with the improved fluidics of the newer phaco machines, the nuclear quadrant can be kept well away from the corneal endothelium with minimal risk to the posterior capsule. This has been described by Paul Regnier as his *hockey stick* phaco technique.

In the approximate 10% of nuclei that are extremely dense, I prefer a Phaco Chop technique, such as the Stop and Chop, as described in this book by Paul Koch, or simply converting the four quadrant technique to a chopping technique. Once each of the quadrants is brought in, chopping can facilitate and accelerate the emulsification of these dense quadrants.

Using the 45° angled, ultraflow 0.3 I/A tip, I have found it to be quite easy to aspirate all of the cortical material, with good access to the subincisional cortical material.

## IOL IMPLANTATION TECHNIQUE

I have long been an advocate of using foldable IOLs, inserted through a small incision to maintain the benefits of small incision cataract surgery, with minimal to no surgically induced astigmatism, rapid vision rehabilitation, and high patient satisfaction. With topical anesthesia, all of this now combines to allow our patients to have vision of good quality immediately following cataract surgery,

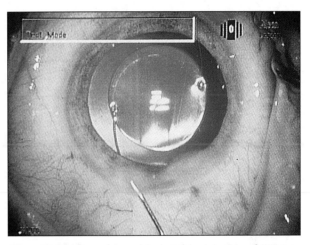

Figure 18-23. Corneal tunnel hydrated by injection of BSS into margins of the corneal tunnel, as well as the roof of the tunnel.

and usually increasing to excellent quality in the first 1 to 2 days following cataract surgery.

The foldable lens of choice for me now is the AcrySof Acrylic IOL, which is available both in a 6 mm diameter, three-piece design, with PMMA haptics, with a high index of refraction (1.55), and the smaller 5.5 mm diameter optic, also in a three-piece design, with the PMMA haptics of the same material, but a thinner edge design. This lens will soon be available in a one-piece, all acrylic design; however, the haptics will be of a traditional design rather than the plate haptic style.

The MA30BA 5.5 mm lens that I am now using is brought to the operating room at the same time as the patient is brought into the operating room. It is kept in its cellophane, shrinkwrapped package in a warm location in the operating room so it will not be cold. When I am ready for the lens implantation, the wagon wheel container is opened, and the lens is removed from the container by grasping the haptic with Kelman-McPherson forceps, dipped in room temperature BSS, and laid on the shelf of the wagon wheel dispenser. The Alcon folding forceps, which has grooves to engage the edge of the optic, is then opened and the optic is appropriately grasped in the folding forceps. When gentle pressure is applied, one can see if the lens appears to be folding correctly, with the fold up or folding down. In the latter instance, the correct fold can be achieved by simply tapping on the center of the optic to reverse the direction of the fold, with subsequent completion of the fold.

The lens is then transferred in a lengthwise manner to the Buratto lens holding forceps (Asico). The incision, which has been previously enlarged to approximately 3.5 mm, is notched open with the 0.12 forceps and the leading haptic is inserted into the incision. It is not necessary to tuck the leading haptic into the optic; however, one should take care that the haptic enters the eye between the jaws of the lens forceps so that it will not be inadvertently crimped. The globe is stabilized during the insertion of the lens by using the closed 0.12 forceps in the paracentesis incision for stabilization.

Once the leading haptic is under the margin of the rhexis and in the bag, the Buratto forceps are turned upward and the lens released with prompt removal of the Buratto forceps, allowing the lens to gently glide out of the forceps and then slowly open. It should be noted that it is very important that both the Alcon folding forceps and the Buratto forceps should be meticulously cleaned by the surgical technician just prior to use to decrease the possibility of any debris from the forceps adhering to the IOL. The trailing haptic can then be placed in the capsular bag in a routine manner with Kelman-McPherson forceps or dialed into place using a Sinskey hook.

It is important that all viscoelastic material is removed. I routinely will slip the I/A tip underneath the implant, as well as in front of the implant, to ensure complete removal of viscoelastic and prevent the possibility of a visco-trapping syndrome.

## CLOSING OF THE INCISION

Once the viscoelastic agent has been removed from the anterior chamber, the sealing of the corneal tunnel is similar to what we have become accustomed to with sealing the scleral tunnel. BSS is injected through the side port so that the eye is firm, but not overly hard, and then the integrity is checked with Weck-cell sponges. If leakage is noted from the wound, a waiting period of 1 minute will usually allow the wound to hydrate and swell slightly to close itself. If additional sealing is required, a small amount of BSS injected into the lateral margins of the corneal tunnel will further hydrate the corneal stroma and seal the incision. No suturing has been required in any of the more than 5000 cases that I have performed using this described technique.

# Chapter 19

# THE IN SITU (FOUR QUADRANT) PHACO FRACTURE TECHNIQUE

*John Shepherd, MD, FACS*

## INTRODUCTION

Phacoemulsification has always been in a state of evolution. Kelman first tried to phacoemulsify in the posterior chamber, but found the anterior chamber phacoemulsification to be safer and more easily taught to beginning surgeons. It has changed in fits and starts ever since. This technique is the present step. Because of decreased funds for research and development, it is conceivable that progress will slow and techniques presented here may change little in the immediate future.

In part, phacoemulsification evolved in order to more easily accomplish the removal of the cataractous lens. But it also was changed in reaction to the convergence of other innovations and techniques, the most important of which was the intraocular lens (IOL).

Initially, the only advantage of phacoemulsification (in the preimplant era) appeared to be the 3 mm incision. The integrity of the posterior capsule was unappreciated. Some surgeons advocated instilling alpha-chymo-trypsin in the anterior chamber and removing the capsule after phacoemulsification! Most surgeons performed a primary posterior capsulotomy at the end of surgery. The 3 mm incision, however, was treasured. It allowed rapid rehabilitation with a contact lens and rapid mobilization.

The introduction of the IOL required extension of this incision, initially to 10 to 12 mm. Later (after adoption of the single plane posterior chamber lens) it was able to be reduced to 6 or 7 mm. These longer incisions were not as effective at or near the limbus as the 3 mm incision, and were gradually moved posteriorly from the limbus to the sclera.

During this period, most surgeons replaced the anterior chamber technique of Kelman with the two-handled iris plane technique popularized by Kratz. The Christmas tree capsulotomy was replaced with the can opener technique. The importance of the posterior capsule was recognized and, following introduction of YAG lasers, few primary capsulotomies were performed.

This method remained pretty much intact from 1978 until 1986. It changed then in response to the advantages and the requirements of a new type of implant—the foldable lens.

The first foldable silicone lens was introduced in 1984.[1] Because of the difficulty in staking haptics to the silicone, it was designed with solid, although thin, haptics. With capsular contraction, a phenomenon not recognized before, this implant bent and bowed forward (Zing). It was redesigned and placed in the sulcus, where it exhibited the tendency to *propeller* and caused pigment dispersion and secondary glaucoma. It was redesigned once more with thicker haptics. This lens (Staar AA4203) was again recommended for bag placement.

Initial results were disappointing. At the time of capsular contraction (4 to 6 weeks postoperatively) one haptic would often fold back the flimsy remnants of the anterior capsule and be pushed off center. Sometimes the capsule split and the implant worked its way into the vitreous cavity. The future of foldable lenses during this period was not promising.

Unnoticed, however, a new method of performing capsulotomies was introduced independently by Howard Gimbel of Canada and Thomas Neuhann of Germany.[2] This proved to be the key for locking this new implant into place.[3] It was rapidly adopted by the small number of foldable lens enthusiasts who, in turn, taught it to many others.

Although capsulorhexis can be used with extracapsular extractions, it is most useful with phacoemulsification. It required, however, some change in technique to remove the nucleus through the small capsular opening

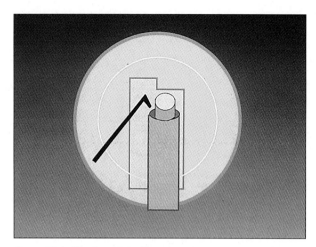

Figure 19-1. Creation of the first groove.

without damaging the capsule edge. Several methods were used during a transition period, but the most useful method became nuclear fracturing.

Nucleofractis or Divide and Conquer was first described by Gimbel.[4] It was modified and more rigidly systematized by Shepherd as the four quadrant or in situ technique.[5] These methods or modifications of them have become the method of choice for most surgeons. Recently, Nagahara has described a chop technique that is very promising.

Because the new implants required only a 3 to 4 mm incision, the wound underwent similar changes. Reducing the length and moving it even more posteriorly allowed us to drop radial sutures and replace them with a *single stitch* horizontal suture. McFarland recognized that even that was superfluous and led the way to adoption of sutureless closures. This was helped significantly by the work of Paul Ernest.[6]

The present technique is therefore a response in large part to the advances of intraocular implants. When the present implants become obsolete, it is probable that the technique of phacoemulsification will also need revision. At present, however, the following is my technique of choice.

## ANESTHESIA

Anesthesia and akinesia have been considered necessary in order to perform cataract surgery in the past. This required general or regional anesthesia.

Most recently, this idea has been reexamined, and many surgeons feel that akinesia is not required in most patients. Furthermore, anesthesia alone can be accomplished by topical medications. This eliminates the orbital injection and its inherent, although rare, dangers. Many surgeons using topical anesthetics have increased the systemic preoperative sedation to almost general anesthetic levels. I have not found this to be necessary. The following is our protocol.

For prevention of infection, the patient begins using one drop of ciloxan four times a day to both eyes the day before surgery. This is repeated the morning of surgery. Because no antibiotic injections are used, we place 4 mg of gentimycin and 10 mg of vancomycin in the 500 cc balanced salt solution (BSS) irrigating solution at the time of surgery.

The patient is received in the preoperative area and dressed for surgery. Usually 5 mg of Valium is given by mouth unless the patient is very old and debilitated, in which a 2.5 mg dose is used. The patient is monitored with electrocardiography, pulse oximetry, and sphygmomanometry until he or she leaves the operating room.

The operative eye is dilated with 1% cyclopentalate and 2.5% NeoSynephrine. These are supplemented with occufen. One drop of each is applied every 5 minutes times four. One drop of 50% solution of betadyne and hypotears is placed in the inferior fornix.

Beginning 20 minutes before surgery, the patient receives one drop of Marcaine 0.75% (injectable) topically to the cornea and this is repeated every 5 minutes, continuing until surgery begins.

The patient walks into the operating room and is positioned on the table. We patch the unoperated eye, believing that this helps prevent unconscious eye movements and blinking. After the usual draping, the lashes are swept back and covered with an adhesive plastic drape. We use a Liebermann type of speculum (Karl Ilg) which allows forcible opening of the palpebral fissure. Care is taken to make sure the lids are open as widely as possible. I believe this helps prevent the patient from trying to blink, preventing unnecessary eye movements.

I try to operate on all patients in the same manner. I sit on the temporal side and rest my ring and small fingers on the patient's malar and temporal bones. I make every effort to make sure that my right forearm is perpendicular to the wound. This is most comfortable if I am sitting 45° to the left. Depending upon the type of operating table used, this may be difficult when operating on left eyes (for right-handed surgeons). I tell the patient that we are beginning the operation and apologize for the bright light, noting that it will dim shortly. Then I usually do not speak to the patient except to correct any movements that he or she may make. Usually, the patient soon forgets that he or she is having surgery, and is quite cooperative about holding the eye steady.

I begin by making a small stab incision about 30° left of where I plan to make the main incision. I use a 1 mm wide diamond knife (Mastel). I then mark the area of the main incision with gentian violet for a width of 3 mm. This defines the length of the incision and also makes it more easily visualized. Using a guarded diamond blade, a 0.20 mg deep, perpendicular incision is made just inside the conjunctiva at the temporal limbus.

The diamond blade is then extended. This blade, which is 3 mm wide, is placed in the depth of the first incision and pushed forward about 1.5 mm to 2.0 mm and then the anterior chamber is entered. The knife is retracted.

The anterior chamber is filled with viscoelastin until the chamber deepens. A bent 25 gauge needle is used to perforate the anterior capsule near the visual axis. The needle

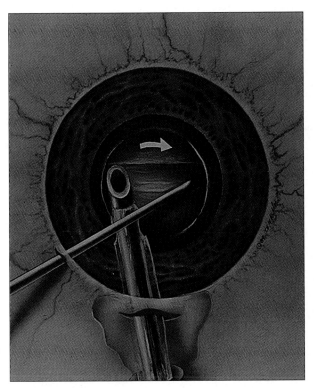 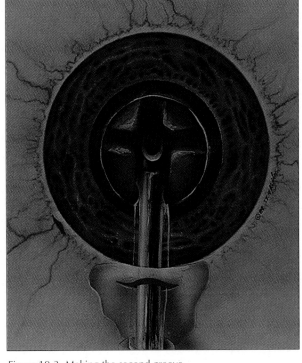

Figure 19-2. Rotation of the nucleus.

Figure 19-3. Making the second groove.

is swept counterclockwise, creating a flap in a spiral manner. A Utrata forceps is used to finish the capsulorhexis. I think the ideal capsulotomy size with a solid haptic silicone lens is 5 to 6 mm. It should be centered on the visual axis. The most common cause of the tear going peripherally is increased vitreous pressure, and this can be prevented by adding viscolelastin to the anterior chamber.

Hydrodissection is performed only to facilitate rotation of the nucleus. We use a 23 gauge McIntyre/Binkhorst cannula which is curved. This same cannula is used later to remove 12 o'clock cortex. We irrigate to the right side nearest the incision first until we see a fluid wave dissect under the nucleus. The cannula is then pressed down on the nucleus which forces the fluid around the sides. This is repeated to the left of the incision. By placing this fluid as close as possible to the anterior capsule, one may free most of the cortex so that less cortical clean-up is needed (Fine's cortical cleavage hydrodissection).

I see no advantage to hydrodelineation of the nuclear or cortical lamellae. I prefer to handle the nucleus as one piece and fragment it by complete fracture lines through and including the epinucleus.

At present I am combining the classical four quadrant nucleofractis technique with a modification of the Nagahara Chop technique.

We use a 30° or 45° phaco tip with the vacuum set at 100 and the aspiration at 26. I prefer a peristaltic aspiration pump.

The tip is placed into the wound bevel-down and rotated bevel-up as the iris is passed. With a Sinskey hook in the left hand to stabilize the nucleus, the phaco tip is used to sculpt a two tip wide groove from 12 to 6 o'clock. This tip goes only slightly under the inferior capsule rim and does not approach the periphery of the capsule. This sculpting is gradual and care is taken not to occlude the tip or burrow into the nucleus. It is shaved off in layers. The bottom of the groove is usually at the level of the posterior Y suture. Sometimes the red reflex is used to judge the depth of the groove. Care is taken to ensure that the groove is bowl-shaped—deeper centrally and more shallow as the periphery is approached. The peripheral capsule must be avoided! The groove ends just slightly beyond the capsulorhexis edge, safely away from the peripheral capsule.

After this groove is completed, the nucleus is rotated clockwise by pressing forward with the phaco tip to the left wall of the groove (closest to the incision) and pushing clockwise. With the Sinskey hook on the right wall of groove, (farthest from the incision), pressure is applied to rotate the lens in the same direction. This creates enough force to break any remaining adhesions.

In the classical four quadrant technique, we would then sculpt another groove perpendicular to the first and slightly deeper. (This is easily done because of increased visibility into the depth of the groove.) Then the phaco tip is placed against the left wall of the groove holding it in place. The Sinskey hook is placed against the right wall near the base and pushed, fracturing the nucleus. This is a cross action method which creates adequate force without wide separation of the nuclear sections. Rotation is facilitated by foot Position 1 (irrigation). Fracturing is facilitated by foot Position 0, which relaxes the posterior

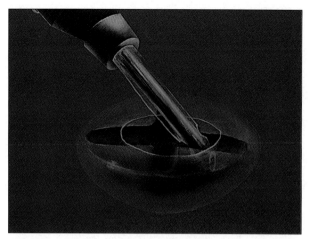

Figure 19-4. Completion of the second groove.

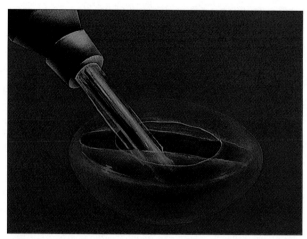

Figure 19-5. Fracturing the first quadrant.

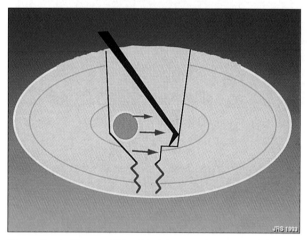

Figure 19-6. Chop modification following formation of the first groove—fracture into two hemisections.

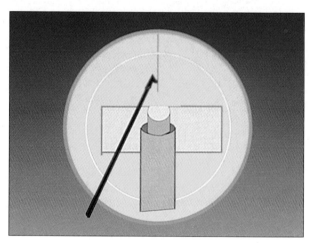

Figure 19-7. Rotate and burrow into the distal hemi-section.

capsule, making it difficult to tear.

The nucleus is then rotated 90° and the fracture repeated until the nucleus is divided into four fragments.

Recently we have modified this technique using Nagahara's Phaco Chop.

In this modification, we start identically by making a two phaco tip wide groove and fracturing it. Then rotate 90° and, instead of sculpting, burrow into the inferior hemi-section near the base and stabilize it with tip left in place. The Sinskey hook is placed under the inferior anterior capsule as far as the equator of the nucleus. It is pressed posterior and pulled toward the phaco tip. This causes the anterior one half or two thirds of the nucleus to separate. The hook and the phaco tip are then separated causing a fracture to occur. This is repeated until all four quadrants are created. This is faster than the classical four quadrant technique and relies less on posterior pressure on the lens diaphragm, which may cause some discomfort to a topically anesthetized patient. Hard nuclei can be fractured into six or eight fragments.

Using the preformed groove allows enough room to remove the quadrants safely in the posterior chamber and avoids the crowding of the original Nagahara technique.

These techniques are safe in that they confine all the sculpting to a period of time in which the nucleus protects the posterior capsule. Even as each quadrant is removed, the remaining quadrants keep the capsule pushed well posterior until only the last remains. Care should be taken to keep the second instrument between the capsule and the last quadrant, avoiding damage to the posterior capsule. This was best described by Paul Koch (see Stop and Chop).

## CORTICAL CLEANUP

In almost all cases, some amount of cortex will remain in the periphery of the capsular bed. I begin removing it by manually removing a wedge shaped segment at 12 o'clock. I use Gill's technique with a 2 cc syringe and a 25 gauge cannula. This is easy if done first while the remaining cortex holds the anterior and posterior capsules apart. Following this, I use a curved irrigation/aspiration (I/A) tip (0.3 mm) to strip the cortex completely. In this technique, the anterior cortex should be grasped first and by

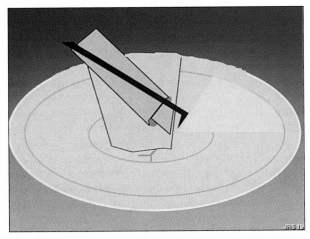

Figure 19-8. At the side of the engaged phaco tip, impale the nucleus with a chopper or hook.

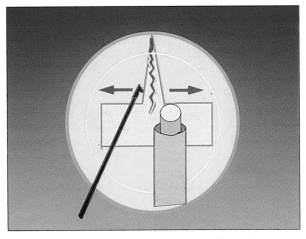

Figure 19-9. Separate the two, creating two quadrants. Then repeat on the other section.

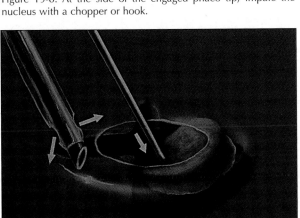

Figure 19-10. Mobilization of the first quadrant.

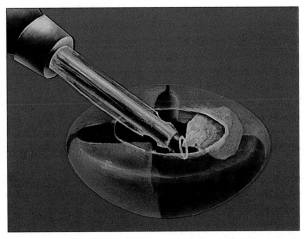

Figure 19-11. Phacoemulsification of the first quadrant.

*wiggling* the tip, the cortex is stripped from its capsular adhesions. I make a point to use a chalazian type of curette (Shepherd-Rensch capsule polisher MorningStaar Instruments) sharpened on both the anterior and posterior surfaces to polish the anterior and posterior capsule all the way to the fornix. Removal of a significant amount of lens epithelial cells in this manner prevents much of the capsular fibrosis that is responsible for complications such as lens decentration and opacification of the posterior capsule.

## IMPLANTATION OF THE IOL

My lens of choice is a foldable silicone lens. Of the two types, I prefer the solid haptic (Staar 4203c) over the three-piece silicone lens with conventional haptics. The latter is used as a backup in case of a broken capsule or zonular tear.

I reinflate the bag with viscoelastin and inject the lens with the MicroStaar injector. The solid haptic silicone lens must be placed in the bag with an intact capsulorhexis. If there is any question of the integrity of the anterior or

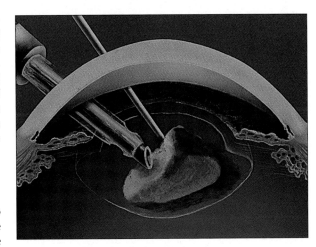

Figure 19-12. Removing the last quadrant.

posterior capsule, a three-piece haptic lens is chosen. Following insertion, the viscoelastin is removed with the I/A handpiece and replaced with BSS. We then check the integrity of the wound. If it is watertight, we are finished. If it leaks, we inject a small amount of BSS into the corneal stroma at each end of the incision. This creates corneal swelling, sealing the wound.

The eye is left unpatched, and the patient is given a topical steroid to use four times for 2 weeks, and the patient continues to use the antibiotic (ciloxan) for 3 more days. We no longer use a shield or restrict any activity. I see the patient the following day and then 2 weeks later. If all is well, the patient is discharged at that 2 week visit.

# SPECIAL SITUATIONS

## Small Pupil

The presence of a small pupil alone is not a serious problem. However, when this small pupil is combined with a dense, hard nucleus, a deep set eye, or high myopia, it can ruin the surgeon's day (and also the patient's).

It is necessary to analyze each patient and try to anticipate any problems. If the nucleus is soft and no other problems are observable, one may operate by retracting the iris with one hand and performing a capsulorhexis with the other. Capsulorhexis is the key to this surgery and no effort should be spared in performing it perfectly.

The four quadrant technique is ideal for small pupils because it can be performed only on the center of the cataract and a large pupil is not necessary. Following fracture, each quadrant can be brought forward of the iris and phacofragmented in the anterior chamber. This can be much more difficult in a high myope or a patient with a hard nucleus. Operating blindly may cause capsular rupture, zonular dialysis, or in the worst case, even loss of the nucleus into the vitreous. When these problems are found in combinations in the same patient, I prefer to use the new pupil retractors. They take about 3 to 5 minutes to place, but convert a difficult case into a routine one.

## Torn Zonules

Zonular dialysis is found in varying degrees in a number of patients. It is probably the result of a combination of factors: preexisting trauma, surgical technique, and anatomical variation. The dialysis can range from the very mildest form in which no frank subluxation is found and the only clue may be a small strand of zonules, or vitreous coming from anterior to the capsule. This only needs treatment by amputation of the strand. It is necessary to recognize it, however, for failure to do so may result in a peaked pupil and possibly vitreous traction.

More severe cases will include subluxation of the capsule. This can be recognized or at least suspected prior to surgery by careful biomicroscopy. One should observe for iridodynesis particularly in Marfan's syndrome or in post-trauma patients. Once the area of dialysis is identified, the surgeon should avoid any maneuver that causes increased traction on the adjacent zonules. This may necessitate manual removal of cortex and very careful polishing of the posterior capsule.

Placing the IOL is of paramount importance. It should be a modified C loop and the haptic should be pointing directly toward the dialysis with the haptics and optic completely within the capsulorhexis. If the IOL is placed in this position, it will stay centered and also keep the capsulorhexis centered.

The most important factors are capsulorhexis and IOL placement.

## Hard Nuclei

Dense nuclei are removed with about the same technique as the others, only with more patience. A 45° tip is more important here and somewhat prolonged sculpting is necessary. It is necessary to sculpt more deeply in order to fracture the quadrants, and we usually make all four grooves before we begin fracturing. A larger amount of the nucleus can be phacoemulsified before the fragments are mobilized, and therefore protect the endothelium.

Some nuclei are so dense that they preclude use of the phacoemulsification technique. These are not always apparent prior to surgery. The surgeon needs to constantly reassure himself that the method is proceeding according to plan, and if not, consider converting to extracapsular removal of the nucleus before a surgical mishap occurs. This depends on experience, and must be learned over a lifetime.

# REFERENCES

1. Mazzocco T. Progress report: Silicone IOLs. *Cataract*. 1984;1(4):18-19.
2. Gimbel H, Neuhann T. Development, advantages, and methods of the continuous circular capsulorhexis technique. *J Cataract Refract Surg*. 1990;16:31-37.
3. Shepherd J. Continuous-tear capsulotomy and insertion of a silicone bag lens. *J Cataract Refract Surg*. 1989;15:335-339.
4. Gimbel H. Divide and conquer nucleofractis phacoemulsification: Development and variations. *J Cataract Refract Surg*. 1991;17:281-291.
5. Shepherd J. In situ fracture. *J Cataract Refract Surg*. 1990;16:436-440.
6. Ernest P, Kiessling A, Slavery K. Relative strength of cataract incisions in cadaver eyes. *J Cataract Refract Surg*. 1991;17:668-671.

# Chapter 20

# DIVIDE AND CONQUER NUCLEOFRACTIS TECHNIQUE

*Howard V. Gimbel, MD, MPH*
*Michael T. Furlong, MD*

## INTRODUCTION

In 1986, I coined the term Divide and Conquer for my technique of in situ phacoemulsification. These techniques evolved because of my observation that a cataract that has been systematically divided and fragmented, rather than impaled by the phaco tip in a random fashion, is more easily conquered. To describe this fashion of fracturing or fragmenting the nucleus into pieces, I coined the term *nucleofractis*, which comes from the prefix nucleo (nucleus) and the Greek suffix fractis (to fracture). Divide and Conquer nucleofractis (DCN) now describes my technique of phacoemulsification.[1]

This radial fracturing of the lens, as well as its lamellar separation by hydrodissection and hydrodelineation into nucleus, epinucleus, and cortex, is somewhat analogous to other objects in nature. For example, a log can have many lamellar separations of bark and annular rings corresponding to the cortex and the epinucleus being separated by lamellar hydrodissection. However, the core of the log is also split with radial fractures, many of which are seen as natural cleavage planes as the wood dries. Likewise, the watermelon has radial as well as circumferential cleavage planes.

When sculpting through the nucleus of the cataract, one often can see the natural radial cleavage planes in the nucleus of the lens corresponding to the Y sutures seen on slit lamp examination. While the radial fractures often follow these natural cleavage planes, the instruments can easily create other radial cleavage planes.

The differing densities of cataracts have spawned two different methods of sculpting that I use as broad variations of DCN: Trench, Multidirectional, and Crater Divide and Conquer.

## TRENCH DIVIDE AND CONQUER (TDC) NUCLEOFRACTIS

### Employed in Soft to Moderately Hard Nuclei

After the continuous curvilinear capsulorhexis (CCC) is completed, hydrodissection and hydrodelineation are performed.[2] This will allow free rotation of the nucleus and epinucleus, thus enhancing the efficacy of DCN. Stress on the zonules is also minimized while rotational maneuvers are being employed. The trench technique is performed by sculpting a deep trough or trench slightly to the right of the center of the lens (for right-handed surgeons) using a 30 or 45° phacoemulsification tip. Stabilization of the lens during the trench creation is accomplished by using a second instrument (a cyclodialysis spatula or nucleus rotator) through a paracentesis incision and resting it on the central anterior surface of the lens.[3] When the trench is judged to be sufficiently deep, the nucleus can then be fractured into two pieces by placing the phaco tip and the second instrument against opposite walls of the trench and forcing the nuclear sections in opposite directions. The instruments must be held deeply in the groove and the fracture should propagate from the center to the superior and inferior rims. The phaco instrument should always be kept on irrigation only (foot Position 1) during this initial fracture. When a complete hemisection is accomplished, the phaco tip is then buried deeply into the left section at 5 o'clock, and by moving the tip away from the larger nuclear mass a second crack is made, separating a pie-shaped section of nucleus. The second instrument is held

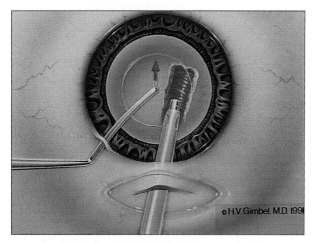

Figure 20-1. Initial trench creation using a second instrument to stabilize the lens.

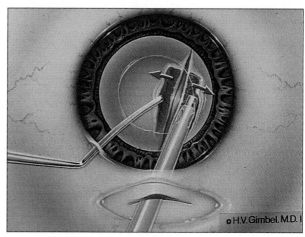

Figure 20-2. Bimanual fracturing technique.

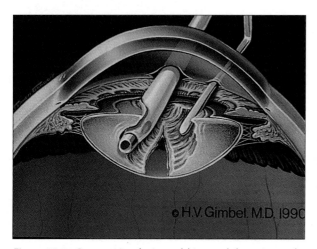

Figure 20-3. Cross-sectional view of bimanual fracturing technique.

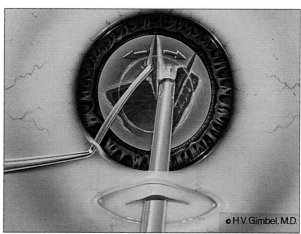

Figure 20-4. Second nuclear fracture creating pie-shaped piece.

adjacent to the phaco probe, and a small down and away force relative to the phaco tip will usually facilitate fracturing. In hard nuclei, the second fracture is made approximately 30° from the first, but this angle should be increased to 60° for softer nuclei. This difference in size corresponds with the ease of phacoemulsifying these wedge segments later in the procedure.

After gentle rotation, additional fractured segments are created in manageable phacoemulsification pieces, with smaller segments needed for denser nuclei. Several rotations and fracturing may be necessary for both heminuclear sections. The separate sections may be brought into the center of the capsular bag after each one is fractured, or they may be left in place until all fractures have been performed. Maximal capsular bag distension is maintained if the latter technique is employed, reducing the chances of inadvertent posterior capsular rupture.

The second instrument assists by stabilizing the lens during cracking and even provides an equal and opposite force that increases the control of the fracture. Appropriate positioning of the nuclear fragments is also facilitated by the second instrument. It is also very help-ful to place it immediately posterior to the mouth of the phaco probe when removing nuclear segments to restrict inadvertent aspiration of the posterior capsule. This is especially true during removal of the last few segments when the capsule's movement is most susceptible to the turbulence caused by aspiration flow. Phacoemulsification of the fragments is usually performed at the iridocapsular plane. Only aspiration or short bursts of ultrasound (U/S) should be used to grasp lens pieces while they are in the capsular bag to limit the risk of breaking the capsule during phacoemulsification.

## Downslope Sculpting

In the past, I attempted a slight variation in the traditional sculpting method used with DCN. By nudging the lens inferiorly with the second instrument, the upper central part of the nucleus could be sculpted deeply—directly parallel and close to the posterior capsule. This afforded early access to the posterior pole of the lens for effective fracturing.[4] The use of capsule anatomy is analogous to manipulating batter in a mixing bowl. By tipping the bowl up on one side, the batter will shift downward, cre-

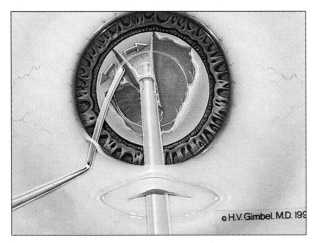

Figure 20-5. Additional pie-shaped pieces are created.

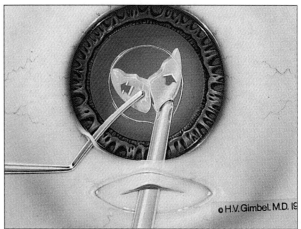

Figure 20-6. The remaining nuclear piece is fractured and emulsified.

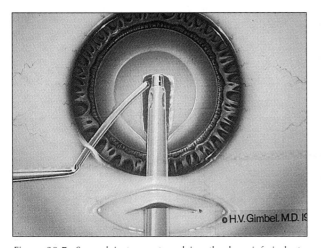

Figure 20-7. Second instrument nudging the lens inferiorly to allow very deep sculpting centrally.

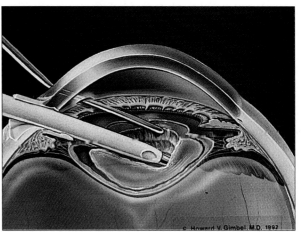

Figure 20-8. Cross-sectional view of downslope sculpting.

ating a deeper concentration and easier accessibility with a spoon. Similarly, with the lens nucleus nudged toward the 6 o'clock position, the surgeon can sculpt very deeply down the slope of the posterior curvature of the lens. I have termed this method *downslope sculpting*.

The key to downslope sculpting is to nudge the lens inferiorly with the second instrument to allow deep central sculpting. Although sculpting is completed very deep, one avoids impaling the posterior capsule because nuclear material is always ahead of the tip. Downslope sculpting thus facilitates sculpting to the posterior pole of the lens where instruments can be held to obtain the first fracture.

Fracturing can follow a number of patterns, including the standard trench method, which can be followed by the creation of an L-shaped fracture. An alternative method is to first create a horizontal fracture, thereby facilitating a similar L-shaped split.

Downslope sculpting has made any pregrooving of the lens unnecessary in all but very dense nuclei.[5] One simply needs to get deep into the center to fracture through the radial fault lines of the lens. With traditional sculpting techniques, the deepest part of the sculpting will end up inferiorly to the center of the lens. If one rotates the lens 90° with each quadrant's sculpting, the plate of nuclear material deep in the center or posterior pole of the nucleus will impede complete fracturing to the center and the sections will tend to hang together at the center. However, with downslope sculpting, complete and efficient fracturing and subsequent emulsification can be accomplished by sculpting deep and fracturing through the entire posterior plate of the nucleus.

## MULTIDIRECTIONAL DIVIDE AND CONQUER (MDC)

Downslope multidirectional nucleofractis is begun by debulking the superior part of the lens (or temporal part of the lens if the approach is from the side). The technique usually involves a trench or a trough sculpted slightly to the right of the lens at the center. Nudging the nucleus inferiorly with the second instrument, downslope is accomplished sculpting very deeply to the posterior pole of the lens. The upper central part of the nucleus can be sculpted

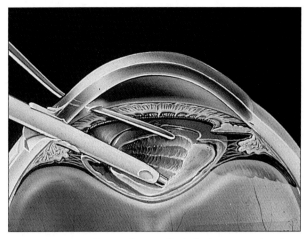

Figure 20-9. Very deep sculpting affords facilitating nuclear fracturing.

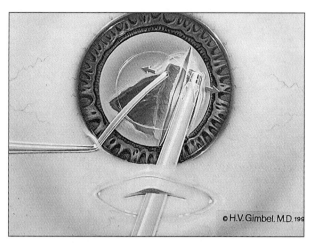

Figure 20-10. Standard trench fracture.

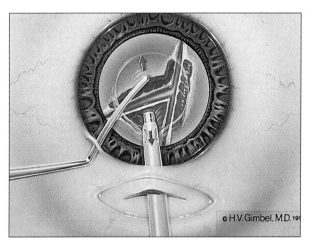

Figure 20-11. L-shaped fracture.

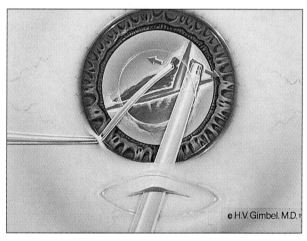

Figure 20-12. Horizontal fracture followed by L-shaped fracture.

very deeply and affords early and effective fracturing. The Kelman tip works very well for this side-to-side movement, allowing for a deep groove horizontally. The phaco tip is then used to stabilize the upper portion while the second instrument pushes inferiorly against the wall, creating a horizontal fracture. A vertical fracture is then created by pushing to the right of the vertical trough with the phaco tip and to the left with the second instrument.

## CRATER DIVIDE AND CONQUER (CDC)

### Employed in Moderately Hard to Very Hard and Even Dense, Brunescent Nuclei

In the case of a dense nucleus, the standard trench may not debulk the nucleus sufficiently to permit easy fracturing. Hydrodissection is performed, which is followed by sculpting a deep crater into the center of the nucleus, leaving a peripheral rim that can later be fractured into multiple sections. The posterior plate of the nucleus must be included in the creation of the crater, otherwise fracturing will be more difficult. A shaving action is used to sculpt away the central nuclear material. Lens rotation is usually required to enlarge and deepen the crater when central lens material becomes inaccessible to the phaco probe due to the initial angle of attack. Again, the Kelman tip is very helpful in these circumstances. The size of the crater should be expanded for progressively denser nuclei. Enough of the dense material must be left in place to allow successful fracturing into sections.

The depth of the crater can usually be judged by the increasing brightness of the red reflex as the sculpting is carried deeper and deeper. Once the depth and width of the crater is judged to be adequate, the two-handed technique is used to create a fracture in the nuclear rim. The nucleus is then rotated and a second fracture is made. This process is continued, leaving the fragments in place, until several manageable pieces are left. This gives maximal distension of the capsular bag, minimizing the chance of inadvertent cutting of the posterior capsule with the phaco tip. Individual sections are then brought

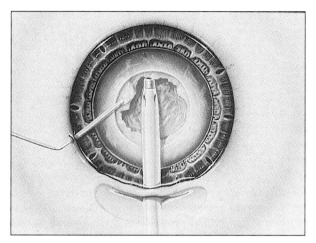

Figure 20-13. Deep and wide crater creation.

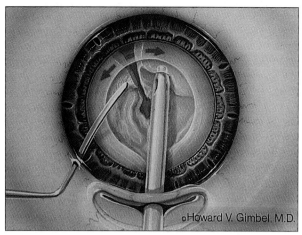

Figure 20-14. Bimanual fracturing technique.

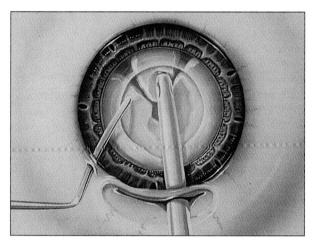

Figure 20-15. After nuclear rotation, additional fractures are created.

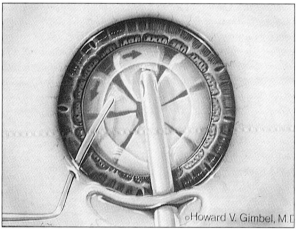

Figure 20-16. Individual sections are brought into the center for emulsification.

to the center for phacoemulsification. Alternatively, the first section may be isolated and emulsified to allow space for subsequent fracturing.

## SMALL PUPILS

The most important goal in small pupil cataract surgery is to limit serious surgical complications. Relatively complication-free surgery in small pupil cases can be achieved with phacoemulsification techniques. These techniques also help to attain other goals such as the use of a small incision, the minimal use of pupil enlarging surgery, and certain verification of in-the-bag placement of a posterior chamber intraocular lens (IOL). This placement, verification, long-term stability, and centration can be virtually assured by obtaining and maintaining a CCC opening in the anterior capsule. The lens nucleus, even though dense and large, can be fractured into small segments and removed by emulsification through relatively small capsule openings, small pupil openings, small scleral incisions and small conjunctival incisions. These are important considerations in many glaucoma patients who have small pupils from long-term miotic therapy and who have had or may in the future require filtering surgery.

### Challenges of Phaco: The Small Pupil

I developed the downslope sculpting method in small pupil cases to quickly reach the posterior pole of the nucleus for efficient fracturing. The lens is nudged inferiorly using a second instrument and the phaco tip sculpts down the concave posterior capsule toward the posterior pole, parallel to the capsule as opposed to perpendicular to it. Once the pole is reached, the two instruments are held deep in the center. The spatula pushes inferiorly while the phaco tip pushes superiorly to create a horizontal fracture in this case.[6] The two instruments are repositioned to create a vertical fracture. The fractured segments can remain in the bag to stabilize it or be removed piece by piece. Notice how the second instrument holds back segments while other segments are emulsified in the center of the lens. As well, the spatula brings nuclear material to the phaco tip to be emulsified. The phaco tip itself stays mainly in the center of the lens.

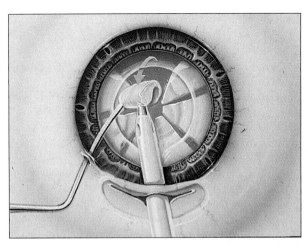

Figure 20-17. Alternatively, the first section may be isolated and emulsified to allow space for subsequent fracturing.

Once the inferior hemisection has been emulsified, the superior hemisection can be brought up to the center of the lens with the second instrument, and further fractures can be created. These small pupil cases demonstrate the distinct advantage of nucleofractis techniques in that the phaco tip does not have to be put under the iris or under the small openings in the capsule. As such, there is little risk of iris or capsule flowing unexpectedly with the lens material into the tip of the phaco port. One should use a lower flow when the pupil is small. This may reduce efficiency, but certainly will increase safety. Again, notice how epinuclear material now is brought to the phaco port using the second instrument. The phaco port itself does not go searching for this material in a small pupil case such as this.

## Challenges of Phaco: Intumescent Lens

The nucleus in an intumescent lens can be safely and efficiently fractured and phacoemulsified using my downslope sculpting technique. In intumescent cases with primary, small capsulorhexis openings, the nucleus is nudged inferiorly with a second instrument. The upper portion of the nucleus is sculpted very deeply because the sculpting is done parallel rather than perpendicular to the posterior capsule. This nudging maneuver allows the phaco tip to get very deep into the nucleus for subsequent fracturing. The phaco tip should be maintained centrally to avoid stress on either the small capsulorhexis rim or a can opener margin. Mechanical stress to the ring of the can opener with the use of the phaco handpiece, or by a second instrument, should be avoided. This is where the downslope sculpting nucleofractis is advantageous for safe emulsification, because the phaco tip always stays in the center of the lens. The second instrument is used to rotate, maneuver, and help fracture the nuclear rim.

The depth of the sculpting is quite easy to gauge in an intumescent lens due to the whiteness of the nucleus and the red reflex exposed during fracturing. In performing phacoemulsification out near the periphery or up near the capsule in the epinucleus, low flow and low vacuum should be used so that a sudden breakthrough with a high flow and high vacuum can be avoided. This will avoid engaging the equatorial capsule with the phaco tip. The intumescent lens is usually easy to fracture and quite often the lens will fracture spontaneously with only an attempt at rotation.

## PHACO SWEEP

Another variation on the theme of nucleofractis is a technique I call Phaco Sweep.[7] In traditional sculpting techniques, the phaco probe is moved from the superior to the inferior portion of the nucleus to create a groove. By using the phaco probe in a lateral motion (nasal to temporal and back again), the central nucleus can be sculpted quickly and deeply while maintaining constant visualization of the tip of the instrument. We prefer to use a 30° Kelman phacoemulsification tip to perform phaco sweep. With this tip, the removal of lens material is more efficient and easier to perform. However, this technique is also possible with standard straight tip phacoemulsification handpieces. The engineers at Alcon explain this difference on the basis of a three-dimensional propagation of the U/S wave front from the bent Kelman tip. Standard handpieces tend to direct their U/S power primarily in the forward direction, somewhat limiting their cutting efficiency for this technique.

As sculpting proceeds to deeper layers, the phaco tip is moved in a lateral sweeping motion. It is important to avoid occlusion of the tip during this procedure. The lens is stabilized inferior to the groove with a second instrument through the paracentesis. After lateral sculpting is sufficiently deep, a horizontal fracture is created as the upper portion of the nucleus is stabilized with the phaco tip while the second instrument pushes against the inferior wall of the groove. Multidirectional nucleofractis may then proceed as described in this chapter, after the nucleus has been rotated 90°, to create multiple wedge-shaped sections. These pieces are then emulsified within the central pupillary zone. Phaco sweep is a variation of downslope sculpting, which enhances visualization of the phaco tip and results in increased safety for the removal of central nuclear material. In addition, the motion of the probe remains parallel to the posterior capsule, diminishing the risk of its inadvertent rupture.

## POLAR EXPEDITIONS

Deep sculpting of the posterior pole of the lens facilitates the fracturing of the nucleus because it provides for safe and efficient segmentation, and removal of the nuclear segments by taking advantage of the natural fault lines of the lens. The natural lens has lamellar planes that lend themselves to hydrodissection and hydrodelineation, but lens fibers are oriented in a radial fashion, creating the familiar Y suture lines. It is these radial bulk lines that one can take advantage of in nucleofractis techniques.

Deep sculpting allows one to obtain the mechanical advantage required to effectively fracture through the entire lens. After hydrodissection and hydrodelineation, one attempts to fracture the hard nucleus through its entirety. The expedition to the posterior pole can be accomplished with forward sculpting or phaco sweep lateral sculpting to thin the posterior plate before fracturing is attempted. Once the posterior pole is reached, the segments fracture very easily with the two-handed technique—even without a Phaco Chop instrument—because the segments are small. When the lens material is brunescent, the Phaco Chop instrument is used to fracture these segments in the crater chop technique. Deep central sculpting is recommended in these dense nuclei—even with crater chop—so that the segments are smaller and more easily managed.

A second instrument is used to manage the segments to keep them down within the lens and from floating up to the cornea. The Kelman MicroTip with the Mackool sleeve is very efficient for the removal of epinucleus. The vacuum and aspiration flow rate are reduced for epinucleus removal when doing irrigation/aspiration (I/A). I use surgeon control of aspiration which allows one to grasp the material at low vacuum, and also allows efficient control of lens material when engaged by the port.

The sculpting should be deep enough to go right through the nucleus into the epinucleus. The bent Kelman tip facilitates this deep sculpting. The parameters for the Legacy with the Mackool system are as follows: U/S power is 40% for sculpting, and 50% to 60% for segment removal, and then 40% again for epinucleus removal. Aspiration flow rate varies in foot Position 2 and 3, from 23 to 27 cc/min; the vacuum is 250 to 340 mm Hg for the nucleus removal, and only 210 for epinucleus removal.

Downslope sculpting toward the posterior pole is used for the multidirectional Divide and Conquer technique. The upper part of the nucleus is removed, and, with phaco sweep polar expedition, involves sculpting of the posterior pole before the horizontal fracture. The lens is stabilized and nudged inferiorly, and the sculpting is done with forward passes until the surgeon is deep in the lens. Then phaco sweep is used to delicately sculpt through the deepest part of the nucleus to the epinucleus before the horizontal fracture is made.

This horizontal fracture is a combination of separation and sheering. The second instrument pushes toward 6 o'clock, and the phaco tip pushes down and away so that these opposing forces result in the splitting of the nucleus as the horizontal fracture. Then the multidirectional fracturing is accomplished without rotating the lens. With the natural fault lines in the lens, this can be accomplished very easily without the chopping technique through the use of two-instrument separation. The fracturing is enhanced by not only separation but again by sheering (pushing down on one segment) down and away so that it is two planes. The upper hemisection can be rotated 180° for similar fracturing, or it can be simply slid down into the central part of the capsule and approached from the equatorial side, and fracturing accomplished.

In Trench Divide and Conquer, polar sculpting is limited to a central trough or trench. This works best in a very soft nucleus where one has to maintain most of the nuclear, which is firm enough to fracture. The nucleus is nudged slightly inferiorly and stabilized with the second instrument. Then the polar expedition for the posterior pole of the lens begins. The trench has to be wide enough to allow the phaco sleeve to get down into the nucleus. Once deep enough, the fracture is obtained with the two instruments. The segments are broken away, similar to the other nucleofractis techniques. Once the fracture is through the posterior plate of the lens, the fractured segments fracture completely without being tied together at the apices, and small segments are easier to manage than large segments. Only low U/S power is necessary for these small nuclear segments to be emulsified. With the new technology of the Alcon Series 2000 and the Mackool system MicroTip and max vac cassette, the chamber remains deep and stable with the lack of postocclusion surge. The different memory settings on the machine also allow one to quickly change from one parameter to another.

## REFERENCES

1. Gimbel HV. Divide and conquer nucleofractis phacoemulsification: Development and variations. *J Cataract Refract Surg.* 1991;17:281-291.
2. Gimbel HV. Continuous curvilinear capsulorhexis and nucleus fracturing: Evolution, technique, and complications. *Ophthal Clinics of North America.* 1991;4:235-249.
3. Gimbel HV. Trough and crater divide and conquer nucleofractis techniques. *Eur J Implant Ref Surg.* 1991;3:123-126.
4. Gimbel HV. Downslope sculpting. *J Cataract Refract Surg.* 1992;18:614-618.
5. Gimbel HV. Evolving techniques of cataract surgery: Continuous curvilinear capsulorhexis, Downslope sculpting and nucleofractis. *Seminars in Ophthal.* 1992;7:193-207.
6. Gimbel HV. Nucleofractis through a small pupil. *Can J Ophthal.* 1992;27:115-119.
7. Gimbel HV, Chin PK: Phaco sweep. *J Cataract Refract Surg.* 1995;493-496.

# Chapter 21

# PERSONAL PHACOEMULSIFICATION TECHNIQUE

*Kunihiro Nagahara, MD*

## PREPARATION

The pupil is well dilated preoperatively by the use of Neosynephrine and tropicamide at 5 minute intervals in four sets before entering the operating room.

### Anesthesia

My routine cataract surgery is performed under topical anesthesia with 4% Xylocaine eye drops. Before entering the operating room, the patient, in the supine position, is anesthetized once by topical anesthesia in both eyes. Once the patient is relaxed on the reclining operating chair and before the scrub, the anesthetic eye drops are again inserted into both eyes. During this procedure, the nurse uses a lid retractor or a finger to lift the upper lid. The patient is instructed to look down in order to place the eye drops in the upper cul-de-sac. This technique helps the patient feel comfortable during the scrub. It is important that the patient feel as little pain as possible during the scrub, because pain would cause the patient to close his or her eyes, therefore making the surgery more difficult.

### Draping

The patient is routinely prepped and draped. A Hogi waterproof cataract drape with a hole is placed over the face, and a Hogi plastic drape covers the eye to keep the eyelashes well away from the globe. After the drape is cut, a standard Kratz wire speculum is placed in the eye, and the plastic is folded back under the upper and lower lids to seal off the lid margin.

## PHACOEMULSIFICATOR

I use three phacoemulsification machines: Diplomat; Allergan, Legacy; and Alcon, Protégé; Storz.

I use Diplomat in routine cataract surgery because the handpiece is equipped with the Zero tip and silicone sleeve. The Zero tip, which I designed, has no bevel, but it has the inside cutting sharp edge. Not only does it have the same shaving capability, but the Zero tip has more aspiration power than the 45° ultrasound (U/S) tip. The infusion fluid consists of 500 mL of (balanced salt solution) BSS Plus with 0.1 mL epinephrine.

## INCISION

I do not use the bridle suture under the superior rectus tendon to fix the eye, because this seems to be uncomfortable for the patient. Instead of the fixation suture, the microscope is mounted with the fixation red light to control eye position during surgery. The conjunctiva is grasped with forceps and a small peritomy is created along the limbus at the 12 o'clock position. Light cautery is used at the operative site.

My routine self-sealing incision for implanting a 5.5 mm single piece polymethylmethacrylate (PMMA) lens is a 3 mm long tunnel, flanged 5.5 mm at its base with a 6.0 mm entry into the anterior chamber. I use a trifacet diamond knife to make a 5 to 5.5 mm straight external incision, which is 3 mm posterior to the anterior limbus and approximately half the thickness of the depth of the sclera. Two side port incisions are made through the limbus at approximately the 10 and 2 o'clock positions using the same diamond knife. The external incision is tunneled upward to the posterior limbus with a rounded diamond knife, keeping the same depth. The anterior chamber is entered just inside of the clear cornea with a 3 mm slit diamond knife in order to make internal incision. This internal incision is extended up to 5.5 to 6 mm with a slit diamond knife or crescent shaped diamond knife before implanting the IOL.

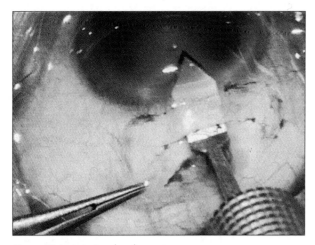

Figure 21-1. Anterior chamber entry.

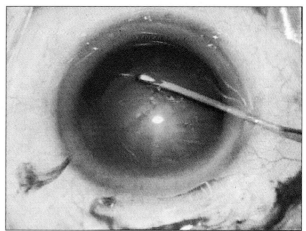

Figure 21-2. CCC with needle.

Table 21-1
### MACHINE SETTINGS DURING PHACOEMULSIFICATION

|  | Type of pump | U/S control | U/S power | U/S vacuum (mm Hg) | U/S flow rate (cc/min) | Tip |
|---|---|---|---|---|---|---|
| Diplomat | Peristaltic | linear | 70% | 110 | 24 | 0 |
| Legacy | Peristaltic | linear | 60% | 150 | 25 | 15, 30 |
| Protege | Venturi | linear | 50% | 150 | --- | 0, 15, 30 |

## CONTENTS OF THE CHAMBER FOR THE CAPSULOTOMY

Viscoelastic material, usually Opegan (low molecule sulfate-sodium hyaluronate, Santen Ophthalmics), is instilled into the anterior chamber from the side port. This puts a slight tension on the anterior capsule and protects the corneal endothelium when a needle is used for the anterior capsulectomy. The aqueous fluid is easily exchanged with the low molecule versus the high molecule viscoelastic material. Therefore, they have more of a chance to contact and protect the corneal endothelium. On the other hand, when I use the forceps, I inject the high viscosity material (Healon, Pharmacia) in order to keep the depth of the anterior chamber.

## CAPSULOTOMY

A continuous circular capsulorhexis (CCC) is performed with a 27 gauge disposable needle as cystotome which is introduced into the anterior chamber through the 10 o'clock position side port. The capsulorhexis is made first with a small tear at the center of the anterior capsule. The lateral movement and gentle tearing make the capsule flap. This flap is turned over and the rhexis is controlled in a circular fashion.

The CCC is 5.5 to 6 mm in size and always larger than the diameter of the IOL optics. The opacification of the posterior capsule is prohibited by adhesion between the anterior capsule edge and the posterior capsule.

## HYDRODISSECTION/ HYDRODELAMINATION

Hydrodissection is carried out with a 27 gauge blunt irrigating needle under the edge of the capsulorhexis, and a water fluid wave is seen as it proceeds under the nucleus and cortical bow. We can judge the size of the nucleus by the hydrodelineation and use of the chopper becomes more comfortable. After the hydrodissection is completed, the nucleus spins easily in the capsular bag.

## EMULSIFICATION FOR NUCLEUS OF HARDNESS 2

The U/S tip is inserted into the anterior chamber and removes the epinucleus inside of the CCC. After CCC, hydrodissection is completed. The epinucleus can be removed effectively with the use of weak U/S energy in addition to aspiration. If the epinucleus is thick and it cannot be removed, the dividing technique becomes more difficult because the U/S tip cannot reach the center of the nucleus. This removing procedure is not necessary for a dense cataract with a little epinucleus.

The phaco chopper is introduced through the side port incision and the U/S tip is driven toward the center of the nucleus. The Sinskey hook improved the length of a point of the phaco chopper by 1.5 mm; it can chop the nucleus from the equator toward the center. Even the short and pointed Sinskey hook can chop the soft nucleus, but use of the phaco chopper is effective at Grade 3 or

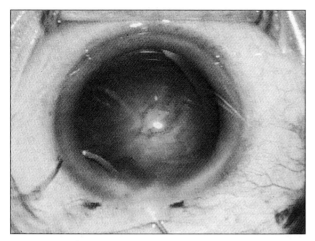

Figure 21-3. Hydrodissection.

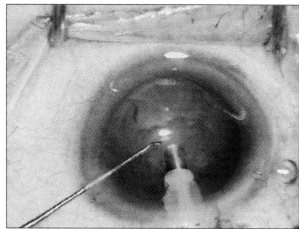

Figure 21-4. U/S tip driving.

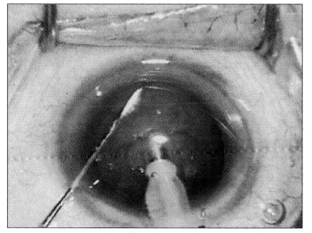

Figure 21-5. Phaco chopper on the equator.

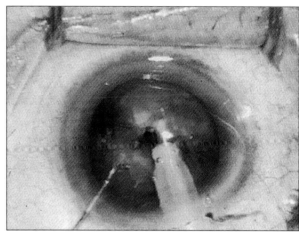

Figure 21-6. First chopping.

more hardness of the nucleus. When the U/S tip is driven, the nucleus is slightly dislocated to the 6 o'clock position with the phaco chopper.

I always use the Zero chip and not other types of the U/S tip, such as the 45 or 30°, depending on the hardness of the nucleus. The U/S power output is controlled with a linear mode to hold the center of a nucleus exactly. It is necessary to pay attention to the soft nucleus because the Zero tip will penetrate the nucleus easily with use of high vacuum and U/S energy.

After the U/S tip holds the nucleus exactly, I put the phaco chopper on the equator of the lens nucleus at the 6 o'clock position. When the anterior capsulotomy is small, pay extra attention not to injure the anterior capsule. I allow the nucleus, which is caught by the U/S tip, to dislocate a little above and make space between the nucleus equator and the capsule, and I insert the chopper there. It is easy to insert the chopper when the equator of the nucleus moves to the inside of the CCC. I draw the chopper toward the U/S tip and chop the nucleus into two pieces. After the first chop is completed, the nucleus is rotated 90° and the inferior half is chopped in half. The two quarter pieces are gently aspirated and phacoemulsified in the capsular bag. All steps of emulsification are accomplished in the center of the capsular bag to prevent corneal endothelial damage and posterior capsule rupture. I chop the soft lens nucleus into four pieces. But, in cases of a hard nucleus, residual nucleus fragments may enter the anterior chamber and injure the corneal endothelium. In that case, it is safe to make small nucleus pieces.

## PHACO FOR NUCLEUS OF HARDNESS 4

The epinucleus in the hard nucleus is very thin. It has a dual structure, which consists of the soft shell and the hard core. The hard nucleus is thicker than the usual nucleus, and the posterior pole side is sticky and hard to chop. To have success in the phaco chop, the U/S tip should catch the core of the hard nucleus and the point of the chopper should go over the equator in order to arrive at the posterior pole side. Taking a point of the phaco chopper over the equator and into the posterior pole side is easy. But it is difficult to hold the core of the hard nucleus with the point

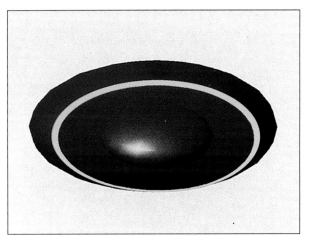

Figure 21-7. The posterior pole side is sticky and more difficult to chop.

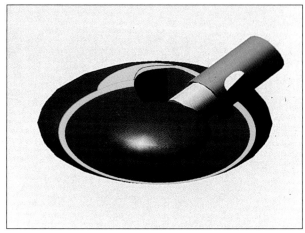

Figure 21-8. The crater is made on the soft shell nucleus, and the U/S tip is driven into the core of the nucleus.

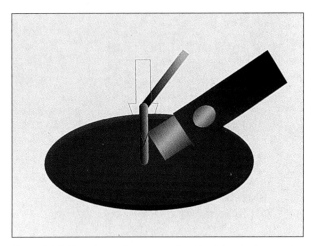

Figure 21-9. The phaco chopper need not be taken to the equator of the nucleus.

Table 21-2

**MACHINE SETTINGS DURING EPINUCLEUS REMOVAL CORITCAL ASPIRATION**

| | Vacuum (mm Hg) | Flow rate (cc/min) | Control |
|---|---|---|---|
| Diplomat | 500 | 30 | Flow rate linear |
| Legacy | 500 | 24 | Flow rate linear |
| Protege | 500 | | Flow rate linear |

of U/S tip. It is impossible to catch a core of the hard nucleus simply by removing the epinucleus and driving the U/S tip into the center of the nucleus. In order to catch the core of the hard nucleus, the crater should be made on the soft shell nucleus, and the U/S tip should be driven into the core of the nucleus (Creator Phaco Chop.)

When the chopping is performed, there are cases when the crack doesn't reach to the posterior pole; the nucleus is then sticky even if the tip holds the core of the nucleus and the chopper catches the equator. In such cases, the chopper should be replaced to the deepest part of the crevasse and should separate the nucleus to complete the phaco chop. The hard nucleus pieces which are chopped are fan-shaped and have sharp edges. They easily turn within the capsular bag, and there is fear that they will hurt the posterior capsule. In such a situation, the point of the fan-shaped nucleus should be held first with the U/S tip and brought to the iris plane that emulsified it.

## Epinucleus Removal Cortical Aspiration

The epinucleus is removed with the U/S tip at the end of the procedure. Aspiration of the cortex is performed using a straight I/A needle with a silicone sleeve even if the cortex is at the 12 o'clock position.

The residual cortex is removed easily in the large CCC cases. So making the large CCC is the key to success for easy removal of the cortex. Otherwise, it is left at the end of the procedure and removed along with the viscoelastic material After I/A cleanup, the posterior capsule is polished with the same I/A tip with low flow rate.

## Enlargement of the Incision

The capsular bag is reinflated with a high molecule viscoelastic material. The crescent shaped diamond knife is then introduced through the wound to enlarge it for insertion of the IOL.

## IOL IMPLANT

The 5.5 mm one-piece PMMA lens is routinely inserted with the two-handed technique. I use the Kelman Mcpherson forceps and a Sinskey hook. The anterior scleral lip is elevated with the forceps. The leading haptics are introduced into the anterior chamber and under the anterior capsule at the 6 o'clock position with the Kelman Mcpherson forceps. The optics are pressed downward with the Sinskey hook, and the trailing haptics are introduced under the anterior capsule at the 12 o'clock position by the compression technique.

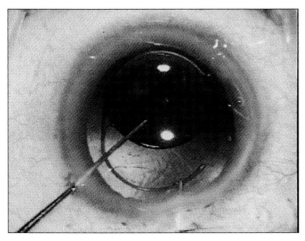

Figure 21-10. Bimanual IOL implant.

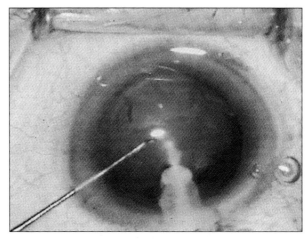

Figure 21-11. The sign of the Karate Phaco Chop.

## Viscoelastic Material Removal

Following implantation of the lens, the viscoelastic is removed with an I/A handpiece, first from in front of the lens and then from behind the lens. The anterior chamber is reinflated with BSS through the side port incision until the chamber is deep and the globe is firm. The wound is then checked with Weck-cell sponges to insure the self-sealing even with firm pressure and manipulation of the globe.

The conjunctive is pulled back into place. If the patient is diabetic, the lower cul-de-sac is injected with 1.5 mL depomedrol in the sub-Tenon's space. The eye is patched with gauze and the patient can leave the operation room.

## PHACOEMULSIFICATION IN PARTICULAR CASES (KARATE PHACO CHOP FOR SMALL PUPIL)

I devised this method to reinforce a weak point of the Phaco Chop technique. In the Phaco Chop technique, we need to take the chopper to the equator. But when mydriasis is poor, the chopper under the iris cannot be seen. The Karate Phaco Chop technique overcomes this weak point, allowing the chopping procedure to be performed within the pupil.

The chopping direction with the Phaco Chop technique goes from the equator to the center of the nucleus, while the Karate Phaco Chop goes from the anterior pole to the posterior pole. This is effective for a small pupil because the phaco chopper need not be taken to the equator of the nucleus. It is difficult to divide a soft nucleus, and therefore better to perform the usual Phaco Chop technique. The Karate Phaco Chop is effective for the hard nucleus, Grade 3, or more. One can see that the Karate Phaco Chop is effective when white smoke rises up while the U/S tip is driven into the nucleus. After shaving the epinucleus, drive the U/S tip into the center of the nucleus. It is important to hold the nucleus with the tip closely and drive the tip deeper than the Phaco Chop technique. The chopper is stabbed in the nucleus just above the U/S tip and these instruments are separated from side to side to chop the nucleus. A point of the chopper needs to arrive at the same depth as the U/S tip. After the first division is completed, the nucleus piece is rotated and the U/S tip is driven into the wall of the crevasse; the chopper is then stabbed for the second chopping.

## CONCLUSION

The two-handed technique for dividing the nucleus is more effective than the single-handed technique.

But the divided nucleus pieces easily come into the anterior chamber and injure the corneal endothelium.

As a result, operation time and U/S time do decrease, as do the corneal endothelial cells. I use enough viscoelastic material to protect corneal endothelial cells.

The starting point of thought to divide the nucleus along its anatomical structure was the Divide and Conquer, and the technique that simplified it is the Phaco Chop.

# Chapter 22

# PHACOEMULSIFICATION: MODIFIED PHACO AND MINI CHOP

*Ronald M. Stasiuk, MD*

## PHACOEMULSIFIER IN USE

The Prestige by Allergan is my current phacoemulsifier of choice, as it is user-friendly for both surgeon and nursing staff. Furthermore, it provides an excellent balance of responsive phaco power, vacuum, aspiration, and fluid dynamics. Alcon's Legacy 20,000 and Storz's Premiere are also excellent units.

My routine phaco tip is the straight 45° needle for most cases, but for hard nuclei, I prefer the Barrett Microflow needle. It provides additional phacofragmentation compared to a conventional needle, with a larger cavitation-wave. Also, the tip temperature remains cooler, thereby preventing thermal wound burn, even with prolonged phacoemulsification.

The curved Kelman phaco tip is also an excellent phaco tip which allows deeper and longer grooving, especially in the subincisional region. However, caution is needed when the tip is close to the posterior capsule in order to avoid a posterior capsule tear.

The new Proficient phaco needle by AMO has a longer stroke length than the original Profinesse needle and, consequently, provides greater cutting power. It is available in the 21 gauge format, which allows a smaller size incision.

## CORNEAL INCISION

### Incision Instruments

I perform the majority of my phaco surgeries with clear corneal incisions and use the following instruments:
- Speculum—Leiberman style 14 mm by Karl Ilg (#13-108).
- Fixation—Modified Thornton ring by Impex (#XRK-129T) or Asico (#AG 2760).
- Incision—The initial preset groove of 300 µm and 1 mm side ports is made with the Osher 1 mm diamond knife (HUCO #4 1316).

The clear corneal tunnel incisions made from the temporal approach with the HUCO 3.0 mm diamond knife (#1377) or with the 2.7 x 3.2 mm HUCO diamond blade (#51406). The clear corneal incision is my first choice for the majority of cases combined with soft foldable implantation.[6]

### Size and Location

The incision is mostly located at the temporal cornea or on the steeper meridian. However, superior corneal incisions may result in greater surgically-induced astigmatism and endothelial cell loss, so this is rarely employed.[13] The size and architecture of the clear corneal suture wound are based upon Ernest's recommendations and the dimensions of the trapezoidal diamond blade.[9] A two-plane incision is preferred with an initial 250 to 300 µm vertical groove at the peripheral cornea for a length of 3.0 mm, with a HUCO preset crystal sapphire blade.

A new 3D diamond knife (Rhein) has been designed by Dr. I Howard Fine to give very consistent and clear corneal incisions, which may eliminate any wound architecture variations and the need for *dimple down* maneuvers[17]. The clear corneal tunnel incision is made from the temporal approach with the HUCO 3.0 mm diamond knife (#41377) or with the 2.7 x 3.2 mm HUCO diamond blade (#51406). It is important that the diamond blades are thin, well cut, and carefully maintained. Metal knives do not give quality or consistently good self-sealing corneal incisions.

The trapezoidal diamond blade is inserted with the blade parallel with the iris to create a corneal tunnel of 1.5 to 2.5 mm length, with entry into the anterior chamber when the shoulders of the trapezoidal blade just enter the corneal tunnel.

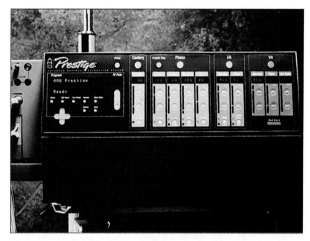

Figure 22-1. Prestige Phacoemulsifier.

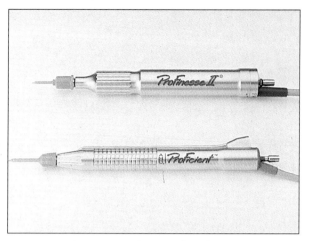

Figure 22-2. The AMO Proficient and Profinesse phaco handpieces with tips.

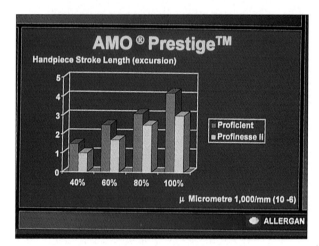

Figure 22-3. The Proficient handpiece by AMO shows a greater stroke length than the older Profinesse handpiece.

## CONTENTS OF THE CHAMBER FOR THE CAPSULOTOMY

Amvisc Plus (Chiron) or Healon GV (Pharmacia) are the preferred viscoelastics for capsulotomy. These maintain a deeper anterior chamber and allow a safer capsulotomy. Extra viscoelastic should be used if a radial tear is likely with a peripheral capsulotomy, so that the anterior capsule and zonules are relaxed. Air bubbles should be avoided to enhance visibility, and extra microscope magnification should be used in cases of the white or dark-brown cataract. The incision is self-sealing and is combined with insertion of soft foldable implants.

## CAPSULOTOMY

### Instruments

I prefer to use the Utrata style capsulorhexis forceps manufactured by Moira (#92). Occasionally, a bent 25 G needle is used for capsulotomy.

### Size and Shape

Generally, a circular or slightly oval shaped capsulorhexis is made, with the diameter slightly overlapping the edge of the optic. However, there are some advantages for the diameter to be slightly larger than the optic, as it seals in the lens epithelial cells to the periphery.

### Technique

A capsule forceps is used to puncture the center of the anterior capsule and pull in a small arc toward the periphery to create a small anterior capsular flap. This is grasped to create a circular tear of approximately 5 mm diameter for a 5.5 to 6.0 mm lens optic. It is regrasped every 90° to complete the circular tear from outside to in motion. It is important to fold over the anterior capsule to create the tear and not to pull it.

In cases with a small pupil, the opening should be enlarged if access is inadequate (<4 mm). Pupil enlarging techniques such as division of posterior synechiae centrifugally with viscoelastic, pupil stretch, multiple sphincterotomies, or use of a flexible iris hook should be considered before capsulotomy. In addition, a Kuglin hook can be used to displace the pupil margin to the periphery while performing the capsulotomy. It is important not to allow the capsular tear to extend peripherally behind the iris out of view; otherwise, a radial tear may ensue.

## WHITE OR INTUMESCENT CATARACTS

Visibility presents a major problem for an adequate capsulorhexis. Intumescent cataracts create problems because of a poor view for capsulorhexis, so extra magnification is needed with dim operating theater lights and care. Furthermore, lens milk clouds the anterior chamber with often increased pressure within the capsular bag.[7]

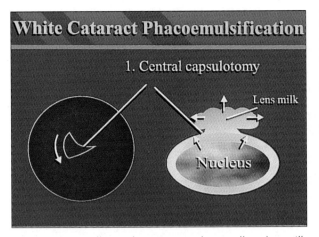

Figure 22-4. A small central anterior capsulotomy allows lens milk to be released and to decompress the capsular bag in a patient with an intumescent cataract.

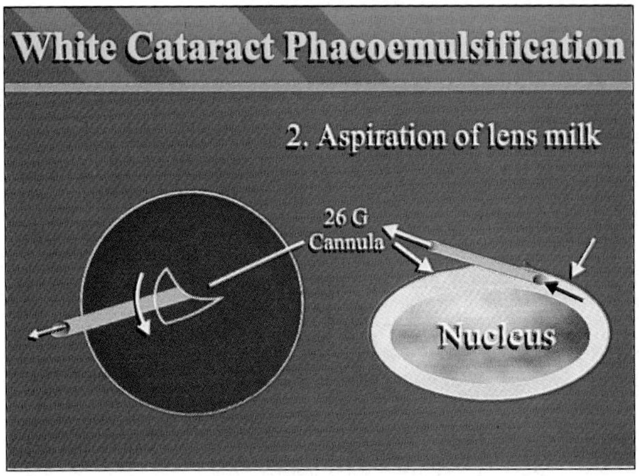

Figure 22-5. A 26 G cannula on a 2 mL syringe is used to aspirate lens milk and soft cortex through a limbal side port in a patient with an intumescent cataract.

## Treatment

- I prefer Amvisc Plus or Healon GV to completely fill the anterior chamber. An air bubble may be a useful alternative.
- Next, the anterior capsule is punctured in the center to release some lens milk and pressure, with a small central capsulotomy.
- Lens milk and some liquid cortex is then aspirated with a 26 G cannula on a 2 cc syringe through the limbal side port, to clear the view and partly collapse the capsular bag. An irrigation/aspiration (I/A) handpiece could also be used for removal of some cortex. Some viscoelastic may be carefully injected into the capsular bag to clear lens milk and give better visibility of the flap.
- Careful capsulorhexis with extra magnification is completed with dim surrounding theater lights.

Some autogenous blood or iris pigment on the anterior capsule may aid visibility of the capsule, or use of a tangentially placed light-source.

- The capsulorhexis is carefully completed. If this is not possible, a can opener capsulotomy could be used with phacoemulsification or ECCE. A secondary capsulorhexis will enlarge the capsulotomy after irrigation aspiration.
- Phacoemulsification is often easy as the nucleus is soft with intumescent cataracts.

For dark brown or black nuclei, similar principles may be applied when performing capsulorhexis as for white cataracts but with a larger capsulorhexis.

## Management of Potential Radial Tears

1. Stop and assess the clinical situation. Relieve any excessive vitreous pressure.
2. Deepen the anterior chamber with viscoelastic, preferably the more viscous type (Viscoat, Healon GV, Amvisc Plus).
3. Grasp the anterior capsular flap close to the tear.
4. Pull the anterior capsular flap centrally.

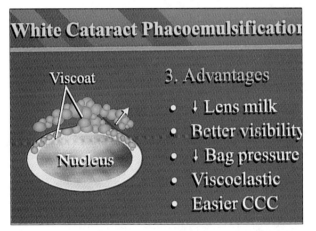

Figure 22-6. Viscoelastic may be carefully injected under the small capsular flap into the bag to clear lens milk and enhance the visibility of the anterior capsule in a patient with an intumescent cataract.

## Management of Radial Tears

Try to prevent this situation with a well-dilated pupil, soft eye, and a good view of the surgical field. Once a radial tear develops, several options are available; the surgeon can complete with a can opener style capsulotomy and perform an ECCE or Maloney style iris-plane phacoemulsification. Also, the surgeon can do a two-staged capsulorhexis and complete with a relieving second radial tear to avoid possible posterior capsular extension.

# HYDRODISSECTION

## Aims

The aims of hydrodissection are to mobilize the nucleus within the capsular bag (hydrodissection), separate the cortex from the anterior capsule (cortical cleavage, I. Howard Fine)[5], and separate the nucleus from the epinucleus (hydrodelamination).

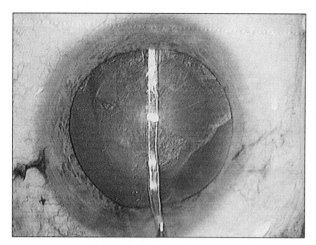

Figure 22-7. Cortical cleavage hydrodissection.

AMO® Prestige™ Settings

| | Sculpting | Quadrants | Epinucleus | IA |
|---|---|---|---|---|
| Power % | 80-100 | 50-100 | 50 | - |
| Vacuum mm Hg | 0-60 | 200-400 | 100-200 | 400-500 |
| Flow Rate cc / min | 24 | 22 | 26 | 24-30 |
| IV Pole cm | 60 | 70 | 70 | 70 |
| Pulse PPS | - | 8-10 | 8-10 | - |

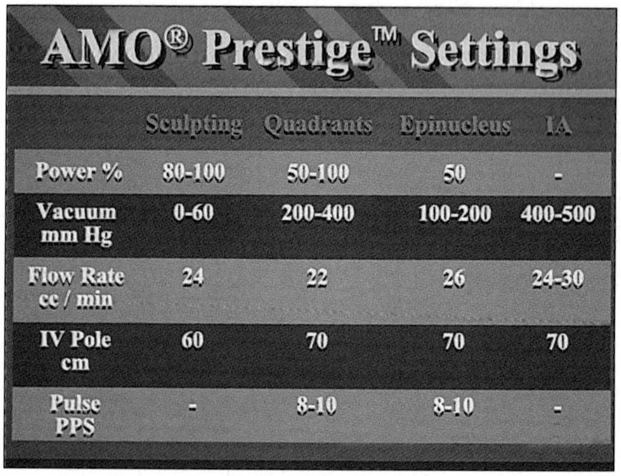

Figure 22-8. AMO Prestige phaco parameter settings.

### Technique

I routinely prefer to use Fine's technique of cortical cleavage in all cases.[5] The advantages are that it allows for a more mobile nucleus. There is no need to remove the epinucleus separately; hence, more safety in routine cases. Viscoat or Vitrax can be used as a *pseudoepinucleus* to protect the posterior capsule in cases of hard nuclei.[12] Also, there is minimal or no I/A of the cortex after completion of phacoemulsification. Therefore, there is less risk of capsular rupture. However, hydrodelamination with the presence of a *golden ring* can be a useful clinical sign for beginning phaco surgeons with a protective outer layer or epinucleus.

## CORTICAL CLEAVAGE TECHNIQUE AND INSTRUMENTATION

I use Visitec 27 G flattened cannula on a 2 mL syringe filled with balanced salt solution (BSS). The cannula is placed under the anterior capsular flap opposite the incision. The anterior capsule is tented upward, and BSS is gently infused until a dissection wave separates the cortex. The nucleus then prolapses forward and partly out of the capsular bag. The posterior lip of the incision is depressed gently with the cannula to allow egress of excess BSS and to avoid excessive increase in intraocular pressure (IOP).

The infusion is stopped and the cannula pushes the nucleus posteriorly back into the capsular bag. A wave of BSS separates cortical fibers from the equator and anterior capsule. This may be repeated and mobility of the nucleus may be tested by rotating it with the cannula or with two Sinskey hooks.

## PHACO FRAGMENTATION TECHNIQUES

1. Soft nuclei—Quadrant Divide without fracture.
2. Medium-hard nuclei—Quadrant Divide with fracture.
3. Hard nuclei (Brunescent, mature)—My modified Phaco Chop and Mini Chop techniques.

### Soft Nuclei

For soft nuclei, I prefer the Quadrant Divide technique without fracture. Instead, I just aspirate each soft quadrant with gentle low power phacoemulsification toward the center. Hydrodelamination may be helpful for beginners where the epinucleus is delineated by a golden ring and provides a landmark and protection to the posterior capsule.

### Medium-Hard Nuclei of Hardness 2

#### *Phase 1: Sculpting*

With medium-hard nuclei, I routinely use the Shepherd-Brint quadrant divide method, using a 45° bevel phaco tip in all cases and a 0.5 mm spatula as a second instrument.[6] The grooves may be made deeper and wider for hard nuclei. The parameters on the Prestige phacoemulsifier are:

- Powe—80%.
- Vacuum—5 to 10 mm Hg.
- Flow rate—24 mL/min.

#### *Phase 2: Division into Pieces*

Each quadrant is then fractured pushing both the spatula and phaco tip parallel and away from each other, with infusion of BSS.

#### *Phase 3: Removal of the Pieces*

Steady aspiration draws the apex of the nuclear quadrant to the center of the capsular bag, where emulsification occurs. The parameters used are:

- Power—80%.
- Vacuum—340 mm Hg.
- Flow rate—24 mL/min.

This is repeated until each quadrant is finally removed in sequence.

Some of the common problems faced and precautions taken by beginning phaco surgeons with the divide technique are:

1. A *poor incision* may result in excessive leakage and shallowing of the anterior chamber. If entry is prema-

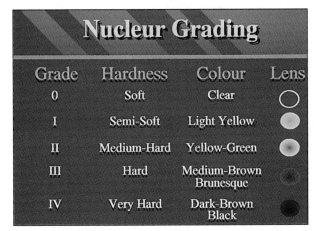

Figure 22-9. This shows grading of nuclei by hardness and color based upon slit lamp microscope examination.

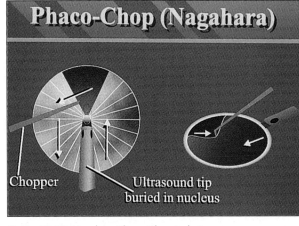

Figure 22-10. Nagahara Phaco Chop technique.

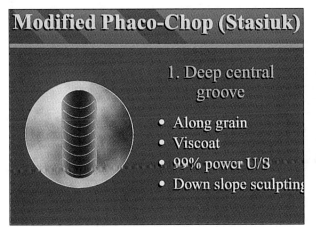

Figure 22-11. Deep central groove with the modified Phaco Chop and Mini Chop technique (Stasiuk).

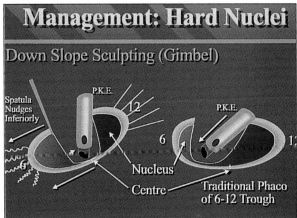

Figure 22-12. Gimbel's technique of downslope sculpting allows for deep grooving and a thinner posterior nuclear plate.

ture, iris prolapse may result in consequent miosis and bleeding. A tunnel incision that is too long may cause corneal distortion and a poor surgical view.

2. A *poor capsulorhexis*, whether it be small or with a radial tear, can result in complications.
3. Make the grooves deeper at the center of the nucleus, so that the nuclear plate fractures easily.
4. *Don't go too peripheral or anterior* with the phaco tip; otherwise, the iris may be engaged or the capsulorhexis may be torn. Stay in the center of the capsular bag.
5. Use *short bursts* of phaco energy rather than long delayed power.
6. *At the end* of removal of the last nuclear quadrant, reduce phaco power and aspiration to the minimum, and watch out for the posterior capsule; otherwise, a hole may eventuate. The spatula may protect the posterior capsule by placing it across the capsule and under the phaco tip.
7. *Avoid* difficult cases if beginning, ie, small pupil, hard nuclei, pseudoexfoliation, and zonular weakness.

## Emulsification for a Nucleus of Hardness 4

### Viscoelastic for Phaco

For routine cases, I prefer Amvisc Plus, as its extra viscosity maintains a deeper anterior chamber during capsulotomy. In addition, there is significant chemical bonding of hyaluronic acid molecules to endothelial receptors to protect endothelium during phacoemulsification. Healon GV would also be an excellent choice.

Both Viscoat and Vitrax adhere to endothelium and afford it protection during phacoemulsification, but visibility may be impaired due to trapping of air bubbles. A well-dilated pupil, a soft eye, and a larger sized capsulorhexis are advantageous. The microscope magnification is increased and theater lights dimmed. In cases of very hard nuclei that are brunesque, mature, or nigra, where the slit lamp microscopy grading is >+3 hardness, I employ my own modified technique of the Phaco Chop and Mini Chop.[10,11,16]

My experiences have shown that the advantages over the traditional Quadrant Divide and the Gimbel Crater Divide methods are that my technique:

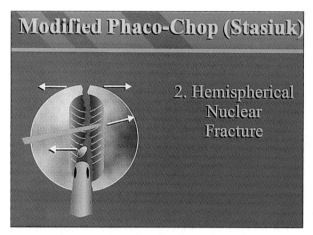

Figure 22-13. Hemispherical nuclear fracture (Stasiuk).

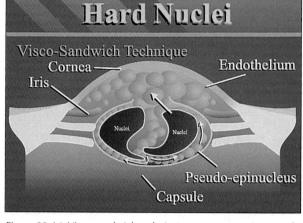

Figure 22-14. Visco sandwich technique protects posterior capsule (pseudoepinucleus), iris, and endothelium during phacoemulsification of a hard nucleus.

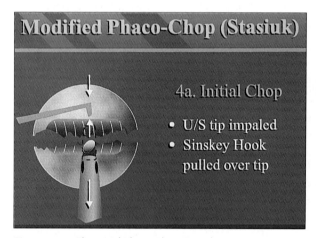

Figure 22-15. The initial Phaco Chop (Stasiuk).

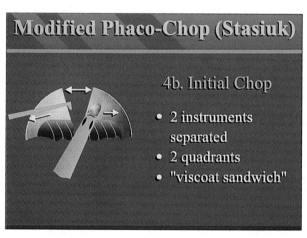

Figure 22-16. The initial Phaco Chop is completed (Stasiuk).

- Is safer.
- Needs less phaco energy and time.
- Has fewer complications such as a ruptured posterior capsule of zonular dialysis.
- Enables the tenacious nuclear plate to fracture easily.
- Easily emulsifies the six to eight small nuclear fragments.
- Has less corneal edema.
- Results in better vision earlier.

The original description of the Phaco Chop technique was introduced by Nagahara in 1993.[11] However, several difficulties were encountered, including the difficulty of impaling the phaco tip into the center of the nucleus. There were problems achieving the complete fracture of the tenacious nuclear plate. In addition, there was insufficient room to maneuver the phaco tip in the presence of a large nucleus. Consequently, I modified the technique which I call *Modified Phaco Chop and Mini Chop*[16]. This was developed independently at the same time Paul Koch described his Stop and Chop technique. Both authors encountered similar difficulties with the Nagahara technique.

My technique, although similar to the Stop and Chop, also employs two other techniques that give more protection and versatility: the Viscoelastic sandwich technique and the Mini Chop technique. The steps are as follows:

1. Phase 1: Sculpting—This phase involves a Deep Central Groove from 3 to 9 o'clock. Using the phaco tip, it is important to emulsify very deep, especially in the center of the nucleus with 90 to 100% power. Gimbel's technique of downslope sculpting helps in this situation to thin out the thick nuclear plate and is aided by use of the Barrett Microflow needle for extra power and cooling of the phaco tip. Vacuum is set up to 60 mm Hg with a flow rate of 24 mL/min with the Prestige phacoemulsifier unit.
2. Phase 2: Hemispherical Nuclear Fracture—The nucleus is fractured into two halves by pushing apart with both instruments deep in opposite directions.
3. Viscoelastic sandwich—Extra Vitrax or Viscoat is injected in between both nuclear hemispheres and underneath to create protection to the posterior capsule (ie, *pseudoepinucleus*).[12]

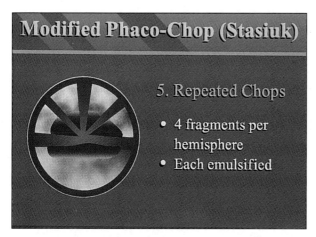

Figure 22-17. Repeat Phaco Chop of each hemispherical nucleus results in three to four pieces.

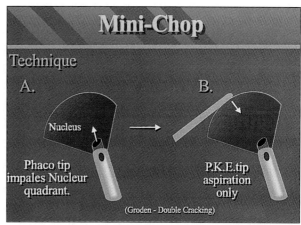

Figure 22-18. Mini Chop technique with initial aspiration of the large nuclear fragment (Stasiuk).

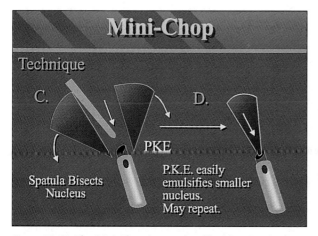

Figure 22-19. The Mini Chop is completed by bisecting the large nuclear fragment with a spatula (Stasiuk).

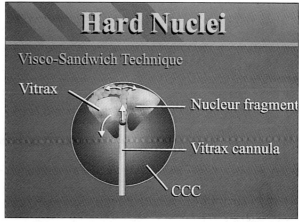

Figure 22-20. Extra viscoelastic may be used to stabilize the final nuclear fragments.

4. Phaco Chop—The 45° phaco tip is used with the silicone sleeve retracted to expose more of the titanium probe tip, so it can penetrate deeper into the nucleus during impalement. Maximum phaco power 100% is used with vacuum set at 340 mm Hg, aspiration flow rate at 22 mL/min, and IV pole at 70 cm. A pulse mode set at 10 pps may be used. The nuclear hemisphere is rotated to the 9 o'clock position and the phaco probe is impaled into its center. The nucleus is then pulled to the center of the pupil to expose more peripheral nucleus to avoid damage to the pupil or capsulorhexis. A Phaco Chop hook with a longer bent tip punctures the mid-peripheral nucleus at 6 o'clock. If it is too peripheral, then the capsulorhexis may be torn. The hook is pulled in to cut the anterior surface of the nucleus over the phaco probe until it is central and then the nuclear hemisphere is fractured into two pieces by spreading them apart (two quadrants).[11]
5. Phase 3: Removal of Pieces—Each of these quadrants is divided into two by repeating the Phaco Chop and then carefully emulsified by short burst of power. The Mini Chop technique, originally described by Groden, is useful to further disassemble the larger nuclear fragments mechanically. The nuclear fragment is held by aspiration only by the phaco tip and crushed into two smaller halves by the 0.5 mm blunt tipped spatula or Phaco Chop hook. Minimal phaco power is needed as most nuclear fragments are phaco evacuated by aspiration.

## VISCOELASTIC SANDWICH TECHNIQUE

Extra Vitrax or Viscoat may be necessary to fill the capsular bag and form a layer over the posterior capsule (pseudoepinucleus) to provide protection from hard jagged nuclear fragments.[12] Furthermore, the nuclear pieces are stabilized and easily rotated by the Viscoelastic sandwich. The corneal endothelium is also protected. The second nuclear hemisphere is removed in the same fashion.

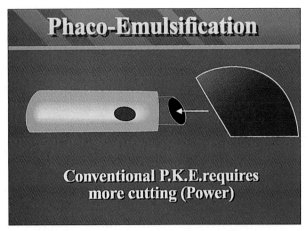

Figure 22-21. Conventional phacoemulsification requires more power.

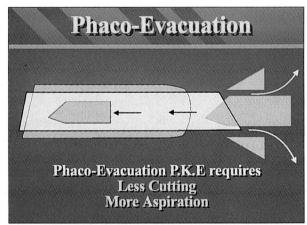

Figure 22-22. Phacoevacuation of smaller nuclear fragments requires less power and mostly aspiration.

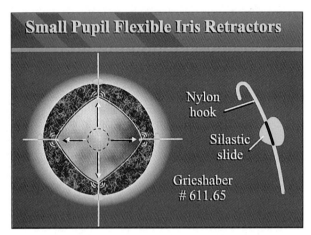

Figure 22-23. Flexible Grieshaber iris retractors may be used in a small pupil to increase exposure of the cataract.

# PHACOEMULSIFICATION IN SPECIAL CASES

## Small Pupil

These cases should only be attempted by experienced phaco surgeons. The most common causes of small pupils are: the use of miotics in glaucoma patients, the presence of pseudoexfoliation, previous iritis and posterior synechiae, trauma, diabetes, and lack of mydriatics.

Management can be subdivided into two groups: preoperative and operative. Concerning preoperative management, miotics should be stopped at least 48 hours before surgery and the glaucoma adequately controlled either medically or with Argon laser therapy. Extra mydriatics for prolonged periods (eg, 1% Cyclopentolate and 10% Neosynephrine) should be used every 15 minutes for 1 to 2 hours before surgery in conjunction with Ocufen. Argon laser Photomydriasis using a double row of laser burns in central iris may help, with settings of 500 µm/200 MW/0.5 sec duration.

Concerning operative management, if the pupil is still <4 mm, pupil enlargement is often indicated even in experienced hands. My preference in management is as follows:

1. Use more viscous viscoelastic (*Viscoat, Vitrax, Amvisc Plus, or Healon GV*) to further stretch the sphincter and divide any posterior synechiae with a cannula in a radial direction toward zonules. Often, this may be sufficient.
2. In cases of a fibrotic pupil, I find the *Pupil Stretch technique* very useful. Here, two iris hooks (Kuglin, Osher finger hook or Sinskey) are used to stretch the pupil toward the angle at 180° apart and repeated at right angles.
   The new Beehler pupil dilator (Moira #19009) utilizes three micro fingers, and one external micro hook may also be useful. Both work well in the elderly on miotics or in pseudoexfoliation.
3. Alternatively, if a thick fibrotic or pigmented ring is attached to the pupil margin, then the fibrotic ring may be carefully peeled off the pupil with forceps and allow further mydriasis.
4. If that still fails, then I'll try multiple small partial *sphincterotomies* (usually six to seven), but not fully across the sphincter muscle, which is about 0.6 mm wide.[3]
5. In younger patients, usually with iritis, stretching is ineffective and glare can be a problem with sphincter surgery. Here, viscoelastic is often effective, but if this fails, then I'll use the four *Grieshaber flexible iris retractors* to create a square pupil through limbal side ports (Grieshaber #611-65).[4]
6. *Radial and sector iridectomies* are rarely indicated. Furthermore, there is a danger of emulsifying iris pillars. Glare can be a real problem and the iris often needs to be sutured with 10-0 Prolene sutures.
7. Concerning *capsular ring-zonular dialysis*, special care is necessary with pseudoexfoliation as often the zonules are loose and the lens may easily subluxate; the capsule is thin and easily torn. In cases of zonular dialysis, insert a capsular ring (Ophtec PC275, 276 or Morcher #14,14C).

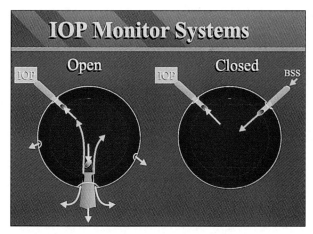

Figure 22-24. Low pressure phaco using an IOP monitor may help reduce high pressure spikes (Gerber, Stasiuk).[1]

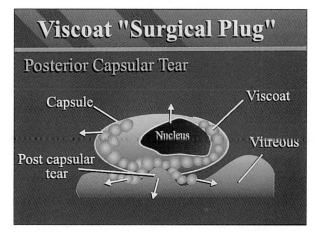

Figure 22-25. Viscoelastic surgical plug technique in a case of zonular dialysis forces the vitreous back into the posterior segment.

## PHACOEMULSIFICATION

I use the same Quadrant Divide technique with several modifications. I work in the center to avoid iris incarceration. Lower power and aspiration settings are used to avoid grabbing iris or capsule. In addition, I feel a bimanual approach is better.

## PHACOEMULSIFICATION IN SPECIAL CASES

### Combined Glaucoma Phaco Surgery

The surgical approach depends upon the severity and IOP level of glaucoma. Trabeculectomy first and then cataract surgery later are used only in advanced and uncontrolled glaucoma as a two-stage procedure. With mild glaucoma and mostly cataract, a standard clear corneal incision (2.7 to 3.0 mm) with a soft foldable lens implant is preferred. In the presence of moderate-severe glaucoma and cataract, I use a fornix-based conjunctival flap, but limbal-based if a Mitomycin soak is used (0.2% for 2 minutes), with a separate temporal clear corneal incision for cataract extraction first.

A triangular 3 x 4 mm *scleral flap* is preferred for more efficient filtration, combined with two releasable corneal sutures. A posterior sclerotomy is done by a *Kelly punch* and a soft foldable lens implant is inserted. In these higher risk patients, an *IOP monitor* may be helpful, utilizing Low Pressure Phaco, which we have developed (Gerber, Stasiuk).[14]

## EPINUCLEUS REMOVAL

In cases of very hard nuclei, the epinucleus may be thin or even absent, but if it is present, removal should be left until all of the nucleus is removed, in order to protect the posterior capsule. The parameters are:
- Power—50%.
- Vacuum—100 mm Hg.
- Flow rate—26 mL/min.

Figure 22-26. Viscoelastic surgical plug technique in a case with a posterior capsular tear.

- Pulse—10 pps.

When the epinucleus is absent, I prefer to use a more viscous viscoelastic such as Vitrax or Viscoat to act as a protective Viscoelastic sandwich. It helps to coat and protect intraocular tissues, especially the posterior capsule, iris, and endothelium during prolonged phacoemulsification times. Furthermore, in situations of complications during surgery such as with a posterior capsular rupture or zonular dialysis, the same viscoelastic may be utilized to act as a *Surgical Plug*. With this technique, vitreous is forced back into the posterior segment by the viscoelastic, thereby enabling a safer completion of phacoemulsification or I/A The viscoelastic tends to remain as a barrier to vitreous, but may need to be replaced if too much is aspirated.

## CORTICAL ASPIRATION

With smaller incision cataract surgery and capsulorhexis, the difficult subincisional cortex is more easily removed by a bimanual I/A technique which I have employed since 1979. With this technique, the aspiration line is separately connected to a plastic handpiece and a

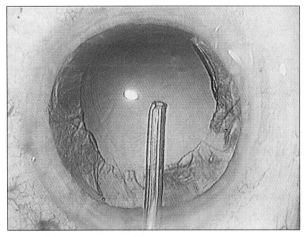

Figure 22-27. The posterior capsule is polished with a Terry polisher to free posterior cortical fibers with viscoelastic.

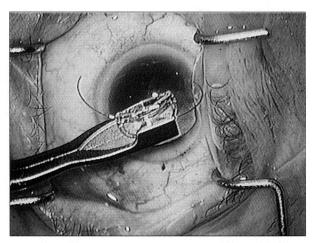

Figure 22-28. An S140 silicone lens implant is folded with forceps.

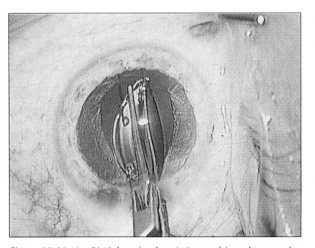

Figure 22-29. An S140 lens implant is inserted into the capsular bag with the leading haptic tucked into the fold of the optic.

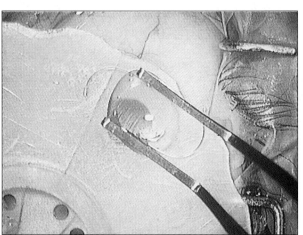

Figure 22-30. An AcrySof MA30BA lens implant is placed on the surface of the wagonwheel with a drop of viscoelastic underneath. A folding forceps then engages the edges of the optic.

curved 23 G Simcoe I/A cannula through the side ports to remove cortex. Infusion is maintained by the Prestige I/A handpiece or separately through the opposite side port with a Buratto infusion cannula.[16] The parameters are:
- Vacuum—400 mm Hg.
- Aspiration Flow Rate—30 mL/min.

Concerning performance, I/A can be eliminated or minimized with efficient cortical cleavage hydrodissection, whereby most of the cortex is removed with phacoemulsification. Any residual cortical fibers may be gently polished off the posterior capsule with a Terry 26 G capsule polisher with an outer silicone tube (Asico #7539) just prior to lens implantation. This can then be evacuated with viscoelastic more safely. The Terry polisher is also useful removing any subcapsular plaques.

Subincisional cortex is best removed with the bimanual I/A technique, where the aspiration cannula and infusion parts are located about 2 o'clock hours away from the incisional site. This gives better visibility and access, rather than using a hooked I/A cannula.

## INCISION ENLARGEMENT

I generally do not enlarge the incision and prefer to use soft foldable implants. The original incision is in the 2.7 to 3.0 mm range. Enlargement is occasionally employed in situations where a hard polymethylmethacrylate (PMMA) lens implant is used in complicated cases or in highly myopic eyes, where a soft implant power is not available. In these cases, the incision is enlarged to 6.0 to 6.5 mm either in the clear cornea or sclera with a diamond knife.

## VISCOELASTIC FOR IMPLANTATION

Amvisc Plus or Healon is preferred for lens implantation using the viscoelastic to inflate the capsular bag, deepen the anterior chamber, lubricate the corneal tunnel incision, and coat the soft lens implant. These viscoelastics provide excellent visibility, deep stable chambers, and are relatively easy to remove with aspiration.

# LENS IMPLANT CHOICE

## Soft Implants

My preference for most cases is to use soft foldable implants, mainly because of the additional benefits of smaller incision surgery without wound enlargement. I also favor Allergan AMO SI40 silicone implants with a higher refractive index and a 6 mm optic size. I like a two-stage insertion technique with slow release. These implants are user-friendly and provide good centration with the firmer PMMA loops, rather than the S130 implants with prolene haptics.

Another preference are the one-piece silicone implants by Staar surgical (AA4203VF or AA4203V) using the MicroStaar injector system (MSI-TR) with the MicroTip cartridge (MTC45) or the Chiron C10uB.

Finally, the AcrySof MA30BA by Alcon (5.5 mm optic) implants provide excellent vision and contrast sensitivity, with a relatively low YAG laser capsulotomy rate.

## PMMA Implants

For scleral pocket incision, I prefer one-piece 5.5 mm round implants by Alcon (MZ30 or Slim Plant). Occasionally, with bilateral multifocal implantation in select patients, I use the Alcon 856X implant. In my personal series of 1200 cases with bilateral 856X implants, about 60% of patients were spectacle independent. For transcleral fixation, I prefer the 7.0 mm Alcon CZ70 BD implant, as it has two eyelets for introducing 10-0 prolene suture to the loop haptics and gives good transcleral fixation. Sometimes in elderly patients, I like the multiflex anterior chamber implant by Alcon (MZA34) as a secondary procedure, which is simpler than transcleral fixation.

# LENS IMPLANTATION

The *S140 lens* implant is folded with the *Fine II folding* (Rhein #05-2333) and *holding forceps* (Rhein #05-2334AL) for insertion. *Polack corneal double-toothed forceps* are excellent for fixation by holding the superior corneal lip and initial opening of the tunnel. Care must be taken with these forceps to avoid scratching the optic with the teeth, by lifting up the superior flap and rotating the handle of the Polack forceps parallel to the IOL holding forceps.

The leading haptic is tucked into the fold of the optic, while the trailing haptic is left free. Viscoelastic lubricates the IOL during its passage through the incision. The folded haptic is then guided into the capsular bag, the optic rotated 90°, and slowly released so that both leading haptic and optic simultaneously unfold. This also works well in cases of a small pupil and ensures placement in the capsular bag. The trailing haptic is then dialed into the capsular bag as a second procedure, with the tips of the holding forceps.

The AcrySof MA30BA acrylic lens requires a different technique. It is removed from the wagonwheel container and is placed onto a drop of viscoelastic on the flat outer surface of the wagonwheel. The outer edges of the optic are slightly depressed posteriorly with open Mcpherson forceps in order to start the fold in the correct direction. Fine notched forceps (Alcon #8065977721) are then used to engage the edges of the optic to hold the lens. The start of folding the optic can be enhanced by pressing the optic on the outer edge of the wagon wheel. Fine holding forceps (Rhein #05-2339-R5001) grasp the folded optic and the lens is then inserted into the incision and into the capsular bag. The leading haptic may be tucked into the fold of the optic with difficulty, in order to avoid kinking of the haptic during insertion. The leading haptic is carefully guided into the capsular bag and released. Once the optic unfolds, the trailing haptic can be dialed into the bag either with a spatula through the side port or with the tips of the holding forceps. The Staar one-piece silicone implant is inserted with the micro-injector and cartridge system with adequate viscoelastic.

# VISCOELASTIC REMOVAL

Conventional viscoelastic Healon or Amvisc Plus is easily removed by the standard irrigation aspiration technique. However, the Quadrant Divide method and extra time may be needed to remove Vitrax or Viscoat.

# NO-SUTURE INCISION

If the clear corneal incision is correctly constructed according to Ernest's recommendation, no suturing will be required. Another advantage of proper wound architecture is that surgically-induced astigmatism is minimized. The wound is tested for wound leak after reformation of the anterior chamber with the correct IOP by use of a dry sponge spear or fluorescein. If a suture is needed, I prefer to use a single box 10-0 nylon suture with the knot buried inside the wound to minimize astigmatism. In cases of wound enlargement to 6 mm, an extra suture is usually required.

# CONCLUSION

Phacoemulsification has evolved significantly with technological developments and improvements in fluid-vacuum dynamics. New advances in phaco tips combined with new surgical techniques, such as the Phaco Chop, together with a variety of viscoelastic agents have made cataract surgery easier and safer. It is important to have a sound basic phaco technique, but it is equally important to have a variety of additional maneuvers to manage more difficult cases, such as the very hard nucleus, zonular dialysis, and posterior capsular rupture.

New soft lens implants and better refractive materials have enabled us to utilize cataract surgery as a refractive procedure, with astigmatic keratoplasty and the use of multifocal implants to correct presbyopia and approach emmetropia.

# REFERENCES

1. Gimbel HV, Neuhann T. Development, advantages, and methods of continuous circular capsulorhexis technique. *J Cataract Refrac Surg.* 1990;16,31-37.

2. Shepherd JR. In situ fracture. *J Cataract Refrac Surg.* 1990;16:436-440.

3. Joseph H, Wang HS. Phacoemulsification with poorly dilated pupils. *J Cataract Refrac Surg.* 1993;19,551-556.

4. Nichamin LD. Enlarging the pupil for cataract extraction using flexible nylon iris retractors. *J Cataract Refrac Surg.* 1993;19,793-796.

5. Fine IH. Cortical cleaving hydrodissection. *J Cataract Refrac Surg.* 1992;19,508-512.

6. Fine IH. Architecture and construction of a self-sealing incision for cataract surgery. *J Cataract Refrac Surg.* 1991;17(suppl):672-676.

7. Gimbel HV, Willirscheidt AB. What to do with limited view. The intumescent cataract. *J Cataract Refrac Surg.* 1993;19,657-661.

8. Gimbel HV. Down slope sculpting. *J Cataract Refrac Surg.* 1992;18,6154-618.

9. Ernest PH, Lavery KT, Kiessling LA. Relative strength of scleral tunnel incisions with internal corneal lips constructed in cadaver eyes. *J Refrac Surg.* 1993;19,457-461.

10. Groden JM. Double cracking. A strategy for hard lenses. *Ocular Surg News.* October 1992;32-33.

11. Nagahara K. Phaco-chop technique eliminates central sculpting and allows faster, safer phaco. *Ocular Surg News.* October 1993;12-13.

12. Rampona DM. Phacoemulsification of the very hard nucleus. *3rd American-International Congress on Cataract, IOL and Refractive Surgery.* May 1993;45.

13. Grabow H B. Results of clear corneal phaco under topical anesthesia—first 300 cases. *3rd American-International Congress on Cataract, IOL and Refractive Surgery.* May 1993;61.

14. Gerber DS, Stasiuk RM, Nave D. "Low Pressure" Phacoemulsification: Adjusted Fluidics in Patients with Advanced Glaucomatous Optic Atrophy. *Ophthalmol.* September 1995:102,9A(suppl):87.

15. Buratto L. Personal Communication. 1996.

16. Stasiuk RM. Modified Phaco Chop and Mini Chop for Very Hard Nuclei. Pre-ASCRS Advanced Phaco Course (Alcon), April 1994 Boston, and *Ocular Surg News.*

17. Fine IH. Personal Communication. Milan conference. 1996.

# Chapter 23

# CURRENT PHACOEMULSIFICATION TECHNIQUE

*Richard Packard, MD, FRCS, FRCOphth*

## INTRODUCTION

Small incision cataract surgery will be 30 years old in 1997. Since that time, the techniques involved have been constantly improving. This improvement has been matched by innovations in phaco machinery and intraocular lens (IOL) materials and design. At every meeting, somebody has put forward a new variation of a technique. The new innovations can be very confusing. This chapter details my current techniques developed over 18 years of experience.

## PATIENT PREPARATION AND ANESTHESIA

### Preparation

Patients are not routinely given any premedication. They will have had a simple drop regime prior to reaching the operating theater as follows:
- G Phenylephrine 2.5%.
- G Homatropine 2%.
- Two drops of each 30 minutes preoperatively.
- G Benoxinate 0.4%.
- Two drops every 10 minutes for 30 minutes preoperatively.

In the operating theater prior to administering any anesthetic, povidone iodine is instilled into the eye. This will be in contact with the tissues for about 10 minutes before being washed out at the start of the operation.

### Topical Anesthesia

The drop regime above is sufficient for topical anesthesia. This technique was not used often in our department until recently because the anesthetists preferred not to give any intravenous sedation, if required, without control of the airway. The advent of intraocular unpreserved lignocaine 1% at the start of the procedure and for hydrodissection has increased the number of patients on whom we can operate without peribulbar injection, because the need for additional intravenous sedation is almost eliminated.

### Peribulbar Anesthesia

#### Medication Mixture
Plain Lignocaine 2% 8 mL mixed with hyalase.

#### Needle
Long shank 23 gauge needle attached to 10 mL syringe.

#### Technique
Three mL are injected inferiorly back from the infraorbital notch and 3 mL superiorly over the supraorbital notch. Both injections point nasally. A mercury bag is then placed on the eye for about 5 minutes—not to soften the eye, but to help spread the local anesthetic.

## PHACO MACHINES IN USE

### Alcon Legacy

The Legacy has just replaced the Series 10,000 Master, which had been in use for 8 years and will soon be fitted with the new high vacuum cassettes. This machine will allow a smaller incision to be used for phaco with the Microseal tip. Also, the new high vacuum cassette will mean higher vacuum levels can be used safely.

### Allergan AMO Prestige

The Prestige has a unique pump monitoring arrangement, which virtually eliminates post occlusion break

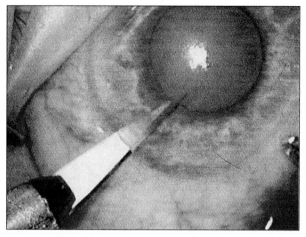

Figure 23-1. Creating a side port.

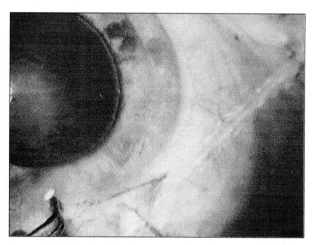

Figure 23-2. The tip of the keratome is buried.

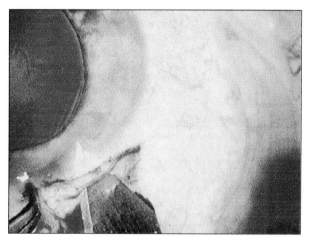

Figure 23-3. The keratome is advanced into the cornea.

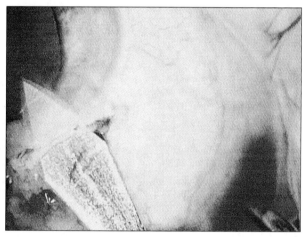

Figure 23-4. The tunnel is completed by entering the anterior chamber.

surge in the anterior chamber by slowing the rate at which the pump regains full speed. This makes it very safe because the chamber does not collapse and intracameral contents are not sucked into the phaco tip.

Both of these machines have a slow rise time to maximum vacuum settings, which is safer when teaching residents in training.

### Tips and Sleeves

Current tips are 30°, which provide the best compromise for sculpting and nuclear fragment removal. These are used with both machines and are covered by silicone sleeves.

## INCISIONS

### Side Port Incision

#### Instruments
Fifteen degree knife, toothed St. Martins forceps.

### Technique

The limbal conjunctiva is grasped with the forceps at about 11 o'clock to steady the eye. The 15° knife is held in the left hand with blade parallel to the iris. The point of the knife is applied to the limbus at the capillary arcade approximately 60° from the chosen position of the tunnel incision. The knife is advanced to produce an incision 1 to 1.5 mm wide. The best way to judge this is to insert the knife until half the blade length remains outside the eye. The incision length should also be 1 to 1.5 mm. It will easily self-seal at the end of the procedure.

*Note*: The incision is made at the edge of the capillary arcade so that the small amount of bleeding will mark its site for insertion of the nucleus manipulator later.

### Scleral Tunnel Incision

#### Instruments
Colibri toothed microsurgical forceps, 15° blade, Alcon phaco slit blade 3.2 mm angled.

### Technique

A small 4.5 mm fornix based conjunctival flap is formed with the forceps and 15° blade.

The flat edge of the slit knife is then used to bare the sclera. No cautery is used, as this may distort the sclera by shrinkage and induce astigmatism. The Colibri forceps grasps the limbus at the left end of the conjunctival opening to steady the eye. The tip of the slit knife is held against the sclera about 1.5 mm behind the anterior limbus 15° above the plane of the iris. The knife is pushed gently forward until the bevel is just covered. The knife is then angulated backward so that the blade is pointing up the slope toward the center of the cornea. The blade is now advanced very slowly, first into sclera and then cornea. The progress of the passage of the knife can be seen clearly. When the tip of the knife is 1 mm into clear cornea, the handle is lifted and the knife advanced again, this time pointing to the scleral spur opposite. When this last is done slowly, a straight entry into the anterior chamber is produced which acts efficiently as an internal valve.

## Corneal Tunnel Incision

### Instruments

Colibri toothed microsurgical forceps, Alcon phaco slit blade 3.2 mm angled.

### Technique

The eye is held with the forceps or a Fine Thornton ring can be used. The blade of the knife is reversed and held vertical to the cornea just inside the limbal arcade. A keratotomy incision is made following the line of the limbus and 60% depth. The blade is then returned to its normal position and applied to the distal edge of the corneal wound pointing toward the corneal dome. After 1.5 mm of slow advancement, the blade is made parallel to the iris for entry into the anterior chamber.

*Note*: Both the scleral and corneal incision can be made in this manner only with a single knife using a blade with a suitable bevel such as the Alcon knife. Other slit knives have a bevel that is too long and too sharp. They tend to cut out to the side.

## Tunnel Position

My incision of choice is the scleral tunnel because it is generally less astigmatogenic. It is also stronger. The corneal incision is only used temporally, the scleral wherever it feels most comfortable.

## ANTERIOR CHAMBER MAINTENANCE

The chamber is now filled with viscoelastic through the side port. In the UK, the choice is between HPMC or a sodium hyaluronate clone. Viscoat is about to be launched in the next few weeks. Provisc (Alcon) (sodium hyaluronate 1%) is what I use at present. I do not think there is much choice among the various sodium hyaluronates; HPMC does not perform as well in the eye, but it is cheaper.

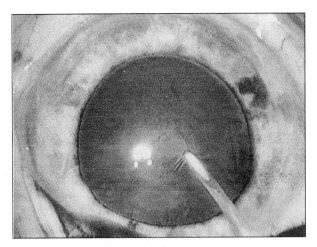

Figure 23-5. Starting the capsulorhexis.

## CAPSULORHEXIS

### Instruments

Straight disposable cystotome, Duckworth and Kent titanium capsulorhexis forceps.

### Technique

The eye is overfilled with viscoelastic as above to flatten the anterior capsule. Refocus the microscope on the anterior capsule.

*Note*: There is much less of a tendency for the capsular tear to move peripherally during the rhexis if the surface is flattened out. If the surgeon is worried about the rhexis getting out of control at any stage of the capsulotomy, more viscoelastic injected into the eye will usually arrest the problem.

The cystotome is attached to the polisher handpiece and inserted through the tunnel. The instrument held in the right hand is steadied by the index finger of the left hand. The capsule in the center of the lens is engaged with the tip of the cystotome and the sharp edge is used to cut the capsule toward 1 o'clock for about 1 mm. The tear is started by dragging the torn capsule first toward 11 o'clock, then 10, then 9, then 8, in a circular manner. The flap of the capsule is laid on top of the adjacent untorn capsule so that it can easily be grasped by the capsulorhexis forceps.

The capsulorhexis forceps having been inserted into the eye are used to grasp the capsular edge. This is then torn in a circular manner, constantly changing the angle of the vector forces by regripping the capsular edge as the tear progresses.

*Note*: The ideal angle of pull to produce the tear depends on both a horizontal and a vertical component. This is particularly important in young eyes with elastic capsules. Do not expect the capsule to tear in the direction in which you are pulling.

Capsules vary considerably in consistency and elasticity. As a general rule, the younger the patient the more elastic the capsules, and these capsules are much more difficult to control. The angle of pull is often at an obtuse

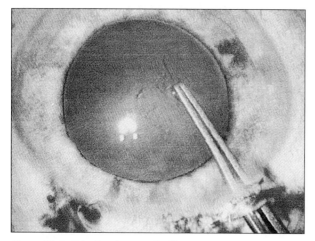

Figure 23-6. Gripping the capsular flap.

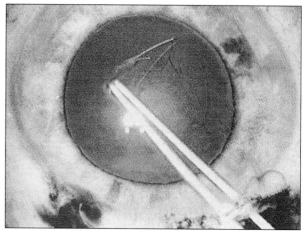

Figure 23-7. Tearing the flap using capsulorhexis forceps.

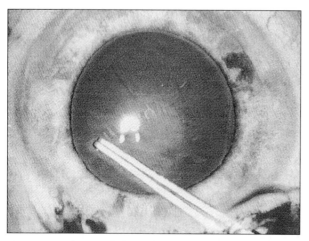

Figure 23-8. The capsulorhexis flap folded over on itself allows a circular tear.

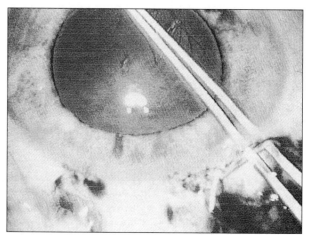

Figure 23-9. Completion of the rhexis.

angle to the direction of tear to prevent drift to the periphery. Aim to make these capsulotomies small (4 mm) and they will probably end up about 6 mm.

## Capsulorhexis Size

The ideal size for a capsulorhexis is between 5 mm and 6 mm. Making it any larger can lead to difficulties with control and is unnecessary. With some implant materials (such as silicone) it is particularly important that the rhexis is not too small at the end of the procedure. A rhexis of 4.5 mm or less may lead to contraction and capsulophimosis. The implant may then decenter and cause the patient to experience glare from the opaque edge of the capsule.

*Note*: If the rhexis looks too small after the irrigation/aspiration (I/A), enlarge it.

### Technique

Inject viscoelastic into the anterior chamber but do not overfill it, as this will put the capsule under tension. Use Vannas scissors to make an oblique cut at the rhexis edge, grasp this new tear with the capsulorhexis forceps, and tear carefully around.

## Reasons for Problems with Capsulorhexis

The most common problem is loss of control of the tear so that it moves peripherally. This may be due most to:
1. Elasticity of the capsule combined with lack of rigidity of the sclera, as seen in younger patients.
2. Excessive pressure from behind the lens.
3. Any other cause for loss of the anterior chamber and escape of viscoelastic.

The cure for all of these is to inject more viscoelastic; if the problem persists, change to a high viscosity viscoelastic such as Healon GV. If the tear appears to stop, this is due to anterior zonular fibers abnormally far forward. Do not persist with the rhexis in this direction or it will rapidly tear toward the equator. Start the rhexis the other way around by making a small cut with Vannas scissors, and then rejoin it at the point where it had previously stopped.

When there is a poor or no red reflex, as in white cataracts or very advanced nuclear cataracts with extreme sclerosis capsulorhexis, can be very taxing. There are a few simple maneuvers which will improve visibility somewhat:

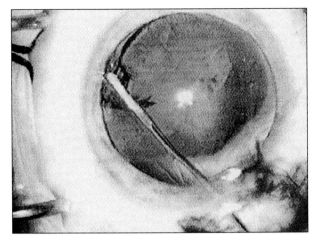
Figure 23-10. Fluid flush with soft cataract.

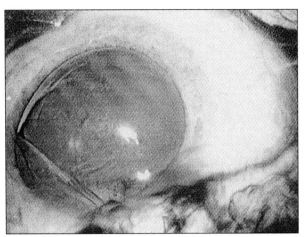
Figure 23-11. Fluid flush seen during hydrodissection.

1. If you don't do so already, sit temporally, as visibility is enhanced.
2. Tilt the microscope so that the light is oblique to the capsule and will reflect from the torn edge.
3. Increase the magnification so that the iris fills your field, and focus accurately. What you lose in depth of field is gained by ease of vision of the capsular edge.
4. In white cataracts, when liquid lens material fills the eye as the capsule is punctured, use the I/A to clear the chamber and suck out anterior cortex. Refill the eye with viscoelastic; your view of the capsule will then be much better.

Small pupils, although they can be enlarged by various means, still make the rhexis more difficult. Viscoelastic may be used to push the pupil open and thus expose more capsule. Also, the nucleus manipulator can push the iris aside in the area where the capsulorhexis forceps are tearing the capsule.

## HYDRODISSECTION

### Instruments
Visitec hydrodissection cannula (with rectangular cross section), 2 mL disposable syringe filled with basic salt solution (BSS).

### Technique
The hydrodissection cannula is placed under the edge of the capsule at about the 3 o'clock position. The capsule is tented up to peel it off the cortex and advanced 1 mm peripherally. BSS is injected rapidly but smoothly to produce cortical cleavage. This is seen as a fluid wave advancing rapidly under the nucleus and epinucleus. The tip of the cannula is then placed on the center of the nucleus and pushed backward toward the posterior capsule. This maneuver has the effect of helping to spread the fluid around the capsule and complete the cleavage. If you feel that the hydrodissection is incomplete, a second injection of BSS can be made at the 9 o'clock position.

Table 23-1
### TECHNIQUE FOR SOFT NUCLEI

| Machine settings | Alcon Legacy | AMO Prestige |
|---|---|---|
| Phaco tip bevel | 30° | 30° |
| Bottle height | 70 cm | 70 cm |
| Vacuum | 100 mm Hg Sculpting and nuclear removal | 35 mm Hg sculpting 260 mm Hg nuclear removal |
| Aspiration rate | 15 mL/min | 18 mL/min |
| Phaco power | 40% linear | 40% linear |

In hard or medium cataracts, it may be difficult to separate nucleus from epinucleus (as in hydrodclineation) and is often not necessary. If it is necessary to get the hard part of a nuclear fragment away from its attached epinucleus during phaco, this can be done with the nucleus manipulator. However, in soft cataracts it is advantageous to clearly see the extent of the nucleus, so that the phaco tip does not inadvertently push through soft nucleus, epinucleus, and capsule. Sometimes with very soft cataracts, part of the nucleus is pushed through the rhexis during the hydrodissection. This does not matter; it will facilitate the aspiration of the soft nucleus.

## LENS REMOVAL

### General Points
- Check that the machine is working satisfactorily before placing the phaco tip in the eye. This includes making sure the machine parameters are those desired.
- Check that the phaco tip is undamaged and that its bevel is at 90° to the irrigation sleeve openings. The exposed tip should be about 1.5 mm beyond the end of the sleeve.
- Check that the foot pedal is comfortably placed.

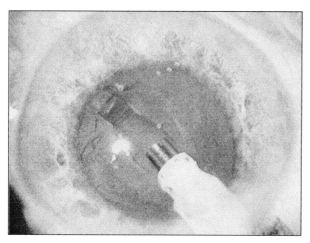

Figure 23-12. Sculpting a trench with microscope focused on its floor.

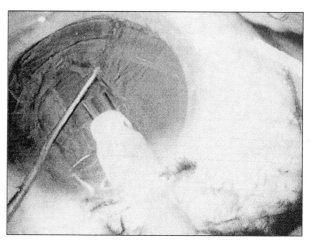

Figure 23-13. Soft Chop.

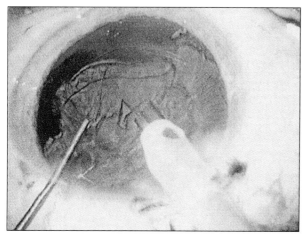

Figure 23-14. Soft segment removal.

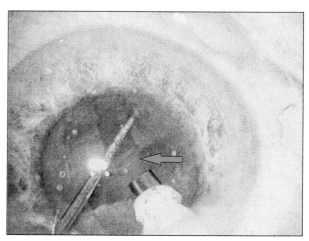

Figure 23-15. Removing residual ridge at the center of the nucleus.

### Instruments

Colibri toothed microsurgical forceps, phaco handpiece, Duckworth and Kent nucleus manipulator.

## TECHNIQUE FOR SOFT NUCLEI

### Emulsification

The Colibri forceps is used to lift gently the edge of the wound, and the phaco tip enters the eye bevel-down. The machine should be in foot Position 0 because the anterior chamber is still deepened by the viscoelastic.

*Note:* If it is not, or if the eye has a shallow chamber, or the pupil is not well dilated and the iris is at risk of damage as the phaco tip enters the eye, redeepen the chamber with viscoelastic. If Viscoat is available and it is being used to protect the endothelium during phaco anyway, this problem will not arise.

Once the irrigation ports are safely in the eye, the foot pedal is depressed to Position 1, allowing the irrigation fluid to deepen the anterior chamber.

- Sculpting—With soft cataracts, it is very easy to pass straight through the lens if too much power is used when sculpting. It should be done with smooth movements, and the edge of the delineated nucleus should not be passed. Make a deep central groove at about 90% depth because even though it may not crack, it will facilitate the pulling of the edge of the lens centrally after it has been chopped.
- Nucleus removal:
1. With the phaco tip in the eye in irrigation mode, insert the nucleus manipulator through the side port incision.
2. Pass the tip of the manipulator (turned on its side) under the rhexis and out to the equator of the nucleus in the 3 o'clock position.
3. Engage the nucleus with the manipulator and pull toward the central groove. As the manipulator reaches the groove, use the phaco tip to separate the two sides of the cut you have made. It does not matter if there is full separation or not.
4. Turn the nucleus with the manipulator and the phaco tip and repeat the slicing at intervals of 2 clock hours. This technique, known as the Soft Slice, will mean that the segments of nucleus even though they are not separated will fold in toward the center of the eye when they are engaged by the phaco tip.

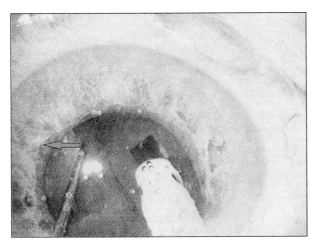
Figure 23-16. Cracking the nucleus.

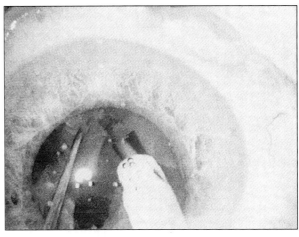
Figure 23-17. Cracking the final quadrant.

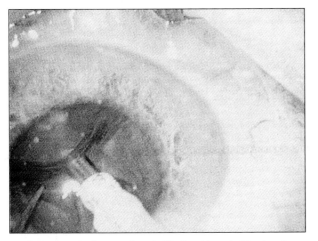
Figure 23-18. The first quadrant is lifted and impaled by the phaco tip.

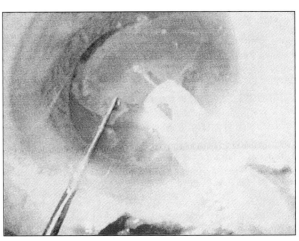
Figure 23-19. Impaled quadrant is brought forward for removal.

5. Bury the phaco tip in one of the segments. No ultrasound (U/S) power is needed for this because of the softness of the nucleus. Allow vacuum to build, and when it has, pull the segment centrally for removal. The nucleus will peel apart along the preprepared cuts. Do this for each part of the nucleus.
6. The epinuclear shell will still be in the eye, but because of the cortical cleavage, hydrodissection will be free to be aspirated. Pass the phaco tip under the rhexis edge into the epinucleus at 6 o'clock, and as vacuum builds pull it centrally for removal. Do not use U/S because this will break occlusion and also punch holes in the epinucleus. Sometimes the manipulator is needed to help the phaco tip engage the epinucleus by moving it from the equator toward the center.

## TECHNIQUE FOR MEDIUM-HARD NUCLEI

This type of cataract is by far the easiest to remove. The nucleus offers some—but not too much—resistance to emulsification, but also has enough substance to allow

Table 23-2
### TECHNIQUE FOR MEDIUM-HARD NUCLEI

| Machine settings | Alcon Legacy | AMO Prestige |
|---|---|---|
| Phaco tip bevel | 30° | 30° |
| Bottle height | 70 cm | 70 cm |
| Vacuum | 150 mm Hg sculpting and nuclear removal | 35 mm Hg sculpting 260 mm Hg nuclear removal |
| Aspiration rate | 15mL/min | 18 mL/min |
| Phaco power | 70% linear | 60% linear |

easy hydrodissection, manipulation, and cracking. It is the ideal type of nucleus on which beginners may learn.

### Emulsification

The eye is entered as already mentioned for the soft cataract.
- Sculpting—In medium-hard cataracts, the nucleus offers some resistance to sculpting. Accordingly,

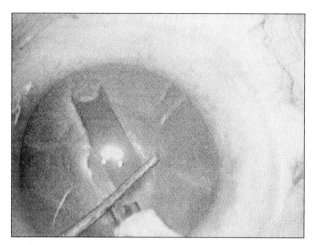

Figure 23-20. White tramlines seen with hard cataract when sculpting.

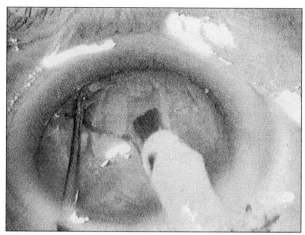

Figure 23-21. Uneven cracking with hard cataract when groove is shallow.

the amount of power needed to emulsify it is that which does not push the nucleus across the eye. It is better to press down with the foot and increase the phaco power than put the superior zonules at risk by pushing at the nucleus. The anatomy of the nucleus should be borne in mind during sculpting. Initially, the anterior cortex is removed widely to expose the hard core. This core is then grooved to a depth of 90% of the nuclear thickness.

*Note:* As nucleus hardness increases, the passes of sculpting should attempt to remove thinner and thinner slivers of nucleus.

*Note:* As the phaco tip advances, it should be slightly elevated to avoid passing straight through the nucleus. It is important to remember that the center of the nucleus is 2.5 to 3.0 mm, but that is because of its elliptical cross section, this reduces rapidly as the phaco tip moves peripherally.

The grooves in the nucleus need not go beyond the edge of the 5.5 mm rhexis. Provided that sufficient depth has been achieved, cracking will occur easily with grooves of this length. It is also important that the grooves are not significantly wider than the phaco needle or cracking will be much less efficient.

Tips for judging the depth in the nucleus when sculpting:
- Remember the diameter of the phaco needle (usually 1.0 mm).
- Remember the anatomy of the lens, with hard central nucleus surrounded by epinucleus and cortex which are softer.
- Watch the change in the red reflex—it gets brighter.
- Refocus the microscope frequently so that the focus is at the plane of emulsification.

When the first groove has been made, the nuclear manipulator is passed into the eye through the side port and placed in the groove. The nucleus is then rotated counterclockwise to present the next area of nucleus to be sculpted. These medium hard nuclei are generally easy to rotate.

Following the fashioning of all four grooves to create a cruciate shape of appropriate depth, the nucleus can be cracked.

*Note:* Although I have used the chopping technique and still do to facilitate the removal of large nuclear fragments, I find that my technique for nucleofractis is the most predictable and consistent, and the easiest to teach our residents in training.

- Cracking:
1. Use the manipulator to move the nucleus so that a groove is placed at the apex of the triangle formed by the phaco tip and the manipulator.
2. These two instruments are then put at the bottom of the groove. The phaco tip stabilizes the nucleus while the manipulator moves to the left. In a medium hard nucleus, little effort should be needed to crack it. The crack should take place centrally but the effect should cause the equator to separate also. This is important for later quadrant removal.

- Quadrant removal:
1. Each quadrant is split in turn, and the manipulator is used to lift the apex of the first quadrant to present it to the phaco tip.

*Note:* If the first quadrant that is approached for removal does not readily detach itself from its position, move to the smallest and try to engage it. Once one quadrant has been removed, the others come easily.

2. Initially the foot pedal is used in Position 3 (phaco mode) to impale the nuclear quadrant on the phaco tip and thus cause occlusion. The foot pedal is now moved into Position 2 (I/A) and vacuum is allowed to build. When you feel that a good grip has been achieved on the nuclear quadrant, it can be moved to the center of the capsulorhexis. In this position, using mostly vacuum assisted by low levels of linearly controlled U/S power, the quadrant is emulsified.
3. The next quadrant is moved into position by the manipulator, tilted up, and emulsified as already described. The remaining two quadrants are dealt with similarly.

*Note:* With the higher levels of vacuum currently being

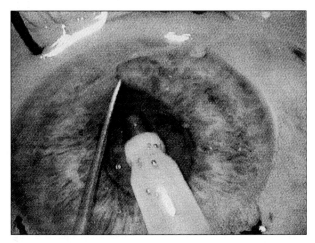

Figure 23-22. Using the second instrument to facilitate sculpting.

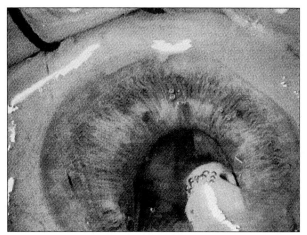

Figure 23-23. Cracking with a small pupil.

used, care must exercised to avoid anterior chamber collapse when occlusion breaks. Two methods are available on modern machines to mitigate this eventuality. With continuous irrigation, even in Position 0 the chamber will always be filled so that the post occlusion break surge is neutralized. The second method is the approach of the AMO Prestige phaco machine. A mechanical model of events in the anterior chamber exists in relation to the pump mechanism. This allows the pump speed to slow to zero after occlusion and maximum vacuum have been achieved. As the piece of nucleus being removed clears the tip and occlusion breaks, instead of the pump accelerating to its predetermined speed, it reaches it after a pause. This allows the anterior chamber to equilibrate without any risk of collapse. This is particularly important with harder cataracts. However, where these mechanical aids are not present, surgeon anticipation of the likelihood of this event has to suffice. The foot pedal has to be lifted immediately prior to the clearing of the port in the phaco tip.

## TECHNIQUE FOR HARD NUCLEI

The hard nucleus presents the phaco surgeon with one of the greatest challenges. The ability of the tip to penetrate the nucleus, often in the face of weak zonules and combined with controlling sharp nuclear fragments in order to avoid damaging capsule or endothelium, requires special skills to avoid problems.

- Sculpting—In order to minimize the movement of the nucleus away from the phaco tip which might put the zonules on the stretch, high U/S power settings are necessary. The use of maximum power on panel control means the greatest possible acceleration of the tip into the hard nucleus. Therefore, it is more efficient and ultimately less power is used. Since adopting this approach, phaco times in hard nuclei have been reduced and nuclear movement largely eliminated.

*Note:* In hard cataracts, the cut edge of the nucleus produces a characteristic white tramline. This will alert the

Table 23-3
**TECHNIQUE FOR HARD NUCLEI**

| Machine settings | Alcon Legacy | AMO Prestige |
|---|---|---|
| Phaco tip bevel | 30° | 30° |
| Bottle height | 80 cm | 80 cm |
| Vacuum | 200 mm Hg sculpting and nuclear removal | 35 mm Hg sculpting 260 mm Hg nuclear removal |
| Aspiration rate | 15 mL/min | 18 mL/min |
| Phaco power | 99% panel then 90% linear | 99% panel then 90% linear |

surgeon when a good red reflex suggested only a moderately hard nucleus.

- Cracking—In hard cataracts, cracking may be relatively easy because the nuclei are sometimes quite brittle. However, the plates of the nucleus often do not part cleanly, therefore it is essential to make sure that the grooves in the nucleus are of adequate depth. The most common cause of cracking difficulties with hard nuclei is due to insufficient depth of the grooves. If problems arise, return to each groove and gently redeepen it. Make sure that all quadrants are well separated before starting to remove them.

- Quadrant removal—Because hard nuclei are also large nuclei, it is often sensible once the quadrant has been well engaged by the phaco tip to take a chopper and reduce the size. This is done by pulling the chopper from the periphery of the quadrant toward the phaco tip. Maintaining occlusion of the tip is vital to avoid hard fragments of the nucleus careering around the anterior chamber. It is important to balance vacuum and power and avoid lens chatter. Even with hard cataracts, once the fragment of nucleus has occluded the port on the phaco tip, surprisingly little U/S power is required

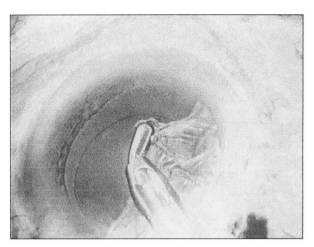

Figure 23-24. Using the I/A tip to pull cortex centrally for aspiration.

to massage it through. Lens chatter causes the nuclear fragments to bounce away from the tip, which has two effects. First, the hard pieces of nucleus will abrade the endothelium, and second, because the machine is working inefficiently and far more power than necessary will be used, it will also take longer. As discussed previously those phaco machines such as the AMO Prestige, which allow high vacuum and have advanced fluidics to minimize postocclusion break surge, improve safety and efficiency in these difficult eyes.

*Note:* There is often little in the way of protective epinucleus in hard cataracts. As proposed by Dr. Michael Colvard, the use of a protective shield, which is slipped between the nucleus and the capsule prior to emulsification, should considerably lessen the risk of capsular rupture.

## Emulsification in Special Situations

### Small Pupil

Modern nuclear disassembly techniques allow much safer phaco than was possible previously in small pupil cases. There are two situations that are commonly found: eyes with small but mobile pupils, and pupils stuck down by synechiae.

If the pupil is not smaller then 3.5 mm and is mobile, overdeepening the anterior chamber will usually allow enough capsule to be exposed to permit capsulorhexis. If not, judicious use of the nucleus manipulator following the forceps around the rhexis will allow it to be completed without pupil modification. The manipulator is used also to move the iris away from the phaco tip in the immediate area where it is working during emulsification. This will allow the grooves for nucleofractis to be cut safely.

*Note:* It is essential to ensure good hydrodissection in these cases, as visibility is so limited.

Pupils which are stuck by synechiae are often very small (1 mm). There is no way that the case can be completed without enlargement of the pupil.

### Enlargement of the Pupil

The instruments used are a viscoelastic syringe with Rycroft cannula, and two nuclear manipulators.

### Technique

1. Synechiae are broken down initially with viscodissection. The viscoelastic cannula is introduced through the side port incision and the tip is placed through the pupil. Viscoelastic is injected gently to free the iris from the anterior lens capsule. This should produce a round but very small opening when the anterior chamber is further deepened with viscoelastic.
2. The two manipulators are then introduced, one through the side port and one through the tunnel incision. They are used to stretch the iris gently from 3 to 9 o'clock and from 6 to 12 o'clock. This will break down existing fibrous tissue, but should not damage the sphincter, so that the pupil often is functional postoperatively. When viscoelastic is then introduced, the pupil will be found to be satisfactorily large.

## COMBINED GLAUCOMA AND CATARACT SURGERY

Small incision cataract surgery lends itself very well to combination with glaucoma filtering surgery to produce a safe, effective operation which has little effect on astigmatism. It works particularly well with foldable IOLs because the wound requires minimal modification.

Instruments for the trabeculectomy: Vannas scissors, St. Martins toothed forceps, bipolar cautery wand, Colibri toothed microsurgical forceps, Alcon angled 3.2 mm phaco slit blade, Crozafon sclerotomy punch, 8-0 Vicryl stitch, and a micro needle holder.

### Technique

1. A conjunctival flap based on the fornix is formed with St. Martins forceps and the Vannas scissors. The conjunctiva is dissected off Tenon's capsule. This is then dissected from the sclera and removed from the area of the trabeculectomy wound.
2. The scleral vessels are gently cauterized using the bipolar wand.
3. A 4 mm vertical groove is prepared using the slit knife 2 mm behind the anterior limbus as previously described. The knife is turned back to its usual position and a tunnel is formed as already described.
4. Phacoemulsification now proceeds normally.
5. After the lens has been inserted and before the viscoelastic has been removed from the eye, the Crozafon punch is inserted through the wound. The distal end of the cutter hooks over the edge of the internal part of the tunnel and the punch is closed. The punch is then removed and the tissue in it removed. The sclerotomy is inspected to see how many bites will be required to produce an adequate opening (usually two). The sclerotomy should be about 1 mm from the proximal lip of the wound and should leak aqueous gently when it is touched with a dry sponge.

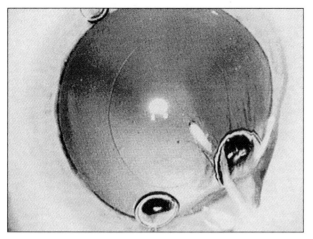

Figure 23-25. Starting the posterior capsulorhexis.

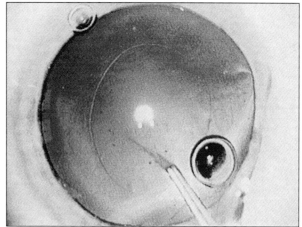

Figure 23-26. Completing the posterior rhexis with forceps.

6. A small iridectomy is made and the viscoelastic removed with the I/A.
7. For closure of the wound use 8-0 Vicryl stitches at each end of the conjunctival wound.
8. Inject BSS through the side port and observe the bleb forming.

## White Cataracts

As previously stated in the discussion of capsulorhexis, these cases are very challenging. However, if the rhexis has been satisfactorily accomplished, there are still a few points worth noting.

The nuclei in these cases are often not only hard but very mobile. In order to maximize control during emulsification, introduce the manipulator early on to stabilize the nucleus. This is particularly important when sculpting.

*Note:* Use of a chopping technique is not recommended in these cases because the capsule can be difficult to see when the chopper is passed to the equator and it is therefore easily damaged.

There is little if any epinucleus or cortex to protect the posterior capsule in the presence of sharp nuclear fragments. Use the same precautions as mentioned in relation to hard cataracts.

## EPINUCLEUS REMOVAL

The main points in relation to persistent epinucleus have been discussed under the section on soft cataracts. However, if there is a bowl of epinucleus, as sometimes occurs with no break in the edge, it can present some difficulty for the surgeon. Here are some suggestions:
- Use the nucleus manipulator to go out to the equator of the capsular bag to pull the epinucleus centrally.
- If this does not work, the manipulator can be used to divide the edge and allow the phaco tip to occlude on one side.
- Finally, if all else fails and the epinucleus refuses to cooperate, use viscoelastic to get under the edge and lift it centrally for aspiration.

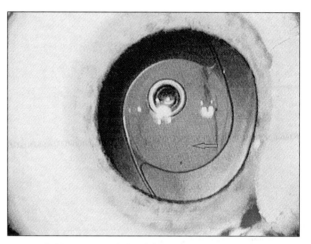

Figure 23-27. IOL optic behind the posterior rhexis.

## IRRIGATION/ASPIRATION

The I/A tip is a 45° tip with 0.3 mm port metal irrigation sleeve. This angulation and size is ideal for I/A in all situations, with the deep anterior chambers generally found with self-sealing tunnels. The advantage of cortical cleaving hydrodissection is that there is relatively little cortex left to aspirate.

Machine settings for both the Alcon Legacy and the AMO Prestige are maximum vacuum 400+ mm Hg, linear aspiration flow 24 mL/min.

Concerning technique, occlusion of the aspiration port is extremely important to achieve efficient cortical removal. Once this has happened, the cortex can be dragged centrally for aspiration.

1. Begin the cortical removal at about the 2 o'clock position and go around the eye segmentally to 10 o'clock. Change the angulation of the tip as you proceed around the eye.
2. Subincisional cortex can present particular problems and can be a common reason for capsular breaks during I/A. Turn the aspiration port toward the 12 o'clock position for access to the superior cortex. When occlu-

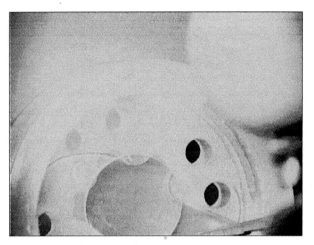

Figure 23-28. Alcon AcrySof MA60 IOL.

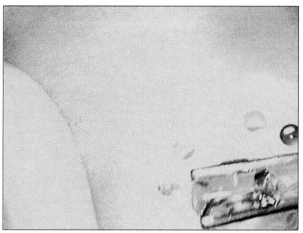

Figure 23-29. Folding the AcrySof lens.

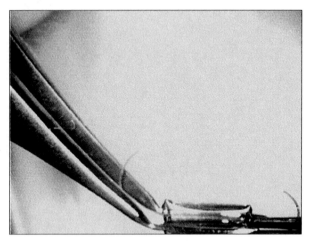

Figure 23-30. Picking up the folded IOL.

sion has occurred, the cortex is pulled centrally by a scooping motion.

*Note:* If the superior cortex does not come easily for whatever reason, leave it in situ until later. When the viscoelastic is injected prior to lens implantation it is used to viscodissect the remaining cortex. The lens is then implanted and with the protection of the posterior capsule by the IOL, the already loosened cortex is easily removed with the I/A.

## CAPSULAR CLEANING

There are sometimes remnants of cortical material which need to be removed from the posterior capsule prior to lens implantation. They can either be polished off using a Kratz scratcher or similar to abrade the capsule gently, or be aspirated off with the I/A in low vacuum mode. If these remnants are not removed they can lead to early capsular wrinkling.

### Capsule Polishing

The instruments used are the Kratz scratcher on irrigation handpiece with free flow irrigation. The technique is a circular movement used on the capsule. A halo reflex from the posterior capsule indicates the correct plane. There is no feeling of contact with the capsule; this is a visual technique.

### Vacuuming the Capsule

The instruments used are the I/A handpiece with phaco machine set with vacuum at 35 mm Hg and aspiration rate at 16 mL/min. Concerning technique, with the settings on the machine at this low level, the posterior capsule can be safely picked up in the I/A port with little or no risk of breaking. Residual cortex and plaque can often be aspirated off by this means.

If there is persistent plaque which does not polish off or cannot be aspirated from the posterior capsule it can be left (for 3 months) for later YAG laser capsulotomy, or posterior capsulorhexis should be considered. This technique allows more rapid visual rehabilitation than delayed YAG, but there are a few surgical points to be considered before undertaking it.

### Posterior Capsulorhexis

The instruments are a straight cystotome as used for anterior capsulorhexis mounted on viscoelastic syringe, and a capsulorhexis forceps. Concerning technique:
1. The cystotome is introduced and the anterior chamber gently filled with viscoelastic. Do not overfill the eye, as it will put too much tension on the capsule.
2. The tip of the cystotome engages the capsule centrally and produces a small tear. In young patients with elastic capsules, this can prove surprisingly difficult. Viscoelastic is injected slowly under the posterior capsule to push back the vitreous face.
3. The capsulorhexis forceps grasps the torn edge of the capsule and the tear is started. The posterior capsule is much more diaphanous than the anterior and also more elastic. Producing the posterior rhexis seems to require more pull than the anterior. Aim to produce a posterior rhexis two-thirds of the size of the anterior.

*Note:* It is important to make sure that the rhexis is

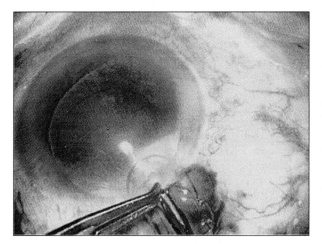

Figure 23-31. Introducing the leading haptic.

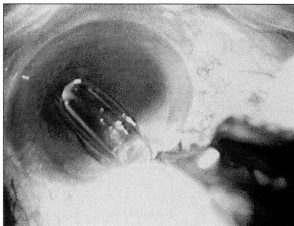

Figure 23-32. Rotating the lens within the eye.

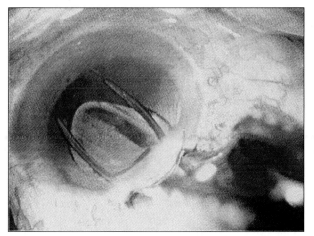

Figure 23-33. Allowing the lens to unfold.

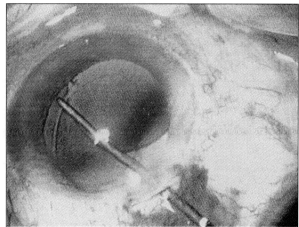

Figure 23-34. Rotating the trailing haptic into position.

truly completed; a radial break at the edge can spread when the IOL is placed in the bag.

When it is anticipated that there may be anterior capsular epithelial cell growth across the anterior hyaloid, an anterior vitrectomy followed by pushing the IOL through the posterior rhexis should be considered.

## IOL IMPLANTATION

### General consideration

The two main considerations are viscoelastic and wound sizing. The eye will need to be refilled with viscoelastic prior to implantation; currently I use Provisc. As previously noted, the choice in the UK is very limited. It is important, particularly with a folding lens, to make sure that the capsular bag is well distended and the anterior chamber is also deep. This will allow easy placement of the IOL and its unfolding with minimum trauma to the ocular contents. In small incision cataract surgery there is now a bewildering array of lenses available in a variety of materials. Some folding lenses can be implanted through unenlarged wounds; often, however, some adjustment of the wound will be necessary. The folding lens which I currently use is the Alcon MA60 AcrySof. This will pass easily through a 3.5 mm opening. The phaco slit knife can be used to ease the edge of the wound and thus enlarge it sufficiently.

### Lens Implant

At present I use only one implant—the Alcon MA60 AcrySof—for all cataracts except high myopes where there is not the dioptric range available. I have stopped using polymethylmethacrylate (PMMA) because it does not fold and therefore denies my small incision. I will no longer use silicone because although on the whole my results were good, the capsular effects and occasional foreign body reaction in the eye are not satisfactory. I like polyHEMA as a material, and have been involved in trials of a new design of lens made of this, but it is not yet commercially available. In my own experience with acrylic (6 years), the results in visual terms as well as the very low capsulotomy rate are impressive. This material also works very well in compromised eyes with uveitis,

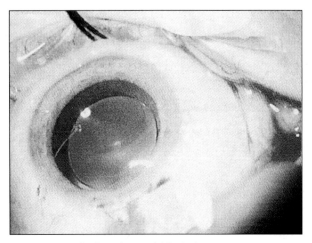

Figure 23-35. Checking the would for leaks.

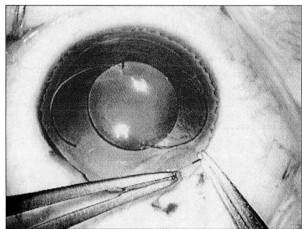

Figure 23-36. Introducing the needle to the bed of the wound.

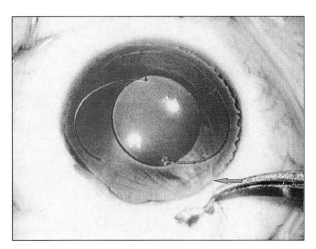

Figure 23-37. Horizontal suture in place.

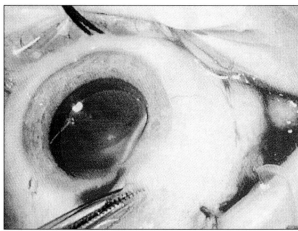

Figure 23-38. Injection of subconjunctival antibiotics.

glaucoma, diabetes, etc. The size and three-piece design mean that it can be used also as a backup lens, and the gentle unfolding of acrylic allows insertion folded even with a capsular break. The lack of capsular contraction that this IOL produces permits me to insert it safely into the bag in the presence of a capsulorhexis break with little risk of decentration.

## Implantation

### Instruments
Angled McPherson forceps, Seibel folding paddles, Duckworth and Kent (Buratto) insertion forceps, Colibri microsurgical forceps, lens dialing hook.

### Technique
1. Open the wagon wheel container for the lens and ask the nurse to squirt BSS onto the lens.
   *Note:* This material is affected by temperature in that if the lens is too cold, it is harder to fold. It is best to place it in a warming cabinet.
2. Move the microscope away from the eye and reduce the magnification. With the McPherson forceps, place the lens on the back of the wagonwheel case.
3. Open the Seibel paddles, press down on the edge of the lens to make sure there is no meniscus of BSS underneath it, and fold the lens. This is done by closing the paddle forceps, having placed the lens in the grooves on the inside of the paddles. The lens can be folded either from 6 to 12 o'clock or 3 to 9 o'clock. I prefer the 6 to 12 fold. Down the microscope, check that the lens has folded in half rather than asymmetrically, which would impair implantation.
4. With the Buratto forceps, grasp the lens along the top of the paddles.
5. Turn the lens so that the straight edge of the folded optic faces the left. This will assure that the haptic which turns on unfolding is outside of the eye, not in the capsular bag.
6. Introduce the distal haptic to the wound which is gripped by the Colibri forceps, and allow it to form a D-shape. Push the optic gently into the eye. As the haptic releases on entering the eye, dip the forceps down to place the distal haptic in the bag.

7. With the optic now in the eye, the hand is rotated so the folded spine of the IOL is superior. The lens is squeezed gently and then released. Normally it drops down into the bag and slowly unfolds. The Buratto forceps can be removed from the eye.

   *Note:* If the lens does not release cleanly, rapidly squeeze it again and release again. Due to the slow unfolding, the forceps can be released faster than the lens regains its unfolded shape.

8. The lens dialing hook now enters the eye and is used to push the optic into the bag if it is not there already. Then with a gentle rotary movement, the lens and its trailing haptic are dialed into the capsular bag.

## VISCOELASTIC REMOVAL

The I/A tip should be used, with the machine set at same settings as for cortical removal. Concerning technique, the I/A tip is introduced into the eye and aspiration is commenced over the center of the optic. It is possible to observe down the microscope the viscoelastic disappearing down the I/A port. In order to remove viscoelastic from behind the implant (which is very important), it is not necessary to go behind the IOL with the I/A tip. Simply press the center of the IOL with the tip and gently move it from side to side. This will squeeze any remaining viscoelastic from under the IOL.

## INCISION CLOSURE

### Closing the Self-Sealing Wound

The hydrodissection cannula attached to a syringe filled with BSS is placed in the side port incision and the eye is reinflated so that it feels quite firm when the center of the cornea is pressed. The watertightness of the wound is tested by placing a dry sponge posterior to the wound and pressing. It should remain dry. In the vast majority of cases, a suture is not required because the tunnel wound and its internal valve close satisfactorily. If the surgery has been complicated and the IOL has been inserted unfolded, or if when tested with a sponge the wound has not sealed properly, a suture will be placed.

### Suturing the Wound

Instruments used for this are a Colibri toothed microsurgical forceps, micro needle holder, Alcon 10-0 nylon suture CU1 needle. The technique starts with lifting the lip of the wound with the Colibri forceps. Viscoelastic is in the eye to retain its firmness. A horizontal pass is made with the needle along the bed of the wound from right to left. The needle is now passed through the upper part of the tunnel from inside out. It is reinserted through the outside of the tunnel again and into the wound to create a horizontal mattress stitch. This is tied into the wound and the ends trimmed. No great tension is needed on the stitch because it generally is acting only to buttress the tunnel.

## CONCLUSION

The conjunctiva is pushed back over the wound by injecting cefuroxime subconjunctivally 5 mm posterior to the tunnel. The drape is then removed and a shield placed over the eye. Postoperatively the patient receives one bottle of G Maxitrol to be instilled four times daily for 2 weeks and then twice daily until it is finished.

# Chapter 24

# PREFERRED PHACOEMULSIFICATION TECHNIQUE: PHACO SLICE AND SEPARATE

*Steve Arshinoff, MD, FRCSC*

## INTRODUCTION

Techniques of dividing the cataractous lens into smaller pieces for easier phacoemulsification have been evolving since 1968, when Kelman first introduced Christmas tree capsulotomy in association with sculpting and cracking. Gimbel introduced more formalized phaco procedures with his trough and crater methods of Divide and Conquer. Over the years, similar variations of this theme developed. Significant departure from these methods began with Nagahara's 1993 Phaco Chop technique, which was unpopular due to it's need for a large capsulorhexis. Paul Koch overcame this problem with Stop and Chop one year later. In 1995, Fukasaku introduced Snap and Split phaco, which has the advantages of eliminating both sculpting and the need to go out to the lens periphery with any instruments. Fukasaku's technique has not gained wide acceptance due to its need for the surgeon to exert considerable stress on the nucleus to achieve a snap, a step that most North American surgeons are not prepared to do. Furthermore, Snap and Split works best on lenses more dense, and therefore more brittle, than those usually seen in a typical North American practice.

Phaco Slice and Separate, the technique that I have evolved from Fukasaku's, retains all of the advantages of the above techniques, but replaces snapping with slicing across the phaco tip-stabilized nucleus with a Nagahara chopper. The chopper is then repositioned to optimally separate the divided lens halves. As the lens is rotated in the capsular bag, small pieces of the nuclear pie (approximately one and one-half clock hours in size) are sliced off, separated, and aspirated into the phaco tip. This technique works with a broader range of lens densities than other chopping techniques, and uses no sculpting and very little phaco time. Furthermore, the phaco time required for a very hard lens is not much more than for a relatively soft nucleus.

## ANESTHESIA

I routinely obtain ocular anesthesia using Astra 1% nonpreserved isotonic Xylocaine injected into the anterior chamber. The patient is given one to two drops of tetracaine upon entering the operating room. After the eye and surrounding facial area are prepped and draped, another one to two drops of tetracaine is administered. The side port incision is made using a 1 mm wide diamond knife with a 30° point, sharp on its bevel and the long side. Following this, approximately 0.3 cc of the Xylocaine is injected, using a 1 cc syringe and a 27 gauge hockey stick blunt canula. This is done in two *puffs*, warning the patient that it may sting a bit.

After the anesthetic injection, a supercohesive viscoelastic is injected through the same side port in order to firm up the eye enough for the creation of the primary incision. Sometimes I reinject about another 0.2 cc of Xylocaine after completing the cortical removal and before injecting the viscoelastic to fill the bag in preparation for intraocular lens (IOL) implantation. The second injection serves two purposes. It assures excellent anesthesia when the IOL stretches the would during implantation, and additionally, it is used to wash any residual cortical cells off the posterior capsule. I learned this anesthetic technique from Dr. James Gills of Tarpon Springs, Florida, and I find it to be much safer and more effective than any of the varied techniques that I used before.

## PHACOEMULSIFIER

My current primary phacoemulsifier is the Chiron Gold. I prefer peristaltic pumps for phacoemulsification because they require less fluid flow through the eye to maintain a stable chamber during phaco, and they are inherently safer during the procedure. Since the independent controllable factor is aspiration rate, whereas vacuum develops only with occlusion and is limited by the maximum acceptable level that the surgeon presets, phaco is a very controlled and gentle procedure. With increasing experience in phaco, I have found that the slower and more methodically the surgeon proceeds, the quicker the operation. When I acquired it about 4 years ago, the Chiron Gold was chosen because of its excellent fluidics, adequate power for very dense lenses, programmability with individual surgeon keys, durability, and ability to use economical resterilizable tubing sets.

Like many other surgeons, I do not always use the same phaco technique. I am fortunate to have been a practicing phaco surgeon during the past 15 years, a period throughout which phaco techniques rapidly changed and evolved. I therefore have considerable experience with most of the techniques that were popular for any period during that time, and feel quite comfortable changing back and forth between different techniques, depending upon the case.

I routinely use a 30° phaco tip (but sometimes 15 or 0°) through a 2.8 mm clear corneal incision. I prefer silicone sleeves because they seal the incision much more effectively, resulting in less fluid leakage from the anterior chamber and, consequently, a more stable anterior chamber throughout phaco. For very hard, hard, and medium lenses I use a technique which I call Slice and Separate, a modification of the Snap and Split phaco technique of Fukasaku of Japan.

This technique has made a huge difference in my surgeries, and even with the densest lenses, I now rarely use more than 1 minute of phaco time, using pulsed phaco with 50% duty cycle. The slicing technique, unlike the Phaco Chop, does not require a large capsulorhexis as the chopper never goes out to the periphery of the lens. It does, however, require meticulous hydrodissection because easy rotation of the nucleus is essential. The slicing technique is much more difficult in softer lenses, where hydrodissection is usually not as complete and the lenses are often too soft to slice. In softer lenses, I use a variation of Paul Koch's Stop and Chop phaco technique. In very soft lenses, I do concentric delamination with hydrodissection and aspirate the lens concentrically, beginning in the middle. All cases are done with phacopulse, 50% duty cycle, five to eight pulses per second, flow rate 20 cc/min, and vacuum limit at 150 mm Hg.

## INCISION

My side port incision is made first using the 1 mm diamond blade as described above. After the application of two drops of topical tetracaine, the eye is stabilized with Castroviejo 0.12 mm forceps, and the blade enters the anterior chamber at about 60° from the intended site of the primary incision. The blade is traversed through the cornea parallel to the iris and sometimes slightly tangential to the limbus. Therefore, the created intracorneal tunnel is longer in order to create a better self-sealing incision.

After injecting the intraocular Xylocaine and filling the anterior chamber with a supercohesive viscoelastic, the clear corneal incision is made peripheral enough to cause a small amount of bleeding but not to elevate conjunctiva on the patient's steepest corneal axis. The 2.8 mm diamond keratome is first drawn across the entry site, not to create a step but just to carefully mark the incision site because stabbing directly occasionally results in a somewhat ragged entry and has a greater tendency to tear the edges. Once a mark is made (about 0.2 mm larger than the intended incision), the keratome is pushed gently through the cornea, again parallel to the iris, attempting to create a roughly square incision. Slight wiggling of the blade makes the incision easier to perform, as entry is easier.

## CHAMBER CONTENTS FOR CAPSULOTOMY

My preferred viscoelastics for capsulorhexis are the supercohesives. When topical or intraocular anesthesia is used, surgery is carried out in an environment of constant positive posterior vitreous pressure since the extraocular muscles are not paralyzed. When the phaco or I/A tips are in the eye, the eye is pressurized by the inflowing BSS to the extent of the bottle height. During capsulorhexis, the anterior chamber is not pressurized except by the elasticity of the viscoelastic device.

The anterior capsule of the lens is a convex surface, much like the surface of a baloon. Once perforated, such a surface with pressure behind it will tend to tear out toward the periphery. This tendency can be completely neutralized if we pressurize the anterior chamber to the extent that the anterior chamber pressure becomes equal to the posterior vitreous pressure, and therefore permit ourselves to operate in a pressure equalized environment. This can only be achieved with the supercohesive viscoelastics: long chain, high zero shear viscosity viscoelastics (like Healon GV and MicroVisc Plus [IVisc Plus], my preferred viscoelastics). Only these *supercohesive viscoelastics* are elastic enough to permit the surgeon to use them to generate pressure.

I fill the chamber with the viscoelastic until I see the pupil dilate slightly and the lens move slightly posteriorly, indicating that I have pressurized the anterior chamber to equalize the posterior pressure which is pressing forward against the anterior lens capsule. I am an ardent proponent of this technique that I have named Pressure Equalized Cararact Surgery. It makes intraocular surgery much easier and safer.

## CAPSULOTOMY

I generally perform my capsulorhexis with a 27 guage needle that I bend myself to achieve a sharper and more vertical tip. I will, in some more difficult cases, use a Utratta forceps but the needle is a bit quicker and simpler. I begin with a puncture in the center of the lens, and then use the edge of the needle like a saw to cut a radius toward the periphery at about the 8 o'clock position. After I'm out about 2 mm from the center of the anterior capsule, I drop the heel of the needle, allowing the sharp tip to engage the capsule. I push the needle into the capsule in a down and out direction, which causes the tear to extend in a spiral clockwise direction.

Once the tear has reached the desired 5 mm diameter, I continue in a circular direction, all the time assuring that the flap is folded over and lying flat on the capsular surface. This yields the best physical tearing angle and allows for the most consistant, central, circular tears. Regrasping is done as necessary, usually about six times during the performance of the capsulorhexis but probably twice that often for a less experienced surgeon or a more difficult case (white lenses, calcified or fibrosed capsule, etc). The developing flap is always dropped into the center, to keep it from obscuring visability and hampering performance of the remainder of the capsulorhexis. Small pupils are done exactly the same way and present no problem, particularly if simple stretching of the pupil is done before the final viscoelastic injection. Smaller capsulorhexises are easier to perform than larger ones with a needle.

The diathermy capsulorhexis devices manufactured by Erbe and Oertli do not generally yield as strong a capsulorhexis as the manually torn ones, since any micro-erratic hand movements during use of these instruments will result in a small jag in the capsulorhexis, which may lead to a radial tear later during nuclear movement within the capsular bag. However, they are wonderful for intumescent, white, crenated, and calcified cataracts, and make these tough cases much easier. Without these devices, forceps, aspiration of cortex first, inverted soft shell technique, and even scissors may be necessary for some difficult cases.

## HYDRODISSECTION/ HYDRODELAMINATION

My preferred phaco technique of Slice and Separate requires meticulous hydrodissection so that the nucleus can be rotated freely. I use a 3 cc syringe filled with balanced salt solution (BSS) and a 27 gauge blunt hockey stick canula. My technique is similar to Fine's cortical cleaving hydrodissection in that I place the cannula under the edge of the capsulorhexis and inject gently as I advance the cannula tip almost to the lens equator. As the cannula is advanced, the force of injection is gradually increased, and the posterior fluid wave is observed. The procedure is repeated 180° away on the other side of the lens, except that this time the lens nucleus is rocked gently and rotated slightly as the fluid is injected, assuring that the nucleus is free for the subsequent steps of phaco. Usually about 1 to 2 cc of fluid are needed for this hydrodissection step to achieve optimal freedom of the nucleus. Hydrodelineation is unnecessary for Slice and Separate phaco, but is useful for nuclei too soft to chop.

## EMULSIFICATION OF NUCLEUS OF HARDNESS 2-4

Personally, hardness 2 means that the nucleus is firm enough to chop but soft enough to make sculpting very easy. Hardness 4 means that the lens is very dense, making sculpting difficult and often causing a flower petal effect with many cracking techniques if the surgeon doesn't go deep enough.

My preferred viscoelastics for all uncomplicated phaco cases are the supercohesive, highly viscous (at zero shear) viscoelastics, Healon GV, and MicroVisc (IVisc) Plus, as explained above. Supercohesive viscoelastics are far superior for space maintenance and make surgery under topical or intraocular anesthesia easy. The viscoelastic used during the phacoemulsification part of the procedure itself is generally irrelevant since the eye is pressurized by the inflowing BSS. The resultant intraocular pressure (IOP) is a function of the bottle height and the presence or absence of any wound leakage as most of the viscoelastic has left the eye by this point. The exception to the irrelevance of the viscoelastic now occurs in the presence of any tissue present in the surgical environment that the surgeon wants isolated from the turbulence of the phaco (eg, the endothelial cells in cases of Fuch's Dystrophy, a frayed piece of iris, or vitreous protruding around a small zonule disinsertion or through a small hole in the posterior capsule). In these cases I perform my Soft Shell technique, where I first inject the dispersive viscoelastic, Viscoat, onto the surface of the lens. Then inject a cohesive, or supercohesive, viscoelastic behind it, such that the cohesive viscoelastic expands to compress the Viscoat up against the cornea or other tissue being isolated in a smooth layer. When the cohesive viscoelastic is aspirated out during phaco, the dispersive Viscoat remains behind, in a smooth layer, to insulate the isolated tissue from the turbulence of phacoemulsification.

The technique of Slice and Separate works as follows: After performing a 4.5 to 5 mm capsulorhexis and good hydrodissection, the phaco tip (30, 15, or 0°) is inserted into the anterior chamber and the prenuclear cortex is phaco'd from the anterior surface of the nucleus within the capsulorhexis. A Nagahara chopper or Fukasaku snapper is present through the side port, and is then used to nudge the nucleus inferiorly. The phaco tip is buried into the nucleus, beginning above and aiming for the center, progressing almost to the center, in depth as well as inferiorly, to the point that the phaco tip comes to rest at just about the center of the lens, and at a depth such that it is covered by a small amount of nuclear material.

The phaco tip is set on 80% power, linear pulse (6/sec), flow rate 20 cc/min, and allowable vacuum maximum at 150 mm Hg. The nucleus is then allowed to stabilize on the end of the phaco tip with the vacuum on.

The Chopper is inserted into the anterior nuclear surface inferiorly, just inside the capsulorhexis, and is drawn to the phaco tip and downward in depth, like a knife, terminating just to the left of the phaco needle with the full depth of the chopper being in the lens. In softer nuclei, the slice must be carried completely past the phaco tip to the proximal capsulorhexis edge, before the slice will propagate. The chopper is then reinserted next to the phaco tip to achieve separation. The Phaco and chopper are now rotated slightly in opposite directions, and pulled gently apart. The nucleus divides into two halves, and the separation is continued until the peripheral aspects of the nucleus come apart.

This method has resulted in slicing across the densest part of the nucleus to allow it to be divided in two by pulling the remaining unsliced, softer part of the lens apart. The nucleus is now rotated about 20° clockwise and the phaco needle is impaled into the nucleus, beginning just before its center and progressing inferiorly and downward as above so that a small wedge is impaled. The phaco chopper is inserted in a similar way, and the small wedge of the left nuclear half is now separated. Extra effort is made to assure that the separation achieved here is complete. This piece is left alone and the procedure is repeated. The second or later wedge is the first one aspirated out by merely depressing the foot pedal slightly and pulling centrally on the impaled wedge after slicing and separating it from the larger nuclear piece to its left. If good separation was achieved and this piece is kept small, it is easily removed. Once this is achieved, there is a lot of space, and the procedure is repeated around the nucleus until it is completely removed.

## PHACOEMULSIFICATION IN PARTICULAR CASES

The only variation necessary in this procedure with varying nuclear hardness is the size of the pieces isolated. The harder the nucleus, the smaller the isolated pieces should be. The same procedure can be used for large and small pupils. For pupils less than 4 mm in size, I dilate them using two hooks of my own design (Arshinoff hooks—Xomed Treace) to stretch the pupil gently, either vertically alone, or in severe cases both vertically and horizontally, and then stabilize the enlarged pupil with a supercohesive viscoelastic. I use the same phaco technique for combined phaco-trabeculectomies as well because pupil size and depth of the anterior chamber are only minor issues using this procedure. It is, however, more difficult in very soft lenses because the first complete slice is often difficult to achieve. In these cases, a single sculpted trough will allow cracking of the nucleus in two, and the procedure can then progress as above.

In cases where the first slice is difficult to achieve, the problem can just be ignored and the surgeon can go on to make the second and subsequent slices, until two successive clean slices are made before attempting to remove the first free nuclear wedge. With practice this becomes easy, and the mental stress on the surgeon due to failure to achieve a perfect slice on the first attempt every time is recognized to be irrelevant.

In extremely soft lenses (congenital cataracts, other young patients, etc), I make no attempt to Slice and Separate. Instead I merely concentrically delaminate the lens into multiple layers with hydrodissection, and then aspirate it with the phaco tip from the center outward. Intermittent brief bursts of phaco are applied just to keep the lens material flowing smoothly into the phaco tip and to keep the vacuum from building up too high during aspiration and phaco of the soft lens material.

## EPINUCLEUS REMOVAL

An epinucleus is only occasionally left behind in these cases. Generally, it spontaneously comes out with one of the last few nuclear segments as a result of the excellent hydrodissection. If a reasonably hard epinuclear shell remains, I remove it by aspirating it with the phaco and applying very brief bursts of phaco energy periodically as it is aspirated to facilitate it's aspiration. I do not change my phaco settings to do this routinely. If a very soft epinuclear shell is difficult to aspirate with the phaco tip, I may leave the remaining parts to be removed with the I/A handpiece.

## CORTICAL ASPIRATION

Cortical aspiration is done with a straight silicone sleeved I/A tip. The silicone sleeved tip is important because it seals the incision, deepening the chamber and allowing easy access into the bag to vacuum out any remaining cortex. I use a maximum vacuum setting of 500 mm Hg and a flow rate of 25 cc/min. Using my phaco technique, remaining cortex almost always consists of a few pieces with frilly edges projecting centrally from the capsulorhexis margin. These are merely vacuumed in succession into the I/A with little difficulty. The underside of the capsulorhexis is then vacuumed and the posterior capsule is vacuumed with the I/A tip resting against it such that the aspiration port is 90° removed from the capsule and aspirating in a direction parallel to the plane of the posterior capsule. The I/A is then brushed along the posterior capsule, using both the vacuum and the physical brushing to polish the capsular surface.

If a problem exists with 12 o'clock cortex, it is easily removed by changing to the 90° I/A tip at the end of the I/A.

## ENLARGEMENT OF THE INCISION

The incision is enlarged to 3.5 mm prior to foldable IOL implantation. My current preferred implant is the 5.5 mm diameter Alcon AcrySof lens. I first inflate the capsular bag and anterior chamber usually with a supercohesive viscoelastic (Healon GV or MicroVisc Plus), and then, with a relatively firm eye, I expand the incision using the 2.8 mm. Beaver keratome is kept in our operating room

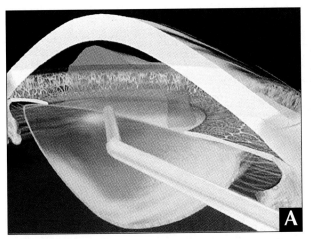 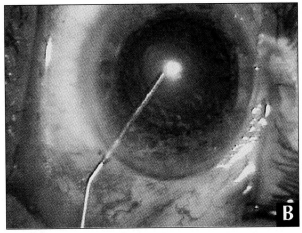

Figures 24-1A, 24-1B. The dispersive viscoelastic is injected first onto the central surface of the lens.

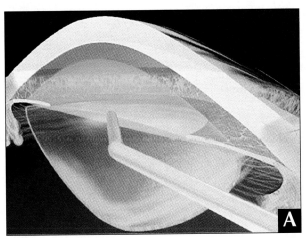 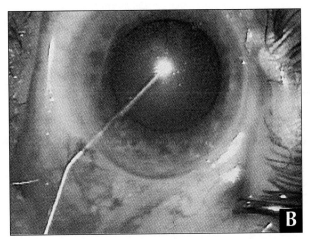

Figures 24-2A, 24-2B. The cohesive viscoelastic is then injected into the center of the dispersive viscoelastic mound, such that the dispersive viscoelastic is pushed up against the corneal endothelium into a smooth layer.

for entry into the anterior chamber through long scleral tunnels, as well as for the purpose described herein. The Beaver keratomes have curved sides without shoulders and so are useful to expand incisions to any size. The curved sides allow the keratome to pass sideways through the corneal incision without the tendency for it to cut outward, which would shorten the tunnel at the sides, an undesirable property of the shouldered keratomes. If a one-piece PMMA IOL is to be implanted for whatever reason, the incision can be further extended with the same keratome without risking tunnel shortening as one proceeds. In these cases, I often lengthen the tunnel somewhat as I go sideways, often extending slightly into the sclera and creating somewhat of a frown effect.

## VISCOELASTIC FOR IOL IMPLANT

I either use a supercohesive viscoelastic to implant the IOL or my soft shell technique. Supercohesive viscoelastics have the advantage of producing maximum stability of the anterior chamber and capsular bag so that while the surgeon is retrieving the IOL and folding it, viscoelastic is not lost from the anterior chamber. This might allow the pressurization of the anterior chamber to decrease, producing folds or wrinkles in the posterior capsule and resulting in greater risk of snagging it with the unfolding haptics of a foldable IOL.

Alternatively the soft shell technique uses the two viscoelastic systems previously mentioned to obtain the optimal benefits of both cohesive and dispersive viscoelastics while avoiding the drawbacks of using either alone. In this technique, the cohesive (Healon, Provisc, MicroVisc, Biolon, Amvisc, Amvisc Plus, etc) or supercohesive (Healon GV or MicroVisc Plus) viscoelastic is injected into the capsular bag and anterior chamber centrally first, until the anterior chamber is about three quarters full. Viscoat or another dispersive (Vitrax, Celugel VSF, Occucoat, etc) is then injected into the center of the capsular bag and anterior chamber until the anterior chamber is full. The purpose of this is that the partitioning of the anterior chamber into two concentric spaces containing fluids with different rheological properties permits the following:

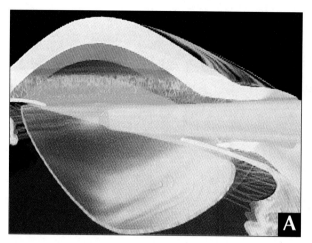 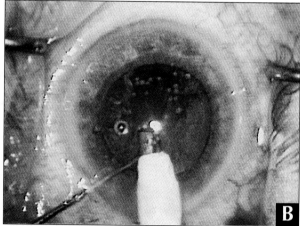

Figures 24-3A, 24-3B. Phacoemulsification and I/A remove the cohesive viscoelastic but not the dispersive one.

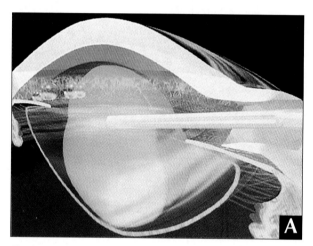 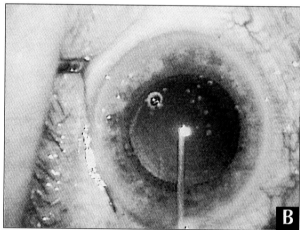

Figures 24-4A, 24-4B. After completing phacoemulsification and I/A, the anterior chamber is filled with cohesive viscoelastic first, followed by the dispersive one, in the reverse order of the above.

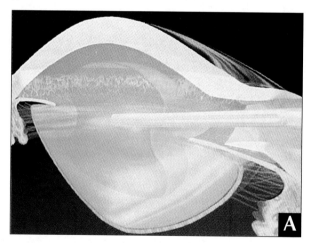 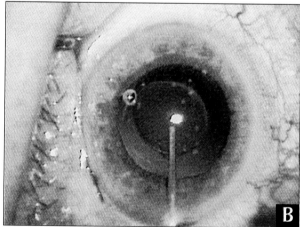

Figures 24-5A, 24-5B. The injection of dispersive viscoelastic into the center of the cohesive one prior to IOL insertion.

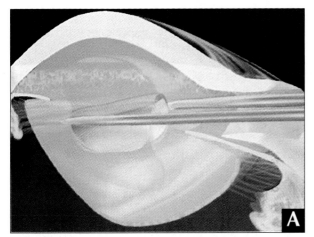 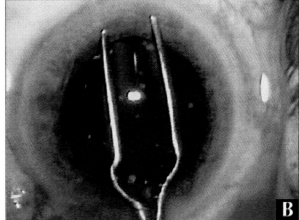

Figures 24-6A, 24-6B. Implantation of the folding IOL into the viscoelastic soft shell.

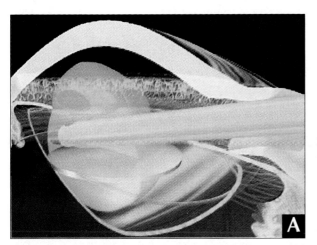 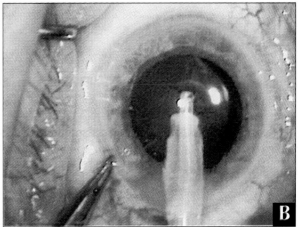

Figures 24-7A, 24-7B. Removal of both viscoelastics after implantation of the IOL is easy because the dispersive viscoelastic is encapsulated with the cohesive viscoelastic.

1. The anterior chamber and capsular bag are stabilized by the enveloping cohesive or supercohesive viscoelastic layer, similar to that achieved using the cohesive or supercohesive alone.
2. The loss of viscoelastic from the anterior chamber is prevented because a cohesive viscoelastic is resting adjacent to the wound, similar to using the cohesive alone.
3. The dispersive viscoelastic is in the center of the anterior chamber and bag where the IOL is going to unfold, allowing easier movement and positioning of the IOL into its desired location, similar to using the dispersive alone.
4. There is a decreased chance of the unfolding IOL snagging adjacent tissues because it is unfolding in a central dispersive fluid environment, while the capsule and anterior chamber are protected and stabilized by the peripheral cohesive viscoelastic.
5. Both viscoelastics can be easily removed because the dispersive viscoelastic is enveloped by the cohesive viscoelastic, similar to using a cohesive alone.

## IOL IMPLANT

My current preferred implant is the 5.5 mm Alcon AcrySof lens. This lens has been associated with a lower incidence of posterior capsular opacification, has a more biocompatible surface than PMMA or silicone, is reasonably easy to use, has PMMA haptics for better centration, and allows implantation through a 3.5 mm incision. I would prefer a smaller incision, but I do not like silicone or hydrogel enough to justify a decrease in incision size by less than 1 mm more.

I fold the lens by picking it up with Livernois paddle pick up and folding forceps and transferring it to MacDonald II forceps for implantation into the capsular bag. I prefer to fold the IOL from 3 to 9 o'clock, such that the haptics are touching but pointed in opposite directions after folding. But I attempt to actually fold the IOL not quite along this axis. Instead, I rotate the grasping folding forceps slightly toward the haptic-optic junctions, so that after folding the haptics do not exactly superimpose but the anteriorly attached haptic points slightly posteriorly, and the posteriorly attached haptic points slightly anteriorly (more like 4 to 10 axis). This decreases the likelihood of either haptic being compressed and distorted when passing through a tight incision, yet allows them to be placed directly into the bag once the anterior chamber is entered, making unfolding and centering easier.

The insertion of the IOL is accomplished merely by placing the folded IOL against the limbus in such a manner that the leading open end of the posteriorly attached haptic folds between the folded sides of the IOL as the optic is compressed against the incision. That way, no haptic tucking is required. The leading optic edge is gently guided into the incision, and for a right handed surgeon, the wrist is externally rotated about 45° to facilitate passage of the IOL through the incision. Once in the eye, the IOL is the rotated back to its vertical position, dropped into the capsular bag, and released, where it opens quite slowly. It is helpful to warm AcrySof lenses slightly before folding to allow for easier folding and decrease the risk of cracking. I ask the circulating nurse to slip it into his or her pocket at the beginning of the case and remove it just prior to insertion.

## VISCOELASTIC REMOVAL

I use my Rock 'n Roll technique to remove viscoelastics. The I/A vacuum is set at 500 (peristaltic machine), and the bottle height is raised to about 75 cm above the eye. The silicone sleeved straight I/A tip is placed on the surface of the IOL, with just enough posterior pressure to push the IOL posteriorly in the bag so that the side irrigating ports direct the flow of BSS into the capsular bag. The I/A tip is rolled from side to side to gently rock the IOL as the BSS causes turbulence in the capsular bag. The IOL is also rocked slightly in the vertical direction. About 25 to 30 seconds of this Rock 'n' Roll is usually sufficient to wash all of the viscoelastic out of the bag, including any that may have been trapped behind the IOL.

## CONCLUSION

Once the case is completed, I routinely hydrate the sides of the clear corneal incision, using a 27 gauge hockey stick cannula on a 3 cc syringe filled with BSS to be certain of an excellent wound seal. Vancomycin 1 mg in 0.1 cc BSS is then injected around the IOL in the capsular bag (technique of Howard V. Gimbel). I use a 27 guage hockey stick cannula on a 1 cc syringe through the side port. The anterior chamber is then firmed up by injecting BSS from a 3 cc syringe with a 27 guage hockey stick cannula through the side port. The wound is tested with the side of the hockey stick cannula on both sides of the main incision and side port and posteriorly to both incisions. Finally, I place Cortisporin drops and Pilopine 4% ointment in the conjunctival cul-de-sac inferiorly. If the patient can be counted on not to rub the operated eye, the eye is not patched.

Patients are treated routinely with Tobradex drops six times a day for 2 weeks postoperatively.

# Chapter 25

# CHOP AND FLIP PHACOEMULSIFICATION TECHNIQUE

*I. Howard Fine, MD*

## INTRODUCTION

Currently, my favorite approach to patients with a cataract is to perform Chop and Flip endolenticular phacoemulsification through a 2.8 mm clear corneal incision, utilizing topical and intracameral anesthesia with implantation through the same incision of a plate-haptic foldable silicone intraocular lens (IOL).

## ANESTHESIA

At this time, my anesthesia involves the instillation, along with dilating drops, of 1 cc of .75% non-preserved Marcaine, repeated 20 minutes later and then once again immediately following the prepping and draping of the patient. After construction of a paracentesis incision with a 1 mm wide trifaceted diamond knife, 0.5 cc of preservative-free 1% Xylocaine is injected into the anterior chamber. The Xylocaine circulates through the anterior chamber, extruding the aqueous humor during the slow administration. Immediately upon completion of this instillation, Viscoat (Alcon) is injected through its cannula into the distal angle in such a way that an expanding wave of viscoelastic forces the anterior chamber fluid out through the paracentesis. This provides a stiff and stable anterior segment.

## PHACOEMULSIFIER IN USE

Approximately 98% of my phacoemulsification cases are performed with either the AMO Diplomax phacoemulsification system or an Alcon 20,000 Legacy phacoemulsification system. The Diplomax has the advantages of high vacuum and downsized tips and also has the most versatile software options. These include occlusion mode, multiple power modulations, and an ability to change programs with the foot pedal which eliminates the need to communicate with a circulator or the surgical assistant. The Diplomax also has options for a second bottle so that one can switch to high- or low-flow systems without waiting for the elevation of the IV pole. The Legacy phacoemulsification system has superb ultrasonic power generation and fluidics. It is capable of downsized incisions and high vacuums and has perhaps the best cutting for techniques that depend on sculpting or grooving.

On the Diplomax, I prefer the 0 or 15° tip utilized bevel-down except for epinuclear removal. On the Alcon Legacy, I prefer a 30°, small incision system tip utilized in the same way with the tapered, downsized sleeve.

## INCISION

I prefer self-sealing, single plane, clear corneal tunnel incisions. Unfortunately, the description of corneal tunnel incisions has become somewhat confused. Based on the description in Hogan, Alvarado, and Widdell's book, *Histology of the Human Eye*,[1] they describe the anterior vascular arcade as extending 0.5 mm into clear cornea anterior to the limbus with its external surface covered by conjunctiva. I will define the limbus to be at the anterior edge of the conjunctival insertion, with the corneal vascular arcade considered to be in clear cornea. I strongly favor a description of corneal incisions that would label as follows:

### Architecture

- Single plane (without a vertical groove at the external edge of the incision).
- Shallow groove (having a groove perpendicular to the corneal surface at the external edge of the

incision up to 400 µm deep).
- Deeply grooved (where the groove perpendicular to the external edge of the incision is greater than 400 µm).

### Location
- Clear corneal (external edge anterior to the conjunctival insertion).
- Limbal corneal (external edge going through conjunctival and limbal tissue).
- Scleral corneal (external edge originating posterior to the limbal tissue).

The eye is stabilized with a 13 mm Fine/Thornton Ring (Mastel Precision Instruments catalog #23116132 or Katena catalog #K3-6161). At this time, I utilize a Rhein 3-D blade (Rhein Medical catalog #05-5082) 2.8 mm wide. This blade has been designed specifically to have different bevel slopes on the anterior and posterior surfaces so that forces of tissue resistance will naturally direct the blade as it is advanced in the plane of the cornea.[2] Perfect incisions can be rapidly and reproducibly constructed. One simply touches the point of the blade at the site where the external incision should be located. Then, the blade is pushed in the plane of the cornea without any attempt to applanate it to the surface of the eye or to dimple down the tip before entering the anterior chamber. Three things occur:

1. The external incision is linear from the perspective of the surgeon.
2. The length of the tunnel incision through the cornea is 2.0 mm because without any dimpling down, the tip enters the anterior chamber through Descemet's membrane 2 mm central to the external incision.
3. From the surgeon's perspective, the incision in Descemet's membrane appears to be a straight line as well. Although the external and internal measures look straight to the surgeon, they follow the dome of the cornea and are therefore arched.

## CONTENTS OF THE CHAMBER FOR THE CAPSULOTOMY

I prefer to use a highly retentive viscoelastic, specifically Viscoat, which gives me maximum stability of the anterior chamber during capsulorhexis. Because of its bulk retention, I also prefer Viscoat during endolenticular phacoemulsification. It remains in the anterior chamber in the presence of irrigation and aspiration (I/A) accompanying phacoemulsification and affords greater cushioning of the corneal endothelium from sandblasting by nuclear material.

I prefer to perform capsulorhexis utilizing a pinch-type forceps, thus avoiding the necessity for a bent needle to start the capsulorhexis. The Rhein capsulorhexis forceps (Rhein catalog #05-2326) has downward-pointing tips at the end of the blades of the forceps, and the arc of the blades is curved so that one can reach over the anterior dome of the nucleus without elevating the superior lip of the incision.

The technique for performing the capsulorhexis is to push down on the capsule with the forceps open, close the forceps allowing a pinching of the central anterior capsule, pull in any direction which creates a flap tear, and then guide the flap tear in a circular continuous curvilinear capsulorhexis (CCC). The capsulorhexis can be widened by allowing the arc to extend out beyond the starting point of the continuous curve. In addition, following the completion of a small continuous curvilinear capsulorhexis, by snipping with a scissors in an almost tangential manner, a new flap can be created which one can tear in a larger continuous curvilinear manner.

In the case of narrow pupil, I like to use a Beehler pupil expander (Moria catalog #19009), but on occasion will use the Rhein capsulorhexis forceps to tear a capsulorhexis that is larger than the size of the pupil. By relying on the flap at the tear point to continuously tent up the iris, I can see where it is tearing through the overlying iris.

In the case of an absent red reflex, there are a variety of techniques which help a surgeon make the capsulorhexis. Among the most important are:
1. Turning overhead lights off to remove disturbing reflexes from the corneal surface.
2. Increasing magnification.
3. Turning the focus speed switch on the microscope down so that focusing is as slow as possible and the carriage movement can't possibly go through the focal plane without one's knowing.
4. Shining a pars plana retinal illuminator in the non-dominant hand obliquely over the limbus in such a way as to illuminate the capsule flap from the side.

In most cases, any one or a combination of these techniques has enabled me to achieve a CCC in the absence of a red reflex.

## HYDRODISSECTION/ HYDRODELINEATION

I continue to utilize cortical cleaving hydrodissection.[3,4] After tenting up the anterior capsulorhexis, fluid is injected through a cannula in such a manner that it goes posterior to the cortex, between the capsule and the cortex. After completely surrounding the posterior aspect of the lens, the fluid becomes trapped by the firm cortical/capsular adhesions in the lens fornix. If one continues to irrigate, the nucleus will be blown out of the bag. However, as one continues to gently irrigate, the capsulorhexis appears to enlarge as the nuclear mass moves forward. At that point, one can stop the irrigation and utilize the long shaft of the cannula (McIntyre cannula, Katena catalog #K7-5150) to depress the lens against the posteriorly loculated fluid. This increases the pressure in the posterior aspect of the capsule and forces the fluid circumferentially around the equator of the lens, rupturing cortical/capsular connections and allowing the fluid to exit through the capsulorhexis. This is accompanied by radial linear striations within the cortex as the cortical fibers are washed centrally, in addition to a snapping back of the capsulorhexis to its initial non-bulging diameter.

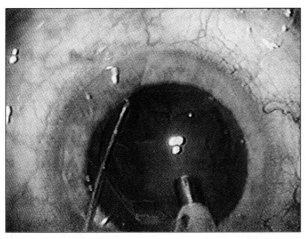

Figure 25-1. The nucleus is supported with the chop instrument in the left distal portion of the golden ring and lollipopped in burst mode with the phaco handpiece.

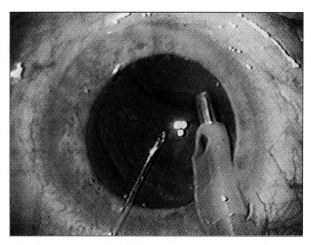

Figure 25-2. Following scoring and chopping of the nucleus, the endonucleus is completely subdivided into two halves.

Hydrodelineation is performed as I have described previously.[4,5] The McIntyre cannula is aimed midway between the center of the lens and the equator of the lens toward the central plane of the nucleus, until the nuclear complex starts to move away in response to the push of the needle. At that point, the direction of the needle is turned tangentially and a back and forth motion creates a tunnel in the nucleus. The needle is backed halfway out of the tunnel and fluid is irrigated into the empty tract. This allows fluid to find the plane of least resistance, which is almost always the juncture of the compact endonuclear mass and the epinuclear shell. In most instances a golden ring is achieved, but on occasion a dark circle or arc of the circle is noticed. One can approach the edge of the arc with the same needle in the same manner and extend the arc one or several quadrants by additional injection. Occasionally one has to inject two, three, or four times in order to achieve circumferential delineation of the epinuclear shell from the endonucleus. At this point, if cortical cleaving hydrodissection and hydrodelineation have both been achieved, the nucleus should spin quite easily within the capsular bag.

In general, the combined volume for cortical cleaving hydrodissection and hydrodelineation is approximately 0.8 mL of balanced salt solution (BSS). During these *hydro steps* it is important to keep the heal of the cannula leaning against the posterior lip of the incision a little bit in order to allow exit of fluid or viscoelastic from the anterior chamber so that the anterior segment of the eye is not over-pressurized.

## EMULSIFICATION FOR NUCLEUS OF HARDNESS 2+ TO 3+

For emulsification of 2+ to 3+ nuclei, I use the Chop and Flip phacoemulsification technique.[6] Following the *hydro steps*, the phacoemulsification handpiece (in continuous irrigation) is brought into the eye and the anterior epinucleus exposed by the continuous curvilinear capsulorhexis is aspirated. I then utilize a Fine/Nagahara chop instrument (Rhein Medical catalog #08-14503R) through the side port incision, sliding it across the surface of the nucleus in contact with the nucleus. This reflects the capsulorhexis and anterior capsule and pushes it in the distal left quadrant until the vertical element of the chop instrument drops into the golden ring. The instrument is then pulled a little toward the surgeon and elevated just slightly to stabilize the lens. In burst mode (which provides the highest impact, lowest cavitational energy available to drive the phaco tip into the nucleus) and high vacuum, the nucleus is lollipopped. Once the nucleus is lollipopped, the vertical element of the chop instrument is moved through the endonucleus toward the side of the phaco tip, following the direction of the groove in the top of the horizontal element of the chop instrument which indicates the direction of the cleat in the vertical element. The nucleus is scored by pulling the chop instrument in the proper direction, toward the side of the phaco needle. Then, as that position is maintained, the chop instrument is pulled to the left and slightly down while the phaco tip is pulled to the right and slightly up. In almost all instances, this creates a chop that divides the endonucleus completely into two.

The nuclear complex is rotated. The chop instrument is again placed in the left distal epinuclear ring and the hemi-nucleus is lollipopped by the phaco tip. The nucleus is once again scored and chopped in such a way that at the completion of the chop, a pie-shaped segment of endonucleus is occluding the tip of the phacoemulsification handpiece. Utilizing burst mode and the chop instrument to control the epinuclear location of the pie-shaped segment of nucleus with maximum control and minimum chatter, the chopped segment is slowly removed from the eye. The nuclear complex is rotated again, and this process is repeated until one whole hemi-nucleus has been removed. The second hemi-nucleus is rotated into position, lollipopped, scored, and chopped in several pieces, each time allowing a pie-shaped segment to be stuck to the phacoemulsification tip where it can be removed

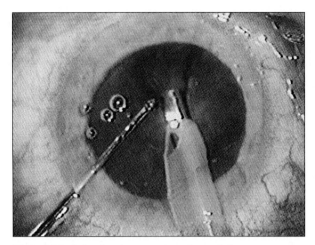 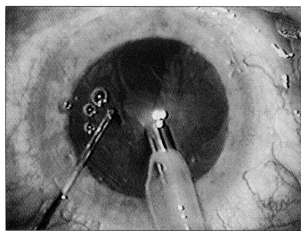

Figure 25-3. Following the second scoring and chop maneuver, a pie-shaped segment of the nucleus remains lollipopped by the phaco handpiece, ready to be removed.

Figure 25-4. Appearance of the endonuclear mass following removal of the first pie-shaped segment.

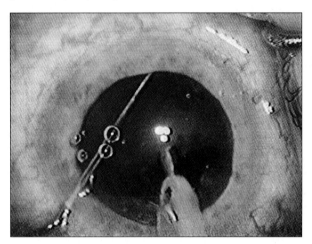 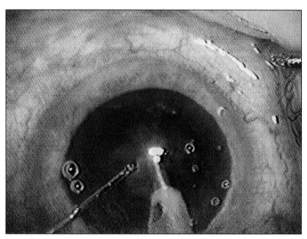

Figure 25-5. The second hemi-nucleus is stabilized and lollipopped, ready to be scored and chopped.

Figure 25-6. Maintaining an endo-epinuclear position of the pie-shaped segments as they are mobilized in burst mode and high vacuum.

under the proper parameters of flow, vacuum, and burst mode phaco, completely within the epinuclear space.

Following the complete dismantling of the nucleus by scoring and chopping, and the complete evacuation of the segments under the proper parameters, one is left with the intact epinucleus.

This is the most efficient technique of dismantling the nucleus that I have ever used. It enables me to entirely abandon the process of sculpting, which is associated with an increased use of ultrasound (U/S) energy and possible sandblasting of the endothelium by nuclear debris created during that process. The chop technique, as utilized in my procedure, is characterized by an increased use of mechanical forces (ie, chopping), a decreased use of U/S energy (by not grooving), and the use of vacuum as an extractive tool. We no longer extract nuclear material by utilizing U/S energy to create a nuclear emulsate which is then suctioned from the eye. Instead, we pull nuclear material out of the eye with high vacuum assisted by bursts of phaco power to modify the shape of the segment so it continues to not only occlude the tip but to move down the tip and out of the eye.

The efficiency of this technique allows me to do average nuclei with phaco powers around 15% at effective phaco times of under 20 seconds. In Chop and Flip phacoemulsification, a great deal of attention is paid to keeping the pie-shaped segments down in the epinuclear shell and not allowing them to chatter, especially in the vicinity of the cornea. This is particularly easy to achieve in burst mode where the high vacuum maintains the piece at the tip and where the chop instrument can keep it down in the epinuclear shell while continuously fragmenting it, so as to facilitate its further dismantling and evacuation from the eye.

## PHACO FOR NUCLEUS OF HARDNESS 4+

I utilize Viscoat for the 4+ nucleus for the reasons given previously. I still prefer to do Chop and Flip phacoemulsification if I can, but I may have to do Crack and

Flip phacoemulsification[5] or a combination like Stop and Chop[7] in which I do some grooving initially. I use very low vacuum and flow and try to shave rather than allow tip occlusion during the grooving process. I do not groove out into the periphery nor too deeply, but try to gain a good purchase on the nucleus and then try to chop rather than crack.

If I am unable to chop, I do a vertical groove that is as deep as I can make it centrally, extending no further than just outside the margins of the capsulorhexis. In almost all instances with a groove like this I can crack. I may use several maneuvers for cracking, first snapping the anterior segment of the groove centrally and then moving toward the edge of the groove to snap it more peripherally and more deeply.

Once the nucleus is divided into hemi-nuclei, I will try to chop each of the hemi-nuclei. However, if this is unsuccessful or if the nucleus is unstable because of its size and hardness, I will perform secondary grooves and crack and chop as the need arises.

The hard nucleus used to be a contraindication for phacoemulsification, but today it can be addressed by a variety of endolenticular phaco techniques. It is specifically in these cases that the new modalities with better cutting, higher vacuum, and power modulations become so useful. The hard nucleus is especially easy to groove with high cavitation tips like the Kelman tip on the Alcon Series 20,000 Legacy system which allows for oblation of nuclear material in advance of contact of that material by the phaco tip. One can do grooving in both forward and backward movements of the handpiece in the meridian of the incision. Then, in a maneuver similar to the Phaco Sweep by Howard Gimbel, one can groove perpendicular to the initial groove so that non-rotational grooving is possible. This can be combined with non-rotational cracking. It is frequently useful to groove into more than four quadrants in order to have smaller, more manageable pieces to mobilize. The epinucleus is very thin and hard and will not flip. Attempts to flip it uniformly result in fracturing of the epinuclear structure into three separate pie-shaped segments following the lines of the posterior Y suture. Each segment flips as it fractures so that the maneuvers to remove the epinucleus in rock-hard nuclei are exactly the same as in less hard nuclei.

Emulsification takes place as was previously indicated. A major difference between a 4+ nucleus and a less dense nucleus is that I make considerably smaller pie-shaped segments in the harder nucleus and therefore there are many more of them.

# PHACOEMULSIFICATION IN PARTICULAR CASES

## Glaucoma Triple

For combined cataract/glaucoma surgery, I frequently do a scleral tunnel incision superiorly and perform phacoemulsification with a Chop and Flip technique. After utilizing a Crozafon/De Laage punch (Moria catalog #18069) to bite off the corneal lip of the incision without ever cutting vertical grooves in my flap, my limbus-parallel straight groove incision serves as the exit filtration site. I usually use a running suture to reattach conjunctiva to the limbus, after having performed a peripheral iridectomy. At this point, I have not utilized releasable sutures nor have I felt the need to since there are no sutures in my incision at any time.

## Pseudoexfoliation

There are a variety of special techniques that are useful in the presence of pseudoexfoliation to minimize the likelihood of zonular dehiscence or loss of nucleus. I prefer to use an endocapsular tension ring which creates circumferential distribution of forces around the zonular apparatus such that one cannot concentrate forces by pulling on the capsule in any location. Instead of stressing adjacent zonules only, the capsular ring causes distribution of those forces to the entire zonular apparatus, adding greater safety for all intraocular manipulations that may take place.

In this instance especially, I like to use the Rhein capsulorhexis forceps that pinch the capsule to initiate the tear rather than a needle which cuts the capsule because it is possible to rupture zonules with any downward pressure of a needle if there is any capsular fibrosis.

If grooving, it is important to concentrate on elevating the nucleus as best as possible by stabilizing the nucleus and elevating it with the second handpiece through the side port incision. Once grooves have been made adjacent to the side port, elevation of the nucleus is done easily with a Sinskey hook through the side port. Therefore, I do a pattern of four superficial grooves early in the procedure in order to give me that type of leverage.

It is important to perform cortical cleaving hydrodissection very carefully, utilizing injections in several different quadrants and being quite delicate when depressing the nucleus to allow for rupture of cortical/capsular connections.

The greatest single threat in pseudoexfoliation is cortical cleanup which can present enormous challenge to zonules adjacent to the area of cortical stripping. If an endocapsular ring is not inserted prior to phacoemulsification, one should consider implanting the IOL with polymethylmethacrylate (PMMA) haptics prior to cortical aspiration so that the haptics can stabilize the bag. Post implantation cortical cleanup takes longer but is safer, though not quite as safe as an endocapsular ring.

## Post-Trauma

Patients who have had previous eye trauma should be carefully examined for the possibility of zonular damage. However, on occasion zonular weakness or partial dialysis does not become evident until the time of surgery. This is another indication for the use of the endocapsular ring which stabilizes the position of the lens capsule and allows surgery to proceed almost as though there were not a compromised zonular apparatus.

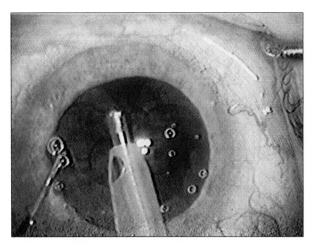

Figure 25-7. Beginning of the aspiration and emulsification of the distal roof and rim of the epinucleus, showing cortex streaming over the floor of the epinucleus in the same location.

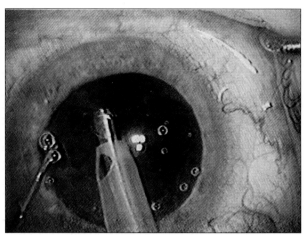

Figure 25-8. Continuing trimming and cortical cleanup in the distal portion of the epinuclear bowl.

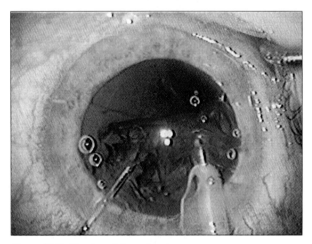

Figure 25-9. Flipping of the epinucleus.

## Small Pupils

Small pupils used to be a relative contraindication for phacoemulsification. However, with the multitude of pupil-expanding techniques available, such as hooks or expander rings or the Beehler pupil expander (an elegant, atraumatic, simple instrument to use), it is no longer reasonable for one to proceed in phacoemulsification with less than adequate visualization due to failure to address the small pupil. In a less than fully dilated pupil, it may be necessary to employ more manipulation than usual to bring the nuclear segments into view for consumption, but adequate visualization can almost always be achieved today.

## Filtering Blebs

Post filtration patients are especially suitable candidates for temporal clear corneal phacoemulsification because the existing filtering bleb is not at all challenged by the surgery and the likelihood of post surgical inflammation, scarring of the bleb, or surgical trauma injuring the bleb is highly unlikely.

## High Myopes

In these patients, there is a great tendency for the lens iris diaphragm to move posteriorly during surgery. A great deal of care must be taken to not press down on the nucleus but to stabilize it, as in cases of pseudoexfoliation, and try to keep it as high in the anterior segment as possible. Care also has to be taken in these patients with proper lens selection. Certain lens styles should be avoided so that the possibility of an oversized bag being too large will not occur.

## EPINUCLEUS REMOVAL

I continue to remove the epinucleus and the cortex in the manner previously described (that is trimming[8] of the epinucleus, with mobilization of the cortex at the same time, followed by flipping of the residual epinucleus and removal from the eye).[9] The epinuclear shell is trimmed as follows[6]: The distal roof and/or rim is purchased by the phaco tip in foot Position 2 and pulled centrally in foot Position 2 until the phaco tip fully clears the edge of the capsulorhexis. Small bursts of power at this point result in a biting off of the epinuclear lip and cause the cortex in that location to stream over the epinuclear floor and into the phaco handpiece. The epinucleus is rotated so that the new roof and rim of epinucleus become available in the distal location. Once again, the epinucleus is purchased in foot Position 2, brought centrally, and then with small bursts of phaco power and moderate vacuum, the nuclear rim is evacuated with cortical material flowing over the epinuclear shell and mobilized at the same time. When the roof and rim of three-fourths of the epinuclear shell have been trimmed, the residual one-fourth is rotated to the distal position, purchased by the phacoemulsification tip in foot Position 2, and pulled toward the incision. At the same time, the second handpiece is pushed into the center of the epinuclear floor toward the distal periphery of the capsule, resulting in anti-parallel forces which allow the epinucleus to flip upside down,

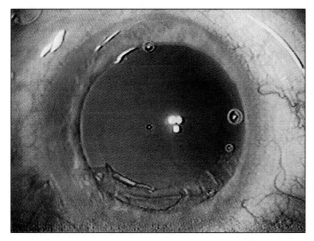

Figure 25-10. Appearance of the capsule following phacoemulsification and viscodissection of residual subincisional cortex to the capsular periphery with some draping over the capsulorhexis edge.

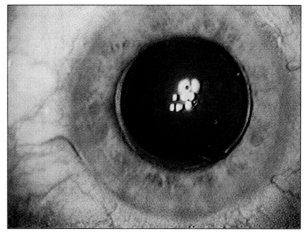

Figure 25-11. Immediate postoperative appearance of the eye following foldable IOL implantation through a 2.9 mm clear corneal incision.

### Table 25-1
#### OMS DIPLOMAX

|  | Sculpt/phaco 1 | Chop/Quad phaco 2 | Trim/Flip phaco 3 | I/A |
| --- | --- | --- | --- | --- |
| ASP | unocc/occluded 16/16 | unocc/occluded 20/30 | unocc/occluded 32/26 | 10 |
| VAC | threshold/limit 20/20 | threshold limit 20/125 | threshold/limit 20/70 | 500 |
| POWER | 70% unocc/occluded cont/pulse 33% | 40% unocc/occluded cont/pulse 80 msec Burst | 60% unocc/occluded pulse 33% | N/A |

#### HI VACUUM

| Sculpt/Phaco 1 | Chop/Quad phaco 2 | Trim/Flip phaco 3 | I/A |
| --- | --- | --- | --- |

|  | | | | |
| --- | --- | --- | --- | --- |
| ASP | unocc/occluded 16/16 | unocc/occluded 26/30 | unocc/occluded 32/26 | 10 |
| VAC | threshold/limit 30/30 | threshold/limit 50/250 | threshold/limit 40/90 | 500 |
| POWER | 70% unocc/occluded cont/pulse 33% | 60% unocc/occluded 80 msec Burst | 60% unocc/occluded 60 msec Burst | N/A |

*Continuous irrigation in all models.

#### VITRECTOMY SETTINGS

|  | Vitrectomy |  | Foot positions |
| --- | --- | --- | --- |
| ASP | 14 | 1 | Irrigation |
| VAC | 250 | 2 | Cutting |
| CUT RATE | 500 | 3 | Aspiration |

*Foot control may be changed by highlighting SIDE VIT (F3). Pedal then controls I/A. Hold right side pedal to cut, let off to stop.

removing it from its proximity to the posterior capsule. It can now be removed from the eye by aspiration or low powers of phacoemulsification.

## CORTICAL ASPIRATION

In general, if there is residual cortical material following flipping of the epinucleus and mobilization of the epinucleus, I use viscodissection of the residual cortex. Injection of viscoelastic under the posterior cortex causes anterior cortical fibers to drape over the capsulorhexis and forces posterior cortical fibers into the capsular fornices. Implantation of the foldable IOL is then accomplished. The residual cortex, whose firm adhesions to the capsule at the capsular fornix have been disrupted by cortical cleaving hydrodissection, is easily mobilized along with residual viscoelastic. I generally utilize the phaco handpiece for this, but on occasion I use a Rhein side port aspirator (#003588) with a bent tip through a side port.

## ENLARGEMENT OF INCISION

It is rare for me to enlarge the incision since I almost always use a 2.8 mm diamond knife. However, if I do enlarge it, I tend to use a metal keratome. The 3-D Rhein

Table 25-2
## FINE PHACOEMULSIFICATION PARAMETERS

| | Phaco settings | | | | I/A surg vac control | |
|---|---|---|---|---|---|---|
| | Sculpt U/S Mem 1 | See below pulse Mem 1 | Trim pulse Mem 2 | Flip pulse Mem 3 | Cortical cleanup | Viscoat removal |
| ALCON 20,000 LEGACY with Kelman Tip Chip/Quad | | | | | | |
| Power | 80 | 50-70 | 50-70 | 50-70 | | |
| Aspiration, Cont flow | 16 | 16 | 16 | 16 | 16 | 30 |
| Vacuum | 0-6 | *80/100/120 | 100 | 50 | 500 | 500 |
| Mode | Cont | Pulse 8/sec | Pulse 8/sec | Pulse 8/sec | I/A Cont | I/A Cont |
| ALCON 20,000 LEGACY with High Vacuum Cassette Chop | | | | | | |
| Power | 60 | **40/50 | **40/50 | **40/50 | | |
| Aspiration, Cont flow | 12 | **14/16 | **16/18 | 12 | 16 | 30 |
| Vacuum | 40 | **160/220 | **120/140 | 100**/180 | 500 | 500 |
| Mode | Cont | Pulse **4/8 sec | Pulse **4/8 sec | Pulse **4/8 sec | I/A Cont | I/A Cont |
| ALCON 20,000 LEGACY with 0.9 mm Small Incision Chop | | | | | | |
| Power | 60 | 50 | 50 | 50 | | |
| Aspiration, Cont flow | 12 | 16 | ***12/16 | 16 | 16 | 30 |
| Vacuum | 60 | 230 | ***230/244 | 120 | 500 | 500 |
| Mode | Cont | Pulse 8/sec | Pulse 8/sec | Pulse 8/sec | I/A Cont | I/A Cont |

*Nucleus 1-2+/3+/4+
**Nucleus 1+/Nucleus 2-4+
***Nucleus 4+
I. Howard Fine, MD

blade is designed for cutting in a forward direction, and I tend not to utilize it when it is necessary to move the knife to one side or the other.

## VISCOELASTIC FOR IOL IMPLANTATION

The viscoelastic I use for IOL implantation is most frequently Occucoat (Storz) because of its ease of removal from the eye and its low cost. However, for implantation of foldable acrylic lenses, which have PMMA or acrylic haptics and open much more slowly, I will utilize Viscoat because it enhances the stability and expansion of the space compared to other viscoelastics.

## IOL IMPLANT

I prefer the Staar plate haptic (VF4203) lens with fenestrations to secure better in-the-bag fixation, and a UV blocker. In my experience, this is absolutely the easiest lens to implant. It goes through a bevel-down cartridge directly from the package into the capsular bag without touching any aspect of the surface of the eye.

The lens is folded by placing it in the cartridge and then closing the cartridge before inserting it into the injector. I tend to use a bevel-down insertion with some rolling oscillations of the tip as it is insinuated into the incision while the eye is stabilized with a Fine/Thornton ring, without ever having to purchase the superior lip of the incision by a forceps. The lens can be delivered in one motion, directly into the capsular bag, by bringing the cartridge into the eye close to the distal margin of the capsulorhexis. As the leading plate comes out of the cartridge, one can back the cartridge away so that the edge of the leading plate stays just under the margin of the anterior capsulorhexis. Finally, when the trailing haptic is deposited in the eye, advancement of the rod in the injector forces the trailing haptic downward into the capsular bag. If the trailing haptic should be deposited on the iris rather than into the capsular bag, I simply bring the I/A handpiece with a 0.2 mm aspiration port into the eye and depress the posterior haptic into the capsular bag as I begin my I/A of residual viscoelastic and cortex. If I use a three-piece foldable IOL, I prefer an injector rather than forceps for implantation.

For removal of residual viscoelastic and cortex, I prefer a 0.2 mm port because it is easier to catch wispy filaments of cortical material and occlude the tip with this compared to a 0.3 mm opening. The bottom of the tip has been sandblasted, so if desirable, I can polish the posterior capsule by going under the plate haptic lens as I irrigate and aspirate.

## FINAL TEST OF THE INCISION

For a final test of the incision, I usually reconstitute the anterior chamber and occasionally use stromal hydration of the incision and side port. If there is any question about the integrity of the incision, I will utilize fluorescein to be certain that there is no spontaneous leakage of fluid from the eye as seen by the green color on the yellow fluorescein. In addition, I also depress the posterior lip of the incision with my finger to be sure that it is actually tight.

## SUTURE IF NECESSARY

If it is necessary to place a suture, I will place a single radial 10-0 nylon suture relatively loosely, recognizing that it has almost no effect on inducing astigmatism because we are suturing the roof of a tunnel to the floor of the tunnel rather than side to side suturing with compression of the lips of the incision.

## CONCLUSION[6]

Chop and Flip represents a major shift in utilization of power to dismantle the nucleus. The same hydrodelineation and hydrodissection steps are utilized. However, with this technique, we are vastly emphasizing the expanded use of mechanical forces (eg, chopping) and the expanded use of vacuum. We are using vacuum as an extractive technique with U/S energy being utilized mainly to lollipop the nucleus and shape segments of nucleus that are occluding the tip into pieces which can be easily evacuated by the vacuum. We need phaco power to help shape the nuclear material in such a way that it occludes the tip. There is a change in emphasis, however, in that we are no longer converting the nuclear material into emulsate which is suctioned from the eye, but rather shaping the nuclear material with U/S energy so that the vacuum can participate in the extraction of the nuclear material. I believe that this is the direction in which we are headed at this time. It is hard to know whether or not anterior chamber or supracapsular techniques will be as safe as the endolenticular techniques, but if they prove to be, they will have the added advantage of being somewhat easier to perform.

## REFERENCES

1. Hogan MJ, Alvarado JA, Weddell JE. *Histology of the Human Eye*. Philadelphia, Pa: WB Saunders Co; 1971:118.
2. Fine IH. The Rhein 3-D diamond blade. *EyeWorld*. 1996;1:2,24.
3. Fine IH. Cortical cleaving hydrodissection. *J Cataract Refract Surg*. 1992;18:5,508-12.
4. Fine IH. Hydrodissection and hydrodelineation. In: Steinert RK, ed. *Cataract Surgery: Technique, Complications, & Management*. Philadelphia, Pa: WB Saunders Co; 1995.
5. Fine IH, Maloney WF, Dillman DM. Crack and flip phacoemulsification. *J Cataract Refract Surg*. 1993;19:6,797-802.
6. Fine IH. Small incision cataract surgery: Phacoemulsification. In: Yanoff M, Dueker D, eds. *Ophthalmology*. Mosby. In press.
7. Koch PS, Katzen LE. Stop and chop phacoemulsification. *J Cataract Refract Surg*. 1994;20:566-570.
8. Fine IH. A spectrum of clear corneal phaco techniques. In: Long DA, ed. *New Orleans Academy of Ophthalmology: Anterior Segment and Strabismus Surgery*. Kugler; 1996.
9. Fine IH. The chip and flip phacoemulsification technique. *J Cataract Refract Surg*. 1991;17:3,366-371.

# Chapter 26

# PERSONAL PHACOEMULSIFICATION TECHNIQUE

*James Davison, MD, FACS*

## ANESTHESIA

I use topical, intracameral anesthesia on virtually all patients. The topical component consists of preoperative drops of Marcaine 0.75%. This is given starting 15 to 20 minutes prior to surgery, a total of five to 10 drops. The drops are given about 3 minutes apart. It is important to keep a folded towel over both of the patient's eyes, so that the patient doesn't stare and allow his or her cornea to dry out.

Intracameral Lidocaine 1% preservative free is given, 0.5 to 1.5 cc into the anterior chamber just after entry with a diamond blade but prior to instillation of viscoelastic. The total contact time is probably 3 to 4 seconds prior to the viscoelastic instillation, but this is enough to give a complete anesthetic block to the intraocular tissues. It is important to inject this fairly slowly as a rare patient may feel a little pressure sensation or even stinging with rapid instillation of Lidocaine into the anterior chamber.

## PHACOEMULSIFICATION MACHINE

I use a Legacy 20,000 on all cases. The tip is a 45° straight tip. I usually prefer the larger standard 1.1 mm diameter tip over the newer 0.9 mm tip, except for very small eyes. The larger tip seems to be somewhat faster in its evacuation of nuclear material. The smaller tip will provide better visualization of nuclear detail, especially in small eyes. I use the 45° straight small tip as well.

The Legacy is used because it gives the most exquisite control over vacuum, aspiration flow rate, and phacoemulsification energy. All three parameters are closely regulated in a very predictable, precise fashion and because of this the integration of these three variables is more accurately accomplished. Load compensation is particularly helpful in the emulsification of very firm lenses. It makes conventional extracapsular cataract extraction virtually unnecessary.

## INCISION

A clear corneal temporal incision is used on virtually all cases. The only time I use a corneoscleral incision is when an acrylic intraocular lens (IOL) is not available in the power needed. The clear corneal temporal incision is accomplished with a Diamatrix blade, model 2490 (Brown Universal Cataract Knife). It is accomplished free hand by first making a groove, which is 3.2 mm in length and 300 μm deep. The blade is then extended, a paracentesis is created, and a full thickness stromal extension of the incision is produced for a combination of the phacoemulsification tip. The incision is 2.8 mm wide for the 0.9 mm phaco tip, and 3.0 mm wide for the 1.1 mm phaco tip.

These incisions are extended at the conclusion of phacoemulsification for implantation of the Alcon AcrySof acrylic foldable IOL. The incisions are made prior to the instillation of viscoelastic so that intracameral anesthesia can be more effective and the tissue less distorted during incision creation. The ultimate length of the shelf of the standard self-sealing incision is approximately 1.75 mm. The location is always temporal as only 0.2 diopters (D) of keratometric relaxation is accomplished overall in this technique with a 3.2 mm long incision (unpublished, personal data).

## CONTENTS OF THE CHAMBER FOR THE CAPSULOTOMY

I use 1% sodium hyaluronate for virtually all anterior capsulotomies. Viscoat can be used in extraordinary situ-

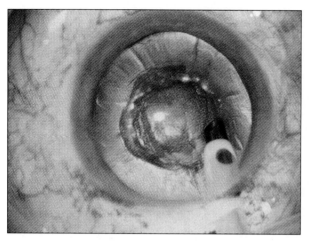

Figure 26-1. Soft nucleus—If quadrants fail to separate, a bowl is created using the lower vacuum memory for sculpting.

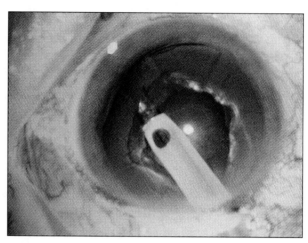

Figure 26-2. Soft nucleus—Phacoemulsification energy is used to bore the tip into the nuclear substance. With occlusion accomplished, intermediate level vacuum builds to a maximum of 80 mm Hg and is used to draw the peripheral nucleus centrally.

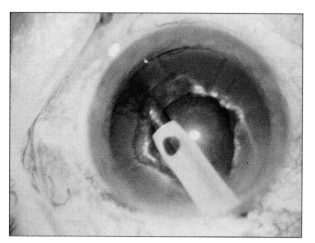

Figure 26-3. Soft nucleus—The occulsion is broken as the last portion of the peripheral nucleus is aspirated. Because the occulsion is broken after the material has been drawn away from the capsule, no capsule is aspirated and the remaining rim of peripheral nucleus falls back.

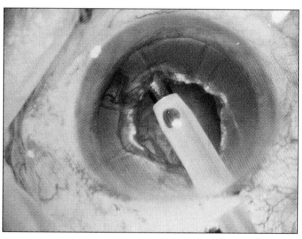

Figure 26-4. Soft nucleus—After rotation of about one clock hour, a new piece of nucleus is in position to be accessed.

ations, but tends to be more difficult to see through and is more slippery as to make anterior capsulotomy by cystotome method actually a little more difficult. The situations when we would use Viscoat would include zonular disruption or other anatomic changes which might make vitreous present. It is important to slightly overfill the anterior chamber to try to make the anterior capsular surface flat. This is especially important as patients are more youthful because their intraocular pressures (IOPs) are slightly higher, and because the elasticity of tissues and the lens contents will want to come forward, tending to spiral the capsulotomy peripherally.

In these situations it may be appropriate to reinflate the anterior chamber several times during the anterior capsulorhexis process. It is always good to reinflate in anticipation of the peripheral extension rather than in response to it.

## CAPSULOTOMY DETAILS

My standard capsulotomy is accomplished with a pre-bent needle cystotome. I start centrally and sweep to the left and toward myself peripherally, accomplishing the ultimate peripheral extension within the first 3 clock hours. The diameter of the finished capsulotomy should be approximately 5 to 6 mm (using a 5.5 mm acrylic IOL). It is important to make the capsulotomy circular so that contraction forces are balanced.

In a pediatric case, it may be necessary to use Utrata forceps if the capsulotomy starts to extend peripherally (in these cases it is helpful to visualize the intended opening as 3 mm as this will ultimately results in a 5.5 to 6 mm opening). If you try to make the opening 6 mm, it will actually be larger when we are finished.

For intumescent lenses, it is helpful to evacuate the liquid contents of the lens bag after initial puncture and

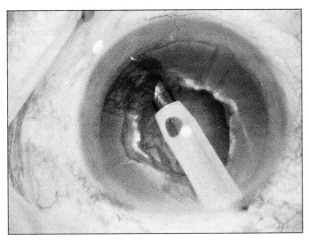

Figure 26-5. Soft nucleus—Very low level phacoemulsification combined with increasing vacuum allows this piece to be drawn centrally.

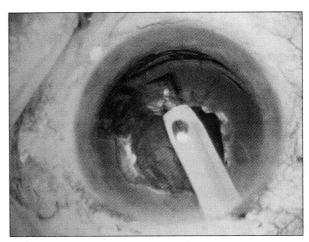

Figure 26-6. Soft nucleus—Occulsion has been broken again and the remainder of the nuclear rim has fallen back into position. As occulsion is broken, there is a sudden gulp of aspiration that occurs. No capsule is encountered because the tip aperture is well away from the capsule. Also, the direction of the aspirated fluid comes from the open left side of the side facing oriented 45° tip.

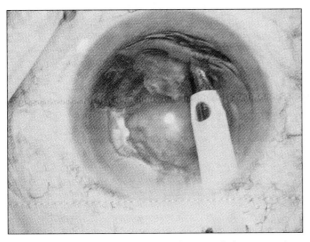

Figure 26-7. Soft nucleus—The 45° phacoemulsification tip best separates pure nonocculded phaco energy from occluded phaco assisted vacuum aspiration. Deeper sculpting can be more safely accomplished without inadvertent occlusion so that the overlying nuclear fragment will fold over the shallow sculpted portion and break off into the tip when it is later used to occlude and aspirate it.

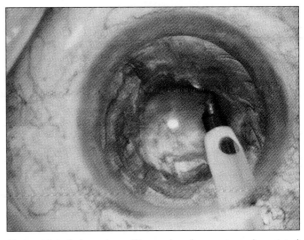

Figure 26-8. Soft nucleus—The nuclear fragment can be rotated further to access it on the surgeon's left or the tip can be rotated to access it on the surgeon's right. This is especially handy if there is a capsular defect on the left side.

replace it with viscoelastic. If visualization is poor, high magnification and continuous movement make visualization better. A moving flap can be visualized where a stationary one will become obscure. If movement isn't seen, one must assume that the capsulotomy is gone peripherally and the capsulotomy should be stopped and converted to a can opener style.

In an extremely intumescent lens with weak zonules or an older patient, a wide can opener style capsulotomy may still be the most helpful.

For management of a small pupil, especially in cases of pseudoexfoliation, I use Grieshaber hooks or the Graether pupil expander. This is particularly true in pseudoexfoliation cases when one might expect capsular contraction syndrome after a capsulotomy of even moderate size. For example, even if the pupil is 4 mm and a 4 mm capsulotomy might be adequate, in a pseudoexfoliation case it is nice to make the pupil even larger so that a 5.5 to 6 mm capsulorhexis can be accomplished to diminish the chances of capsular contraction syndrome.

## HYDRODISSECTION/ HYDRODELAMINATION

Hydrodissection is very much preferred over hydrodelamination. Hydrodelamination only creates an extra step with a peripheral nuclear layer which must be removed separately.

Hydrodissection is accomplished with a 30 gauge can-

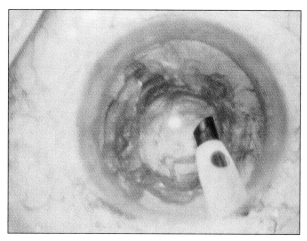

Figure 26-9. Soft nucleus—Deeper sculpting is again accomplished after another two or three clock hours' rotation.

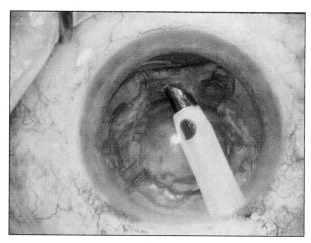

Figure 26-10. Soft nucleus—Material can be drawn centrally with the tip.

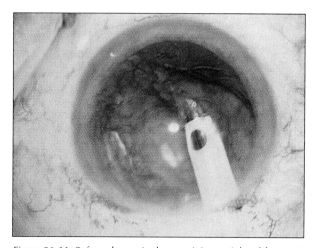

Figure 26-11. Soft nucleus—As the remaining peripheral fragment gets smaller, more of it wants to volunteer itself for aspiration when the tip is occluded. This results in a dislocation and a flipping of the posterior fragment. While this new presentation is fast, it risks damage to the capsular bag and corneal endothelium.

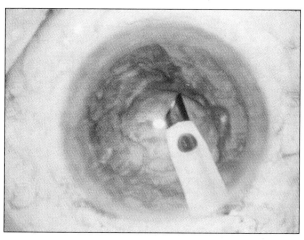

Figure 26-12. Soft nucleus—Instead, the volunteering material is pushed back into place and another rotation accomplished with deeper sculpting used again.

nula placed just under the anterior capsular flap. Fluid is gently injected under this flap until a wave is seen coming around peripherally. If no wave is seen, for whatever reason, this process can be accomplished 180° away, and one can assume that a wave will have been created and just missed. A 30 gauge cannula allows for a fine stream of fluid without excessive volume, making chances for capsular and iris problems lower. Total volume used is approximately 1 to 1.5 cc. These maneuvers are done to the right or left. It is unnecessary to do this in a subincisional fashion.

## PHACOEMULSIFICATION TECHNIQUE

Phacoemulsification is accomplished under the initial protection of 1% sodium hyaluronate. If Viscoat is used one must make sure to evacuate enough Viscoat centrally to establish inflow of fluid and outflow of material through the phacoemulsification tip. This is needed to prevent wound burn.

Phacoemulsification is accomplished in firm lenses by first sculpting across the surface of the lens to improve the red reflex overall. A deep groove is then created with the 45° tip. The lens nucleus is rotated 90° and a groove, approximately two phacoemulsification tips' width, is created again. The lens is rotated multiple times so that the peripheral nucleus can be accessed after initial groove creation, and the 45° tip can be used to remove as much nucleus in a non-occluded state peripherally as possible. (Settings for the sculpting with the 1.1 mm tip are phacoemulsification power 90%, vacuum 18 mm of Mercury, and flow rate 18 cc/min of water; settings for 0.9 mm tip are phacoemulsification power 90%, vacuum 50 mm of Mercury, and flow rate 14 cc/min.) After this, the nucleus is cracked into four quadrants in cross-handed, windshield wiper type fashion; ie, a cyclodialysis fashion (which is a 0.5 mm spatula which has been modified

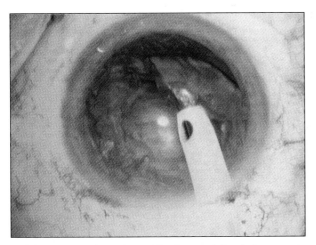

Figure 26-13. Soft nucleus—The last peripheral fragment is engaged and brought centrally.

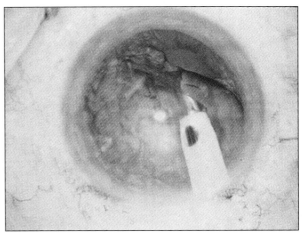

Figure 26-14. Soft nucleus—Aspiration is safely accomplished in this central location.

down to 0.4 mm) is used to push the right handed nuclear fragment peripherally away from the other fragments in a fashion that would be parallel to the arc formed by the equator of the lens. The phacoemulsification tip can be turned on its side and used to push the left handed fragment away from the right. A tearing motion is seen, which starts peripherally and extends centrally, as the posterior nuclear fibers are torn. This is done four times. The phacoemulsification tip is then turned on its side and the deeper, firmer pieces of nuclear material are removed in the non-occluded state. This is accomplished with multiple rotations with the lens nucleus.

For removal of the lens quadrants, the settings of the phacoemulsification machine are changed to reflect the chief operational force of vacuum and the secondary use of phacoemulsification (1.1 mm, phacoemulsification tip, phacoemulsification power max 70, vacuum 150 mm of Mercury, and flow rate 18 cc/min) (0.9 mm phaco tip, maximum phacoemulsification power 70, vacuum 230, and flow rate 14 cc/min), and the phacoemulsification tip is turned on its side and applied to the flat surface of the remaining nuclear fragment, which is distal and left of the surgeon. The occlusion occurs and the fragment is withdrawn from the periphery rolled centrally. It is rolled centrally, by rotating the tip slightly so that the 45° aperture position changes from a side orientation to a face-up orientation to present the nuclear piece to the large area of central safety in the anterior segment. The material is then allowed to collapse into the phacoemulsification tip with newer fragment portions constantly being placed into the distal left position with the cyclodialysis spatula. Each quadrant is removed in a similar fashion.

For an extraordinarily soft lens which doesn't crack, four grooves are converted into a bowl and the material merely is aspirated with the phaco tip in a side-oriented position. The settings for the soft nuclei are for a 1.1 mm tip, phacoemulsification of 50% max, vacuum 80 mm of Mercury, and flow rate 18 cc/min. The settings for the small tip are maximum phaco power 50%, maximum vacuum 170 mm of Mercury, and flow rate 14 cc/min.

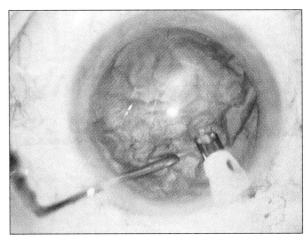

Figure 26-15. Soft nucleus—All of the peripheral nucleus has been removed, leaving a small posterior disc of nuclear material which is pried forward into the iris plane by the cyclodialysis spatula.

## EPINUCLEUS REMOVAL

If an epinuclear layer is left, it is inadvertent. It can be removed sometimes easily with the phacoemulsification tip, sometimes more safely with a 0.3 mm irrigation/aspiration (I/A) tip crushing its substance in a back and forth fashion over the 0.3 mm aperture. The I/A is accomplished with a 0.3 mm straight aspiration tip. With the capsulotomy the appropriate size, no curved tips or extraordinary manipulation is necessary. We usually start with subincisional cortex but this is not essential. If a small strand of cortex remains or pseudoexfoliation is present in larger wedges of cortex which seem to stress the capsular support system, a 0.2 mm tip can more easily isolate these remaining strands. It is easier to build the vacuum with the smaller port to occlude and draw material centrally where it can be aspirated. If material is still inaccessible, a bimanual system can be used, using the cyclodialysis spatula to hold up the anterior capsular leaflet while using the I/A tip, either the 0.3 to 0.2 to go underneath. If some peripheral cortex still remains, the IOL can be

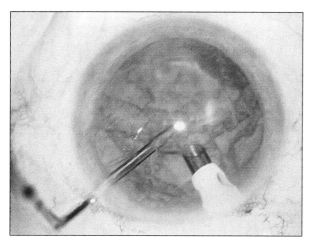

Figure 26-16. Soft nucleus—Phacoemulsification energy can be engaged when the fragment is supported in a central location and the tip aperture faces up, well away from important structures.

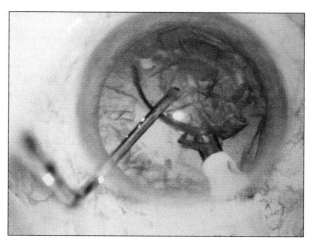

Figure 26-17. Soft nucleus—The cyclodialysis spatula supports the fragment and protects the posterior capsule until after the last piece is aspirated.

placed and rotated very carefully so the peripheral haptic loosens the remaining cortex and it becomes available to the easier occlusion and drawability of the 0.2 mm tip after the IOL has been placed. Settings used are surgeon control of aspiration, 500 mm of vacuum maximum, and 50 cc/min aspiration flow rate.

For capsular vacuuming, a 0.2 mm straight tip is always used. With sweeping motions the capsule can be easily vacuumed at the settings 11 mm of vacuum mas and 11 cc/min of flow rate. In high myopes or persons with distended concave posterior capsules, the bottle can be lowered to 40 to 50 cm above the eye so that capsular concavity is less pronounced.

## ENLARGEMENT OF THE INCISION

Enlargement of the incision is accomplished with Diamatrix diamond blade, as mentioned above.

## VISCOELASTIC FOR IOL IMPLANT

Normally 1% sodium hyaluronate is used because of its good visibility and its easy evacuation. If a capsular rent is present, it would be appropriate to try to tamponade the rent with a more retentive viscoelastic, ie, Viscoat, but this is certainly the exception.

## IOL IMPLANT

I use the Alcon AcrySof acrylic foldable IOL in all cases I possibly can. In cases of less than 10 D (where these lenses are not available), I prefer a one-piece polymethylmethacrylate (PMMA) IOL, approximately 12 mm to 12.5 mm in overall length and 5.5 mm in diameter. For higher than 30 D, usually piggy-back PMMA IOLs are used. For those patients requiring 9 D of power, I will usually round up to use a 10 D acrylic IOL just because of the extra deep anterior chamber and the advantages of the acrylic IOL.

The advantages of the acrylic IOL are numerous. First, it goes through a small clear corneal temporal self-sealing incision. Second, it has a substantially lower posterior capsulotomy YAG rate. Third, it seems to produce less postoperative inflammation both in the anterior segment and substantially less cystoid macular edema than not only PMMA lenses, but especially lower than the incidence with silicone lenses. This lens has an additional advantage of being able to be used in the case of anterior radial capsular tears (versus plate haptic IOLs), and it is particularly useful in cases of imperfect capsulorhexis.

The method of folding is a standard method using standard Alcon instruments. The lens is wet prior to complete folding. The instruments are cleaned before the first use of every day, and they are cleaned and polished with a wet sponge to remove oxidants, which would otherwise be imprinted on the IOL surface. The lens is fed into the anterior chamber with the leading haptic, which is compressed ever so slightly with instillation of the trailing haptic. I make an effort to not distort the haptics any more than necessary to preserve structural symmetry and help promote improved optic centration.

## VISCOELASTIC REMOVAL

Three-tenths mm I/A tip is used with the settings of 500 mm of Mercury Max Vac and 50 cc flow rate. First, balanced salt solution (BSS) is run through the handpiece so that all air has been removed. The tip is then inserted into the wound and slightly underneath the proximal optic edge to gain access to the viscoelastic, which is posterior and underneath the optic. The lens is tilted up slightly and the viscoelastic removed without difficulty. After the posterior viscoelastic is removed, the tip is left in the anterior chamber but placed on the anterior surface of the optic, and the rest of the viscoelastic is removed from the anterior chamber.

## FINAL TEST OF THE INCISION

The final test of the incision is accomplished in the following sequence. With the 30 gauge cannula, the incision is hydrated by injecting BSS into the corners of the wound at mid-stromal level. The paracentesis site is injected in similar fashion. It is helpful actually to do this first so that any flakes of cortex which have been sequestered in this site can be flushed into the anterior chamber and the I/A tip reintroduced for removal of the flakes if needed. The eye is slightly over-inflated; a sponge is simply used to press down on the wound and compress it. With the pressure on the wound, one can easily see if the wound is going to be self-sealing, as the eye will remain firm and fluid will not be lost. The 30 gauge cannula is then inserted into the paracentesis site allowing some fluid to escape. With a sponge, by tactile sensation, the incision again is pressed all the way across its surface gently until the eye is normal pressure and indents fairly easily. However, it should still be firm enough to be normal and ensure apposition of the wound edges. With this initial overcompression and then decompression, wound edge approximation is thorough and self-sealing qualities are ensured.

Rarely does a self-sealing wound not adequately seal. In this case, one or two 10-0 nylon sutures can be placed into the wound as needed. The knot buried on the corneal side and the sutures can be removed anywhere from 1 to 14 days later.

## CONCLUSION

The wound is always placed temporally because this is the most efficient and safe place a phacoemulsification IOL should be placed. If astigmatic errors exist greater than 2 D preoperatively, especially with-the-rule, one can perform transverse astigmatic keratotomy at the end of the IOL procedure.

Similarly, if macular epiretinal membrane exists, conversion at the conclusion of this procedure can be accomplished easily to pars plana vitrectomy (a retrobulbar block is used in these cases).

If a combined glaucoma procedure has been anticipated, the IOL can be placed in clear corneal fashion as described above and then a standard trabeculectomy performed superiorly.

# Chapter 27

# PERSONAL PHACOEMULSIFICATION TECHNIQUE

*Harry B. Grabow, MD*

## ANESTHESIA

Topical anesthesia using sterile non-preserved 4% lidocaine, 0.5% tetracaine, or 0.5% proparacaine is my preferred method for routine cataract procedures. The lidocaine solution is manufactured in the USA in single use glass ampules. It is drawn up into a syringe by a nurse and administered in sequence with the dilating drops: tropicamide 1%, phenylephrine 2.5%, flurbiprofen, and then the lidocaine. This sequence is repeated three times over 30 minutes. In the operating room a few additional drops of the lidocaine are administered prior to prepping to the unoperated fellow eye. This produces a blunt corneal reflex bilaterally, as the patient will be instructed to keep both eyes wide open during the operation to minimize orbicularis squeezing on the speculum on the operated side.

During the procedure, stabilization of the globe is necessary when making the diamond-blade incisions and the capsulorhexis. This is achieved by having the patient fixate on the microscope light. I have lowered the intensity from 5 out of 6 on my Zeiss-CS system to 4. The fiberoptic coaxial light makes a rectangular reflex on the cornea. I know the patients are fixating with the fovea when they describe the light as a *rectangle*. The diamond keratomes require counter-pressure which is achieved with a blunt instrument at the limbus 180° away from the keratotomy site. Motility during phaco is easily controlled with two instruments in the eye.

The topical drops anesthetize the cornea and conjunctiva, but have no intraocular effect. As in a case of secondary anterior chamber implantation, the undilated iris is sensitive and manipulation causes pain. The dilated iris has no sensation. The same appears to be true regarding the ciliary muscle. Manipulation of the zonule, such as occurs with chamber deepening on insertion of the phaco tip or with rotation of the nucleus, can cause pain, a phenomenon I call *ciliary proprioception*. Surgeons who use cyclopentolate report that their topical patients rarely complain of discomfort, as this agent has a good cycloplegic effect. In those cases where supplementation is desirable for patient comfort, propofol is administered intravenously in 10 mg increments. This produces a transient hypnosis with amnesia that clears rapidly in minutes.

Some surgeons achieve intraocular ciliary analgesia by injecting non-preserved lidocaine into the anterior and/or posterior chamber. Usually, only 0.5 cc is necessary and it must be injected before viscoelastic is instilled, as the viscoelastic can coat the intraocular surfaces and block the effect of the lidocaine. Some patients may feel the lidocaine as a burning upon injection, which is thought to be due to its acidic pH. This sensation can be reduced by diluting 2% lidocaine with an equal volume of balanced salt solution (BSS). Injection of intraocular lidocaine in the presence of an opening in the posterior capsule or zonule has produced temporary pharmacologic amaurosis, similar to the effect of retrobulbar injection.

I use topical anesthesia on 98% of my cases. The remaining 2% receive peribulbar and are disqualified from topical according to the six *D's of Disqualification*. Three are systemic: deafness, dysphasia, and dementia. Three are ocular: dense cataract (that will not transmit the rectangular light image to the retina), degeneration of the macula (with only parafoveal fixation), and dysfunctional motility (not allowing the patient to move or stabilize the eye onto centric fixation). In addition, small pupil cases requiring a pupillary enlarging technique may be performed more comfortably with a block; however, intraocular lidocaine may also produce adequate analgesia.

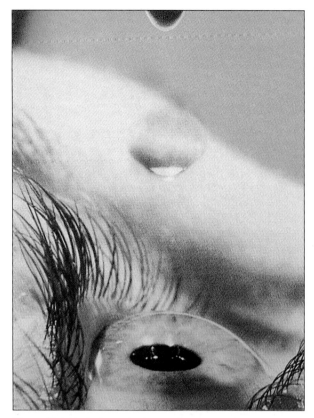

Figure 27-1. Topical anesthesia.

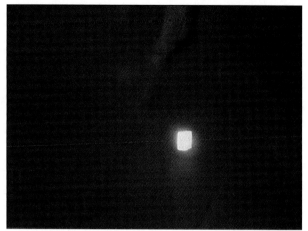

Figure 27-2. Coaxial light reflex for subjective fixation during topical anesthesia.

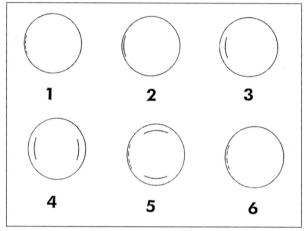

Figure 27-3. Six steps to sphericity.

## SIX STEPS TO SPHERICITY

Since beginning phacoemulsification and foldable lens implantation through 3.0 mm sutureless clear corneal incisions in 1992, and after a 4000 case experience, I have become comfortable and familiar with the astigmatic effects of this cataract incision. Its predictability has allowed the development of a systematic approach to preexisting astigmatism. The system involves six combinations of four variables:

1. Ungrooved uniplanar clear corneal incisions.
2. Grooved biplanar clear corneal incisions.
3. Astigmatic keratotomy (AK).
4. Toric intraocular lenses (IOLs).

The system is designed to be used with temporal clear corneal incisions only and—for the purposes of this system and its application to astigmatism reduction—*temporal* is defined as within 30° of the horizontal axis. I do not choose to perform unsutured clear corneal phaco and foldable incisions obliquely or superiorly, as I believe incisions at these axes have demonstrated higher degrees of corneal endothelial cell loss (Hoffer & Grabow) and an increased risk of early postoperative infectious endophthalmitis. Though many American and European surgical colleagues have safely and successfully mastered *on-axis* oblique and superior incisions, even with unsutured 5.0 mm incisions for polymethylmethacrylate (PMMA) lenses, all of my cataract incisions are now temporal, not only for the aforementioned reasons, but also for efficiency and ergonomics. It has simply become easier now to be temporal.

### Step 1

The first step to sphericity is applied to spherical eyes. In these cases, we want the postoperative corneal curvature to match the preoperative curvature. Therefore, a simple, single-plane, very peripheral temporal stab incision is used. This incision is astigmatically neutral, usually resulting in either no change in astigmatism or no more than a 0.37 D induction with-the-rule.

### Step 2

For mild astigmatism against-the-rule of 0.50 to 1.25 D, a two-step grooved incision is used. The groove depth used in this system is 300 µm. However, depths of 400 µm (Williamson) and 600 µm (Langerman) can be used. Obviously, the deeper the groove, the greater the effect. In addition, as with all incisional keratorefractive procedures (radial keratotomy [RK] and AK), age is a factor. The 60-year-old cataract patient might result in only a 0.50 D change in cylinder, whereas the 80-year-old would get a 1.25 D shift *from the same incision*.

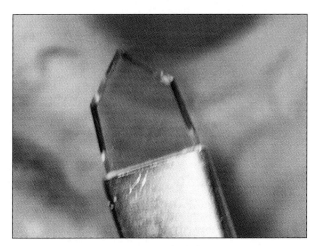

Figure 27-4. Williamson trapezoid blade, 2.5 mm x 2.9 mm (Diamatrix).

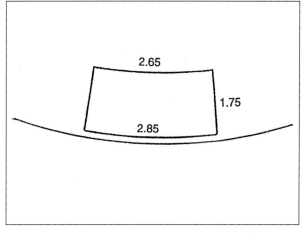

Figure 27-5. Trapezoid clear corneal incision dimensions (Williamson).

## Step 3

For moderate against-the-rule astigmatism of 1.50 to 3.00 D, the same two-step grooved incision is used; however, it is moved 0.5 to 1.0 mm centrally on the corneal surface. Moving the vertical groove centrally effectively reduces the optical zone of the *AK portion* of the two-step phaco foldable incision, thereby increasing its effect. Again, the effect is age-related.

## Step 4

For high degrees of against-the-rule astigmatism, 3.00 to 6.00 D, the two-step incision is used, as in Step 3. However, an AK incision is added across the cornea 180° away for more effect. For 4.00 D, the full-thickness phaco incision would be placed at an optical zone of 8.0mm. An AK incision would then be added at the 8.0 optical zone (180° away) and two additional AK incisions (a pair) at the 7.0 mm optical zone. For 6.0 D of astigmatism, a triple set of incisions may be desired, especially in a younger patient, at optical zones of 6.0, 7.0, and 8.0. *Note:* the full-thickness grooved phaco incision moved in on the cornea can be very powerful in the elderly over 80 years of age. Also, remember that with-the-rule astigmatism is visually preferable to against-the-rule astigmatism. Therefore, overcorrection of against-the-rule and undercorrection of with-the-rule is recommended.

## Step 5

For oblique-axis or with-the-rule astigmatism, the astigmatically neutral, single-plane, ungrooved T-CCI is used and the appropriate AK incisions are placed on-axis. I prefer to make all of my AK incisions first, before entering the eye with the phaco-foldable incision, as the eye is more firm and the incision depths are more reliable.

## Step 6

This is the ultimate step that I have been privileged to incorporate into my astigmatic armamentarium (as I have been one of the investigators in the USA) and which will eventually add to and replace many of the previous

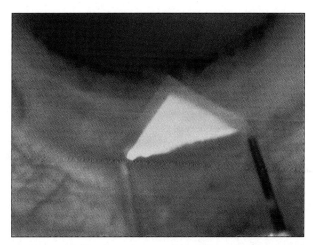

Figure 27-6. Self-sealing, clear corneal incision: 1.75 mm stromal tunnel.

steps in this system of astigmatism management: the toric IOL. In the USA, Staar will soon have available (pending the FDA's expected approval in 1997) 2.00 D and 3.50 D models for approximately 1.00 to 1.25 D and 2.00 to 2.50 D of cylinder, respectively. We will be able to use these alone or in combination with AK to ultimately have the simplest, safest, and most predictable method of reducing astigmatism in our cataract patients.

## CLEAR CORNEAL INCISIONS

For approximately 80% of cases in which no correction of astigmatism is planned, a 2.65 mm single plane stab incision is made in the temporal clear cornea, using a 2.5 mm x 2.9 mm Williamson trapezoid blade (Diamatrix). The intracorneal tunnel is ideally 1.50 to 1.75 mm long. Making the tunnel shorter improves visibility but risks wound leak. Making the tunnel longer produces a better seal but also results in visually disabling striae during instrumentation.

The blade is first advanced in the stroma in a plane parallel to the corneal curvature until the angles of the

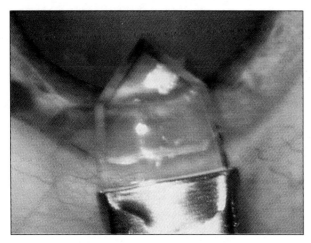

Figure 27-7. Self-sealing, clear corneal incision: trapezoid 2.5 mm x 2.9 mm.

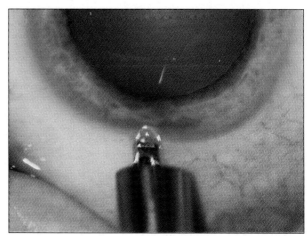

Figure 27-8. Step one of the two-step grooved biplanar clear corneal incision: 300 µm groove with guarded Williamson step blade (Diamatrix).

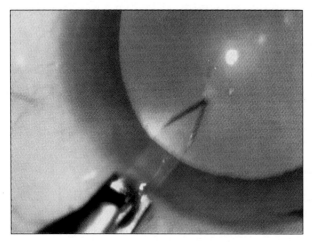

Figure 27-9. Side port 1.0 mm paracentesis with Williamson *step* blade (Diamatrix).

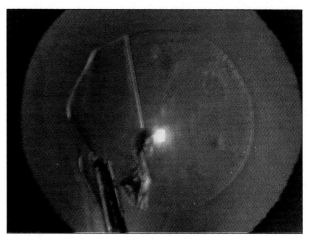

Figure 27-10. Anterior CCC with Utrata forceps.

shoulders reach the external opening. The point of the blade is now approximately 1.50 mm into the clear cornea and is now angled downward in order to perforate Descemet's membrane. Once into the anterior chamber, the blade is turned flat, parallel to the plane of the iris, and further advanced until the angles of the shoulders now reach the internal opening being created. This makes the internal keratotomy 2.65 mm and enlarges the external keratotomy to 2.85 mm.

The remaining 20% of cases have surgically correctable astigmatism. Some of these patients may receive a two-step grooved incision. A 300 µm clear corneal groove is made temporally, first using a Williamson *step* blade (Diamatrix). The same blade is then fully extended and used to make the 1.0 mm side port. Viscoelastic may then be injected to replace aqueous. This serves to produce a firmer eye for the primary keratotomy and to prevent chamber collapse on entering. The primary keratotomy is then made using the William *trap* blade (Diamatrix) in similar fashion to the single-plane stab incision.

## CAPSULORHEXIS

An anterior continuous central circular capsulorhexis (CCC) is made on every case. With the patient fixating on the microscope light, a curvilinear capsulotomy is made with a bent 25 G needle (Visitec, #1610A) mounted on the viscoelastic syringe through the primary keratotomy incision. After making a central puncture of the capsule, the needle tip is drawn toward its point of entry into the eye, curving to my right, and stopping short of the imaginary circle to be created. Utrata capsulorhexis forceps are then used to complete the capsulectomy, regrasping approximately every four *clock hours*.

The ideal capsulorhexis is 5.0 mm in diameter for a 6.0 mm optic. I believe that the margin of the capsulorhexis should cover the edge of the IOL optic by 0.5 mm. This allows symmetrical concentric contraction postoperatively, in order to avoid asymmetric IOL decentration which can occur with larger openings. Larger openings at surgery are easier to phaco through and give better postoperative visibility of the peripheral retina. However, they also risk extension to the equator by catching an

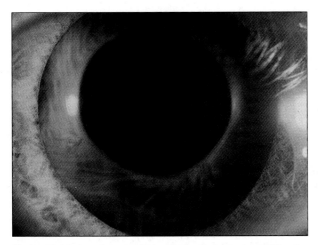

Figure 27-11. Anterior capsulorhexis, 6 months postop, with minimal and symmetrical fibrotic contraction.

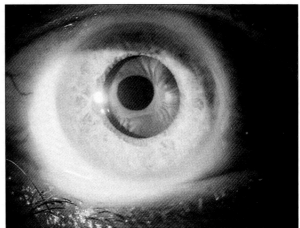

Figure 27-12. Anterior capsulorhexis, 1 year postop, with slightly eccentric excessive fibrotic contraction requiring YAG laser capsulotomy.

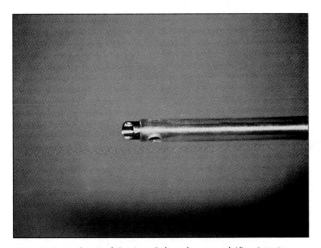

Figure 27-13. Surgical Design *Cobra* phacoemulsification tip.

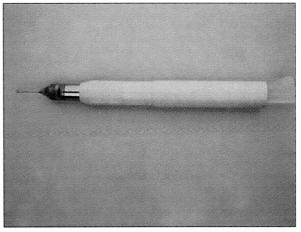

Figure 27-14. Surgical Design lightweight magnetostrictive phacoemulsification handpiece.

anteriorly inserted zonular fiber and by allowing more anterior displacement of the lens due to posterior pressure. Openings smaller than 4.0 mm are more difficult to phaco through and may contract postoperatively, requiring YAG laser enlargement.

## CORTICAL CLEAVING HYDRODISSECTION

A 30 G cannula angled at the hub is used for cortical-cleaving hydrodissection with BSS, a technique defined by I. Howard Fine. The tip of the cannula is placed through the primary incision and under the anterior capsule to my left. The capsule is slightly elevated and BSS is injected. A posterior dissection wave is observed to advance from (my) left to right and the nucleus is observed to expand the capsulorhexis and split the prenuclear cortex. At this point, injection is stopped if in situ phaco is intended. Otherwise, continual injection results in partial hydroexpression of the nucleus, which can be fully expressed for rapid anterior chamber phaco.

Preferring in situ phaco, the nucleus is then tamponaded back into the bag with the side of the cannula.

Hydrodelamination is no longer performed, as the intention is to have all of the cortex removed with the epinucleus using the phaco tip. Therefore, leaving the cortex adherent to the epinucleus and the epinucleus adherent to the endonucleus aids in mechanical cortical-cleaving because the whole cortico-epiendonuclear complex is rotated together during four quadrant grooving.

Occasionally, for soft cataracts, hydrodissection will be intentionally continued until hydroexpression occurs (ie, one pole of the nucleus is pushed anteriorly through the CCC). The 30 G cannula is then used to dial the nucleus completely out of the bag for anterior chamber phaco.

## FOUR QUADRANT PHACOFRACTURE

Phacofracture has been my preferred technique since it was described by John Shepherd in the 1980s. It is different from the Divide and Conquer technique of Gimbel or the Phaco Chop technique of Nagahara in that

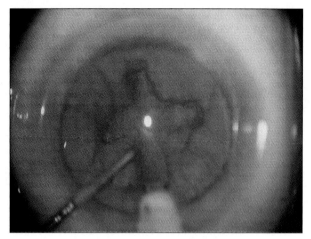

Figure 27-15. Grooved nucleus ready for four quadrant fracturing.

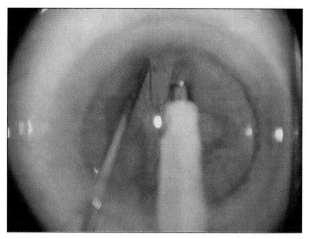

Figure 27-16. Direct parallel instrument phaco fracturing of the floor of the grooves.

Shepherd fracturing is performed following pregrooving, whereas the former techniques involve fracturing without pregrooving. This technique is applicable to all degrees of nuclear sclerosis, with a few modifications for very soft and very hard nuclei.

The procedure begins with a longitudinal groove initially, slightly less than the diameter of the capsulorhexis in length. A 30° maxi Cobra phaco tip is used on a Surgical Design Ocusystem II$^e$ art magnetostrictive handpiece with the power set at 30%. The vacuum is -25 mm Hg and the flow at 8 cc/min for sculpting. These are changed to vacuum -150 mm Hg and flow 24 cc/min for removing quadrants.

The groove width varies according to the hardness of the nucleus. For 2+ and 3+ nuclei, the groove is made approximately one and one-half times as wide as the phaco tip. This is standard and is the most common nucleus. Very soft nuclei can be grooved in two different ways: either very narrow—the width of the phaco tip—for four quadrant fracturing, or very wide—more than twice as wide as the phaco tip—for two quadrant (bisection) fracturing. Very advanced nuclei (4+, brunescent, or nigra) also require very wide grooves—more than twice the width of the phaco tip.

The grooves are sculpted without occlusion of the phaco tip. When the depth of the groove becomes deeper than the width of the phaco tip, the length of the groove may be extended by careful tip occlusion toward the periphery under the anterior capsule. It is not necessary to groove all the way to the equator of the nucleus to achieve fracturing. It is actually dangerous because the lens is thinner and softer out in the periphery and it is easy to perforate the equatorial capsule. Less phaco power and, therefore, less aspiration and vacuum, should be used when extending grooves under the anterior capsule.

The depth of the groove necessary for successful fracturing of the floor of the groove also varies with different degrees of nuclear hardness. Very soft and very hard nuclei require the deepest grooves, probably 95% deep, whereas medium nuclei fracture well at 80 to 85% depth.

A smooth floor with a good red reflex is usually a good indication that it will fracture. Philippe Crozafon states that the fracturing instrument must be placed at the bottom of the grooves, on the floor, to achieve effective separation of adjacent quadrants resulting in floor fracturing. I usually prepare all four grooves before any fracturing, although fracturing can be performed when each groove is ready.

I perform direct parallel instrument fracturing using a blunt, cylindrical, polished Barraquer iris spatula in my left hand and the phaco tip in my right hand. In order for these instruments to be parallel in a groove, their respective clear corneal entry incisions are 45° apart. Following fracturing of the nucleus into four quadrants, the blunt Barraquer spatula is used to lift the central apex of the first quadrant off the posterior cortex of the capsulorhexis opening, where it is safely engaged by occlusion by the phaco tip. The quadrant is then fully emulsified, and the process is repeated until all quadrants are removed.

At the beginning of the emulsification of the final quadrant, the blunt tip of the Barraquer spatula is placed below the fragment in the center of the posterior capsule. In this way, the capsule is held down and away from the elevated aspiration forces of the phaco tip to avoid inadvertent aspiration of the capsule when the final piece of nucleus clears the tip.

## V-GROOVE TRIFRACTURE

Charles D. Kelman and, more recently, Aziz Anis have described this technique, which results in removing the nucleus in three pieces instead of four, which may reduce ultrasonic time.

Only two grooves are made, creating a V. The floor of each groove is then fractured, dividing the nucleus into three pieces. The piece in the center of the V is removed first and each remaining third is then removed. A chopper can be used to create the divisions and to further subdivide each third.

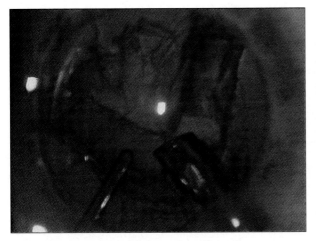

Figure 27-17. *V-groove* ready for nuclear trifracturing.

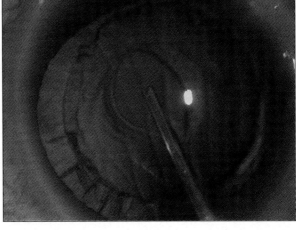

Figure 27-18. Beginning of post-phaco cortical cleaving viscodissection.

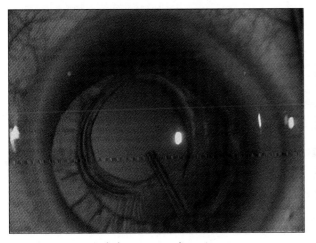

Figure 27-19. Cortical cleaving viscodissection.

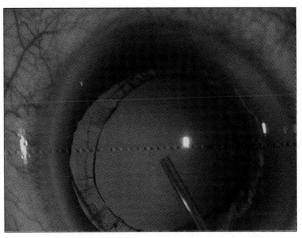

Figure 27-20. Cortical cleaving viscodissection completed; all cortex deposited into capsular equatorial recess.

## Supracapsular Phacoemulsification

Soft nuclei are often dislocated into the anterior chamber, not by the tumbling technique (Phaco Flip of David Brown), but by hydroexpression and dialing. A capsulorhexis of at least 5.0 mm facilitates nuclear dislocation.

Emulsification can then be performed from the *outside-in* on the whole intact and undivided nucleus using a *carousel* technique. The aspiration is set at 24 cc/min and the vacuum at 150 mm Hg. The phaco tip is placed under the nucleus, away from the corneal endothelium. The 30° bevel is turned central and is occluded by the posterior surface of the equator of the nucleus. As the lens is emulsified, it rotates like a carousel, becoming progressively smaller in diameter.

This technique is ideal for soft nuclei and in cases of a weak zonule in which endocapsular emulsification may place dangerous stress on the zonule. Although this technique often results in ultrasonic times of less than 1 minute, it is not recommended for hard nuclei or eyes with either corneal guttata or low endothelial cell counts.

# CORTICAL CLEAVING VISCODISSECTION

Following completion of phaco, all cortex may have been simultaneously removed during phaco or easily after phaco with the phaco tip in approximately 50% of cases due to successful cortical cleaving hydrodissection. In the cases in which adherent cortex remains, indicating a failure of cortical cleaving hydrodissection, the cortex is not subsequently removed by the automated irrigation/aspiration (I/A) tip (as had been done in the past), due to the risk of breaking the exposed, unprotected posterior capsule. Rather, viscoelastic is injected into the capsule between the remaining cortex and the posterior capsule in such a way as to cleave off the cortex from the center of the posterior capsule, depositing it in the equatorial recess. This is accomplished by placing the tip of the cannula through the center of the posterior cortex, on the posterior capsule, and then injecting the viscoelastic (regular Healon or Amvisc), which cleaves off or dissects off the posterior cortical fibers and pushes them centripetal-

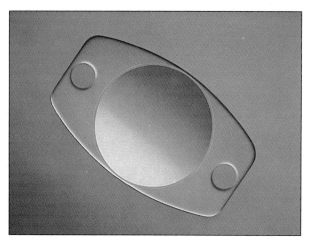

Figure 27-21. Staar 4203VF one-piece, plate-haptic, foldable, silicone, aphakic, capsular bag IOL.

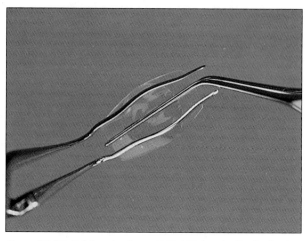

Figure 27-22. Folding the Staar 4203 IOL longitudinally for forceps implantation.

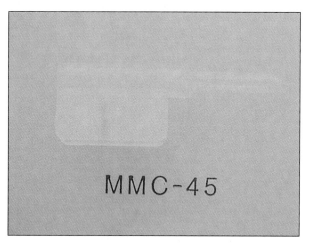

Figure 27-23. Staar 45° beveled cartridge for injection of the 4203 plate-haptic IOLs and the three-piece polyimide loop-haptic IOLs.

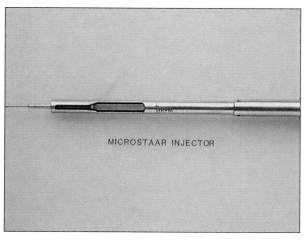

Figure 27-24. MicroStaar® injector for implantation of both Staar plate-haptic and polyimide-looped foldable IOLs.

ly (peripherally) toward their sites of origin at the equator of the bag. The capsule at this stage contains both the cortex and the viscoelastic and is ready for the next step, IOL implantation.

## IOL IMPLANTATION

My implant of choice is the Staar 4203VF one-piece, plate-haptic, silicone, foldable IOL for all cases of cataract with keratometric cylinder less than 1.00 D. Since 1987, I have implanted more than 7000 of these IOLs. For eyes with preoperative keratometric cylinder of 1.00 D or greater, which may be confirmed by corneal topography, I prefer to use the Staar 4203T toric IOL in order to reduce or eliminate the effect of the corneal astigmatism. Not only do these lenses result in minimal surgically induced incisional astigmatism (0.12 D average for scleral-pocket incisions and 0.37 D average for temporal clear corneal incisions), but they also have one of the lowest YAG rates of current IOL designs, 4% after 2 years and 8% after 4 years.

The spherical lens, model 4203VF has a 6.0 mm symmetrical biconvex optic of constant center thickness which is currently manufactured in powers from +9.50 to +30.50. The planar plate haptics have an overall diagonal length of 10.8 mm and an enlarged fenestration of 1.15 mm in diameter. This opening allows for capsular fixation of the IOL by fibrotic adhesion of the anterior and posterior capsules. Although the lens may be implanted with folding forceps, almost all surgeons who use this lens prefer to inject it. The 45° beveled oval cartridge and the MicroStaar injector allow for one-step implantation through a 2.8 mm scleral incision or a 3.0 mm corneal incision. James Carty injects the lens through a 2.5 mm corneal incision without introducing the cartridge tip into the incision.

The IOL is loaded into the cartridge by the scrub technician while I complete phaco. The cartridge is first prepared by filling the tip and coating the folding chamber with viscoelastic. The IOL is then transferred from its package with a titanium cylindrical-bladed silicone lens forceps and placed longitudinally into the folding chamber. The folding wings are then brought together, rolling

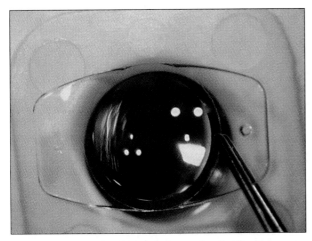

Figure 27-25. Cylindrical-bladed titanium lens holding forceps for safe transferring and loading of silicone IOLs.

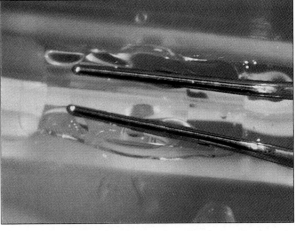

Figure 27-26. Loading of the Staar 4203 plate-haptic IOL longitudinally into the folding chamber of the cartridge.

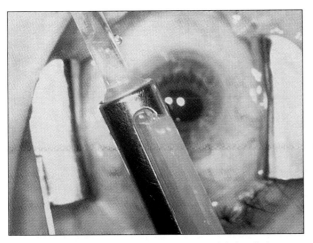

Figure 27-27. Cartridge with viscoelastic and folded (rolled) IOL in MicroStaar injector.

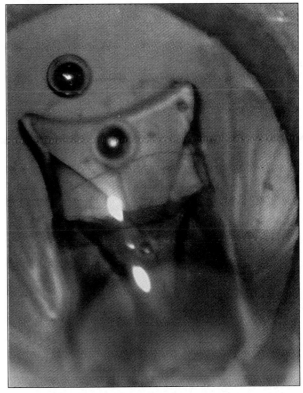

Figure 27-28. Leading haptic of Staar 4203 being injected into capsular bag through intact anterior capsulorhexis.

the lens into a cylinder, and the loaded cartridge is placed into the injector.

Following evacuation of the bag with the phaco or (in the event there is cortex remaining) cortical cleaving viscodissection, the cartridge tip is inserted through the unenlarged 3.0 mm or 3.2 mm clear corneal phaco incision into the anterior chamber. The injector piston is advanced, causing the implant to move forward and ejecting the viscoelastic from the cartridge tip. The emerging leading plate haptic is directed through the anterior capsulorhexis and unfolds in the bag. The optic follows next, and the trailing haptic is directed into the capsule by rotating the cartridge tip, allowing the haptic to emerge from the cartridge and unfold by its own internal elastic memory. The empty cartridge is then removed from the eye.

## POST-IMPLANTATION CORTICAL ASPIRATION

The capsule now contains the implant, viscoelastic substance, and, in the event of incomplete or failed cortical cleaving hydrodissection, residual cortex. The automated I/A tip with the 0.2 mm port is placed inside the anterior chamber for the first (and only) time in order to remove both the viscoelastic and the cortex. The optic and plate haptics of the IOL serve as a rigid barrier to protect the posterior capsule from the aspiration forces of the I/A tip, thereby preventing inadvertent tearing of the posterior capsule. Once all cortex is removed, viscoelastic trapped behind the optic may be removed with the I/A tip with the aspiration port safely facing anteriorly.

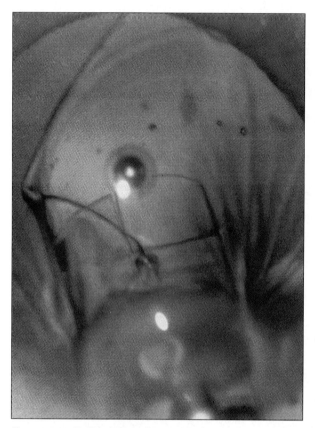

Figure 27-29. Trailing haptic of Staar 4203 being guided into capsular bag through anterior capsulorhexis by rotation of the cartridge tip.

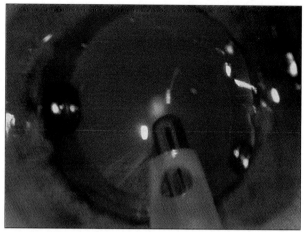

Figure 27-30. Post-implantation cortical aspiration.

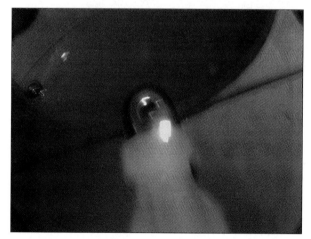

Figure 27-31. Removal of viscoelastic from capsular bag behind IOL to prevent entrapment syndrome.

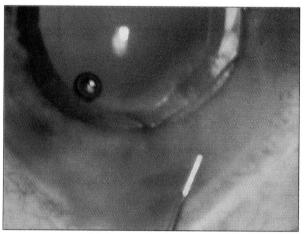

Figure 27-32. Temporary closure of sutureless clear corneal incision by stromal hydration with BSS.

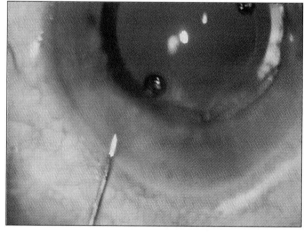

Figure 27-33. Stromal hydration of 1.0 mm side port incision.

## WOUND CLOSURE

The self-sealing, sutureless, temporal clear corneal phaco incision is now closed by first injecting BSS into the corneal stroma at each end of the incision. This technique was first devised by I. Howard Fine, and swells the external corneal lip of the incision for several hours. BSS is then injected through the 1.0 mm side port paracentesis to deepen the chamber and close the door internally, applying aqueous pressure against the self-sealing internal corneal lip. The superficial stroma of the 1.0 mm side port incision is then hydrated. This concludes the procedure, which averages 8 minutes.

## INTRAOPERATIVE ANTIBIOTICS

Subconjunctival injections are not administered, as the eye only has surface topical anesthesia and the conjunctiva has not been violated with the clear corneal incisions. Rather, gentamicin 8 mg and vancomycin 20 mg are injected into the 500 cc infusion bottle of BSS Plain solution, along with 0.5 cc of non-preserved epinephrine.

## POSTOPERATIVE ROUTINE

No pad or shield is placed over the eye, which has full lid and extraocular motility following the topical anesthesia. The patient is instructed not to rub the eye and may resume normal activity that afternoon. For medicolegal reasons, since the patient may have received intravenous sedative medication, driving an automobile is not recommended until the next day. As no miotic is used, the pupil may remain dilated for several hours, usually returning to normal function by late afternoon or early evening of the operative day.

Immediately following removal of the lid speculum and drape, the head of the stretcher is raised. The stretcher is rolled into the recovery area where vital signs are taken and the patient is offered a beverage and sweet roll. We instruct the patients to be NPO after midnight before surgery, except for certain vital early morning oral medications which may be taken on arising at home, with sips of water only. Systemic anticoagulant medications, such as Coumadin and aspirin, are continued. The risk of retrobulbar hemorrhage is zero, as no needles are used in the orbit. The risk of hyphema is zero, as no incision is placed in the vascular sclera or iris.

No eyedrops are prescribed on the day of surgery, as we want the patients to avoid any periocular or global pressure. Tobradex (tobramycin and dexamethsone) drops are begun at home four times a day, 2 days before surgery and are resumed from the same bottle on the first postop day. These are continued for 4 weeks on a schedule tapering each week, four times a day, three times a day, two times a day, and finally, daily in the fourth week.

# Chapter 28

# PERSONAL PHACOEMULSIFICATION TECHNIQUE

*Tsutomu Hara, MD*

## ANESTHESIA

Only topical anesthesia induced with 0.5% tetracaine hydrochloride eyedrops (Tetocain, Kyorin Pharmaceutical Co) is used. These eyedrops are installed four times every 30 minutes starting 2 hours preoperatively. When patients cannot control their ocular movement, a sub-Tenon's injection of 0.1 mL of 2% lidocaine hydrochloride (Xylocaine, Fujisawa Pharmaceutical Co) is administered to the area around the superior rectus muscle followed by placement of a bridle suture. When the ocular movement is beyond control or painful, retrobulbar anesthesia using 3 mL of Xylocaine or peribulbar anesthesia using 6 mL of Xylocaine is induced. In such cases, 0.1 mL of adrenaline diluted 1,000 times is added to 20 mL of 2% Xylocaine solution to make 2% Xylocaine containing adrenaline diluted approximately 200,000 times. Using this solution, the injection is administered 20 minutes preoperatively and the surgery is performed without the high vitreous pressure associated with a completely painless condition.

## PREFERRED PHACOEMULSIFICATOR

I use the Legacy 20000 (Alcon Japan Ltd, Tokyo, Japan). I have used Alcon products since the Cavitron 8000 was introduced, and the results have been sufficiently reliable to choose the current machine. The Legacy maintains the anterior chamber depth well and rarely causes bubble formation. Usually a 1.2 mm regular straight tip is used, with a 15° apex. A new 0.9 mm straight U/S tip is more efficient, especially when the surgeon encounters a nucleus harder than +4°.

## INCISION

The incision serves two purposes: first, tight sealing of the wound, and second, correction of the presurgical astigmatism. For the latter, suture tightening at the weak meridian is not recommended because the results are so unstable. Simultaneous astigmatic keratotomy also is not recommended because many reports have been published indicating that a rupture can occur following radial keratotomy after impact with an air bag during a car accident. Astigmatic keratotomy should be done at least 3 months postoperatively. The last option is flattening of the steep meridian using a self-sealing incision without a suture. The incision for the primary wound is made using a 3.2 mm wide-angled diamond Lance blade (Katena). For the side port, a 1 mm straight diamond knife (Mikura Diamond Knife, Inami Co) is used.

A 3.5 mm wide linear incision 1 mm from the limbus flattens the corneal curvature at the incision meridian by 0.5 diopter (D) (surgically induced astigmatism is 0.5 D). A 3.5 mm wide limbal incision induces 0.75 D astigmatism. A 3.5 mm wide clear corneal incision induces 1.0 D of flattening of the incision meridian. A 6.0 mm frown incision central width, 1 mm with both ends 3 mm from the limbus, or a 6 mm wide linear incision 2 mm from the limbus flattens the incision meridian by 1.0 D. A 6 mm limbal or linear clear corneal incision flattens the incision meridian by 3 D. At present, there is no practical incision that totally prevents surgically induced astigmatism. Therefore, if the presurgical astigmatism is 0, the best choices are a 3.5 x 1 mm incision and a foldable intraocular lens (IOL). Even with this combination, 0.5 D of post-surgically induced astigmatism is induced. When a 3.5 mm wide linear incision is located 2 mm from the limbus, the surgically induced astigmatism is less, but phaco tip movement is considerably restricted. Therefore, a 3.5 mm wide incision 1 mm from the limbus is the practical limit.

In this technique, the conjunctival flap becomes problematic. If a fornix-based conjunctival flap is created and bleeding is halted using a wet-field bipolar coagulator, the

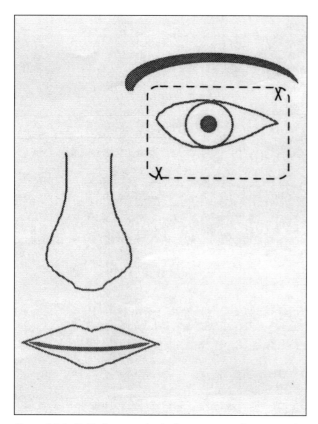

Figure 28-1. Peribulbar anesthesia for rare cases that cannot be controlled by eyedrops or sub-Tenon's anesthesia. The patient's eye is maintained at the primary position. The injection needle should be perpendicular to the skin surface 3 mL for each X point. The injection should be administered 20 minutes preoperatively.

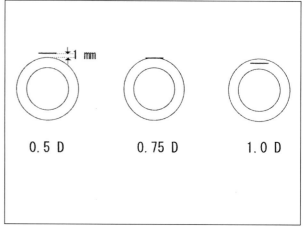

Figure 28-2. The flattening effect of the 3.5 mm wide incision on the incision meridian.

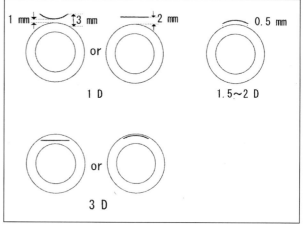

Figure 28-3. The flattening effect of the 6.0 mm wide incision on the incision meridian.

surgery proceeds without bleeding. However, conjunctival healing is not as rapid and perfect as that in the following procedure (developed after long-term trial and error).

I penetrate the conjunctiva using the 3.2 mm wide angle diamond Lance blade, dissect the scleral flap, and penetrate the anterior chamber. Hemorrhage from the conjunctiva and scleral surface is minimal and does not prevent the continuation of the procedure. The conjunctival incision is not sealed. Because there is no conjunctival preparation, and there is only a 3.0 mm linear slit, the postoperative conjunctival healing proceeds extremely smoothly and there are no obstacles to future surgery. However, this technique has a limitation. During phacoemulsification, the irrigating solution easily penetrates under the conjunctiva and in most cases 180 to 360° high chemosis occurs. Although this resolves completely by the next morning, this procedure cannot be used in no-patch surgery.

In patients under 30 years of age, an IOL with a rigid polymethylmethacrylate (PMMA) optic must be selected, because the long-term stability of this lens has already been proven compared to the relatively new soft IOLs. Subsequently, the minimum incision length is 6 mm. The relationship between incision type and surgically induced astigmatism differs from surgeon to surgeon.

First, each surgeon should determine his or her own formula, then create a wound based on that formula, monitor the results carefully, and modify the original formula.

A steep meridian is not always in an easily accessible area. If the surgeon can use both hands, he or she can sit at the 12 o'clock position and shift slightly. I am naturally right-handed, but have trained my left hand by writing medical records for 8 hours a day for more than 10 years. However, after reaching 60 years of age, I invested in a chair that rotates around the patient's head. Careful consideration is required before adopting this system, because it may limit the rotation of the operating microscope for the surgical assistant or TV monitoring camera, or force the rearrangement of peripheral tools.

## ANTERIOR CHAMBER CONTENTS FOR CAPSULOTOMY

One percent sodium hyaluronate is used. At present, Opegan-hi (molecular weight, 1,900,000-3,900,000; Santen Pharmaceutical Inc), Opelead (molecular weight,

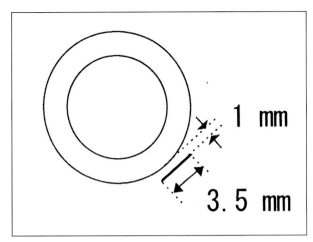

Figure 28-4. Of the practical incisions used today, the 3.5 x 1 mm linear incision suppresses surgically-induced astigmatism to the least degree. (Surgeon's view.)

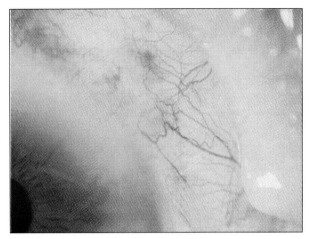

Figure 28-5. The 3.5 x 1.0 mm incision 7 days postoperatively.

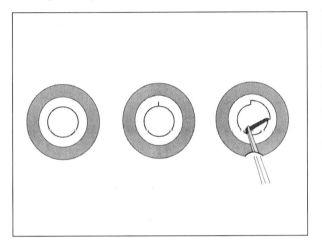

Figure 28-6. The second CCC after IOL implantation.

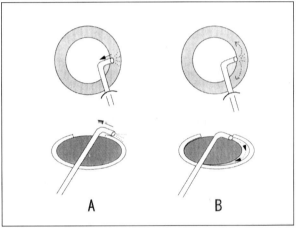

Figure 28-7. Secure hydrodissection. Liquid dissects the same plane in all areas.

1,530,000-2,130,000; Senju Pharmaceutical Inc) or Healon (molecular weight, 1,900,000-3,900,000; Pharmacia & Upjohn) can be used. There is no discernible difference among these sodium hyaluronate products.

## CAPSULOTOMY

A linear incision is made radially from the center with a bent 25 gauge disposable hypodermic needle, and with forceps, a capsular flap is pulled in clockwise to create a circle 5.5 mm in diameter. However, in case of significantly high vitreous pressure, the rhexis is sometimes completed with only a needle to avoid an intraoperative shallow anterior chamber by preventing minimum leakage of the viscoelastic material.

When the continuous circular capsulorhexis (CCC) is distorted toward the periphery, it is important to maintain sufficient anterior chamber depth by injecting viscoelastic material into the anterior chamber. When the CCC is too small, after IOL implantation, a small oblique cut is placed at the 5 o'clock capsular window rim and creation of the CCC can be resumed. The rim of the 6 mm IOL optic helps to form an adequate CCC of accurate size.

Various iris expanders can be used for small pupils. Superior and inferior iridotomies 1 mm long are an easy, practical method considering the postoperative fundus examination. Do not aggressively adhere to the maintenance of a small round pupil. A resultant small pupil following iris suturing prevents postoperative fundus examination or photocoagulation.

For mature cataractous eyes, a small dot incision is placed at the center of the anterior capsule. The milky contents are washed out with repeated irrigation. After all fluid contents have been washed away, CCC is started. Another method is the creation of a puncture at the inferior anterior capsule with Nd:YAG laser shots; the puncture allows the contents to leak into the anterior chamber. Because this procedure may produce acute glaucoma when it is performed more than 12 hours preoperatively, the entire schedule should be strictly timed.

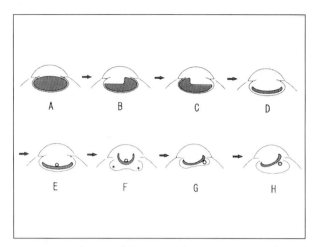

Figure 28-8. Phacoemulsification and aspiration for a nucleus of hardness 2. (A, B) The lower cataract is thinned. (C) The lens is rotated. (D) The lower cataract again is thinned; then the big ball becomes a big plate. (E) The center of the plate is held with a spatula and the irrigation is stopped. (F) Following aqueous humor leakage, both sides of the plate float. The narrow space should not be overlooked. (G) The spatula is moved to the space and the posterior surface of the big plate is held. (H) Irrigation is resumed; then the peripheral part is bitten. A large plate becomes a small plate and can be bitten safety.

## HYDRODISSECTION/ HYDRODELAMINATION

Balanced salt solution (BSS) is used with a 10 mL syringe with a bent two-step needle. The key factor in hydrodissection or hydrodelamination is that the dissected planes from all of the CCC edges should be matched. To accomplish this, the needle is moved slowly on the anterior capsular surface from the periphery to the CCC edge by spreading liquid from the syringe. Immediately after the syringe passes the CCC margin, the liquid invades the space between the capsular bag and the surface of the lens contents.

## EMULSIFICATION FOR NUCLEAR HARDNESS 2

Viscoelastic for phaco—Any economical 1% sodium hyaluronate products can serve as viscoelastic materials to maintain the anterior chamber depth.

Phaco technique of choice—Divide and Conquer (Gimbel) or Phaco Chop (Nagahara) is sometimes difficult. First by thinning, change a ball to a plate and then shorten the plate diameter.

- Phase 1—Sculpting. Phaco power of 60% and vacuum of 66 mm Hg are used throughout the emulsification of a nucleus of hardness 2. First, thin the inferior nucleus. If done carefully, the cortex at the equator can be removed safely in most cases. The nucleus then can be rotated and thinned.
- Phase 2—Division into pieces. Dividing a soft nucleus is sometimes difficult.
- Phase 3—Removal of the pieces. After sculpting, the central groove is pressed gently with a U/S tip and irrigation is stopped. This makes the anterior chamber shallow, because the central part of the thinned lens is pressed by the tip. Both sides of the peripheral cortex and the nucleus float anteriorly like open wings and a space is created between the lens content and the posterior capsule. The spatula is then rapidly moved from the anterior center of the thinned lens to the posterior surface of the floating lens content and irrigation is resumed. The crucial time when a space appears between the lens and the posterior capsule is short, but it occurs in most cases. Careful attention must be paid to this. If the irrigation is discontinued for too long, corneal endothelial damage occurs as a result of the flat anterior chamber.

## PHACO FOR A NUCLEUS OF HARDNESS 4

Viscoelastic for phaco—It is unnecessary, and any economical products previously described can be used.

Phaco technique of choice—Divide and Conquer or Phaco Chop and other numerous modifications are performed. Basically, the first division is done by Gimbel's method, after which Phaco Chop is performed. It is safe to make a deep groove at first instead of attempting a chop initially. A new 0.9 mm wide straight U/S tip (Alcon) is effective for removing a hard nucleus. Because of its small diameter, the apex of the tip is easily and completely blocked by the lens material. Then, as a result of a subsequent high negative pressure in the suction tube, the lens follows extremely smoothly.

- Phase 1—Sculpting. The parameters used for a nucleus of hardness 4 are 90% power and 110 mm Hg vacuum throughout emulsification. First, sculpting is done at the center. The width of the groove is 1.5 times the width of the sleeve and the depth is as deep as possible within a safe range.
- Phase 2—Division into pieces. With a U/S tip in the right hand and a Castroviejo spatula in the left hand, the surgeon first divides the inferior part of the groove. The nucleus then is rotated for 90° and Phaco Chop is performed.
- Phase 3—Removal of the pieces. After confirming that the nucleus has been completely divided into four to six free quadrants, the equator of each quadrant is bitten and pulled to the central area, then fragmented cautiously at or under the iris plane. The U/S power must be maintained at a very low level when initiating this procedure because the tip may bounce the quadrant. After confirming that the tip has bitten the block well, the U/S power can be increased, with care taken so that the U/S tip does not penetrate the block and damage the iris or posterior capsule.

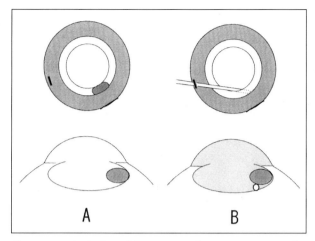

Figure 28-9. Aspiration of the cortex at the incision site. (A) The cortex remains at the incision site. (B) Pressing the posterior capsule posteriorly allows the remaining cortex to be easily aspirated.

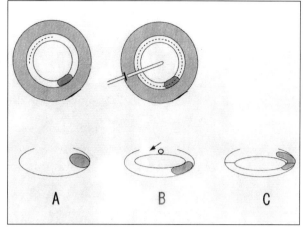

Figure 28-10. (A) The cortex remains. (B) After IOL implantation, the center of the IOL is held and the viscoelastic material is allowed to leak through the incision. (C) A part of the cortex under the IOL appears on the IOL surface. Cortex aspiration can be done easily.

## PHACOEMULSIFICATION IN SPECIAL CASES

For a small pupil, a flexible iris retractor (Grieshaber & Co) or a Greather small pupil expander is used. A short iridotomy done in all four directions on the pupillary margin is a practical choice. It is noteworthy that an upper iridotomy or iridectomy, even if it is a sector, does not reduce the postoperative visual function because of partial occlusion by the upper lid.

In a combined glaucoma/phaco operation, a hard IOL with a 6 mm optic is used so that the width of the incision is 6 mm. For safety, the conjunctival flap should be limbal based. After making a 4 mm limbal-based triangular scleral flap at the center, both ends are enlarged to 6 mm for a conventional self-sealing incision. A penetrating incision is added in the internal lip under the scleral flap, the peripheral iridectomy is done through the incision, and, finally, three radial knot sutures of 10-0 nylon are placed.

Recently, reports have appeared about patients with a subluxated cataract who underwent phacoemulsification followed by IOL implantation after temporary placement of a capsular ring in the bag. However, the remaining Zinn's ligaments may be damaged afterward and induce future IOL dislocation. Therefore, in such cases the IOL should be fixed in the ciliary sulcus even if phacoemulsification can be completed uneventfully.

## EPINUCLEUS REMOVAL

The parameters of the phacoemulsificator are 60% power and 66 mm Hg vacuum pressure.

## CORTICAL ASPIRATION

A straight or bent tip is used at 60% power and 66 mm Hg vacuum pressure. Moderately experienced surgeons sometimes break the posterior capsule during cortex aspiration. It is essential not to chase the cortex excessively, especially at the incision site. Two safe procedures are available. First, the spatula can be inserted through the side port and the posterior capsule placed at the incision site. The cortex then can be easily aspirated without posterior capsular incarceration. Second, the remaining cortex at the incision site can be easily removed after IOL insertion. In such cases, the inferior part of the optic is held with a Castroviejo spatula to prevent IOL tilting or dislocation during aspiration of the cortex located between the capsule and the IOL optic in the superior area.

Creation of another wide wound inferiorly to accommodate insertion of an aspirating machine to remove the remaining cortex in the superior area is unnecessary. Intraoperative cleaning of the inner anterior capsule has no clinical relevance at present. The anterior capsule is best unpolished, because incomplete polishing may provide the area where the metamorphosed lens epithelial cells proliferate easily. A small amount of remaining lens fibers usually disappears during postoperative one week because of the macrophages. Therefore, extensive posterior capsular polishing is useless. When posterior capsule polishing is necessary, it is best done without irrigation. A small amount of viscoelastic material is injected into the anterior chamber. After the polishing needle is inserted into the anterior chamber, following aqueous humor leakage, the posterior capsule bulges forward and becomes convex, which facilitates polishing. The proper amount of viscoelastic material is a key point. Performing a primary capsulorhexis of the central posterior capsule in an elderly patient is not an indispensable procedure.

## ENLARGEMENT OF THE INCISION

A hockey stick type diamond knife (KM510 angled crescent knife, KOI,) is used to enlarge the 3.2 mm incision to 6.0 mm in cases of PMMA IOL insertion. When a soft IOL is implanted, the wound is enlarged to 3.5 mm

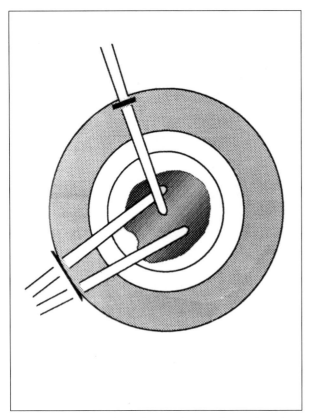

Figure 28-11. If the soft acrylic IOL does not flatten after releasing the IOL forceps; the top of the IOL is pressed backward with the spatula.

with a Lancet knife (3.5 mm wide-angled Alcon Ophthalmic slit knife, Alcon).

## VISCOELASTIC FOR IOL IMPLANTATION

As described previously, any 1% sodium hyaluronate product can be used.

## IOL IMPLANTATION

I use a 12 mm long foldable lens with 6 mm acrylic optic (AcrySof, Alcon) or an 11 to 13 mm long IOL with a 6 mm PMMA optic (Menicon Co). Both are Sinskey type and their loops are angulated forward 15°. All patients under age 30 receive hard IOLs. In patients over age 30, foldable IOLs are used for the cases with 1 D or less of preoperative astigmatism, and hard IOLs are used for those with more than 1 D. In patients who have preoperative astigmatism of more than 1 D, using a soft IOL defeats the benefits of a small incision.

AcrySof lenses are inserted with their accessory forceps. They should be maintained at approximately 30° to 40°C in the attached thermal unit to prevent crack formation, which is often induced at low temperature at the center of the optic. The lens should be folded slowly. Generally, instructions demand application of a coat of viscoelastic material on the IOL surface at insertion. However, this has little effect because when the surgeon begins to insert the IOL, the intracameral viscoelastic material immediately leaks outward through the wound and immerses the IOL surface. Excessive viscoelastic material on the IOL surface is rubbed off at the wound edge during insertion. After insertion, if the optic is unfolded too slowly, the top of the bulging optic is pushed backward gently using a Castroviejo spatula. The upper haptic is inserted by rotating the optic with an IOL manipulator or bending the upper haptic with forceps. The haptic's location is basically horizontal.

## VISCOELASTIC REMOVAL

In uneventful cases, viscoelastic material in the anterior chamber is removed by an infusion/aspiration (I/A) tip at a vacuum pressure of 500 mm Hg. When vitreous loss has occurred and the vitreous strand is repositioned without vitrectomy, the I/A tip is not used. The viscoelastic material remaining in the anterior chamber is carefully aspirated by syringe and exchanged with BSS bit by bit. Repeating this procedure, the viscoelastic material is removed without trapping the vitreous strand in the wounds. If some vitreous fiber incarceration occurs with deformation of the round pupil, a spatula or irrigation needle can be used to reposition the strand.

## SUTURING

After injecting sufficient BSS into the anterior chamber, the anterior chamber depth is confirmed for 10 seconds. When it is almost flat or very shallow, only one radial knot suture of 10-0 nylon at the center of the wound is required. If a self-sealing incision with lamellar keratotomy is performed, even if it is converted to extracapsular cataract extraction and the incision is enlarged to 10 mm, three radial knot sutures are sufficient. If an adequate anterior chamber depth is not maintained with three sutures, this indicates that the lamellar keratotomy was insufficient.

## CONCLUSION

Recently, many surgeons have been performing cataract surgery during the early stages of cataract development, while patients still have good vision, to maintain the quality of life. However, care should be taken. When complications occur, patients usually compare pre- and postoperative visual acuity levels. Early surgical intervention resulting from physician competition should be avoided not only for patients but also for surgeons.

# Chapter 29

# PERSONAL PHACOEMULSIFICATION TECHNIQUE

*Paul S. Koch, MD*

## ANESTHESIA

The patient usually receives no preoperative sedation, although a very nervous patient may receive 5 mg of oral diazepam (Valium).

Just prior to entering the surgical suite, the patient receives one drop of 0.5% Proparacaine. Once in the surgical suite, the speculum is used to separate the eyelids and a small corneal stab incision is made. The anterior chamber is then irrigated with approximately 0.25 to 0.50 cc of 1% unpreserved lidocaine, available in the USA as Xylocaine-MPF (Astra). The eye is anesthetized within 2 or 3 seconds and the effect lasts for 30 to 45 minutes.

## PHACOEMULSIFICATOR

I use the Storz Premier phacoemulsification machine for several reasons. The Venturi pump is, in my opinion, the most sensitive and precise pump available for phacoemulsification. It is an *on demand* pump and it is simple to vary the vacuum levels directly. In the USA, the Venturi pump is the only one used by vitreoretinal surgeons when working at the macula because of its delicate precision. Naturally, this benefit carries over into those cases where vitrectomy is required subsequent to a phacoemulsification procedure, because my phacoemulsification machine is also the vitrectomy machine of choice.

I use a 30° angled tip for balance between aspiration and cutting.

## INCISION

I use only metal blades. A 15° blade is used to make a corneal stab incision, and then the anterior chamber is firmed with viscoelastic. The primary phacoemulsification incision is placed in the temporal corneal periphery. The tip of a 2.65 mm keratome is used to make a partial-depth vertical incision, and then the keratome is used to dissect a tunnel approximately 2 mm into clear cornea before entering the anterior chamber.

## CONTENTS OF THE CHAMBER FOR THE CAPSULOTOMY

The purpose of the viscoelastic at this stage of the operation is to maintain the chamber for the capsulotomy. I like to use Occucoat (2% methylcellulose) (Storz), because of its economy and availability in large volume.

## CAPSULOTOMY

I use capsulorhexis forceps with a sharp tip. The tips are placed on the anterior capsule and poked through it. The forceps are pulled toward the incision and then pushed slightly to the right, causing the rip in the anterior capsule to become curved. The edge of the anterior capsule is then grasped with the forceps and torn in a counterclockwise direction, regrasping the flap approximately every 3 clock hours. The capsulotomy is approximately 6 mm in diameter.

When there is difficulty with the capsulotomy, it is almost always because of an imbalance between vitreous pressure and anterior chamber pressure. If the anterior chamber pressure is low, the nucleus moves forward, putting tension on the zonules, which then tries to pull the capsulotomy peripherally. The best way to avoid difficulties with the capsulotomy is to use enough viscoelastic so that the anterior chamber is as flat as possible.

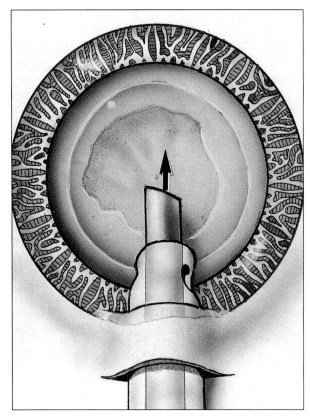

Figure 29-1. Dr. Nagahara's Phaco Chop after capsulorhexis and hydrodissection; the phaco tip is sunk into the nucleus as close to the incision as possible.

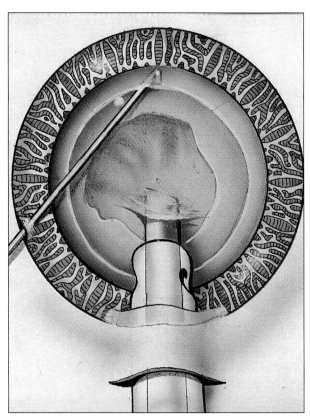

Figure 29-2. The chopper is introduced into the eye through the side port incision and sunk into the nucleus at 6 o'clock. I made my choppers by modifying Sinskey hooks; I broke off the tip and bent the shaft at an angle of 90° for about 1.5 to 1.75 mm of its length (from the tip to the beginning of the curve). Then I bent the straight part to 45° about 15 mm from the end so that the handle was in a comfortable position in respect to the supraciliary arch and the nose.

If the pupil is very small, the capsulotomy can be made only about as large as the pupil. The edge of the iris will serve as a cutting board, limiting the size of the capsulotomy.

Cases of white cataracts are a bit difficult because when the anterior capsule is punctured, the explosion of liquid cortex can cause a spontaneous tear in the capsule which extends all the way to the equator. To prevent this, the anterior chamber should be filled with a viscoelastic first to tamponade the anterior capsule and restrict the expulsion of its contents. Once the anterior capsule is punctured, the white liquid cortex should be irrigated gently from the bag using a small irrigation cannula. As this is being done, the dark cataract begins to appear beneath it. The capsulotomy can be performed more easily over this darker reflex. It is also helpful to use extremely high magnification in order to see the edges of the capsule during this maneuver.

## HYDRODISSECTION/ HYDRODELAMINATION

When hydrodissection fails, it is usually because of adhesions under the incision. I have eliminated this problem by using the viscodissection cannula described by Dr. Lief Corydon. The tip of the Corydon cannula is angled backward about 150°. It slips nicely through a small phacoemulsification incision and permits hydrodissection directly under the incision.

Once in the eye, the tip of the cannula is slipped under the superior anterior capsule and lifted up toward the cornea, tenting the capsule upward. As a result, when the fluid is irrigated it separates the cortex from the capsule, leaving very little, if any, cortex remaining after nucleus removal. This technique, known as cortical cleaving hydrodissection, was originally described by Dr. I. Howard Fine.

## EMULSIFICATION FOR NUCLEUS OF HARDNESS 2

I continue to use the Occucoat (2% methylcellulose) (Storz).

Phacoemulsification is performed using the Stop and Chop phacoemulsification technique. This a procedure which combines the nucleus preparation techniques (trench or crater) described by Dr. Howard V. Gimbel, with the nucleus rim segmentation technique described by Dr. Kunihiro Nagahara (Phaco Chop). I have found this to be a simple, safe, and reproducible means for

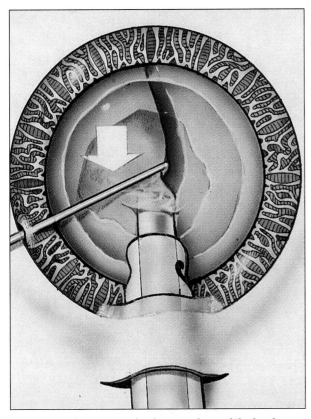

Figure 29-3. The U/S tip is fixed in one place, while the chopper is pulled toward it. This way the nucleus splits into two parts, which are held together by the posterior plane alone. If the chopper is too short from the curvature to the tip, good separation can be difficult. I find that the best length is 1.5 to 1.75 mm.

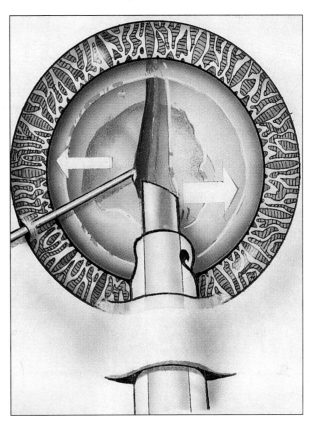

Figure 29-4. When the chopper has been pulled completely toward the phaco tip, the two instruments should be separated, the chopper toward the left and the U/S tip toward the right. In this way, the two halves of the nucleus are separated.

emulsification. Space is prepared in the middle of the cataract, so when the nucleus rim is segmented, there is space in which to manipulate it within the confines of the capsule bag. Next, the posterior plate is separated, permitting nucleus segments to be pulled away from the fornix. Finally, each nucleus half is chopped, with each motion being directed into the middle of the bag, eliminating any stresses on the capsule or zonules.

- Phase 1—Sculpting. The power is always set for 80% maximum and is adjusted by me using foot switch control. The vacuum setting, using the Storz Premier Venturi System, is set as low as possible, 30 mm Hg. In large pupils, sculpting is performed by passing the phaco tip from the incision to the distal location, going progressively deeper with each pass. The tip is also moved one tip-width to each side, giving a sculpt line of approximately three tip-widths in width.
- Phase 2—Division into pieces. The *chopper* is a modified lens hook with a length of 1.5 mm from bend to tip. It is placed into the anterior chamber and pulled against the left side of the sculpted trench while the phaco tip is pushed against the right side of the sculpted trench. This separates the nucleus into two halves. The vacuum setting is then increased to 150 mm Hg and the nucleus is

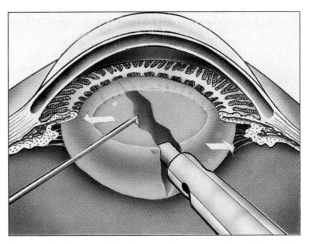

Figure 29-5. By separating the two instruments the nucleus splits right through, including the posterior plane. The nucleus is split into two, with almost no need for U/S power.

rotated approximately 90°.
- Phase 3—Removal of the pieces. The phaco tip is placed in the nucleus about one-third of the way from right to left. It is impaled there, using a burst of phaco power for penetration, then just aspiration to hold it there. The chopper is placed in the nucle-

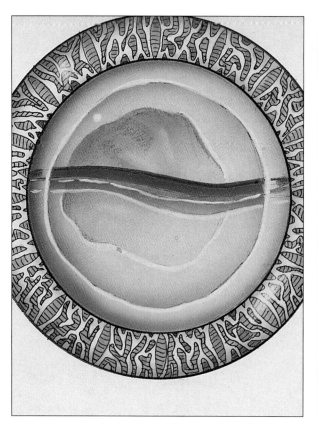

Figure 29-6. Once the first fracture has been completed and the nucleus has been split into two, the nucleus is rotated through 90°.

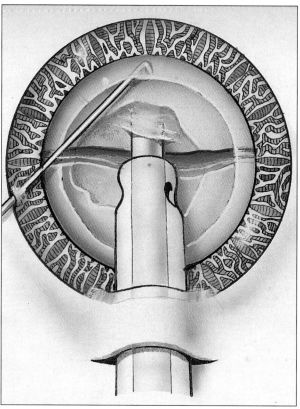

Figure 29-7. Now the two halves are split into quarters. The U/S tip is once again sunk into the denser, more internal part, while the chopper is stuck into the peripheral part, which is the softer part of the distal hemi-nucleus.

us periphery and then pulled toward the phaco tip. As the instruments reach each other, the chopper and the phaco tip are separated, effectively chopping off a triangular wedge of nucleus, which, because it is already impaled on the phaco tip, can be emulsified without any further manipulation. This step is repeated six to eight times until the entire nucleus is removed.

## PHACO FOR NUCLEUS OF HARDNESS 4

I continue to use Occucoat (2% methylcellulose) (Storz). The technique continues to be the Stop and Chop Phacoemulsification technique, but this time it is modified by performing a step I call repeated nucleus bisection.

- Phase 1—Sculpting. The phacoemulsification power is increased to 100% maximum and the vacuum is maintained at the lowest possible setting, which in the case of the Storz Premiere Venturi System is 30 mm Hg. The amount of sculpting performed is considerably greater than is the case with softer cataracts. With the very dense cataracts, I try to remove as much of the hard center of the nucleus as possible, because this is the only time when the nucleus is held securely below the level of the anterior capsule. I try to remove all of the nucleus within the diameter of the capsulorhexis. This is what Dr. Howard Gimbel calls the *crater*.
- Phase 2—Division into pieces. After completion of sculpting, I make one additional sculpt to the periphery at 6 o'clock, rotate the nucleus 180°, and repeat so that there is a division line from top to bottom. I pull the nucleus to the left with the chopper and push to the right with the phaco tip, separating the cataract into two halves.
- Phase 3—Removal of the pieces. Here the technique is different than with the softer cataracts. If we try to chop a hard cataract by going one-third of the way from right to left, as we do with softer cataracts, the nucleus will simply pivot on the phaco tip. This prevents easy chopping. The one way to ensure an efficient chop is to balance the nucleus on the phaco tip by placing the tip exactly in the middle of the nucleus half. We can then chop the nucleus in half, creating the first bisection. Each quarter is treated the same way, balancing its middle on the phaco tip and chopping it in half. Continuing this method, repeated bisection, allows us to chop a very hard cataract into a number of smaller segments which can be emulsified rather easily.

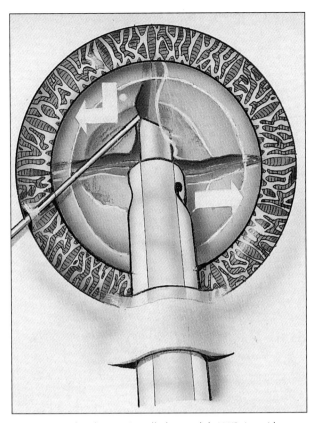
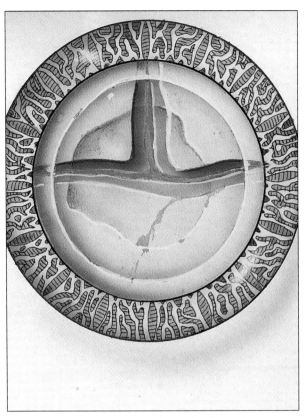

Figure 29-8. The chopper is pulled toward the U/S tip, with separation of the distal hemi-nucleus. When the chopper reaches the phaco tip, it is pulled to the left, while the tip is pushed in the opposite direction, toward the right. The distal hemi-nucleus is split completely into two quarters.

Figure 29-9. Now one half of the nucleus has been split into quarters. No U/S power has been used except for small, short bursts required to sink the tip prior to every chop.

## PHACOEMULSIFICATION IN PARTICULAR CASES

### Small Pupils

The technique is modified to compensate for the proximity of the inferior pupil. Hydrodissection must be thorough and complete, because if there are any tensions when rotating the nucleus, they can go unnoticed because of the limited visibility. Sculpting is modified because standard 12 to 6 sculpting brings the phaco tip close to the inferior pupil. Low flow is essential to prevent unintended aspiration of the pupil. The phaco tip is kept above an imaginary line between 3 o'clock and 6 o'clock and moved back and forth while digging a well into the nucleus. Once the tip is very deep into the nucleus, it can be directed toward 6 o'clock, but it must be kept deep in the nucleus, keeping a cushion of nucleus between the tip and the iris. Once a tunnel has been made, the softer tissue on its surface can be unroofed, turning the tunnel into a grove. From then on, the procedure continues exactly like Stop and Chop in cases with large pupils.

Very hard cataracts behind small pupils are treated much the same way as soft cataracts behind small pupils, except that the amount of sculpting is much greater. I try to make a crater instead of a trench because of the density of the cataract, then separate the cataract into halves and perform repeated bisection on each nuclear half. If the pupil is too small to permit adequate visualization, I stretch the pupil using a Beehler Pupil Expander (Moria), which stretches the pupil in four directions at one time.

### Combined Glaucoma/Phaco Operation

If I have to combine phacoemulsification with a glaucoma procedure, I work from the top rather than from the side. I make a limited space conjunctival flap and work my way to the sclera. I dissect a 5 x 5 mm scleral flap and then enter the anterior chamber using my keratome. Phacoemulsification is performed as previously described and the foldable lens is implanted. Miochol is used to constrict the pupil and then the trabeculectomy block is excised using a punch. A peripheral iridectomy is performed and then the scleral flap is sutured followed by watertight closure of the conjunctival flap.

### Epinucleus Removal

The hydrodissection technique described previously rarely leaves epinucleus behind, but when it does, I use the phacoaspiration mode of the Storz Premiere machine. This turns the phaco tip into a surgeon-controlled aspiration tip, with linear control of the vacuum level. If the

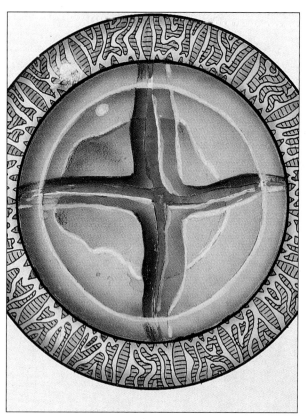

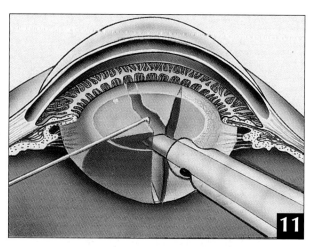

Figures 29-10, 29-11. The nucleus is rotated through 180° and the other inferior half is split in exactly the same way. Now the nucleus is split into four parts which can be emulsified. At this point, there were problems. The only split between the nuclear quadrants was the *chop* line and the pieces slotted together like pieces of a jigsaw puzzle. It was therefore difficult to separate them sufficiently to proceed with the emulsification.

foot is pushed to the right, a preset burst of phaco power is activated. I set the machine for a maximum vacuum level of 160 mm Hg. I aspirate the epinucleus and tease it out of the fornix, using as much vacuum as I need. Sometimes the epinucleus is aspirated without difficulty, but sometimes it needs to be emulsified. In these cases, I turn my foot to activate the phaco power, preset at 8%. This helps removal of the nucleus while preserving excellent followability.

## CORTICAL ASPIRATION

The thorough cortical cleaving hydrodissection obtained with the Corydon cannula usually leaves little cortex in the eye. When I have to remove it, I use a 0.3 mm tip. The linear aspiration setting is 450 mm Hg. I place the tip under the anterior capsule until the cortex is held securely, then tease and peel the cortex off the fornix and posterior capsule to the middle of the pupil, and increase aspiration to remove it at that point. It is my feeling that peeling it off gives cleaner capsules than immediate aspiration. The cortex under the incision is removed by tilting the tip in order to grasp the cortex directly. If this does not work, I remove the straight tip and substi-

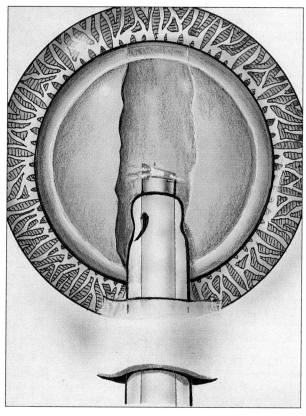

Figure 29-12. The only difference between the Phaco Chop and the Stop and Chop is the sulcus; the groove allows more room for moving the nuclear fragments when emulsification begins. In the majority of cases, I carve a groove with a uniform thickness, from the center toward the bottom, similar to Gimbel's *trench Divide and Conquer*. With very hard nuclei, I carve the center of the cataract first, as Gimbel teaches us in his *crater Divide and Conquer*. But we do not wish to remove the whole hard internal nucleus; a reasonably hard cataract is required to support the phaco tip during the chop.

tute a 90° tip, which allows me to reach under the capsule very easily. The posterior capsule is cleaned using a Nightingale curette. This is essentially the same as a chalazion curette, but with the solid dome cut off. The curette

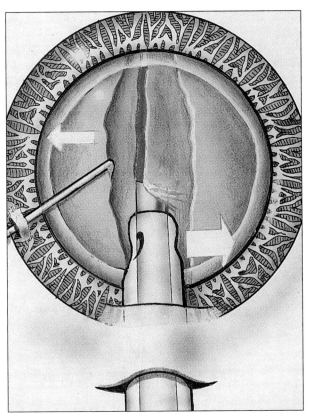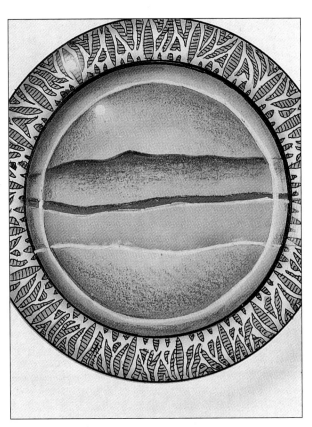

Figure 29-13. The chopper is sunk in, pushing against the left wall. I pull it toward the left while pushing the phaco tip toward the right. Separation of the nucleus is obtained with the standard nucleofracture approach. I stop at this point. From now on I continue with the chop.

Figure 29-14. After the first nuclear split, I rotate the nucleus through 90° to prepare the first chop.

slips through the incision very nicely without causing any wound gaping and allows a very safe way to thoroughly clean the posterior capsule.

## ENLARGEMENT OF THE INCISION

I enlarge the incision from 2.65 to 3.2 mm in order to insert the intraocular lens. I reinsert the 2.65 mm keratome and push gently to one side to enlarge the incision.

## VISCOELASTIC FOR IOL IMPLANT

I continue to use the Occucoat as described in previous sections.

## IOL IMPLANTS

I previously used a plate silicone lens, but I switched to a three-piece silicone lens because of its greater range of uses. The three-piece lens can be used if the anterior capsule is broken, and it can be placed in the sulcus if the posterior capsule is broken. I use the three-piece lens manufactured by Staar and inject it through the Staar injector. My staff folds the lens in the cartridge and loads the injector for me. After I enlarge the incision of 3.2 mm, I place the injector in the eye and screw it to push the lens forward. As the inferior haptic is released from the injector, I rotate the handle clockwise slightly to be sure the haptic goes into the bag. As the optic comes out, I rotate the injector slightly counterclockwise so the superior haptic will slip directly into the bag. If the superior haptic does not go into the bag spontaneously, I use a lens hook to rotate it the rest of the way. If I am injecting the lens over a torn posterior capsule, I manually cut a Sheets' Glide to 3 mm and place that through the incision and into the sulcus, so as the lens unfolds there will be no risk of it falling through the posterior capsular opening.

## VISCOELASTIC REMOVAL

I use a 0.3 mm I/A tip and linear vacuum set at maximum 450 mm Hg. I place the aspirator directly on top of the intraocular lens (IOL) and press on the lens as I aspirate the viscoelastic to try to express any residual contents from the capsular bag. Sometimes, especially in cases when the capsulotomy is small, viscoelastic remains trapped by the optic. In these cases, I place the aspirator under the IOL and aspirate the viscoelastic from the bag.

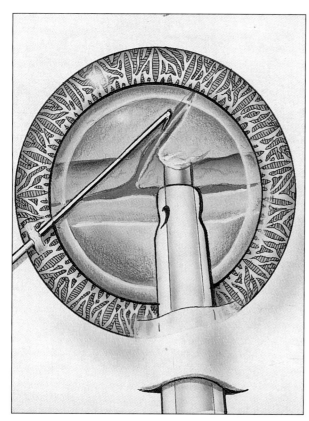

Figure 29-15. The chopper is sunk into the periphery and the U/S tip at about one-third of the distal hemi-nucleus; I pull the chopper toward the tip. That way we obtain about one-third of the hemi-nucleus. One can see that a fragment of nucleus remains attached to the phaco tip, without any further need for manipulations. The surgeon just has to emulsify and the piece will be removed.

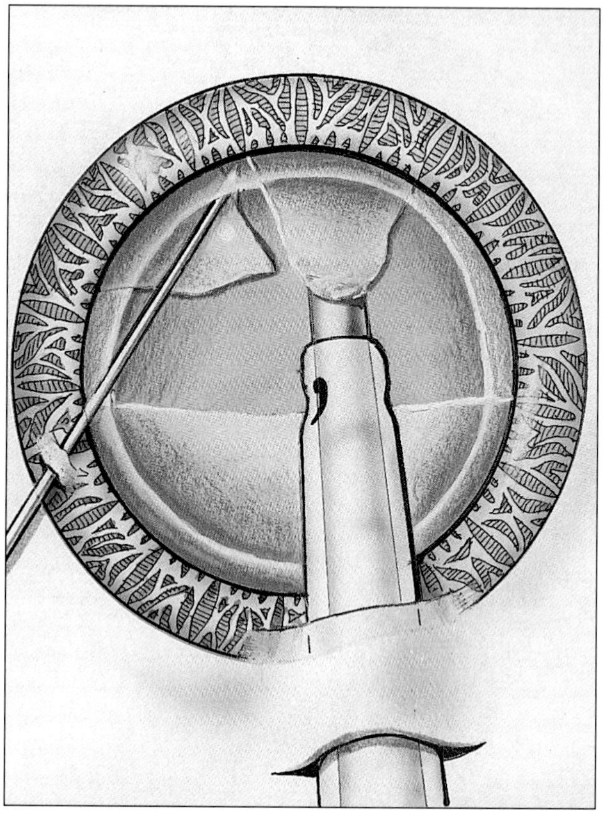

Figure 29-16. I then move on to the rest of the nucleus. The U/S tip is sunk in slightly toward the left, breaking off another piece. Again, it can be seen that this fragment is attached to the U/S tip and can therefore be emulsified with no further maneuvers.
In a typical cataract, I split each half into three small pieces for a total of six pieces. I split very soft nuclei into just four pieces, if absolutely necessary. I split very hard nuclei into eight or more pieces.

## FINAL TEST OF SUTURE KEEPING

The stroma alongside the primary incision and the side port incision are lightly irrigated with balanced salt solution (BSS). This forms a fairly secure seal, and I gently press with a Weck-cell to confirm that the incision is secure.

## EVENTUAL SUTURE

If the incision does not seal by itself, a single 10-0 nylon suture is placed and rotated so the knot is buried.

## CONCLUSION

It has been my goal to simplify phacoemulsification as much as possible. Each of the steps I have described have been defined over a period of time to make the operation as easy to perform as possible. The use of intraocular lidocaine eliminates needles, ocular pressure, decompression devices, ecchymosis, and superficial hemorrhages. Eliminating the needle also reduces patient apprehension. Operating from the side improves visibility and eliminates conjunctival cutting, bleeding, and cautery. Beginning the capsulotomy with the tip of the forceps eliminates the use of a cystotome. Hydrodissection using a Corydon cannula gives superb cortical cleaving hydrodissection, especially in the subincisional area, promotes easy nucleus rotation, and eliminates most of the residual cortex. The Stop and Chop technique is simple and reproducible. It is adaptable to small pupils and very dense cataracts. In dense cataracts, we break the cataract using repeated bisection. Cortical aspiration is rarely necessary, but when it is, subincisional cortex removal is facilitated by using a 90° tip. Injecting a silicone lens eliminates the clumsiness of holding instruments and permits preparation of the lens by the operating room staff. Sealing the incisions with BSS is effective and usually eliminates the need for sutures, which naturally eliminates the need to remove sutures following surgery.

I try to stamp out inflammation following surgery as quickly as possible. I begin using Prednisolone 1% every 2 hours for the first week and then slowly taper off the drops over the next 4 weeks.

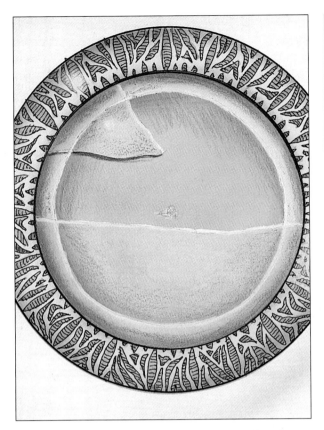 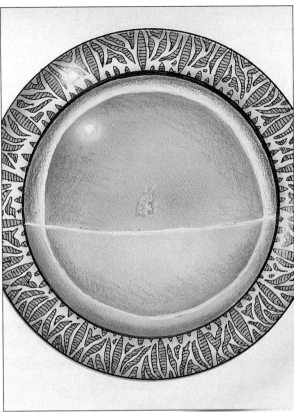

Figure 29-17. The last small fragment remains free and can be easily removed. It is not attached to the phaco tip so I have to approach it to be able to emulsify it.

Figure 29-18. The second half of the nucleus is rotated downward. Alternately, it can be pushed gently downward without rotating it. This cataract is particularly suitable for soft nuclei, which are more difficult to rotate.

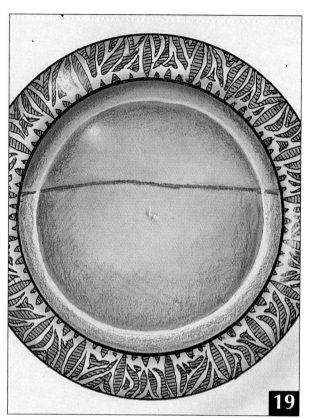

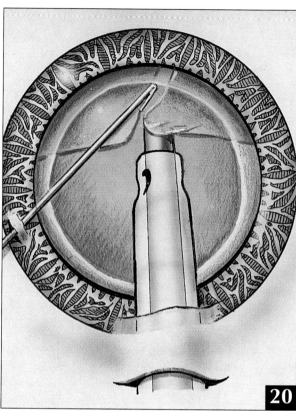

Figures 29-19, 29-20. Following rotation, the same maneuvers are repeated. The phaco tip is sunk into the solid walls of the internal nucleus at about one-third of the half. The chopper is sunk into the peripheral nucleus and pulled toward the phaco tip. When the two instruments are close together, the chopper is pulled toward the left and the phaco tip is pulled toward the right. In this way a fragment of the nucleus is detached, which will stay attached to the phaco tip. It is then emulsified with a short shot of U/S.

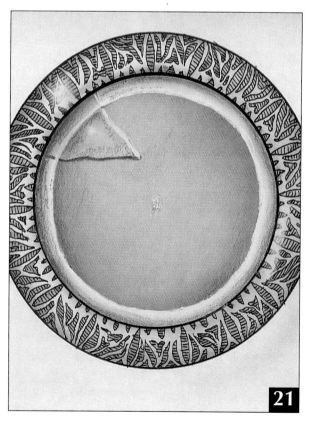

Figure 29-21. Finally, the phaco tip is placed under the last fragment to remove it easily. It should be noted that during the entire procedure, no nuclear segment is lifted or turned over. The nucleus is just rotated through 360° and the fragments are removed one by one only after the division. I feel that the Stop and Chop procedure is the safest, easiest, most accurate, and most repeatable phacoemulsification technique. It exists thanks to the efforts of Dr. Gimbel who taught us how to split the nucleus, and thanks to Dr. Nagahara who taught us how to perform the Phaco Chop.

# Chapter 30

# PERSONAL PHACOEMULSIFICATION TECHNIQUE

*Hiroko Bissen-Miyajima, MD*

## ANESTHESIA

For almost all cases (98%), topical 4% Xylocaine is applied 5 min and 1 min before surgery. For complicated cases, which need reconstruction of anterior segment and iris suture at the end of surgery, peribulbar anesthesia of 1.5 cc 2% Xylocaine with epinephrine is added.

## PHACOEMULSIFICATION IN USE

Alcon Series 20000 Legacy is used. The most important thing during phacoemulsification is anterior chamber maintenance. Legacy can give us a very stable and deep anterior chamber even with a higher setting of vacuum or flow rate. Its superior followability makes the procedure very effective; thus the movement of a U/S tip or an I/A tip is minimal and a stretch to the incision site is avoided. Also, Legacy changes the image of peristaltic pump due to its quick response time.

For the shape of the tip, I routinely use a Kelman tip (curved 30°), since the curved tip provides better cutting efficiency. The top of the tip is curved down so the surgeon does not need to hold the handpiece steep, which opens the wound and causes wound leakage. I prefer the tip with a smaller diameter. MicroTip and Mackool tip allow smaller incision size and better manipulation even in cases with a small pupil. The Mackool tip allows for a very tight incision and does not cause wound burn due to its outer ring inside the sleeve.

## INCISION

Ninety percent of cases are done by temporal clear corneal incision. For MicroTip, 2.75 mm keratome is used. For Mackool tip, I use 2.6 mm keratome which comes with high vacuum cassette. This is a single step incision; however, the angle of the keratome is changed three times. Entering the cornea is steep which makes a half thickness groove. Then the keratome is made parallel to the corneal curvature to achieve 1.5 mm tunnel. Finally, the keratome is pushed again steeply to make a dimple and perforate into the anterior chamber. The final figure of this incision is similar to hinged incision. This controlled technique can be done only with steel keratome; diamond keratome is too sharp for this manipulation.

In cases of more than 2 diopters (D) with-a-rule astigmatism, I make the scleral self-sealing incision superiorly. The same keratome is used. For scleral tunnel, Alcon's crescent knife is used.

## CONTENTS OF THE CHAMBER FOR THE CAPSULOTOMY

While performing a capsulotomy, I use viscoelastic material, such as Healon (Pharmacia & Upjohn) or Provisc (Alcon).

Some people recommend lower molecular viscoelastics. I feel more comfortable using one type of viscoelastic material through the whole surgery. I have no problem manipulating the anterior capsule under these viscoelastic materials.

## CAPSULOTOMY

Continuous curvlinear capsulorhexis (CCC) is made with a bent 27 gauge disposable needle connected to the irrigation line. The size of the CCC is 5 mm around. In cases of narrow pupil, I make a small CCC with the same technique. It is helpful to be able to see the edge of the anterior chamber during phacoemulsification. If the CCC seems to be too small after intraocular lens (IOL) implantation, I will widen with Utrata forceps. In cases with red reflex absence or with a mature cataract, I try CCC with Utrata forceps while noting the radius of the cut capsule.

## HYDRODISSECTION/HYDRODELAMINATION

Cortical cleaving hydrodissection is routinely performed. In cases with a small pupil, I may add hydrodelamination. During phacoemulsification, hydrodelamination may occur unintentionally; however, to avoid residual epinucleus, hydrodelamination is not performed.

I use a disposable 27 gauge blunt needle with 3 cc syringe. The amount of balanced salt solution (BSS) is approximately 0.5 cc.

## PHACO FOR NUCLEUS OF HARDNESS 2

### Viscoelastics for Phaco

There are no additional viscoelastics since the anterior chamber is already filled with viscoelastics at the time of anterior capsulotomy. The phaco technique of choice is Phaco Chop for soft to 4+ nuclei.

### Emulsification

- Parameters—MicroTip or Mackool tip (high vacuum casset)
- Maximum power—50%.
- Aspiration flow—Position 2: 25 cc/min; Position 3: 20 cc/min.
- Vacuum limit—200 mm Hg.
- Bottle height—75 cm.

During the procedure, I usually do not change the settings since the Phaco Chop technique does not need central sculpting, and holding power is essential.

Surface cortex is at first aspirated for visualization. I do not perform central sculpting except with very hard blunescent nuclei. The U/S tip digs into the center of the nucleus and holds with Position 2 of the foot switch, which can easily occlude the tip with the nucleus. The lens is chopped with a phaco chopper from the 6 o'clock to 12 o'clock position. Then the lens is turned 90° and a second chop is made in the same manner. For 1+ to 3+ nuclei, I make four sections of nucleus. The first quarter of the quadrant is then aspirated and emulsified. The lens is turned again and the next quarter of the quadrant is easily made by divided manner with the phaco chopper. Only half of the size of the lens remains, and it is chopped into two pieces. Each quarter of the quadrant is aspirated and emulsified. For aspiration of quadrant pieces, the holding power is also necessary, and high vacuum is helpful.

## PHACO FOR NUCLEUS OF HARDNESS 4

### Emulsification

- Maximum power—90%.

The other parameters are the same as phaco for a nucleus of hardness 2.

For a very hard nucleus, I make central sculpting a rather wide area, so that a dense nucleus will not move around and touch the corneal endothelium. After sculpting, the lens is chopped into six or eight pieces instead of four pieces in same manner. During this procedure, a phaco chopper is also used to keep away the nucleus fragment from corneal endothelium.

## PHACOEMULSIFICATION IN PARTICULAR CASES

### Small Pupil

I prefer to use the curved tip of Dr. Charles D. Kelman, especially in a case with a small pupil. Since the top of the tip is curved down, one can keep the tip away from the iris. I do not use an iris retractor. If the pupil is wider than diameter of the phaco tip, phacoemulsification is possible with help of some hook. With the phaco chopper or any type of hook one can stretch or protect the iris. A tip with smaller diameter, such as MicroTip or Mackool tip, is very helpful.

### Corneal Opacities

In the past, if a cataract was accompanied by corneal opacity, the use of phacoemulsification was not encouraged. But with a stable anterior chamber and efficient emulsification, phacoemulsification has become much safer, and with help of viscoelastics, one can protect corneal endothelium during the procedure. I get a high percentage of cataract patients with corneal disease because there is an eye bank as well as a corneal transplant center in the hospital where I practice.

I always try CCC; however, if corneal opacity is too dense, I convert to a can opener technique. For these special cases, I try not only hydrodissection, but also hydrodelamination to loosen the lens fragments for better manipulation. If the lens fragments are not free from the capsule or epinucleus, additional viscoelastics are injected to delaminate. During phacoemulsification, if one has a problem manipulating nuclear fragments, viscoelastics can be added anytime. If the surgeon is patient enough to repeat this procedure, phacoemulsification is possible even with dense corneal opacity and can provide the big advantage of small incision surgery.

## EPINUCLEUS REMOVAL

- Parameters—Same as phaco for the nucleus.

Since hydrodelamination is avoided, the epinucleus is usually aspirated with the nucleus quadrant. Even if a thick epinucleus remains, a MicroTip or Mackool tip can act like I/A cannula since the aspiration port is smaller and makes effective aspiration of the epinucleus. Also, with a high vacuum setting, once the tip is occluded with the epinucleus, most of the epinucleus comes to the aspiration port at once.

## CORTICAL ASPIRATION

- Aspiration flow—25 cc/min.
- Vacuum limit—500 mm Hg.

A curved I/A cannula with a silicone sleeve is used. I put the tip under the edge of CCC and move it along the capsule opening. With this technique, most cortex comes together, and minimum movement of the I/A tip is required. The cortex at the incision site can be easily aspirated with a curved tip. However, the disadvantage of not using a second cannula from another side port is the effect on the incision site.

For cleaning of the posterior capsule, the capsule vacuum mode is used and safely cleaned with I/A tip. If obvious opacity remains even after this cleaning, posterior CCC is made with a Utrata forceps following IOL implantation.

## ENLARGEMENT OF INCISION

I am mainly using a foldable IOL and enlargement is necessary to implant the AcrySof lens (Alcon). The MA30, whose optic diameter is 5.5 mm, can be implanted through 3.2 mm incision; however, I prefer to implant an MA60 whose optic diameter is 6.0 mm. A 4.1 mm keratome (Alcon) is used and can enlarge the incision with a very smooth cutting edge.

## VISCOELASTIC FOR IOL IMPLANT

Healon (Pharmacia & Upjohn) or Provisc (Alcon) is used. Among these two materials, there is no big difference in the ability to keep the anterior chamber. For the AcrySof lens, I prefer to have a very deep chamber and viscoelastics of high molecule.

## IOL IMPLANT

- A foldable IOL is preferable for clear corneal incision.
- AcrySof is mainly used, then silicone IOL.
- Acrylic, Alcon, AcrySof MA60BM, diameter 6.0 mm.
- Silicone, Allergan AMO, SI30, diameter 6.0 mm.
- A PMMA IOL is implanted if the IOL power is not suitable with a foldable IOL, such as very low power.

The reason I prefer the AcrySof is the low rate of capsular opacification (both anterior and posterior) and less postoperative inflammation.

## METHOD OF FOLDING AND INSERTION

- AcrySof—For the folding lens, use folding forceps; for insertion of the AcrySof, use forceps (PMS).
- Silicone—Fine's holding block is used to fold, and Fine's universal II forceps is used to hold the lens.

## VISCOELASTIC REMOVAL

I/A MAX mode is used.

From the incision site, the I/A cannula is inserted and put over the IOL, and viscoelastics are aspirated for 10 seconds. At the end of aspiration, the IOL is slightly pushed with the I/A cannula to release the remained viscoelastics behind the IOL.

## FINAL TEST OF SEALING INCISION

Fulfill the BSS into the anterior chamber from aside port incision. Check if any leakage comes through the incision. If the incision is sealed, hydration is not performed.

## CONCLUSION

The techniques of CCC and hydrodissection have made cataract surgery more safer and effective. With the introduction of a new series of Legacy, our abilities have spread to very complicated cases where phacoemulsification was not possible before. Also, a smaller incision with a foldable IOL showed its great advantage, and with AcrySof, postoperative complication has reduced. These new technologies have made both surgeons and patients very pleased.

# Chapter 31

# PERSONAL PHACOEMULSIFICATION TECHNIQUE

*Robert H. Osher, MD*

## ANESTHESIA

I have worked with one nurse anesthetist for more than a decade and she gives a wonderful retrobulbar block. Since I have not encountered any problems with her technique, there has been little motivation to change to a different method of anesthesia. In cases with a high risk of bleeding, topical anesthesia is used.

## PHACOEMULSIFIER IN USE

I use the Alcon Legacy 20,000 because of its remarkable versatility and reliability. I have had this machine in each of our four operating rooms for the past 2 years with a stellar track record for performance. The tip selection depends upon the type of cataract—a 30° round (30R+ Alcon) in routine cases and a 30° Kelman tip for the yellow or brunescent nucleus.

## INCISION

The incision that I prefer is a posterior limbal approach in the majority of cases. This incision is placed where the access to the globe is optimal depending upon the anatomy of the bony orbit. Of secondary importance is the axis of the steepest meridian of curvature, although I routinely perform astigmatic keratotomy for more than 2 diopters (D) of preexisting cylinder. I am comfortable with the clear corneal incision if the patient has a preexisting filtering bleb, scleromalacia with rheumatoid arthritis, ocular cicatricial pemphigoid, or is on anticoagulant therapy. The incision is constructed with an initial vertical groove using a guarded diamond knife (Duckworth & Kent 5-600) followed by an anterior dissection into clear cornea with a trifaceted diamond knife (Storz E0108). The incision length varies between 3.5 to 6.0 mm depending upon whether an acrylic, hydrogel, or polymethylmethacrylate (PMMA) lens insertion is planned.

## CONTENTS OF THE CHAMBER FOR THE CAPSULOTOMY

After the anterior chamber has been entered, Healon GV is injected into the eye. This viscoelastic agent is my first choice because of its superior chamber deepening characteristics and its bubble-free visibility.

## CAPSULOTOMY

The capsulorhexis is performed with a 22 gauge needle between 5.5 and 6.5 mm in diameter. Although more difficult to perform, I believe that a larger rhexis is safer and facilitates the surgical procedure, while minimizing the likelihood of postoperative problems. Yet the diameter of the rhexis is deliberately reduced in the pediatric eye because the elasticity of the capsule encourages the edge to run toward the periphery. A smaller rhexis is also helpful in cases with preexisting zonular dialysis. The rhexis is initiated approximately 110° opposite the incision entry, more central to ensure finishing outside of the starting point. The continuous tear is only modified in a white cataract where the initial puncture is even more central. If the lens is white and firm, I try to complete the rhexis with minimal disengagement of the capsule, but may need to switch to either a forceps or a mini can opener which will be enlarged and converted to continuous tear at a later point in the procedure. If the lens is white and intumescent, I will aspirate the soft cortex through the initial puncture in order to lower the intralenticular pressure and reduce the tendency for the rhexis to run. If the lens is white and Morgagnian, the liquefied cortex is aspirated and the lens bag is refilled with Healon GV. Occasionally, a scissors is necessary to complete the capsulotomy in this type of cataract, but the initial puncture should be placed near the incision since introducing the scissors allows cutting away from (not toward) the incision site. The same rules apply to the leathery fibrotic capsule.

## HYDRODISSECTION

The hydrodissection is accomplished with a 27 gauge cannula (safer than a 30 gauge) on a 3 cc plastic syringe placed under the edge of the capsule in several locations. The injected stream of balanced salt solution (BSS) is gentle, while applying intermittent downward pressure on the lens to facilitate the posterior fluid wave. Very limited hydrodissection is recommended in cases with zonular dialysis or posterior polar cataract when there is a risk of either posterior misdirection of BSS or capsular rupture.

## PHACOEMULSIFICATION TECHNIQUE

My phacoemulsification technique, known as Slow Motion phaco, takes advantage of the reduction of all parameters, which I have advocated since developing this technique in 1984. The aspiration rate is set between 20 and 25 cc/min, the vacuum is reduced to 10 mm Hg, and the phaco power is surgeon-controlled with a maximum of 60%. The infusion is continuous and the bottle height, which is adjusted with an automated foot switch, is set so that a single stream projects from the limbus to the mid pupil as the handpiece parallel to the iris is held just above the incision. The reduced infusion means minimal turbulence inside the eye and the Healon GV remains in the anterior chamber throughout most, if not all, of the emulsification. The surgeon must remember to check the phaco functions before entering the eye, and then to remove a small quantity of viscoelastic material just above the surface of the lens to ensure good fluid exchange at the tip in order to avoid the possibility of a thermal burn. Yet the benefit of Slow Motion phaco is maximum safety, because neither the iris nor the posterior capsule moves toward the tip. Moreover, the corneas appear crystal clear in the majority of eyes on the first postoperative day.

The specific technique depends upon the hardness of the nucleus. If relatively soft, a one-handed rotational technique is easily performed. If hard enough to crack, a row of anterior cortex is cleared to get the phaco tip below the level of the capsulorhexis. Then a long, deep central groove is sculpted. The nucleus is divided into hemispheres with the Osher Nucleus Chopper (Storz E612) and rotated 90°. On memory 2, the vacuum is elevated to 25 mm Hg and the hemisphere is either chopped or divided into quadrants. The nuclear segments are again rotated 180°, chopping or dividing the remaining hemisphere. The apex of each quadrant is tipped anteriorly and emulsified. If the nucleus is hard, the Kelman tip is used and memory 3 is requested, in which the vacuum is elevated to 50 mm Hg with a concomitant slight elevation in the bottle height. If an epinucleus remains, it is aspirated with the phaco tip. There are many variations of this overall theme, but this technique allows safe and efficient emulsification regardless of the pupil size, zonular integrity, or cataract type.

## CORTICAL ASPIRATION

The cortex is removed with a 0.3 mm I/A tip with an aspiration rate of 16 cc and a vacuum ceiling of 400 mg Hg. The rise time is surgeon-controlled by the foot switch accelerator. The fundamental principles include grasping only the most proximal portion of the anterior cortex, stripping as the vacuum builds, and rotating the port away from the posterior capsule as the cortex is aspirated. I strongly recommend initially removing the cortex closest to the incision. By doing so, the cortical bowl serves to keep the capsular bag open during the removal of the most difficult cortex. By contrast, if the subincisional cortex is left until last, the capsular bag will tend to close further, adding to the difficulty of this task. If the subincisional cortex cannot be safely removed, a J-shaped 27 gauge cannula (Storz E4420) is used to remove the cortex after the capsular bag has been filled with Healon GV in preparation for the lens implantation. A dry cortical removal with the chamber filled with Healon GV is occasionally necessary if there is a capsular tear, zonular dialysis, or extensive positive pressure. The size of the cannula is dependent upon the viscosity of the viscoelastic agent. Residual wispy ribbons of cortex are best removed with a smaller gauge cannula for occlusion of the tip.

## CLEANING OF THE POSTERIOR CAPSULE

Once the cortex has been completely removed, I prefer to vacuum the posterior capsule unless the capsule is extremely thin (posterior polar cataract) or inordinately loose. The aspiration rate is set at 5 cc/min and the vacuum is set at 11 mm Hg, increasing to 13 mm Hg if a capsular plaque is present. The central capsule is always vacuumed first, to prevent an uncontrolled capsular tear, as in the rare instance of a burred tip. Occasionally, I will use a 27 or 30 gauge cannula to vacuum off a dense plaque. Another trick, called the minimal aspiration technique, is useful when the posterior capsule is especially fragile or spidery. I will vacuum during a staccato depression and release of the foot pedal, preventing the vacuum from building up too high as the tip is moved back and forth quickly across the posterior capsule.

## ENLARGEMENT OF THE INCISION AND IMPLANTATION OF THE IOL

After filling the capsular bag with Healon GV, the wound is enlarged to 3.5 mm with a diamond keratome if a 6.0 mm hydrogel or acrylic optic is to be implanted. I prefer a foldable IOL with PMMA haptics in the majority of my cases. If a larger 6.0 mm PMMA optic has been selected for any number of reasons, the wound is enlarged with the trifaceted diamond knife and the incision size is confirmed with the Osher Internal Caliper (Storz #2419). The soft lens is folded from 6 to 12 o'clock using an Osher platform with titanium mushrooms (Duckworth & Kent) with the Seibel-Osher Folding Forceps (Duckworth & Kent) and inserted with a titanium Osher Lens Forceps (Storz). Once the leading haptic and the optic are within the capsular bag, an Osher Y-Hook (Storz E0577) is placed into the crotch of the trailing haptic/optic junction and rotated into the bag. A one-piece PMMA lens is implanted by controlling the trailing haptic with an Osher Biangle Hook (Storz E0573MNI), which is placed into the eyelet and released in the bag. Regardless of the IOL type, the optic is rotated until the lens appears to be well-centered.

## VISCOELASTIC REMOVAL AND CLOSURE

Complete removal of the viscoelastic is especially easy with Healon GV. I place a 27 gauge cannula on a 3 cc plastic syringe filled with 1 cc of BSS solution behind the optic and aspirate the Healon GV, which readily follows itself into the cannula until all is gone. I reinject a portion of the viscoelastic in front of the optic to deepen the anterior chamber before withdrawing the cannula. Miochol is instilled to constrict the pupil and confirm optimal centration of the IOL. The watertightness of the 3.5 mm wound is confirmed and the incision is left sutureless. A single horizontal 10-0 nylon suture is passed to assure a watertight closure of the 6.0 mm incision. A miniature I/A tip (Storz E4973) is placed into the anterior chamber and the remaining Healon GV is completely removed and exchanged for BSS solution. The conjunctiva is reapproximated with the coaptation cautery and any elevated tissue is trimmed flush to prevent a foreign body sensation on the first postoperative day.

## CONCLUSION

In conclusion, my practice is limited to cataract practice by referral only and I have a high percentage of one-eyed or otherwise challenging patients. I believe that the procedure described above offers the patient an extremely safe, modern, yet time-tested operation.

# Chapter 32

# PERSONAL TECHNIQUE FOR CATARACT SURGERY

*Donald N. Serafano, MD*

## INTRODUCTION

In 1976, I began doing cataract surgery. At that time, intracapsular extraction was the most popular technique. Extracapsular was done by some progressive surgeons, and phaco was done by very few. Intraocular lens (IOL) implants were of the iris suture or Binkhorst two-loop or four-loop design. Over the past 20 years, phaco machines have been updated, phaco techniques have changed, new IOL designs have made the implantation safer, and outcomes have improved. Today we are discussing topical anesthesia, fine points of fluid dynamics, viscoelastics, and foldable lens designs. The excitement of cataract surgery continues for me and I do not see an end in sight. As long as there are surgeons, patients, research, development, and biomedical engineers, we will make progress for the sake of better patient care.

## ANESTHESIA

Topical anesthesia is surgeon dependent. If the surgeon feels comfortable talking and reassuring the patient, then 95% of patients will tolerate being awake and aware of the surgical procedure. Pain is not a factor; it is psychological. The surgeon must be confident of his or her ability and the patient must feel confidence in the surgeon. With this in mind, I have written my current protocol for cataract anesthesia.

## PHACOEMULSIFIER, TIP, AND SLEEVE

I use the Alcon Legacy 20,000, MicroTip and sleeve, MaxVac cassette, or Mackool system.

The Legacy has easy, reliable set up for operating room personnel. The memory is capable of many settings for each surgeon. The dynamic range of fluidics allows for vacuum from 10 to 300 mm Hg with safety. Emulsification takes place at relatively low powers. My average power is from 18 to 25%. This dynamic range of fluidics lets the surgeon individualize the settings based on the phase of cataract removal, ie, sculpting, quadrant management, and chopping, and also individualize the settings based on the grade of the nucleus.

My tip choice is the 45° bevel with a 20° bent Kelman MicroTip. This allows for visibility and maneuverability in the anterior and posterior chambers. The sleeve fits closely to the tip so that insertion is safe and Descemet's membrane is not damaged.

## INCISION

Diamond blades cut tissue cleaner and are more exact than stainless steel. My initial groove is near clear cornea, temporal approach. The corneal groove is made 300 μm in depth. A side port is made. Then viscoelastic is placed in the anterior chamber. For a MicroTip a 2.8 mm diamond keratome is used, and a 2.6 mm diamond keratome is used for the Mackool tip.

This type of incision is later opened to 3.5 mm for IOL insertion. Vector analysis demonstrates that 0.8 D of predictable with-the-rule astigmatism is induced. There is very little variation in the direction and magnitude of the surgically induced corneal astigmatic vector.

## CONTENTS OF THE CHAMBER FOR THE CAPSULOTOMY

For continuous curvilinear capsulorhexis (CCC), it is important to have the pressure in the anterior chamber exceed the vitreous pressure. This will keep the anterior capsule flat in the iris plane and prevent the CCC from tearing peripherally because of posterior pressure. In order to accomplish this, I use Viscoat, which is a highly retentive viscoelastic that stays in the anterior chamber.

## CAPSULOTOMY

With the anterior chamber filled with Viscoat, the corneal groove is opened with the diamond keratome. A preformed 25 G cystotome is used to open the capsule from center to periphery in a curved arc. Once the radius and curve are established, an Utrata forceps is used to complete the CCC. This is best accomplished by swinging the peripheral tear around the radial length that was first established. The CCC should be 5 to 6.5 mm in diameter. If the CCC tears peripherally and cannot be retrieved, then scissors may be used to finish the rhexis. With small pupils, it is best to first enlarge the pupil using either stretching techniques, sphincterotomies, or iris retractor hooks. If the rhexis is too small, it is possible to enlarge the CCC after the IOL is in the capsular bag by doing a secondary CCC. Make a cut with scissors into the edge of the capsule and use a Utrata forceps to create a larger CCC.

## HYDRODISSECTION/ HYDRODELINEATION

I consistently do hydrodissection to free the nucleus from the capsular bag. The only exception is a congenital posterior polar cataract, because hydrodissection can tear the posterior capsule (if the posterior chamber is too adherent to the lens material. A 26 G cannula either round or flat attached to a 5 cc balanced salt solution (BSS) filled syringe is used for dissection and delamination. If the nucleus is Grade 3 or 4, then the lamellae may no longer exist, making delamination impossible. However, in a Grade 1 or 2 nucleus, delamination creates an epinuclear layer that protects the posterior chamber during emulsification of the nucleus.

## VISCOELASTIC FOR PHACOEMULSIFICATION FOR A NUCLEUS OF HARDNESS 2

During phaco I want a viscoelastic that protects the endothelium. Viscoat does remain as a protective barrier during emulsification regardless of the fluidic Parameters. After making the side port incision, I replace the aqueous with Viscoat. It is rare that additional Viscoat is necessary during phaco, except when a Viscoat *sandwich* is created around a nuclear fragment that can potentially damage the endothelium or the posterior capsule.

## PHACO TECHNIQUE

Normal approach is a type of Divide and Conquer technique. The MicroTip and MaxVac cassette or Mackool system are preferred.
- Phase 1—Sculpting. I create a groove proximal to distal within the delaminated nucleus as deep as possible. The bent Kelman tip allows for subincisional grooving. The width of the groove is adequate for the tip and sleeve. Phaco sweep is then done right and left to create a cross.
- Phase 2—Division into pieces. A second instrument is used to facilitate cracking into four quadrants. Using the phaco tip and a Drysdale (Katena) spatula, the proximal/distal groove is cracked to create two hemispheres. Then the cross grooves are cracked to create four quadrants. Rotation of the nucleus has not been necessary to this point.
- Phase 3—Removal of the pieces. Choose a quadrant that is completely free and ultrasound (U/S) into the material until the occlusion bell is heard. Then bring the quadrant into a safe central position and emulsify it. This is repeated for each quadrant. When emulsifying the last quadrant, I use pulse mode at eight to 10 pulses. This keeps the last quadrant on the tip instead of moving freely in the anterior or posterior chambers.

## PHACO FOR A NUCLEUS OF HARDNESS 4

### Viscoelastic for Phaco

Again, I use Viscoat for the same reasons as for hardness 2, ie, to coat and protect the endothelium. If the phaco is prolonged because of the size and/or hardness of the nucleus, then additional Viscoat may be added to insure adequate protection.

Phaco technique is either Divide and Conquer and/or Phaco Chop using the 45° Kelman MicroTip and MaxVac cassette or Mackool system. The thermal insulation on the Mackool phaco tip is beneficial with a hard nucleus because higher average phaco power and phaco time will be necessary.
- Phase 1—Sculpting. I create wider grooves with a central crater in order to debulk the nucleus. The grooves usually require rotation of the nucleus several times in order to make the grooves as deep as possible. The grooves are extended more peripherally because there may be no lamellae or epinuclear layer.
- Phase 2—Division into pieces. The Drysdale second instrument and the phaco tip are used to crack the nucleus. The instruments may have to be repositioned several times to complete the cracks and to free the quadrants.
- Phase 3—Removal of pieces. Find a quadrant that is free and tilt the apex of the piece up away from the posterior capsule This can be accomplished by using the phaco tip and a second instrument. When the apex is away from the posterior capsule remove the apex until the quadrant looks crescent shaped. If the equatorial portion of the quadrant is too large, then a Phaco Chop technique is used to divide the remaining portion of the quadrant into smaller pieces. Each piece is emulsified as it is frac-

tured away from the main portion. The same steps are followed for each subsequent quadrant until they are all removed. The last quadrant is the most critical. At this point, the quadrant can tumble and potentially damage the posterior capsule or the endothelium. The phaco can be set to pulse and more Viscoat may need to be added.

## PHACOEMULSIFICATION IN PARTICULAR CASES

### Small Pupil

If a pupil is too small to safely do phacoemulsification (ie, less than 4 mm), then pupil management is the first step before CCC. Buffered epinephrine 0.1 to 0.2 cc is placed in the 500 cc bottle of BSS plus. The pupil is freed of any synechiae with Viscoat and the Viscoat cannula. If a larger pupil is desired, pupil stretching can be done with two push-pull instruments such as a boathook (Lester, Kueglen, Fukasaku, etc) creating microtears of the sphincter. To further enlarge the pupil scissors sphincterotomies can be done or if necessary iris hooks may be used. Now the pupil should be at least 5 mm and adequate for safe phaco. The MicroTip, MaxVac, or Mackool systems are excellent for a small pupil because the nuclear particles can be occluded onto the phaco tip and brought into the safe visible center for emulsification.

### Combined Glaucoma/Phaco Operation

My approach is a fornix-based conjunctival flap and superior trapezoid-shaped scleral flap. The entry is into the cornea but not quite as anterior as the self-sealing tunnel. Often pupil management is required. Small pupil phaco techniques are used, and the incision is opened to 3.5 mm for insertion of an acrylic IOL. A peripheral iridectomy is done, the scleral flap is closed with interrupted 10-0 nylon sutures, and the conjunctiva is closed with 9-0 vicryl suture on a BV100 needle. Laser suturelysis is done 3 to 5 days postoperatively if necessary.

## OTHER SPECIAL CASES

### Myopia

The anterior chamber can become very deep with myopia; therefore, continuous irrigation is very helpful in maintaining a constant anterior chamber depth. The irrigation bottle may have to be lowered and vacuum settings adjusted lower accordingly.

## EPINUCLEUS REMOVAL

### Method of Performance

The MicroTip allows for easier occlusion and folding in of the epinucleus. It is important to free the epinucleus so that the subincisional epinucleus can be rotated to a position for tip occlusion and removal. This step requires very little U/S power. The phaco tip serves as a large port I/A. The problem is that the large port also has sharp cutting edges and evacuation of the epinucleus can occur rapidly. Careful attention of the position of the posterior capsule is necessary. If it is perceived as too dangerous to remove the subincisional epinucleus, then stop and withdraw the phaco tip and finish with the I/A handpiece and tip.

## CORTICAL ASPIRATION

### Type of Tip

I am currently using a metal sleeve with a 45° I/A tip. This allows for easy entry and good visibility; however, the incisional leakage is greater than with the silicone sleeve. This may result in slightly shallower chambers during I/A.

### Method of Performance

If possible, I prefer to remove the more difficult subincisional cortex first while there is still cortex holding the rest of the bag slightly open. Then I remove cortex in an orderly fashion going around the clock until it is removed. Use the flow to bring the peripheral cortex to the tip and strip toward the center of the capsular bag.

### *I/A at the Incision Site*

Try to take this early. If it is not possible to remove the cortex, then the tip can be changed to a 90 or 120°, or the cortex can be removed after the IOL in placed in the capsular bag.

## CLEANING OF THE POSTERIOR AND ANTERIOR CAPSULE

I use cap vac setting with the 45° I/A tip. The setting is 9 to 12 cc/min flow and 9 to 12 mm Hg vacuum. If there are excessive cells on the anterior capsule, an attempt is made to vacuum and clean away these cells.

## ENLARGEMENT OF THE INCISION

### Instruments

An Alcon short cut 3.5 mm satin finish keratome is used to enlarge the incision for IOL insertion. The short cut blade does not have a sharp point; therefore, an inadvertent second opening cannot be made since the tip of the blade cannot cut into the corneal tissue.

### Method of Performance

After I/A and cap vac have been completed, Viscoat is placed into the anterior chamber and capsular bag. The 3.5 mm short cut blade is placed into the previous corneal anterior chamber entry point. The blade must be parallel to the plane of the iris; then it is advanced until the widest portion of the blade is in the internal opening of the anterior chamber entry site.

## VISCOELASTIC FOR IOL IMPLANT

I use Viscoat as a viscoelastic for an IOL implant because the Viscoat stays in the eye during insertion of the IOL and maintains the capsular bag opening. Since volume in the eye is being replaced by the IOL and the insertion forceps, a retentive viscoelastic is important. Less retentive viscoelastics will rush out of the eye when the IOL and forceps are inserted.

## IOL IMPLANT

### Type of IOL

My primary IOL is a foldable. This allows for the largest optic size through the smallest incision. The Alcon acrylic gives excellent visual acuity and the lowest YAG rate of any IOL on the market today. In a study that I have conducted with 157 patients, my YAG rate is zero with up to 20 months follow-up.

#### Method of Folding and Insertion

I prefer to fold in a longitudinal format, ie, 12 to 6. I do not tuck the haptics. I insert the leading haptic under the distal anterior capsular rim. The lens is then rotated and slowly released from the forceps. Once the IOL is clear of the forceps, the forceps is removed and the trailing haptic is rotated into the capsular bag with a push pull instrument such as a boat hook. The position of the IOL is checked and found to be secure.

#### Instruments for Folding and Inserting

I place a small amount of viscoelastic on the side of the IOL wagon wheel delivery system. The IOL is then placed on the viscoelastic. A paddle forceps is used to pick up the IOL, and it is folded slowly. A cross action insertion forceps is used to pick up the IOL out of the folding paddle forceps. This insertion forceps is then used as described in the method of insertion.

## VISCOELASTIC REMOVAL

### Method and Performance

I use the metal sleeve I/A with the 45° tip. The tip is placed over the IOL and foot Position 2 is used. By pressing down on the IOL with the tip, viscoelastic from behind the IOL comes around the IOL and into the anterior chamber, where it is removed with the I/A. It takes 40 to 50 seconds to remove all the Viscoat.

### Final Test of Self-Sealing Incision

After Viscoat removal, 0.5 cc miostat is used in the anterior chamber to insure lower intraocular pressure (IOP) during the immediate postoperative period. A syringe with BSS plus with a 30 G cannula is used for stromal hydration at the edges of the incision. Through the side port, the same cannula is used to wash out the anterior chamber and fill it with BSS Plus until the IOP feels normotensive. The side port incision may also need stromal hydration. The incision is checked with a cellulose spear. If the anterior chamber stays at a constant depth and there is no leakage, the case is completed. In the event that there is a leak or shallowing of the anterior chamber, a single radial suture of 10-0 nylon is used for the closure. The knot is rotated and buried.

## CONCLUSIONS

Virtually every year the method of cataract surgery is modified in some way, either by a personal observation, choice of instrument, parameter adjustment, communication with another surgeon, articles, or attendance at meetings. Communication and teaching are necessary functions in medicine. The patients have the most to gain.

# Chapter 33

# CURRENT TECHNIQUE FOR PHACOEMULSIFICATION AND IMPLANT OF INTRAOCULAR LENSES

*Bo Philipson, MD*

## ANESTHESIA

My standard technique used to be *sub-Tenon flush anesthesia*. First, the conjunctiva is anesthetized with two to three drops of topical tetracaine. Approximately 2 mL lidocaine 20 mg/mL and adrenalin 12.5 µm/mL are then injected into the nasal lower quadrant via a small cut made with Vannas scissors in the conjunctiva and the tenons capsule 5 to 10 mm from the limbus. The injection is given through a blunt needle; therefore, the risk of perforation is nonexistant. The surgery can be started immediately and the patient will not feel any pain. The patient can move the eye with relative freedom, but sometimes there is akinesia which causes diplopia for a few hours following surgery.

Today I use a clear corneal incision with topical tetracaine (0.5%) anesthesia combined with Lidocaine 10 mg/mL. In these cases, 0.1 mL lidocaine is given intracamerally through the side incision.

## PHACOEMULSIFICATOR

I currently use one of three different phacoemulsifiers: Allergan´s Prestige, Alcon´s Legacy, and Universal. They are all worthy of merit. The Prestige and the Legacy are more modern with greater computerization and a larger range of vacuum. My first love, however, is the Universal. It is the most cost-effective and meets the needs of the surgeon once one is familiar with it. I use the phaco tip at a 45° angulation with a regular silicone sleeve. Although the high angulation may make it more difficult to occlude, it allows better visibility of the tip.

## THE INCISION

I use both foldable and nonfoldable intraocular lenses (IOLs). The size of the incisions required for these lenses are 3.2 and 5.2 mm, respectively. For the folded IOLs, the placement of the incision depends on the eye (left or right) and whether or not astigmasim is to be corrected. In the right eye, if there is mimimal or no astigmatism, the incision is temporal, in the clear cornea, and about 2.5 mm long. If astigmatism is to be corrected, the incision is made on the steep meridian as a corneoscleral tunnel incision. At times a corneal incision is required on the opposite side on the 7 mm diameter. Depending on the astigmatism, the incision is 0.6 mm deep and 1 to 3 mm long, according to Dick Lindstrom's nomogram.

In the left eye, if there is minimal or no astigmasim, the incision is made in the nasal quadrant between 10 and 11 o'clock. The incision is started 1 to 2 mm into the sclera under a peritomy and ends approximately 2 mm into the cornea. Astigmatism in the left eye is corrected following the same technique as discussed for the right eye.

For the nonfoldable 5.0 mm IOLs, I use a 5.2 mm corneoscleral incision starting approximately 1 to 2 mm into the sclera under a small fornix-based flap. First, a shallow, slightly curved frown incision is made. The tunnel is then created with a crescent knife in the middle of the cornea, and the perforation into the anterior chamber is performed with a 3.2 mm lancet knife about 2 mm into the clear cornea. Before the IOL is inserted the incision is extended with a 5.2 blunt lancet knife.

I usually use ultrasharp disposable steel knives made by Alcon. Although diamond knives may be sharper when new, I find that they do not last as long as expected. There is no disadvantage in using steel knives, and they are more than adequate when one is familiar with their use. For astigmatism correction I use a very thin diamond blade made by Mastel.

## CONTENTS OF THE ANTERIOR CHAMBER FOR THE CAPSULOTOMY

During all surgeries the anterior chamber is filled with a viscoelastic substance (VES). Healon is my first choice in most cases. In patients less than 50 years old and in complicated cases such as absence of red reflex or shallow anterior chamber, I use Healon GV due to its high viscosity.

## CAPSULOTOMY

The capsulotomy is started with a 20 gauge needle, the tip of which is angulated, attached to a syringe filled with balanced salt solution (BSS). I start the rhexis in the center and move to the right and toward myself, in a clockwise fashion. When a flap of the capsule is free, I stop the rhexis and remove the needle. A capsulorhexis forceps (Katena Utrata K5-5081) is then introduced. The flap of the capsule is grasped near the rhexis edge and the forceps is moved in a clockwise fashion. New grasps are taken three to six times or more frequently if there is pressure from behind the lens, always near the edge. If the edge of the rhexis moves peripherally, the anterior chamber should be refilled with Healon GV, a new grasp taken close to the edge, and the force of forceps directed more towards the center.

Capsulorhexis should always be performed slowly and in a controlled fashion. The edge of the rhexis should be visible at all times during the procedure, which may require widening the pupil, high magnification, washout of opaque cortical material, and/or substitution of the cortex with viscoelastic material. The optimal diameter of the rhexis is 5 mm. See section *Phacoemulsification in Particular Cases* for the discussion of the management of the small pupil.

## HYDRODISSECTION

Hydrodissection is performed to make rotation of the lens within the capsule possible. To accomplish this, I flush BSS through a thin blunt needle in different directions under the capsule. The wave of BSS should be seen in the posterior side of the lens. The lens can then be wriggled to break any attachment between the capsule and the lens substance. Rotation of the nucleus is tested and the hydrodissection repeated if the nucleus cannot be rotated.

## EMULSIFICATION FOR NUCLEUS OF HARDNESS 2

### Viscoelastic for Phaco

The choice of viscoelastic depends on the elasticity of the capsule and the degree of risk for tears of the capsule toward the lens equator. In patients with a relatively soft nucleus, my choice is Healon for patients who are over age 50 and Healon GV for patients younger than 50 years. The phaco technique I choose depends on my ability to rotate the nucleus. If it is possible to rotate the nucleus, I use a Divide and Conquer technique as described below. Occasionally I use hydrolineation although I usually do not need it. In a rare case in which it is not possible to rotate the nucleus, I will proceed by sculpting the nucleus and lifting the epinucleus. This is aided by injecting viscoelastic under the cortex to avoid being too close to the posterior capsule when aspirating the cortex or epinucleus into the phaco tip.

- Phase 1—Sculpting. The sculpting is performed under a low vacuum (0 to 20 mm Hg) with normal setting for power and flow. I create two grooves crossing at 90° angles, rotate the nucleus, and make the grooves deeper. While increasing the depth of these grooves, care must be taken not to touch the posterior capsule.
- Phase 2—Division. The division of the nucleus is accomplished with a nucleus rotator inserted through the side port and the phaco tip. I position the instruments deep into the middle of the groove, between the center and the periphery. The rotator is pressed to the left and the phaco tip to the right until the nucleus is cracked. I then rotate the nucleus 90° and repeat the procedure until the nucleus is separated into four pieces.
- Phase 3—Emulsification and removal. The vacuum is set at 100 to 250 mm Hg, depending on the type of phaco unit used. I use a two-handed technique, controlling the nucleus fragment with the rotator spatula in my left hand and directing the phaco tip with my right. The phaco tip touches a quadrant of the nucleus to occlude the aspiration and increase the vacuum, making it possible to move the nuclear fragment toward the center. To create the emulsification needed to occlude the tip, the power of emulsification may be increased when the fragment is in a safe position well away from the capsule. During most of the emulsification the phaco tip is kept with the bevel-down, and the nucleus rotator is used to prevent fragments of the nucleus from coming too close to the endothelium and to move the pieces toward the phaco tip.

## PHACO FOR NUCLEUS OF HARDNESS 4

### Viscoelastic for Phaco

When the nucleus is very hard I prefer using Healon GV, especially if the pupil is small and exfoliation can be seen indicating that the zonula are weak.

- Phase 1—Sculpting. I perform sculpting in the hard nucleus in a similar fashion as I do with the softer nucleus, but with several differences. The power is set at 100%, the vacuum is set at 20 mm Hg, and the flow is at normal setting. Each stroke with the phaco tip is shallow in order to minimize the movement of the nucleus and to prevent breaking the zonula, and the grooves are made very deep centrally in order to make cracking easier.

- Phase 2—Division. I perform cracking in these cases in a similar manner as previously described; however, the grooves must be made deeper. Sometimes I perform the cracking under the protection of a viscoelastic.
- Phase 3—Emulsification and removal of the pieces. The vacuum is set at 100 mm Hg or higher to facilitate occlusion. I begin emulsification in that quadrant of the nucleus which is easiest to move. The phaco tip approaches the central edge of the quadrant as the quadrant is lifted with the nuclear rotator. As phacoemulsification proceeds it is important to avoid the endothelium and iris with both the phaco tip and nuclear fragments, and therefore, it should be performed in a slow and controlled manner. To achieve this, it is best performed in the center of the capsular bag.

## PHACOEMULSIFICATION IN PARTICULAR CASES

In cases involving a small pupil, I begin by using Healon GV as viscoelastic, overfilling the pupil to help widen it. The pupil is then stretched with two instruments (usually a nucleus rotator and lens hook) pulling in opposite directions. If posterior synechia are present, they are broken with either the viscoelastic or a spatula. When a fibrotic membrane is present in the margin of the pupil it may be dissected and cut free. Another option is that small incisions may be made in the sphincter with more viscoelastic used to widen the pupil. If the pupil is too small or if the zonula are defective, as in severe exfoliation cases, I use four Grieshaber iris retractors. Each retractor is placed at 90° angles to each other through a small limbal incision. Care should be taken not to apply too much pressure on the iris by pulling on the retractors, just enough to create a sufficient pupil. If the lens appears unstable after the capsulorhexis, I apply the retractor hooks on the edge of rhexis to stabilize the lens during the remaining surgery.

## COMBINED GLAUCOMA/PHACO SURGERY

Regarding the incision, in most cases I use the same one for both procedures, a triangular scleral flap 5 x 5 mm and a scleral-corneal tunnel incision with one suture at the end of surgery. An ordinary corneo-scleral tunnel incision without a suture can also be used. Sclerectomy and peripheral iridectomy are always performed. Initially, the conjunctiva is opened at the limbus in order to make a fornix-based flap. At the end of surgery, this flap is sutured with 10-0 nylon in continuous and tight fashion.

In these cases, I generally use an IOL with heparin surface modification like the Pharmacia Upjohn 809, which is 5 mm in diameter. If a foldable silicone IOL is used, I prefer a temporal incision for the phaco and a separate superior site for the trabecelectomy.

## EPINUCLEUS REMOVAL

In most cases, the epinucleus is removed in the same manner as the cortex. Occasionally, when the epinucleus is thick, it can be moved forward with the rotator and then safely aspirated with the phaco tip. I always try to stay well away from the posterior capsule. In most cases, I aspirate the non-nucleus material with the irrigation/aspiration (I/A) tip.

## CORTICAL ASPIRATION

The I/A tip I most often use is the Stortz-Sheet-McPherson E 1807, which is curved at a 45° angle. First, the cortex is aspirated downward, then on the sides, and last, close to the incision. The cortex is aspirated first at the rhexis and on the anterior capsule. When occlusion is noticed, the tip is moved toward the center. The cortex is then stripped away from the capsule as it is aspirated. If the capsule is engaged, the I/A tip should not be pulled at all. The aspiration should be stopped, and the tip should be moved to engage the cortex in another area. The posterior capsule usually does not need any extra cleaning. If it is needed and the I/A tip is very smooth, the remnants may be aspirated. If minor plaques are left, they can be loosened with the blunt tip used to inject viscoelastic before inserting the IOL. Ultimately, the anterior capsule may be left containing some epithelium. It is very time-consuming and difficult to remove all cellular debris from this area, and I think few surgeons are successful in mastering this procedure.

## ENLARGEMENT OF THE INCISION

If an incision must be enlarged I use a keratome. For the smaller incisions required by the foldable silicone IOLs, I use a disposable 3.2 mm instrument (Alcon 8065-9932-61). For the 5 mm IOLs, I use a 5.2 mm instrument with a blunt tip (Alcon 8065-9656-61).

## VISCOELASTIC FOR THE IMPLANT

I use Healon or Healon GV, the same viscoelastic used earlier in the surgery, for the insertion of the implant. In rare cases in which the anterior chamber is shallow or the capsule is ruptured, I use Healon GV. The viscoelastic is injected into the anterior chamber and the capsular sac from the position farthest from the incision site to avoid trapping aqueous in the anterior chamber.

## IOL IMPLANT

As a standard IOL, I use a heparin surface modified polymethylmethacrylate (PMMA) one-piece IOL

(Pharmacia 809). This IOL has a 5 mm optic diameter and capsular C haptic which centers very well. Also with this IOL, the 5.2 mm corneo-scleral tunnel incision does not need suturing. This lens is extremely biocompatible and I use it in about 20% of my cases. In the other 80%, I use silicone IOLs; most often the three piece Allergan SI 40 NB with PMMA haptics which can be inserted through a 3.5 to 4.0 mm incision, depending on the diopter and the ensuing thickness. I also use plate IOLs such as the Staar AA4203 VF with an inserter. This IOL can be inserted through the 3.2 mm incision.

If sulcus placement is needed, I use the Pharmacia 722 C which has an overall diameter of 14.5 mm. For transscleral fixation, I use Pharmacia 722 Y with the same diameter. Both lenses are one-piece PMMA IOLs with heparin surface modification. The 722 Y has two holes in the haptic which are excellent for the purpose of suturing, if necessary.

## VISCOELASTIC REMOVAL

The viscoelastic, Healon, or Healon GV, is aspirated with the I/A instrument. The tip is lightly pressed against the IOL while aspiration is performed in different directions. Due to its high viscosity, great care should be taken when aspirating Healon GV to ensure that all visible substances have been evacuated.

## FINAL TEST OF SELF-SEALING INCISION

I complete the surgery by injecting cefuroxime (Zinacef) 1 mg into the lens capsule with a blunt needle through the side port incision. The anterior chamber is then further filled with BSS to give a good intraocular pressure (IOP). I inspect the incision for integrity while the BSS is injected and while light pressure is exerted with a blunt instrument. Very rarely a suture is required. If so, a radially placed 10-0 nylon suture which can be removed a few weeks after surgery is used. If the conjunctiva has been opened, the opening is reduced by applying cauterization. Finally, when the surgery is complete, an eye pad is applied which can be removed after approximately 6 hours. The eye is examined the day after surgery and after 3 weeks, at which time reading glasses are prescribed.

# Chapter 34

# PHACOEMULSIFICATION WITH LENS IMPLANTATION: CURRENT TECHNIQUE

*Thomas Neuhann, MD*

## INTRODUCTION

In the almost 30 years since Dr. Charles D. Kelman first developed phacoemulsification, this technique has become the universally accepted optimum solution for the removal of the cataractous lens in conjunction with the implantation of an artificial lens for the correction of aphakia. This development has been made possible through a continuous process of improvement and development not only of phacoemulsification itself, but numerous techniques around it—from the dramatic technical improvements of the phaco machines to hydrodissection techniques, capsulorhexis, nuclear fraction techniques, viscoelastics, and foldable lenses—to name just a few. This process is far from being completed; it is ongoing. Therefore, any description of a current technique can only be a *snap shot* in time, which, however, does not devaluate it. In this sense, the following description should be understood.

## PREOPERATIVE PREPARATIONS

### Premedication

I do not routinely administer any psychopharmacological premedication. Only obviously extremely nervous patients and those who require it actively by themselves will receive an oral dose of an anxiolytic with little sedative properties, such as chlorazepam derivatives.

Since preoperative antibiotic eyedrops are highly controversial from microbiological and hospital hygiene standpoints, and since their efficacy has never been scientifically established, I no longer apply them routinely. The perioperative infection prophylaxis is discussed later.

### Anesthesia

The patient is under continuous surveillance by an anesthetist throughout his or her stay in the surgical unit. The patient brings to surgery the results of a recent general medical exam of specifications worked out in cooperation with the anesthesia department. He or she receives a venous access, electrocardiogram (ECG), and pulse oxymeter monitoring.

Our routine anesthesia is peribulbar in the vast majority of cases. General anesthesia is used only in patients who cannot cooperate or who require it by themselves. This is a very rare occurrence. After an extensive trial period, topical and intracameral anesthesia have not been so overwhelmingly or enthusiastically preferred that patients have recommended them as first choice. However, these modalities are used in patients who spontaneously express fear or dislike of the injection if they otherwise meet the criteria for topical anesthesia. Under these circumstances, it accounts for under 10% of our cases.

For peribulbar anesthesia I use a 27 gauge sharp needle and 5 cc of bupivacain 0.5% with 150 1% hyaluronidase. With the patient in upgaze, the skin is perforated in the lateral third of the lower lid at the lower tarsal border. With the patient returning his gaze into primary position, the needle is then left to find its own way into the peribulbar space, using almost no more forward pushing force than the weight of the 5 cc syringe. Only gentle guidance is used. With the finger tips blocking reflux of the anesthetic into the lower lid, the anesthetic is slowly injected. Prompt upper lid ptosis and globe akinesia together with almost total freedom of pain—only a sensation of pressure is usually reported—indicate the correct position of the needle. This technique provides almost instantaneous anesthesia, as tested with the corneal reflex and globe akinesia from satisfactory to excellent within 5 to 10 minutes. Therefore, any mixtures with shorter acting substances have not ever been necessary with this technique.

The truly peribulbar and not retrobulbar nature of this technique is indicated by the fact that light perception, even vision, is preserved.

With monocular patients, I use shorter acting anesthetics so that their patch can be removed shortly after surgery.

I no longer routinely apply oculopression. This almost totally avoids the occurrence of prohibitively deep set eyes, and it is no longer routinely necessary because of the very limited amount of anesthetic injected into the orbit. What is not reabsorbed by the time of surgery serves as a very gentle lift for the globe into a surgically more comfortable position. Obviously, oculopression is used whenever deemed advantageous in an individual case.

## Perioperative Infection Prophylaxis

A gauze soaked in regular betadine solution is placed over the closed lids. When oculopression is applied, this gauze is placed between the compression balloon and the closed lids. Thus, the betadine imbibes the periocular skin and the lid margins for around 10 minutes. Just before draping the patient, Q-tips soaked in half-strength betadine solution are used to gently mechanically clean the entire conjunctival sack. After draping and placing the lid speculum, the conjunctival sack is finally copiously rinsed with half-strength betadine solution to remove any loose cells, debris, etc, from the previous manipulations. Finally, the irrigation fluid contains 20 mg of Vancomycin and 40 mg of gentamycin per 500 cc of balanced salt solution (BSS).

Finally, draping is performed with a whole body sheet with an integrated adhesive field over the eye. The adhesive field is applied over the widely open lid fissure in such a manner that, cutting it open over the globe, one obtains two large flaps that can be reflected around the entire lid margins with the lid speculum. The drapes contain an integrated fluid collection bag and a malleable integrated retractor to establish breathing space over nose and mouth. Low-flow oxygen supply is delivered underneath the drape. The model of Barraquer-Oosterhuis with solid plates is the lid speculum preferred over all others. It gives the greatest safety against lid margin contamination even in cases of less than perfect adhesive field draping. This speculum unites the advantage of the unique lightness of the Barraquer or Kratz specula with a mechanism that actively retracts the lids and avoids being squeezed by any residual lid force or tight lids.

## INCISION

I practice two basic kinds of incisions:
- A scleral pocket incision.
- A posterior limbal incision.

Scleral pocket incisions are applied mainly when rigid polymethylmethacrylate (PMMA) IOLs are to be implanted. Their construction in detail depends on the astigmatic effect which one wishes to obtain through them. The inner incision is always the same. Its cordlength corresponds to the diameter of the IOL, it is 1:1.5 mm in clear cornea forming a *corneal lip* which Ernest has shown to be the deciding factor for self-sealing properties, and it is parallel to the limbus. The outer incision can take any form between a straight line and a narrow U-shape according to the desired astigmatic effect. With the ends of the incision between 5.0 and 5.5 mm apart, a flattening of the respective corneal meridian of around 1 diopter (D) is obtained. A distance between the incision edges of 6 to 6.5 mm (I do not use larger optics) will result in a flattening of the corresponding corneal meridian between 1 and 2 D. When the incision edges are 4 or less mm apart—achieved by a pronounced *frown* or *U* pattern—induced flattening of the cornea in the respective meridian is below 0.5 D.

Technically, the outer incision is performed at about half scleral thickness with the round dissecting blade, held almost vertically to the sclera. Its rounded design makes for a smooth and regular rounded contour of the incision. The same blade is used to dissect a scleral pocket into the clear cornea, the width of the pocket corresponding to the diameter of the lens to be implanted. The inner incision is then opened with a calibrated keratome, corresponding to the width of the phacoemulsification tip.

Posterior limbal incisions are our primary choice for the implantation of all foldable lenses, which I implant whenever possible. These incisions never exceed 3.5 to 4.0 mm in length. In order to conform closely to the requirements for a self-sealing and deformation-resistant incision as established by Ernest, the depth of the tunnel between outer and inner incision is between 2.5 and 3.0 mm, resulting in a square (or close enough to be considered square) profile in all cases. Since these incisions are astigmatically neutral within 0.25 D, as the results of a large topographically controlled study in our own patients have shown, these incisions are always placed temporally.

Technically, a vertical outer incision is preplaced at the most posterior aspect of the limbus within conjunctiva fixa—the conjunctival insertion, where it is fused with Tenon´s capsule and sclera. The depth of this incision should be about two-thirds of tissue thickness in this place. The horizontal part of this tunnel incision is created directly with a calibrated keratome, which is advanced into clear cornea exactly following the corneal contour at about half corneal thickness, thus creating a *hinge*. At 1.5 to 2 mm into the clear part of the cornea, the keratome is pointed acutely downward, the inner lamellae of the cornea are perforated, and the blade is immediately redirected towards the inner apex of the corneal dome. This will create a perfectly straight inner incision. With this technique, Ernest´s requirements for a self-sealing and deformation-safe tunnel incision can be maintained for all currently available foldable lenses.

Finally, two paracentesis openings are placed at somewhat less than 90° from the incision. As a right-handed surgeon I use the right paracentesis for the capsulorhexis and the left paracentesis for the second instrument during phacoemulsification. Additionally, these two paracenteses openings offer unhindered access to every single aspect of the capsular bag with instruments or cannulas.

## CAPSULORHEXIS

My standard method of performing capsulorhexis is with a custom bent 23 G needle under irrigation without viscoelastics. The needle is bent to form about one-fourth of a circle, its tip being bent approximately 45° away from the bevel. It is mounted on an infusion handpiece which is in turn connected to the infusion line of the phaco system. The needle is introduced through the right paracentesis under continuous irrigation. The capsule is punctured close to the center and an initial curved slit toward the periphery performed with the cutting edge of the needle. The capsule is then lifted from underneath this slit, thus propagating the tear until it reaches the intended capsulorhexis diameter. Now the capsule can be folded over, engaged with the needle tip from its epithelial (back) side, and regrasping as necessary, torn in a circular fashion, until the tear blends into its point of departure.

Performing the capsulorhexis through a paracentesis rather than through the incision offers various advantages. The inner incision, which is so vital for its postoperative tightness, is not compromised by the needle working around it. Working through the paracentesis, the cornea is not deformed, unlike when working through the long tunnel incision. With the needle shaft in the lateral paracentesis, the globe can be continuously positioned and held in a position which provides an optimum red reflex at every moment.

Performing capsulorhexis under irrigation offers the advantage of a freely floating capsular flap which readily identifies its leading tear edge; with viscoelastic, the capsular flap can sometimes be folded over several times which may make orientation difficult in some instances.

Nevertheless, there are a number of situations in which viscoelastics greatly facilitate the performance or completion of capsulorhexis, with or without a forceps technique.

## HYDRODISSECTION/ HYDRODELINEATION

Hydrodissection generally denominates the capsulocortical cleavage, hydrodelineation is commonly used for the cortico-nuclear cleavage by means of the injection of fluid. They fulfill two distinctly different tasks.

Corticocapsular hydrodissection is meant to free the lens contact from its capsular attachment and thereby enable the surgeon to freely rotate the lens matter in the capsular bag without stressing the zonules.

Cortico-nuclear hydrodelineation is meant to demarcate (delineate) the hard inner nuclear part of the lens that necessitates emulsification from the soft cortex, which is amenable to aspiration only.

Which one of these two steps the surgeon will perform will therefore depend on the phacoemulsification technique used. I routinely do corticocapsular hydrodissection. I use a 30 guage blunt curved cannula with which I lift the capsulorhexis margin, sliding alongside the inner capsular face into the fornix. Then I slowly inject BSS which, in this way, will very cleanly dissect the cortex from the capsule. Care is taken to gently press on the lens content but not to over-pressurize the eye when the injected fluid has a tendency to lift it out of the capsular bag.

This will also force the fluid all the way around the entire lens.

## PHACOEMULSIFICATION

The phaco tip is introduced through the incision with its bevel downwards and with reverse flow. This will inflate the chamber immediately upon entry of the tip and thus avoid snagging intraocular structures. As the anterior incision is passed, the bevel of the phaco tip is rotated towards the cornea, thus avoiding stripping Descemet's membrane with the leading edge of the inverted tip. As soon as the infusion sleeve has entered the chamber with both side holes, reverse flow is exchanged for regular infusion.

Emulsification of the nucleus starts by sculpting a deep central hole or groove—oriented 12 to 6 o'clock—in the nuclear center. It is important that this initial nuclear excavation be as deep as possible. In order to get deep enough, this initial sculpting must be as wide as the infusion sleeve in order to prevent the latter from inhibiting the emulsifier from penetrating deeply. The length of the groove is of secondary importance. In no case is it necessary to extend the length of this initial groove beyond the *golden ring* of the hydrodelineated inner nuclear margin.

The next step is the disassembly of the nucleus into two or more parts. For this, I use two basic different techniques.

During cracking, the nucleus is rotated 90° so that the initial groove is now oriented horizontally. This enables the second instrument to be introduced deeply into that groove through the left paracentesis. The phaco tip itself reaches across the second instrument, deeply into the groove also. With the second instrument holding the upper half of the nucleus back, the phaco tip pushes the inferior half slightly away. When both instruments are applied correctly, ie, deep enough in the nuclear groove, a minimal displacement of the two instruments in a cross action manner is sufficient to divide the nucleus into two halves. The inferior half is then purchased with the phacoemulsifier, pulled out into the center, and emulsified, followed by the superior half, which can either be dislodged into the center or rotated inferiorly to be treated in the same way as the inferior half before.

During chopping, for very hard nuclei I prefer a modification of Nagahara's ingenious chopping principle: A curved specula with a drop-like tip is used as the chopping instrument. With or without pregrooving, the nucleus is purchased with the phaco tip and held with suction (at a minimum of -200 mm Hg). From the front surface, the nucleus is penetrated with the chopper exactly at the lateral margin of the phaco tip, which thus creates the necessary counterhold. When the chopper tip has penetrated deeply enough, a slight movement apart from the phaco tip and chopper breaks the nucleus apart. This maneuver is continued so that a number of pie-shaped nuclei sectors are chopped apart. They are left in place in order to keep the capsular bag naturally expanded. Only when the entire nucleus has been broken up into the desired amount of segments does one proceed to aspire and emulsify one segment after the other.

These are, of course, only the basic principles of our main emulsification techniques, which really are applied in countless minor variations, as the individual case dictates.

There is one major difference between classical teaching and my own technique. While classic teaching calls for the avoidance of tip occlusion during sculpting and the application of tip occlusion only for the second stage of aspiration and emulsification of the disassembled nuclear fragments, I opt for tip occlusion right from the beginning. Phaco power is most efficiently applied with occlusion. I therefore try to secure tip occlusion from the very first moment on, which is best obtained by attacking the nucleus surface very steeply—a technique aptly called *downslope sculpting* by Dr. Howard V. Gimbel.

## ASPIRATION OF CORTICAL REMNANTS

For approximately 2 years, for the aspiration of cortical remnants, I have completely converted to the usage of a bimanual system, using separated irrigation and aspiration (I/A) cannulas through the two preexisting paracenteses. This system, introduced many years ago by Dardenne, has been revived and adapted for today's techniques by Brauweiler. My cannulas are both slightly curved, the irrigation cannula possesses two side exits, and the aspiration cannula has one 2.5 mm opening at the concavity of the tip. This system offers the greatest amount of flexibility, versatility, and independence of the site of the ports. Additionally, the irrigation cannula can be used as a second instrument for multiple purposes, such as holding the iris-side, mashing material into the aspiration port, etc. A major advantage of this system is that the problem of subincisional cortex no longer exists. A simple exchange of irrigation and aspiration ports between the paracenteses solves any such problem and thus settles a bewildering array of I/A tips which have proliferated over the years.

Even the most perfect possible *cortical cleavage hydrodissection* cannot guarantee that there will not be any remaining lens fibers or fragments adherent to the posterior capsule. Although one can leave those for spontaneous reabsorption, I prefer to clean the capsule as thoroughly as possible. I have given up all *vacuum cleaning* techniques and have replaced them completely by forced irrigation. Using a syringe with a curved 30 G blunt cannula introduced through one of the paracenteses, the capsule is irrigated at an acute angle close to the adherent cortical remnants. This will hydrodissect them off the capsule, much like flushing dirt off a paved surface with a garden hose. This technique has the major advantage of extreme security because it does not physically touch the capsule with an instrument other than the water jet from the cannula.

## LENS IMPLANTATION

The anterior segment is now filled with a viscoelastic substance (VES). Although it is absolutely possible to restore the anterior segment with fluid or air, I now routinely use a VES. I exclusively use those based on hyaluronic acid. These are not only superior in space maintenance; Stenevi also has shown that the endothelium is physiologically covered by a layer of hyaluronic acid which is depleted during surgery and restored with viscoelastics on a hyaluronic acid basis. By using such viscoelastics, I therefore combine optimum mechanical properties with the reconstitution of physiologic circumstances.

When implanting rigid lenses, one should not overinflate the anterior segment because this necessitates the implantation at a very pronounced downward angle. The anterior segment should be filled just enough to create an open bag inferiorly. The superior bag may even be collapsed by the viscoelastic, thus creating a *viscoelastic glide* as advocated by Crozafon.

For the implantation of soft foldable lenses, full inflation of the anterior segment is advisable since the loss of some of it during the implantation process is unavoidable.

Of all methods for implanting foldable lenses, those using an injector are theoretically preferred over those using a folding forceps. The major reason for this is the complete sequestration of the implant from the outer eye by the injector, thus minimizing the danger of picking up any contamination from the ocular surface. This technique is today routinely available only for plate-haptic lenses.

Of all the countless refined devices for the folding of lenses, I prefer the simplest one. I routinely fold my lenses over a tying forceps in a free hand manner.

There are two interesting exceptions; both concern acrylic lenses.

I like to fold the Alcon AcrySof lens with my fingers. The body temperature makes the lens soft and pliable, and it therefore greatly facilitates foldability. It is grasped with a tying forceps and implanted.

The Memory-Lens is special in that it needs no folding at all. It comes prerolled and can be implanted without the help of any instrument that holds it in its folded position.

At the current level of quality of most IOLs available on the market, it is difficult to make a choice of preference based on uncontradictable superiority of performance. I currently implant silicone as well as acrylic foldable lenses. At my current level of experience, it is difficult to uphold the notion of a *gold standard* for PMMA lenses. Current silicone and acrylic foldable lenses have a performance record, which is at least as good as that of PMMA lenses. The only dimension that is lacking with the newer materials is that of track record over longer periods of time. However, there are no present indications that would even remotely indicate the possibility of inferiority to PMMA. Therefore, I currently implant foldable lenses wherever they are available for the individual patient. PMMA lenses are my choice, wherever foldable lenses are not available, mainly in cases of extreme refractions (>30 D or <10 D).

I tend not to implant silicone lenses, especially not with plate-haptics, in cases with loose zonules.

As an additional implant, I freely use capsular expansion rings wherever zonular laxity seems to be a factor.

## CLOSURE

As outlined in the incision chapter, closure is really not an issue in current practice because I attempt to construct my incisions as self-sealing and in such a way that they are resistant to deformation by the application of outside force.

The self-sealing nature of incisions so constructed is potentially compromised by the deformation incurred by the passage of instruments through those incisions during the course of the surgery. It is in order to counteract these tissue deformations, that it is advisable to swell paracenteses and main incisions by means of stromal hydration. I test every individual wound by point pressure to the posterior aspect of the incision. If it withstands point pressure at normal IOP, I leave the wound unsutured. With rare exceptions, this is the case for all small incisions. For the larger incisions, I will routinely use a suture for all straight or close-to-straight frown incisions because they will always leak under such test conditions. I use one single stitch in the middle of the incision, which is always sufficient when correctly applied. This suture is removed within 2 to 4 weeks after surgery. In order to avoid undue induced astigmatism, the suture is definitively tied only after pressurizing of the globe to high-normal IOP.

In general, it is my principle to apply a suture, whenever in doubt. I strongly believe that, when in doubt, safety is the highest value.

Recently, a controversy has arisen over how clinically relevant the safety aspect of resistance to point pressure at the conclusion of surgery is. This is and will always be an endless discussion, because it is a very subjective notion.

Personally, as a surgeon and potential patient, I prefer to err on the safe side, especially since this is not associated with any demonstrable disadvantage to either the patient or the surgeon.

## CONCLUSION OF SURGERY

I no longer use subconjunctival injections, drops, ointments, or anything else. A dry patch is applied for the time until the anesthesia wears off. Routine postoperative treatment is prednisolone-acetate eyedrops three to four times daily, replaced by non-steriodal eyedrops at the same frequency whenever there is even the slightest history of a glaucoma. Steroids can probably be completely replaced by non-steriodal eyedrops with no loss of efficiency; at the moment this purely is an economic question. Trials following rigid scientific criteria have shown absolutely equivalent anti-inflammatory efficacy.

## A FEW TECHNICAL DETAILS

As an irrigation solution I use BSS at room temperature. Using chilled solutions in my experience has not had clinically obvious advantages. My solution contains epinephrine (ie, 1 cc of intracardiac epinephrine in 1,000 cc of irrigation solution) 1:1,000,000, Gentamycin 40 mg and Vancomycin 20 mg per 500 cc. This is not the place to discuss the fundamental issue of the addition of antibiotics to the irrigation fluid for infection prophylaxis. In my experience, however, it has drastically reduced the incidence of endophthalmitis from the established frequency of around 1 to 2 per 1000 to no florid endophthalmitits after phacoemulsification in more than 7000 consecutive cases. Under practical circumstances, this is *practical evidence* enough for me to continue this practice.

### Machine Settings

It is absolutely clear that the settings of the phaco machine are of paramount importance for the entire surgical technique and course of an intervention. However, the settings depend highly on the system used, the technique used, personal preferences, and, last but not least, under the circumstances of the individual surgical case. Settings would certainly fill more than a chapter of their own. Nevertheless, certain basic principles of understanding can be outlined here.

#### *Flow*

Phacoemulsification is essentially and by principle a *high flow procedure*, as fundamentally opposed to the *low flow procedure* of vitrectomy. While current discussions may pretend that there is a controversy about this concept, the reality is that much of this controversy is based only on a difference of definitions: High flow in closed system ophthalmic surgery is, by magnitude, 20 cc/minute ± 5 cc/min. Low flow is 1 to 5 cc/min by magnitude. When these orders of magnitude are introduced, most currently at surgical courses and scientific meetings, differences will probably no longer be a matter of discussion.

For the choice of its magnitude, it is important to understand the function of flow. It determines how well and how readily material is brought to the active instrument tip (*followability*). Since phacoemulsification is a technique where the tip is positionally relatively inert—namely in the middle of the anterior segment—while the material is being brought up to it, the flow must be chosen relatively highly. This means an order of magnitude of 20 cc/min ± 5 cc/min.

Vitrectomy is really the opposite; material must not be attracted to the active instrument port in order to avoid undue traction. Therefore in vitrectomy, low flow settings of 1 to 5 cc/min must be chosen.

#### *Suction*

Suction is really a parameter, with the exception of pure Venturi pumps, not directly determined by the surgeon. The setting that is required by the surgeon is really *suction limit*. This setting determines how much suction the machine is allowed to create before quitting the attempt to achieve the preset flow. How high the surgeon will set this limit will mainly depend on the lumen diameter of the aspiration tip. With standard phacoemulsification tips, a maximum suction limit of 100 cc/min is advisable. With tips of specific configurations, which reduce the diameter at its narrowest place, suction limits can be raised up to as high as -200 to -300 mm Hg. With conventional phaco tips, suction limits of over -100 mm Hg are increasingly hazardous. This setting will determine how well a once-aspirated piece of nucleus will stick to the tip (*holdability*), a property of paramount importance in all chopping techniques.

### *Phaco Power*

With the parameter of phaco power, the elongation and the amplitude of excursion of the phaco tip are determined. In the past, the general concept had been that the harder the nucleus, the higher the power needed to be. But I have learned that this is an oversimplification and no longer valid. Increasing the power beyond a certain point—which is to be determined individually in every case and depends on the interaction of many factors, among them the *holdability* function as described above—is more counterproductive than productive. Like life in general, here too *less is more*. The repelling effect of higher powers often overcompensates the destructive efficacy of higher phaco power settings. The more experienced the phaco surgeon becomes, the less high power he or she applies, even in the case of very hard lens nuclei.

Adequate parameter settings of the phaco machines requires a profound understanding of the mechanism of action of phacoemulsification in a very basic way. It is highly advisable that every phaco surgeon take the time and effort to thoroughly understand the physics behind the powerful tool that he uses.

The irrigation system of the phacoemulsifier deserves more attention than it has generally been given in the past. The infusion side of such systems must fulfill two seemingly contradictory goals. It must be loose enough to prevent wound burns by the hot emulsification tip while providing water tightness to the best possible extent. In recent years, Mackool has come up with a system that reconciliates the seemingly contradictory requirements. An outer sleeve of soft silicone conforms to the contour of the incision so perfectly, that no irrigation fluid is lost. An inner second sleeve, meanwhile, isolates the hot tip from the inner wound walls. Any surgeon using phacoemulsification will greatly benefit from the usage of this unique irrigation sleeve system.

Another very helpful and simple property of a phaco machine is the option of continuous irrigation. This option is highly recommendable.

## CONCLUSION

Phacoemulsification, much unlike former surgical techniques, is a highly intellectual technique. Its perfect application necessitates not only a profound engineering and physics understanding, but it also calls for a highly flexible attitude on the part of the surgeon. He must be willing and capable of applying those basically understood principles to the particular circumstances of the individual case. Phacoemulsification is really a mixture of basic intellectual understanding and *a box of tricks*. The art is knowing which tricks to select for each individual case.

Wherein former times manual dexterity was the dominating requirement for successful ophthalmic surgery, today microsurgery of the eye is primarily an intellectual challenge; manual dexterity, however, does not hurt.

# Chapter 35

# THIRTY YEARS OF PHACOEMULSIFICATION: THE EVOLUTION OF MY TECHNIQUE FROM 1967 TO 1997

*Charles D. Kelman, MD*

## INTRODUCTION

According to some commentators, cataract surgery had reached the zenith of perfection in the 1960s. Derrick Vail stated in 1965 that extracapsular cataract surgery had become as "extinct as the buffalo."

Somewhat later, some of our most respected ophthalmic surgeons railed against phacoemulsification as though it has been conceived by Satan himself.

Confronted with the results of a 1994 ASCRS poll which show phacoemulsification as the preferred method of cataract extraction by 86% of ophthalmic surgeons interviewed, one can only be wary of speaking in absolutes where removal of the crystalline lens is concerned.

I began performing phacoemulsification in the posterior chamber. To teach the technique more easily, I went to the anterior chamber and still believe this to be the safest version of the technique. Certainly, it is the only method I recommend for those beginning phacoemulsification. The ease of conversion to standard extracapsular procedure when the nucleus is in the anterior chamber insures a successful completion of the extraction with a technique the surgeon has already mastered.

While my views on anterior chamber phacoemulsification are well known, I have never maintained that there is only one correct way to perform phacoemulsification, any more than I would claim that phaco itself is the end point in the evolution of cataract extraction techniques.

The work of Gimbel and Neuhann in the area of continuous circular capsulorhexis (CCC) in 1984 and 1985 piqued my curiosity. Hydrodissection drew my interest posteriorly, especially in cases of endothelial disease or very soft, difficult to prolapse nuclei. Greater sophistication in all parameters (flow, vacuum, etc) with the newest phacoemulsification machines has given surgeons better control in the posterior chamber. My own efforts in developing curved phacoemulsification tips bode well for the future of emulsification in the posterior chamber.

Though my early (and admittedly less sophisticated) versions of hydrodissection and nucleofractis are documented in the *American Journal of Ophthalmology* and in my personal records of 1967 and 1968, I'm considered, with some justification, a proponent of phacoemulsification in the anterior chamber. Yet it wasn't until 1972, after working in the posterior chamber since 1967, that I perfected a technique to bring the nucleus into the anterior chamber.

Prolapse of firm nucleus through an adequately dilated pupil is relatively simple with the seesaw technique. The potential risks to the iris and posterior capsule with posterior chamber phaco are avoided; a viscoelastic substance (VES) is used to protect the corneal endothelium.

## EVOLUTION OF POSTERIOR CHAMBER TECHNIQUE

My posterior chamber protocol has been evolving with the assimilation of new techniques and technology, as well as the reincorporation of the hydrodissection and nuclear fracturing maneuvers I used in the late 1960s.

My original fractus technique involved the creation of a central trough in the nucleus using a phaco tip with a sharp right angle bend near the tip. I used a modified Ringberg forceps to split the lens in two. Since the angulated tip was awkward to maneuver and had poor followability characteristics, I would switch to a straight tip to complete the emulsification. Due to difficulty of manufacturing a reliable angulated tip (in those days) and the need to change to a straight tip to complete the procedure, I temporarily shelved the technique.

The popularity of the CCC in the 1990s caused a resurgence in phaco techniques that involved nucleus division.

I knew from my early work in phaco that an angulated phaco tip had many advantages over a straight tip for groove creation. However, with my original design, once the nucleus was split in half, a straight tip was required to complete the emulsification.

I needed to design a single tip that would facilitate low vacuum sculpting for groove creation and high vacuum nuclear bonding for completion of the case.

The new angulated tip is a hybrid design that does both jobs well and in addition enhances cavitation effects with resultant lower phaco power requirements. I prefer a version of the tip that is 10% smaller in diameter than a standard tip.

My return to nuclear division began where I left off in the 1960's with a simple bisecting technique. I added a third quadrant, and then a fourth as described by John Shepherd. The V groove is my latest technique for dividing the nucleus. Since there is no need for nuclear rotation, this would seem an easier technique for nuclear fracture that those previously described.

My wound construction, capsulotomy, and hydrodissection techniques are essentially identical regardless of which phaco technique I may use. My selection of a viscoelastic is based upon the condition of the cornea, depth of the anterior chamber, and degree of dilation.

## Wound Construction

I recently modified my technique, which began with a fornix-based conjunctival flap. Currently, prior to flap creation, I use a technique which might be best described as *transconjunctival cautery*. Here methelene blue serves two functions. The first is to improve visualization within the operated eye, the second is to act as an indicator to help me identify areas where I have achieved adequate homeostasis. A wetfield eraser is applied directly to the conjunctiva with adequate irrigation and cauterized areas are indicated by the lack of a methelene blue stain. The cautery serves to eliminate the conjunctiva directly behind the limbus, as if it had been dissected away. I then create a flap 0.5 mm from the limbus with sharp Wescott scissors.

With a lamellar knife such as a Beaver 6600 or an angulated Alcon crescent knife, a groove is made approximately 3 mm posterior to the vascular arcade. A scleral tunnel is then created utilizing the same lamellar knife (The width of this tunnel is dependent upon the incision size required for IOL implantation). Care is taken to insure that the dissection is carried forward into clear cornea.

The anterior chamber is entered with a 2.5 mm angulated keratome (3.2 mm with standard diameter tip/sleeve) held parallel to the iris. The keratome is carefully advanced until the point of the blade is visible just anterior to the vascular arcade. The point of the knife is tipped posteriorly so that a small dimple is seen, and the knife is carefully advanced, in the manner described by Fine, adjusting the angle of the blade so that a straight line is visible on its anterior surface as Descemet's is incised. This assures the successful creation of a self-sealing flap valve.

## Clear Corneal Technique

For many years, starting in 1967, I used a 15° Sharpoint knife to create a shelved limbal keratotomy incision for KPE and PECCE with 6 mm polymethylmethacrylate (PMMA) lenses. Pressure from my colleagues caused me to abandon the corneal approach and turn to the scleral tunnel I described above. A few years later, with foldable lenses becoming the norm, these same colleagues have succeeded in convincing me to go back to a corneal approach with the self-sealing corneal lip incision. At present, I use a modified temporal-superior approach and begin by creating a 1 mm paracentesis (with a 15° metal Sharpoint knife), through which I instill viscoelastic to displace aqueous and firm up the globe. I advance a 3.2 mm diamond keratome until the angles of the blade reach the external corneal. The tip of the blade is tipped slightly down to incise Descemet's membrane and then advanced up to the hub of the blade at the original angle. This results in a tunnel length of 2 mm. At the conclusion of the case, I inflate the chamber through the paracentesis with balanced salt solution (BSS) to seal the corneal flap valve. Should the incision leak at this time, stromal hydration at the wound margins will usually create a seal.

## Capsulotomy

A viscoelastic is instilled and a Kelman cystotome capsulorhexis forceps is used, with the jaws slightly open, to create a small inverted V-shaped tear in the inferior portion of the anterior capsule. The same forceps is utilized to complete a continuous tear capsulorhexis in a manner similar to that described by Gimbel and Neuhann in the mid 1980s.

## Hydrodissection

I prefer to use a 30 gauge cannula on a syringe for hydrodissection of the nucleus. The nucleus is slightly rotated to assure that hydrodissection has adequately cleaved cortical adherences.

# PHACOEMULSIFICATION

## Central Nucleus Bisecting Techniques

A deep central groove is made in the lens to three-fourths depth with a curved high efficiency phaco tip (10% smaller in diameter than a standard tip) using 70% maximum linear power, 20 cc/min flow and 0 to 2 mm Hg vacuum. I use the phaco tip, a cystotome, or a Kelman nucleus rotator to rotate the nucleus 90° and sculpt an additional groove, bisecting the inferior half in softer lenses (and bisect the superior half as well in harder nuclei). This additional groove facilitates the fracture, vacuum-bonding and phacoemulsification of the first quadrant to be emulsified. Viscoelastics are again instilled into the eye to deepen the chamber.

With a Kelman nucleus cracker, the lens is split in half inferiorly and superiorly. With a channel dissected away in the middle of the lens, it is now easy to introduce the phacoemulsifier into each portion of the lens. Emulsification begins using 50% maximum linear power for 1+ 3+ nuclei and 60 to 70% maximum linear power for 3+ 4+ nuclei, 27 cc/min flow and 150 mm Hg vacuum (when using a standard diameter tip flow is set to 25 cc/min and maximum vacuum is set to 110 mm Hg) to draw one quarter of the lens toward the center of the pupil. Following the emulsification of the first pie-shaped quarter of nucleus, the remaining quadrants of the nucleus are very simply and easily vacuum-bonded and emulsified in similar fashion.

## Victory Groove Technique

During the preparation of a groove in the lens with the phacoemulsifier, the lens is rotated somewhat counterclockwise and the groove, instead of being from 12 to 6 o'clock became from 12 to 4 o'clock. During this procedure, I then decided to make a second groove, not perpendicular to the first, but at an angle to it, with the second groove going from 12 to 8 o'clock. Both grooves were then split, releasing a large central portion of nucleus which was then easily emulsified and aspirated. The rest of the lens simply moved easily into the central pupillary area and was also easily emulsified and aspirated. Since that time, I have been using this V groove technique almost exclusively during phacoemulsification and have found that it has greatly simplified the operation, reducing the time necessary to emulsify and aspirate the lens with a much greater degree of safety.

## Reverse Flow Sculpting

The term *zero vacuum* is a misnomer since even with minimum aspiration flow rate, some vacuum will be produced at the phaco tip. In addition, the action of the vibrating phaco tip causes a phenomenon known as ultrasonic pumping. Laboratory experiments have shown that 30 cc/min can easily be ultrasonically pumped by a typical phaco handpiece. Surgeons aware of the problem of achieving true zero vacuum have attempted to overcome this problem by simply removing the aspiration line from the phaco handpiece. This would seem to be an effective method of producing zero vacuum since the disconnected pump is not actually contributing to fluid aspiration. In reality, however, vacuum will still exist at the tip, a result of outflow created by ultrasonic pumping enhanced by the exit of irrigation fluid from the elevated bottle through the bore of the phaco needle. Attempts at clamping off the aspiration line completely result in obscured visualization of the eye due to unaspirated emulsate in the chamber. The absence of coolant flow, as would occur with a clamped-off line, creates a serious risk of overheating the eye. Mindful of this, I decided to take the zero vacuum concept a step further by actually reversing the fluid flow on the phacoemulsifier. Reversing the standard sources of irrigation and aspiration (I/A) causes irrigation from the elevated bottle to enter the eye through the bore of the phaco needle and aspiration fluid to exit the eye through the holes in the silicone sleeve. This makes it impossible to attract the posterior capsule to the phaco tip. Moreover, the fluid outflow from the phaco needle actually tends to push the posterior capsule back, at the same time breaking cortical adherences due to enhanced continuous ultrasonic hydrodissection. Vacuum is produced in this system not at the phaco tip, but at the orifices in the soft silicone sleeve. Emulsate is thus evacuated from the eye, ensuring excellent visualization for the surgeon. Optimum tip cooling is maintained because of the continuous flow of irrigation fluid into and out of the eye. Occlusion is nearly impossible to achieve since both ports of the silicone sleeve would have to the blocked. I can maintain chamber depth and, in many cases, am able safely to sculpt so deeply that mechanical fracture is often unnecessary. Typical machine settings using the mini Kelman tip are 60% maximum linear power, 12 to 14 cc/min flow and 10 mm Hg vac.

## Bowl and Roll Technique

This technique evolved as I sought a way to safely manage a recalcitrant nuclear bowl adherent to the posterior capsule. Although I typically would resort to my PAL technique it occurred to me that a properly designed manipulator could help to lift the bowl off the posterior capsule without resorting to a pars plana incision. The instrument I designed (Storz SP 7-55675) worked so well in complicated cases that I evolved a technique in which I intentionally create a bowl.

After performing a 5 mm capsulorhexis, I use a hydrodissection cannula to free the lens within the capsular bag. The Kelman mini curved phaco tip is used to sculpt a bowl in the center of the nucleus. Viscoelastic is instilled and the Kelman *Wand* is placed in the sculpted bowl. The nucleus is inverted by pushing and then rolling it with the wand. The nucleus is positioned in the iris plane which allows the posterior portion of the lens to be emulsified away from the posterior capsule. This technique should not be used in cases where zonular integrity is in question.

## Irrigation and Aspiration

My I/A is performed using an angulated I/A tip with a 0.3 mm port. In some cases I will use ultrasonic I/A or a larger bore I/A tip to facilitate cortical aspiration. I am currently working on a steerable I/A handpiece to facilitate the aspiration of 12 o'clock cortex. I like a blunt, flattened cannula on a bulb irrigator for capsule polishing.

## Lens Implantation

A three-piece foldable lens is currently my lens of choice for phacoemulsification. This lens, when folded, will pass through a 3.0 mm scleral incision or a 3.2 mm corneal incision. With a silicone lens, in lieu of a specially designed holder or folder, I simply grasp the lens with a Kelman-McPherson forceps, bisecting the optic and perpendicular to the haptics. The posterior surface of the optic is coated with a viscoelastic to facilitate a smoother release of the Kelman-McPherson forceps after folding. A Fine Universal II forceps is used to fold the lens in half, and under viscoelastic the folded intraocular lens (IOL) is placed into the capsular bag through the capsulorhexis.

I slowly open the Fine Universal II forceps to facilitate a controlled release of the folded lens. Too rapid a release can result in posterior capsule rupture since the haptics are directed against the posterior capsule as the lens unfolds.

With an acrylic lens, I use a paddle forceps to fold the lens and then transfer the folded implant to the appropriate insertion forceps. Utilization of instrumentation designed for a silicone lens can result in optic damage when used with an acrylic implant.

When a PMMA lens is used, the incision is enlarged using the appropriate angulated blunted keratome.

Under viscoelastic the IOL is placed into the capsular bag through the capsulorhexis. Typically I rotate the lens 180° clockwise and place the trailing haptic in the bag using a Kuglin hook.

The IOL is checked for proper centration and Miochol is instilled. I aspirate the remaining viscoelastic with the I/A handpiece of the phacoemulsifier.

## Would Closure

With a scleral tunnel, although I construct a potentially sutureless wound which I believe to be a great advantage in the event of and intraoperative complication, I elect in most cases to close the wound with a single 10-0 nylon suture. In clear corneal cases that refuse to seal properly following stromal hydration, I also use a single 10-0 nylon suture. Subconjunctival Garamycin and Solu-Medrol are injected.

# Chapter 36

# BIMANUAL IRRIGATION/ASPIRATION: BURATTO'S TECHNIQUE FOR REMOVAL OF SUBINCISIONAL CORTEX IN PHACOEMULSIFICATION

*Lucio Buratto, MD*

## INTRODUCTION

One of the problems that has to be dealt with in extracapsular cataract surgery is how to aspirate the cortical material below and around the incision. This is particularly valid following phacoemulsification with a corneal or scleral tunnel, especially if the rhexis is small or decentered, ie, with anterior capsule persisting in the area close to the incision.

In order to simplify the procedure, restrict the tension-traction in the tissues, and reduce the severity of the complications, a number of techniques have been developed to expose, capture, and aspirate the cortical material. However, only one, in my opinion, achieves the objectives satisfactorily—in an effective, safe, and rapid manner. I am referring to the technique which uses two separate cannulas: one for irrigation and one for aspiration introduced through two separate side port incisions.

What follows is a brief description of all of the techniques used to remove the subincisional cortex, with examination of the advantages and drawbacks of each.

These will be followed by a detailed description of the technique using two separate cannulas.

## ASPIRATION WITH REGULAR COAXIAL CANNULA THROUGH THE MAIN INCISION

The usual access route to the cortical material is obstructed because of the tunnel floor, the iris, the anterior capsule, and balanced salt solution (BSS) loss from the sides of the cannula itself.

### Verticalization of the Coaxial Tip

When phacoemulsification was first developed, the subincisional cortex was removed using a technique which involved verticalization of the coaxial irrigation/aspiration (I/A) tip.

To correctly perform an operation with an anterior limbal incision, the bottle of BSS is raised so that the depth of the anterior chamber and the capsular space increases. The handle is then brought into a vertical position (which is normally kept almost parallel to the iris plane). The orifice on the tip is brought into contact with the cortex material; capture occurs under low aspiration (80 to 100 mm Hg). Once this has happened, the handle is rotated through 30 to 40° to move the aspirating orifice away from

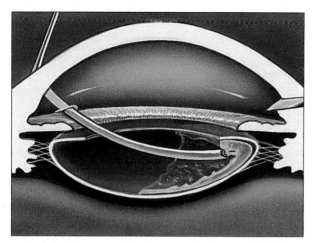

Figure 36-1. Aspiration of the cortex with the cannula connected to a syringe.

Table 36-1
**ASPIRATION CYCLE**

Step 1. Place the hole near the cortical material with the pedal in Position 1 (only irrigation).

Step 2. Place of pedal in Position 2 (I/A) and press it until sufficient vacuum has been reached (linear aspiration) to engage the material in the hole.

Step 3. Wait a few seconds until the occlusion of the hole is achieved and the vacuum rises in the line until the set value is reached.

Step 4. Pull the tip toward the middle of the capsular bag, thereby detaching the material from the capsule.

Step 5. In the middle of the capsular bag, wait until the material is aspirated and the hole disoccluded.

Step 6. Repeat the operation as many times as necessary to complete removal of the cortex.

the posterior capsule. The vacuum is increased slightly (120 to 150 mm Hg), and the tip is rotated through a further 120 to 150° to direct the aspirating orifice toward the surgeon (distant from the posterior capsule). Then the vacuum is increased again (300 to 500 mm Hg) to completely aspirate the cortical mass captured in the orifice.

It stands to reason that with this verticalization, abnormal pressure is exerted on both edges of the incisions—upward on the anterior edge and downward on the posterior edge. The former causes the formation of corneal folds with consequent reduction in visibility; the latter can exert abnormal pressure on the iris tissue.

The maneuver also causes distention of the incision with a consequent increase in BSS loss, reduction in the chamber depth, raising of the posterior capsule, and an increased risk that the I/A tip will capture and rupture the posterior capsule.

If the I/A tip is inside the tunnel, scleral or corneal, and if there is poor mydriasis and a small rhexis, it is almost impossible to use this method successfully (also because the cortex is covered by the rhexis).

## Extension of the Incision

A second technique can be used when the surgeon will implant an intraocular lens (IOL) which requires a wide opening (polymethylmethacrylate [PMMA]). This technique involves extending the incision to the size suitable for the IOL and first inserting the I/A tip at the extreme right to aspirate the cortex situated in the sector on the left, and then on the extreme left to aspirate the cortex on the right.

The technique is difficult. As the incision is wide, a considerable amount of BSS will escape and the chamber will flatten. It is therefore difficult to capture the material, particularly if there is poor mydriasis or small rhexis, or even if the surgeon uses a spatula, introduced through the side port incision, to retract the iris.

## Mobilization of the Cortex with Manual Aspiration

A third technique consists of capturing the cortical material by aspiration exerted by a thin cannula connected to a syringe containing BSS (manual I/A) and mobilizing the mass. In this case, the cannula has an orifice in the tip. The mass is then aspirated with a coaxial I/A cannula inserted through a side port incision.

Some BSS is injected to deepen the chamber; the cannula's orifice then approaches the material. Using the piston of the syringe, the surgeon exerts strong aspiration to occlude the orifice with the material and capture it. The cannula is then drawn toward the center of the chamber in order to detach the cortex from the capsular adhesions or the remainder of the material. When the particular sector of cortex is detached, aspiration is interrupted and the surgeon irrigates slightly to free the orifice and mobilize the material in the chamber. This maneuver is repeated three to four times until enough quantity of material has been mobilized. The surgeon then enters the chamber with a classic coaxial I/A tip and the free material in the chamber is aspirated. This will also increase the visibility if the maneuver of mobilization has to be repeated.

Attempting to aspirate the material inside the syringe is not productive for a number of reasons. It is difficult because this procedure uses a thin cannula and the material will not pass through. Also as the surgeon has to use considerable aspirating force, the passage of the cortical mass can suddenly draw fluid out and flatten the chamber.

This procedure allows the surgeon to capture very small pieces of material in each phase. If there is a large amount of material, this technique will have to be repeated. Nevertheless, if performed patiently, the technique will provide the surgeon with the desired results. It is time-consuming, particularly if there is a large amount of material or if the material is very adherent. In addition, as this technique can be difficult, it should only be used to remove small quantities of cortex.

## Technique Using Viscoelastic

Another technique involves the use of viscoelastic substance (VES) to mobilize and capture the cortex. The procedure involves aspirating all the cortex which can be easily reached and aspirated (the sectors which are distal and lateral to the tunnel), leaving the non-removable

Table 36-2
## I/A USE OF THE TIPS

| Vacuum range mm Hg | Flow mL/min | Material | Tip |
|---|---|---|---|
| 0.2 tip 0-500 | 15-40 | Suitable for threadlike material or small masses | Straight |
| 0.3 tip 0-500 | 15-30 | Any kind of cortical material | Straight or angled |
| 0.5 tip 0-100 | 15-20 | Wise dense cortical masses | Straight |
| 0.7 tip 0-100 | 10-15 | Wide dense cortical masses or epinucleus or soft nucleus | Straight |

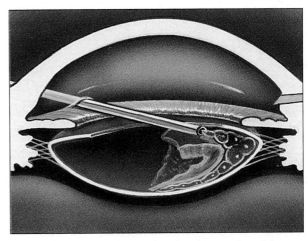

Figure 36-2. The VES is injected between the capsule and the cortex which is detached; it is then aspirated with a coaxial cannula.

material in place. The viscoelastic must be a hyaluronic acid-based material—Provisc or Healon would be a logical choice. Viscoadhesive substances, such as Viscoat or Methylcellulose, are not suitable. The product is injected gradually where there is residual material to try to detach the adhesions between the cortex and the anterior capsule, and between the cortex and the posterior chamber.

The surgeon enters the anterior chamber with the coaxial cannula (without irrigation) and brings the aspiration orifice into contact with the material to be aspirated (the maneuver is simple because VES has created space and widened the pupil, improving visibility). Aspiration is then activated and both the cortex and VES are removed. The maneuver can be repeated if necessary.

The disadvantage of this technique is that several injections of VES are required.

If the cortex is particularly adhesive, rather than repeating the maneuver, the surgeon can implant an IOL and proceed as described below.

### Mobilization Cortex Using an IOL

This technique involves the insertion of an IOL in the capsular bag, even when subincisional masses persist. Do not remove the VES that was injected for the implant (again it should be hyaluronic acid). The lens is rotated in a clockwise direction and the surgeon takes advantage of the mechanical action exerted first by one loop and then by the other which mobilize the masses. They are finally aspirated together with the VES using a coaxial I/A cannula.

This procedure will sometimes reach the objectives rapidly. In other cases, rotating the IOL is difficult because of the presence of the cortex, or because mobilizing the masses is difficult. This technique causes zonular stress through the repeated rotation of the IOL which is not always a smooth procedure.

In addition, it does not always completely remove the residual cortex.

### Technique with the Binkhorst Cannula

Another method consists of using an I/A tip with a curvature of 180° with an orifice at the extremity (Binkhorst); it allows the surgeon to reach the equator of the capsular bag below the tunnel.

Theoretically this works very well. In reality, it presents several problems because the cannula must be large so that the internal lumen (in the zone where the cannula curves) is large enough to aspirate the cortex. The introduction through the main incision involves BSS loss and a reduction in chamber depth. Consequently the cannula can easily contact the posterior capsule which may rupture.

Moreover, the aspiration orifice is at the end of the cannula and the surgeon often has to direct the orifice toward the equator inside the capsular bag. The orifice can therefore snag the equator or the posterior capsule in its attempts to aspirate the cortex.

This will happen very easily if the pupil is narrow or when the equatorial insertion of the cannula is done under conditions of poor visibility.

Another problem with the Binkhorst cannula is that rotation of the cannula inside the eyeball is difficult because of the shape of the cannula itself. The removal of the cannula from a corneal tunnel can also be difficult because the curved part of the cannula tends to stay trapped against the lower edge of the tunnel.

### Technique with a Curved Coaxial Cannula

One huge step forward was the invention and production of angled or curved coaxial cannulas. They are generally angled between 45 and 90° with a slight gentle curve of the body of the tip, which allows the surgeon to reach the cortex positioned at the equator of the capsular bag close to the main incision.

In these cases, the surgeon will normally aspirate the distal and lateral material with a straight coaxial cannula; to remove the subincisional material, the tip is removed and replaced with a curved coaxial tip.

In order to eliminate this phase, some surgeons have stopped using the straight cannula and only use an angled cannula for all the phases of I/A, even though aspiration of the distal sectors can be more difficult. The angled cannulas have considerably simplified the aspiration of the cortex around the incision but this has not

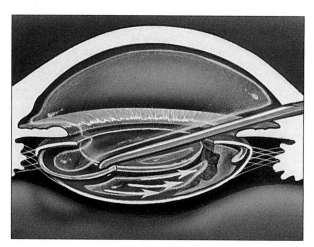

Figure 36-3. The IOL is positioned in the bag and then rotated. In this way, it mobilizes the cortex and is aspirated with the coaxial cannula.

completely resolved the problem, at least where the subincisional is concerned.

In fact, the orifice reaching the cortex cannula must always be brought into a vertical position to a certain degree, and must be angled inside the tunnel. This will cause a certain amount of distortion to the edges, which in turn causes problems of visibility because of the formation of corneal folds. It also induces fluid loss from the chamber with consequent reduction in the spaces in the capsular bag, with problems in capturing and removing the cortex itself.

In addition, it is difficult for the surgeon to remove the cortex in the event of a small rhexis, narrow pupil, or flat chamber, even if he or she uses a spatula to retract the iris.

## SYSTEM USING THE TWO SEPARATE CANNULAS

### Introduction

In view of all these difficulties, I started using an I/A device which has two separate handles—one for irrigation and to keep the chamber shaped, the other to aspirate the cortical masses—using them through two separate incisions.

Initially, the irrigation handle was a Kratz scraper introduced through a side port incision; the other was a common straight aspiration cannula without a sleeve (with the irrigation orifice of the handle plugged). The aspiration handle is introduced through the incision used for phaco.

With time I developed and perfected the system.

I created a system with two different handles, one to be applied to the aspiration tube and one connected to the irrigation. Then I started using the cannulas through two side port incisions leaving the main incision untouched.

I gave special attention to the production of these two cannulas testing a number of thicknesses and a variety of diameters of the irrigation orifices. I tried a single irrigation orifice at the end of the cannula, then one on the side, then two on the side, then one at the end and two on the sides. I tried big orifices and small orifices, positioned at various distances from the end of the cannula. I examined straight and curved cannulas, tested both sanded and smooth, tried ones which had a slightly tapered or cylindrical terminal portion. I also did the same for the aspiration cannula.

### Technical Features of the Two Cannulas

Hundreds and hundreds of operations have been performed using a variety of methods. After all these tests, it emerged that the ideal characteristics of the cannulas are as follows:

- Handles—Titanium proved to be the best material and it is also the lightest. However, stainless steel and aluminum are valid alternatives.
  The internal lumen must be greater than the internal lumen of the cannulas; this will facilitate the aspiration of the cortex with the aspirating cannula, and BSS irrigation with the irrigating cannula. It will also make cleaning the handles easier.
- Cannulas—The surgeon must be able to detach the two terminal cannulas. This will facilitate cleaning and maintain the excellent performance of the cannulas. They can be screwed in (in which case, the surgeon must use a small screwdriver to tighten or release the cannula) or injected/extracted with a rapid lock-in device.
  In the latter case, the surgeon may wish to have a series of different surgical cannulas available, each with different characteristics. They can be replaced in just a few seconds to respond to every clinical requirement. In practice, this does not happen very often.
- The two cannulas must be slightly curved. This facilitates the access to the equatorial material, reduces the movement in the chamber, and avoids exerting excessive pressure on the two side port incisions.
- The two cannulas must have exactly the same diameter so that they can be used alternately through the two side port incisions. The optimal diameter for the cannula is 23 G; 21 G is also good, and 25 G is better especially for extracapsular cataract extraction (ECCE).
- The two terminals must be closed (so the orifices must be positioned along the shaft). This limits the risk of Descemet's membrane detachment when entering the chamber, but above all reduces the risk of rupturing the posterior capsule when one of the cannulas enters a flattened anterior chamber.
- The two terminals of the cannula must be slightly thinner, ie, they should be slightly tapered. This will facilitate their entrance through the side port incisions.
- The end of the aspiration cannula must be slightly sanded. This will allow the surgeon to use the cannula to clean the posterior capsule or to clean the internal surface of the anterior capsule following capsulorhexis.
- There should be just one aspiration orifice, situated

Table 36-3
# POSSIBLE TECHNIQUES TO ASPIRATE SUBINCISIONAL CORTEX

## Technique of tip verticalization

| Technique | Drawbacks |
|---|---|
| Lift BSS bottle. | The posterior capsule is easily captured. |
| Turn the hole toward the material and attempt occlusion. | Tension on the rhexis. |
| Rotate the tip by 180°. | Abnormal pressure on the incision lips. |
| Take the tip to the middle and detach the cortex. | Formation of corneal folds. |
| Wait for removal included by the effect of aspiration. | Reduced visibility. |
| | Divarication of the incision with BSS leakage and imbalance of flow in anterior chamber. |
| | Possible sleeve retraction inside the tunnel with subsequent stop decrease in irrigation. |

## Widening the incision

| Technique | Drawbacks |
|---|---|
| Widen the tunnel to 4-5 mm and insert the tip at the ends. | Most of the problems described above remain, especially if the tunnel is long. |
| Use the right end to aspirate in the left sectors and vice versa. | As leakage increases, the chamber depth decreases. |

## Mobilization of masses with cannula and syringe

| Technique | Drawbacks |
|---|---|
| Capture the capsule with the hole. | The cannula must be thin; otherwise imbalance may be induced in the anterior chamber. |
| Traction toward the center and detachment. | Long and difficult procedure. |
| Mass release. | |
| Repeat the procedure. | |
| Once masses have been accumulated, use automatized I/A. | |

## Mobilization of masses with the IOL

| Technique | Drawbacks |
|---|---|
| Leave the masses and insert the IOL. | Stress on the zonules and the equatorial capsule. |
| Rotate the lens inside the bag and free the masses. | Incomplete mobilization. |
| Then aspirate while removing the viscoelastic. | Incomplete removal. |
| | Difficult IOL removal. |

## 180° bent cannula by Binkhorst

| Technique | Drawbacks |
|---|---|
| Introduce the cannula. | The cannula is big and bulky. |
| Rotate to place it vertically. | It induces lip distortion with BSS leakage and consequent reduction of space inside the bag. |
| Introduce the hole in the capsular fornix. | It is likely to cause capture of the posterior capsule of the rhexis. |
| Capture the mass. | Aspiration and/or blind capture. |
| Aspirate the mass. | |

## Bent and angled cannulas

| Technique | Drawbacks |
|---|---|
| Insert the cannula. | A certain verticalization of the tip inside the tunnel is required. |
| Rotate it until the hole touches the material. | Difficulties persist in case of small rhexis and/or miosis. |
| Capture the material and aspirate it. | |

## Two-handed technique by Buratto

| Technique | Drawbacks |
|---|---|
| Two separate cannulas are used: one for irrigation and one for aspiration. | Two lateral incisions are required. |

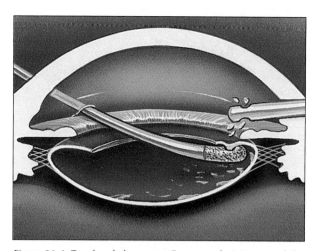

Figure 36-4. Two-handed system—One cannula irrigates and the other aspirates the cortex and the material adhering to the anterior capsule (Asico).

on the concave side of the cannula, about 1.5 mm from the end of the cannula. To clean the posterior capsule with the vacuum technique, the cannula must have an orifice on the convex side.
- The optimal diameter of the aspiration orifice is 0.3 mm. There must be two irrigation orifices; the optimal diameter is 0.5 mm. One of the two orifices must be on the convex side and the other on the concave side. In this way, the irrigation flow is directed toward the chamber angle.

These handles and cannulas are manufactured by Asico.

## Principles for Use of the Two Cannulas

In the two-handed phaco techniques, the surgeon usually only performs one side port incision. However, for the two-handed aspiration of cortex procedure with two different cannulas, a second lateral incision is required.

The two cannulas have been produced to be used alternately through the two side port incisions, so the aspiration of the cortex will be performed in two steps.

In the first phase, the aspiration cannula is introduced through the side port incision positioned on the right of the main opening (while the aspiration cannula enters the incision on the left) and all the cortex in the 180° opposite the entrance point of the cannula is aspirated. Next, the two cannulas are simultaneously extracted and inverted so that the aspirating cannula can remove the residual material of the capsular bag.

In this way, the surgeon can easily reach the entire 360° of the capsular equator and removal of the cortex can be complete even in the sectors below the primary incision.

## Incisions for the Cannulas

The two side port incisions must have their entrance in clear cornea in front of the vascular arches of the limbus. They must be about 70° from the primary incision and are performed with a 30° blade (Alcon 5481). The incision must be almost tangential to the iris plane and be trapezoidal in shape. The external opening (1.6 to 1.8 mm) must be slightly wider than the internal incision (1.0 to 1.2 mm) facilitating the penetration of the cannula. The internal opening must be just slightly larger than the diameter of the cannula to reduce the BSS leakage and avoid the formation of corneal folds.

An opening with these characteristics facilitates the spontaneous closure at the end of the operation.

An incision which is too small will cause the formation of corneal folds, with reduction in visibility, particularly when the aspiration cannula is angled to reach fragments close to the entrance incision.

An incision which is too wide will allow excessive BSS leakage. Thus, the chamber will flatten to a greater extent during the I/A procedure with some problems of spontaneous self-sealing at the end of the operation.

## Technique

The handle fitted with the irrigation cannula is attached to the irrigation tube (a mistake cannot be made as the aspiration cannula will not fit); the same applies to the aspiration handle.

A right-handed surgeon will usually prefer to start with the irrigation handle in his right hand and the aspiration in the left.

Prior to entering the chamber, the surgeon pushes the pedal into Position 1 to remove air from the aspiration handle. He or she should not move into Position 2 because if air enters the aspiration line, the aspiration procedure will be radically changed.

The tip of the irrigation cannula is therefore introduced through the side port incision on the left of the main incision with irrigation open.

As BSS enters the anterior chamber it will deepen the spaces immediately, distend the cornea and the capsular bag, and facilitate the entrance of the irrigation cannula through the other side port incision.

At this point, the irrigation cannula can remain immobile inside the incision while the aspiration cannula is brought to the equator, opposite to the entrance point.

The cannula approaches a fragment of cortex and when contact is made, the surgeon activates the aspiration by pushing the pedal about halfway down.

The cortical material occludes the orifice, the vacuum increases along the aspiration line, and the material sticks more firmly to the orifice. Slowly and gradually, a sector of the cortex detaches from the capsular bag.

At this point, the surgeon moves the cannula toward the center of the chamber.

When the fragment has been freed and the cannula is positioned with the orifice roughly at the center of the anterior chamber, the pedal is pushed down completely so that the vacuum reaches its maximum preset value. This allows rapid aspiration of the captured cortex.

This maneuver is repeated as often as is necessary to remove all the material within reach of the 180° opposite the entrance point of the aspiration cannula.

Then the aspiration cannula and the irrigation cannula are withdrawn and inverted. The aspiration cannula is now introduced through the incision which was previ-

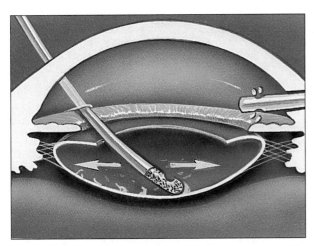

Figure 36-5. Two-handed technique—One cannula irrigates while the other scratches the posterior capsule (Asico).

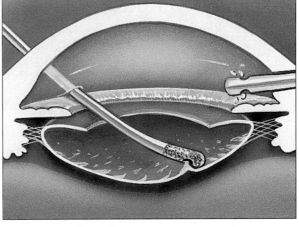

Figure 36-6. Two-handed technique—One cannula irrigates and the other aspirates the residues adhering to the posterior capsule (Asico).

ously used for the irrigation cannula, and it is used to aspirate all the remaining material.

At the end of the operation, the complete closure of the two side port incisions is usually spontaneous. In the event of slight leakage, the edges of the two incisions can be edematized with BSS using a 27 G cannula connected to a disposable sterile syringe.

During the procedure, the surgeon may find it useful:

- To keep aspiration under direct visual control as this will help avoid accidental capture of the anterior or posterior capsules.
- To avoid traction or tension on the incisions because this may cause the formation of corneal folds which will interfere with visibility.
- To wet the cornea frequently so that visibility is always optimal for observing within the anterior chamber.
- To realize that the aspiration of particularly hard masses may be assisted by rubbing the irrigation cannula against the mass which occludes the aspiration orifice.
- To use the cannula, if there is poor mydriasis, as though it were a spatula to move the iris laterally and give a better view of the cortex, aspirating it with the aspiration cannula.
- To remember that if one of the incisions is too wide and allows too much fluid to escape, the problem can be rectified by edematizing one or both of the edges, as is normally done at the end of the operation. Alternately, the tip can be placed obliquely inside the incision in order to partially close the incision.
- To be aware that at the end of cortex aspiration, some filaments may persist. These are difficult to aspirate because they are not large enough to cause occlusion. The surgeon should leave them where they are and mobilize them during or after VES injection using the sanded portion of the aspiration cannula.

## Other Uses of the Two-Handed System

The aspiration system can be used to clean the posterior capsule and this can be accomplished with two techniques:

- The first uses the sanded convex part of the cannula to gently scratch the capsule.
- The second involves the traditional vacuum technique with the usual parameters (vacuum 5 to 30, flow rate 5 to 15, low bottle). This maneuver may be slightly more difficult with the standard aspiration cannula because the orifice is positioned on the concave part of the cannula. For this procedure, a cannula was specifically designed with an orifice on the convex portion.

With suitable mydriasis, it is also possible to aspirate the germinative cells placed under 360° of the internal face of the anterior capsule.

To achieve this, the parameters must be changed with vacuum set at 40 to 50 and flow rate 5 to 10 cc/min.

If necessary, the two-handed system can also be used to remove portions of the epinucleus or small fragments of the nucleus which were inadvertently or accidentally left in the chamber.

For this purpose, the two cannulas must be used in a coordinated manner. The aspirating cannula captures the material, the vacuum is allowed to increase, and when sufficient occlusion has been obtained, the irrigation cannula is used to facilitate removal of the material.

Two different methods can be used:

- The irrigation cannula is rubbed against the aspiration cannula. In this way, the rapid occlusion/disocclusion of the aspiration combined with the mechanical splitting action of the irrigation tip provokes a slow but progressive aspiration of the material.
- The cannula is pushed against the material; it splits, and the penetration of the cannula to occlude the orifice is facilitated. Then more material is captured and the maneuver is repeated several times. It is a procedure which is more suitable for hard material.

The two-handed system allows complete control of the eyeball in surgery with local anesthesia for the non-cooperative patient.

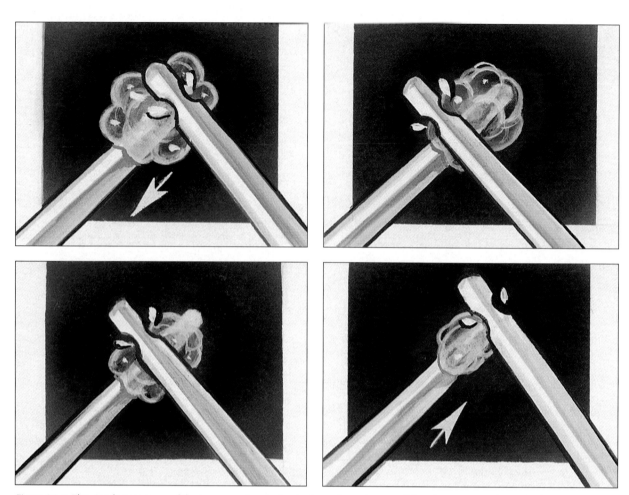

Figure 36-7. The simultaneous use of the two cannulas mechanically ruptures the material and encourages the aspiration (Asico).

The position of the two cannulas, at about 140° from each other, allows the surgeon to move the eyeball in any direction should it be required. This allows for improving the red reflex of the fundus, centering the eye when it has been decentered, and giving a better view of the cortex in some of the sectors which are not easily explorable.

## The Use of the Parameters

Surgeons experienced in performing cataract surgery with automated methods of cortex aspiration know that during the operation, it is important to place the bottle at the right height to obtain a chamber of suitable depth.

They also know that in order to have a chamber with a stable depth, or at least one with minimal fluctuations, the flow rate and vacuum must be set correctly and used in an appropriate manner.

This knowledge can also be applied to the two-handed technique for I/A of the cortex. There are some differences due to the fact that with this system the entire procedure is performed inside an almost totally closed chamber (loss through the main incision is absent and that from the side port incisions is minimal). As a result, almost all the fluid escapes from the aspiration cannula. However, when this is occluded by cortical material, irrigation predominates so the spaces increase because of excess fluid.

On the other hand, when the aspiration tip disoccludes, fluid is drawn rapidly into the tubes (particularly if the tubes are elastic) and there is slight flattening of the chamber. The use of ideal parameters and/or machines fitted with anti-collapse mechanisms allows the surgeon to perform the entire procedure in conditions of maximum safety, with excellent control of the chamber depth.

Normally the flow rate is set at 18 mL/min and maximum vacuum is 400 mm Hg with linear control of the aspiration. Appropriate use of the pedal, flow rate, vacuum, and bottle height will also help reduce fluctuations in the anterior chamber to a minimum.

Here are some examples:
- The system is well-balanced when the cortex has been captured, detached from the capsule, transported to the center of the chamber, and aspirated without the chamber flattening to any great degree. If, on the other hand, the chamber flattens suddenly, it means that excessive vacuum and/or flow rate were used or that occlusion was used for too long which caused the tubes to collapse. The surgeon should then reduce the preset values of vacuum and flow rate, or raise the bottle slightly.
- If the mass is small, its removal will not create any fluctuations in the anterior chamber. If the mass is

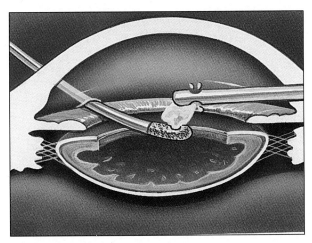

Figure 36-8. Two-handed technique—A small piece of epinucleus or nucleus is captured by the aspiring cannula and is mechanically fragmented using the irrigating cannula (Asico).

large, it may require occlusion for a longer period. When disocclusion occurs, there will be a sudden flow of fluid out of the chamber which will cause it to flatten. To avoid this problem, the surgeon should simply reduce the quantity of material aspirated in every phase.

Alternatively, 75 to 80% of the material can be aspirated under the maximum preset vacuum. The surgeon can then reduce vacuum, just a few seconds before the tip disoccludes (by reducing pressure on the foot pedal), so that when the tip actually does disocclude, the vacuum in the aspiration line is low. This maneuver will prevent mini-collapse of the chamber.

- When the aspiration orifice occludes, the anterior chamber will normally deepen slightly or gradually. However, if the chamber dilates considerably as soon as the aspiration tip occludes (something which frequently occurs in myopic eyes), it means that the bottle is too high, so the surgeon should lower it.

## Use of Two Side Port Incisions

Injection of BSS through a side port incision fills the anterior chamber and produces an increase in internal pressure. This causes the complete closure of the tunnel with the deep flap sticking to the superficial one.

During the bimanual procedure, there will be a very small but negligible amount of fluid loss from the two side port incisions.

In practice, all the maneuvers with the two cannulas are performed in an almost totally closed chamber under positive pressure. This distends the structures of lesser resistance—the cornea and the posterior capsule.

Distention of the cornea will prevent, or at any rate considerably reduce, the formation of corneal folds, with consequent improved visibility of the structures behind it.

Distention of the capsular bag will also distend the posterior capsule and will eliminate any folds in it.

It is unlikely that the capsule will be snagged or cap-

### Table 36-4
### VACUUM TECHNIQUE FOR POSTERIOR CAPSULE CLEANING

Microscope
  High magnification is required.
Tip
  0.3 with moderately retracted sleeve.
Parameters
  Vacuum 5-25 mm Hg; flow 5-15 mL/mm; bottle low.
The cornea
  Must be reflecting and well stretched.
The anterior chamber
  Formed but not deep. Otherwise it is difficult to plat the tip at the right angel (and the posterior capsule becomes too convex posteriorly).
Technique
  The hole is placed touching the capsule.
  The pedal is operated in Position 2.
  The tip hole is occluded (considering the parameters used, it is a moderate occlusion).
  The tip is moved continuously in various directions. If it is kept immobile, the vacuum will have time to increase in the hose and thus the capsule may be firmly trapped inside the hole).
Cleaning mechanism
  The capsule is aspirated inside the hole. Moving the tip continuously, the capsule is taken inside the hole and cleaned.
  Cleaning is accomplished by scratching on the opening rim.
Bottle
  Placed low, so as to reduce the flow and avoid excessive chamber deepening.

tured by the aspiration cannula. The distention of the posterior capsule enlarges the capsular bag and increases the space available for the cannulas, thus facilitating access to the cortex.

All of this allows the surgeon to remove the cortex in a very short amount of time, which will have a positive add-on effect to the final outcome of the operation.

The positive pressure in the anterior chamber will widen the pupil which contributes considerably to improving the visibility of the entire capsular equator and of all the maneuvers inside the anterior chamber.

The stretching of these structures will provide an overall extension of the anterior and posterior chambers (in particular, the capsular bag) and their communication pathway (the pupil) with an increase in the spaces which are useful for the surgical maneuvers, which are thus performed with more precision and safety.

The surgeon can aspirate the cortex while avoiding any contact with the iris, considerably reducing postoperative inflammation and therefore the amount of medical treatment required during follow-up.

However, the use of one of the two cannulas through the main incision (scleral or corneal tunnel) will change the performance of the entire system.

Table 36-5

# I/A OF SUBINCISIONAL CORTEX: TWO-HANDED TECHNIQUE BY BURATTO

**Advances**

| | |
|---|---|
| Both cannulas can be alternatively introduced through both incisions to reach easily the entire 360° of the capsular bag | Thus the entire bag can be thoroughly cleaned. |
| Closed chamber technique | The tunnel incision is closed by the internal pressure. The two lateral incisions are too small to allow a significant amount of fluid to leak out, and, besides, they are obstructed by the cannulas. |
| Positive pressure technique | The increased internal pressure causes relaxation of the chamber, the posterior capsule, and the iris (which induces mydriasis). |
| Corneal stretching | Reduction or absence of fold with consequent improved visibility. |
| Distension of capsular bag and posterior capsule | Erases folds, increases access to the masses, and improves visibility; it widens working spaces for the cannula. |
| It permits moving one cannula against the other | It eases aspiration of hard masses difficult to aspirate. |
| Iris retraction | The irrigation cannula can be used to retract the iris in case of miosis and facilitate working with the other cannula. |
| Quick, easy, and safe technique | It reduces the risk of rupturing the rhexis and/or the posterior capsule. |
| Checking eyeball motility | Especially with topical anaesthesia or under Tenon's capsule, the bimanual technique provides very good control of ocular motility. |

**Drawbacks**

| | |
|---|---|
| Two lateral incisions | Slight corneal trauma. |
| Occasional instability of the chamber depth | During occlusion phases, the chamber tends to widen, as no leaks are present. |

In fact, the tunnel loss had a width ideal for the phacoemulsification tip (2.8 to 3.2 mm), and the introduction of a cannula finer than the phaco tip without the sleeve will cause the incision to open with excessive loss of BSS. This will reduce the depth of the capsular bag and decrease access to the equatorial masses. Removal of the masses themselves will be more difficult because they will remain trapped between the anterior and the posterior capsule. Moreover, with the chamber poorly distended, corneal folds will tend to form.

In other words, the entire procedure becomes more difficult.

## The Two-Handed System for Aspirating VES

This system can be used at the end of the operation to aspirate the VES from both the anterior chamber and the capsular bag.

The technique and parameters will differ slightly depending on the type of VES.

With a cohesive VES (Healon, Healon GV, Provisc), the vacuum will be fixed at 400 mm Hg and the flow rate at 18 mL/min, and the removal occurs gradually but rapidly.

- The aspiration cannula is positioned at the center of the chamber and the vacuum is activated. This allows rapid progressive aspiration of all the material without the surgeon having to look for it. With this maneuver, the surgeon can also remove the VES inside the bag or behind the IOL. If the VES is not removed, the surgeon should use the cannula to exert pressure on the center of the IOL's optic disc and push out the material positioned under the IOL. Alternatively, the surgeon exerts pressure on one side of the disc (about halfway between the attachment points of the two loops), pushing part of the bag. He or she then applies pressure on the other side to remove the remaining portion. During all of these maneuvers, the irrigation cannula stays immobile just inside the incision. Normally, this procedure does not require the cannulas to be exchanged.
- With an adhesive VES (Viscoat, Vitrax, or methylcellulose) the parameters are different (vacuum 500 mm Hg, and a flow rate of 30 mL/min).

As this material adheres to the tissues, the surgeon should use a technique of fragment aspiration. The aspiration cannula must search for the VES in the various sectors because the substance is not spontaneously attracted to the aspiration orifice in the same way as the cohesive product.

The first portion of VES to be removed is situated at the center of the chamber, then the VES inside the bag and behind the lens, and finally the portions in the chamber angle and those that adhered to the cornea.

The irrigation cannula in this case can be a great help. By moving it into the anterior chamber and directing the BSS flow to the various sectors, it will encourage the mobilization and fragmentation of the VES which will facilitate its capture and aspiration.

To remove the viscoelastic materials completely, the surgeon will normally have to exchange the cannulas.

Two maneuvers can encourage the escape of the VES trapped behind the lens. In one procedure the chamber is allowed to flatten during the exchange of the cannulas. This will allow the vitreous to exert upward pressure which will slowly and gradually push the VES out of the capsular bag.

The other procedure involves bringing the irrigation cannula close to the edge of the IOL, directing the flow from one of the two orifices toward the equator of the bag. This will help mobilize the VES in the bag itself, particularly if the maneuver is performed in a number of sectors.

The aspiration cannula can be used to push the optic disc and squeeze out the VES which is behind it.

## Disadvantages of the Two-Handed System

The main disadvantage of the two-handed system is having to perform an additional incision—a total of three as opposed to the usual two.

There is therefore another small lesion of the epithelium, the stroma, and the endothelium, one more than in the classical technique with a main tunnel incision and a single side port incision.

Alternating between occlusion/disocclusion of the aspirating tip can cause a certain degree of imbalance due to the alternating of flattening and deepening of the chamber. Careful adjustment of the parameters of aspiration and flow, the height of the bottle, and the correct use of the pedal will normally reduce these problems to a minimum.

Some surgeons believe that the extra side port incision will encourage postoperative inflammation. However, our clinical experience has shown the complete opposite. The reduced number of manipulations of the iris and the reduction in operating time has been shown to reduce the trauma on the anterior segment quite considerably.

## The Two-Handed Technique in Phaco Without Tunnel and in ECCE

The two-handed aspiration technique with two separate cannulas is ideal for phacoemulsification with self-sealing corneal or scleral tunnels.

However, the technique can also be used in a manner similar to the technique of phacoemulsification without a tunnel, provided that the main incision is closed with a temporary suture to avoid fluid loss.

In the ECCE procedure, it can also be used successfully, but again the incision must be tightly sealed (with five to six interrupted sutures). In this case, two separate incisions are not required for the cannulas as they can be introduced through the two extremities of the main incision and between two sutures (in 8-0 silk or 9-0 nylon).

If the flow rate is not sufficient to widen the spaces in the posterior chamber, the surgeon may find it useful to use a larger irrigation cannula which will allow a greater fluid flow into the anterior chamber.

## CONCLUSION

In conclusion, the technique of I/A of the cortex using two separate cannulas is an easy procedure.

The method is safe and rapid, and gives the surgeon great freedom of movement in the anterior chamber and inside the capsular bag. This system allows the surgeon to clean 360° of the equator and work in a completely closed chamber. It is the elective procedure for any situation in which it is difficult to remove the subincisional cortex, but it is also recommended as a routine procedure to remove the cortex completely from the capsular bag.

# Chapter 37

# FOLDABLE INTRAOCULAR LENSES AND DELIVERY SYSTEMS

*Lucio Buratto, MD*

## INTRODUCTION

Foldable intraocular lenses (IOLs), combined with small incision cataract surgery, are gaining wide acceptance as the standard of care in ophthalmic surgery. Current statistics in the United States indicate that foldable IOLs are used in almost 50% of all cataract surgeries (first half 1996, ASORN, September 1996). This is not surprising for this part of the world, because over 90% of all cataract surgical procedures (Leaming, ASCRS, 1996) are performed using phacoemulsification.

These types of statistics for outside the United States are much more difficult to obtain and validate. However, current estimates place the phacoemulsification procedure at about 35 to 40% and foldable IOL use at about 25% of all implants. Irrespective of which area of the world one is looking at, foldable IOL use is definitely growing very rapidly. The primary reason for this rapid growth is, of course, the increasing number of phaco procedures and the surgeon's desire to maintain the size and integrity of the original phaco incision, rather than enlarging for polymethylmethacrylate (PMMA) implantation. The benefits of combining a foldable with the phaco procedure include:
- Less surgically induced astigmatism.
- Improved self sealing wound.
- Quicker healing.
- Quicker visual recovery.
- Less postop patient management.

Thus, both surgeons and patients benefit from foldable technology.

At the same time, because the acceptance has been so rapid, there is still considerable research and development required to finalize on the material and the appropriate delivery system for foldable IOLs.

## INCISION SIZE

All the benefits of small incision surgery can be realized only if the appropriate materials and delivery systems can be combined without having to compromise any other aspect of the surgical procedure.

A very important aspect of the procedure, in general, is the ability to construct and maintain an incision that is as small as possible at the conclusion of the surgery. There is much discussion about this topic; however, numerous studies have shown that the incision at the end of a case is not the same as the one created at the beginning. The incision actually enlarges at every step of the procedure and the biggest increase comes during the insertion of the IOL. In general, the statistics (in vitro, in vivo, and clinical) indicate that none of the material/delivery systems available today can deliver a lens through an incision or wound size of less than 3.3 mm. The studies go on to conclude that forcing a lens through too small an incision is even more traumatic to the incision than enlarging to a size that does not require a forceful insertion. The trauma can lead to wound instability, stripping of Descemet's membrane, and stromal disruption that *could* affect wound apposition and have subsequent astigmatic impact.

These factors contribute to the conclusion that IOL technology clearly lags behind the current phacoemulsification standards for required minimum incision sizes. The requirements for phaco, in fact, are going even smaller, thanks to new tip technology and the desire to maintain a tightly sealed chamber during cataract removal. Alcon Laboratories has recently introduced phacoemulsification tips that can go through incisions that range from 2.6 to 2.75 mm. There most certainly is some stretching, and even tearing (minimal), of the

Table 37-1
**THICKNESS: COMPARATIVE TABLE FOR VARIOUS MATERIALS* (6.0 MM OPTIC / 21.0 D)**

| Refractive index | Thickness mm material | (Central optic) |
|---|---|---|
| 1.41 | silicone | 1.82 mm |
| 1.43 | silicone | 1.28 mm |
| 1.46 | silicone | 1.18 mm |
| 1.55 | AcrySof | .84 mm |

*Only premarket approved products (USA), as of publication.

wound when these tips are first passed through the incision, and also when there is manipulation of the tip to access the lens material in various quadrants of the capsular bag. However, it is doubtful that these maneuvers enlarge a wound to the size that is actually required for existing IOL technology. In fact, the incision enlargement has been reported to increase only slightly from the original keratome size, especially when compared to the enlargement seen at the conclusion of phaco and then lens implant (Steinert, et al).

## MATERIALS

There is a broad selection of materials available to the international surgeon today. The United States is much more limited in its choices, because only silicone and AcrySof are approved for implantation. The key factor in selecting a lens material should, of course, be that the material is at least as safe and effective as time-proven polymethylmethacrylate (PMMA). There should be no compromise in any area of patient or surgeon concern. This begins with preoperative patient selection, as well as intraoperative handling and performance, and concludes with the short- to long-term performance of the material in all areas of clinical performance.

The oldest materials in the foldable technology arena are the silicones. They have been implanted for a little over 12 years and deserve some recognition for legitimizing the routine use of foldables. At the same time, it is apparent that the silicone materials, designs, and delivery systems all represent a compromise over the PMMA standard.

## CONSIDERATIONS

There is wide acknowledgment that silicone is not a perfect material for intraocular use. Perhaps the only promise that this material really fulfilled is that it could, in fact, be delivered through a small incision. Beyond this very basic requirement, there are a number of additional key criteria that silicone, as we know it today, can never meet. The most apparent material fault is that the refractive index for all silicone materials cannot be manipulated above 1.46. This creates the first area of compromise, because the refractive index determines, for a given diopter, how thick a lens has to be. The thickness of the lens subsequently determines the minimal incision size required for a given material.

In the case of silicone, this disadvantage led manufacturers to reduce the useful optic size (compromising the patient), so that they could still claim a reasonably small incision. The useful optic size for silicone, irrespective of the 6.0 mm label, is shown below:
- 12.0 to 18.0 D    5.50 mm useful optic.
- 19.0 to 21.5 D    5.25 mm useful optic.
- 22.0 to 27.0 D    5.00 mm useful optic.

The only exceptions to these optic size reductions, with silicone, are the Pharmacia (formerly Iovision) product and Chiron (formerly Iolab) product, which have full 6.0 mm optics.

This approach accomplishes the desired incision size. However, it does not provide a full-sized optic to the patient and can lead to disabling glare with even minor amounts of decentration. Spherical aberration with this type of approach is also a commonly reported phenomenon.

The conclusion from this experience should convince IOL manufacturers that the best approach is not *small incision at all costs*, but rather *small size, no compromise*. After all, when one has to sacrifice a number of long-term results for a single short-term benefit, one has to question whether the technology represents an advance or a step backward.

There are a number of hydrogel and hydrogel copolymer products beginning to appear in the international market; however, they have many of the same issue as the silicones with respect to refractive index. This means that they will be difficult to implant through a small wound or that the optic size will have to be reduced to address their innately low refractive index.

There are also a number of *acrylics* being introduced, but again, the refractive index for all of these materials falls below the established standard of PMMA, which is 1.49.

The only material that surpasses PMMA and holds true promise for the future is the acrylic copolymer from Alcon, currently being marketed as AcrySof. The AcrySof material was first implanted a little over 6 years ago, and now follow-up on these patients would indicate that this material has properties, as yet not fully understood, that for the first time demonstrate that one does not have to look at tradeoffs in performance when considering use of a foldable IOL.

Thus, it appears that the area of concentration for IOL research and development would be to understand the mechanism of action for performance improvements that have been observed with AcrySof and to fine-tune these features so that they can be incorporated into current and future lens material research.

Additional areas of compromise have been routinely observed and reported with the silicone group of products.

## PREOPERATIVE

1. Do not implant in patients at future risk for vitreo-retinal procedures. This is due to the fact that many posterior segment surgeons are reporting difficulty observing the peripheral retina due to the non-optical flange that is used in the reduced optic size silicone products. More serious, however, are the reports that it is virtually impossible to see through a silicone lens during posterior segment procedures due to condensation build-up during air fluid exchange (open capsule), and also the affinity for silicone oil adhesion to the silicone IOL during retinal procedures. In many cases, the lens has to be explanted and replaced. PMMA and the acrylics and hydrogels can all be managed in these situations. (Jaffe, et al; Apple, et al.)
2. Patients who are at risk for inflammatory reactions postoperatively should also be avoided, because the material does not appear to be as biocompatible as PMMA. This means that silicone IOLs should be avoided in patients who are prone to uveitis or who are undergoing a combined procedure for glaucoma. AcrySof has been selected in these cases because the results, in certain surgeons' hands, indicate that the material is extremely quiet postoperatively. (Aaberg, et al; Arnold, et al.)

## INTRAOPERATIVE

There are a number of decision points that must be considered during any cataract surgical procedure. One of the final decisions that may have to be made is the choice of an IOL. At the beginning of each case, the plan is already in place, and, if everything goes exactly as planned, the original choice of an IOL can proceed as specified. However, plans should be changed if there is an unexpected event during the procedure, or even if the circumstances are not perfect for the originally planned implant which has been chosen.

1. Torn capsule—Certainly if the tear is substantial and cannot be controlled, the choice of any foldable IOL should be questioned. However, in the presence of a minor capsular tear, an AcrySof lens can be considered because it is so much easier to control and opens inside the eye in a very gentle manner. The use of a silicone lens would definitely be contraindicated. However, if an implant is used, one can safely assume that either PMMA or AcrySof could be implanted according to the surgeon's preference.
2. Asymmetric capsulorhexis—This is another situation where silicone is contraindicated. The primary reason is that the silicone materials have shown a tendency to create traction, retraction, and contraction of the capsular bag. This is evident in the rather high number of cases of capsular phimosis as well as significant decentrations and anterior capsule retraction over the optic edge (behind the lens optic).
3. Improperly sized capsulorhexis—An improperly sized capsulorhexis has been identified as contributory to capsular phimosis, as well as lens dislocation with silicone IOLs. These dislocations can result in either a posterior or anterior displacement of a single haptic or foot plate or complete displacement of both haptics/plates and the optic. The theory as to why this occurs is related to the fact that silicone generates very high levels of fibrotic activity which, in turn, creates asymmetrical forces in the capsular bag that the lens is unable to counteract.

This, combined with the fact that there is little potential for long-term fixation due to no adhesion to the capsule, creates a lens which is not stable through the postoperative time period. AcrySof has adhesive qualities that ensure early and long-term positive fixation in the capsule in addition to adhesion to the capsulorhexis margin, thereby eliminating the potential for capsular phimosis or capsular displacement.

4. Ciliary sulcus placement—In situations that call for placement in the ciliary sulcus, the silicone foot plate lens is contraindicated, because it has a fixed diameter overall length, and it would not remain stable, centered, or provide adequate fixation for that location. A multi-piece silicone lens with prolene haptics would also be ill-advised, due to the fact that the prolene would be in direct contact with the vascular tissue of the ciliary body. AcrySof, if using the 6.0 mm optic which has an overall length of 13 mm, would provide the same type of support and performance seen with a PMMA equivalent type of lens.

In summary, the AcrySof lens is a good choice, regardless of preoperative patient selection considerations or unanticipated intraoperative situations. Silicone use must be reconsidered in a variety of situations. This necessity eliminates silicone consideration in a rather broad range of patients and surgeries and rules out its consideration as a routine use IOL design or material.

## DELIVERY SYSTEMS

Delivery systems today are of two main types: forceps and injectors. Depending on the mechanical behavior and the surgeon's clinical preference, these choices allow for a variety of implantation techniques and options. Silicone plate haptic lenses are almost always, of necessity, used with an injector delivery system.

Table 37-2
### COMMERCIALLY AVAILABLE MATERIALS*

| | | |
|---|---|---|
| AcrySof | High refractive index, copolymer | 1.55 |
| PMMA | Industry standard | 1.49 |
| Clariflex | Low refractive index acrylic | 1.48 |
| Memory Lens | Low refractive index, acrylic/hydrogel | 1.47 |
| Phacoflex | Low refractive index, silicone | 1.46 |
| Various | Low refractive index, silicone | 1.41-1.44 |

*From the Multinational Companies.

## The Injector

There have been, and continue to be, continual improvements in the area of injector technology. At the same time, these systems are still not totally predictable or reliable. Most of the attempts at improvement have been directed at reducing incision size. However, even though there have been many years of work on this system, the incision sizes are still no better than what can be achieved with a standard forceps.

The infatuation with the injector delivery type of system seems to be based on two surgical requirements that apply to a very small segment of today's cataract surgery practice. These requirements are speed and ease of use. Speed is only a plus with the injector system if one allows the assistant to do the actual loading of the cartridge and then the injector. If the surgeon performs this him- or herself, the time savings versus forceps are non-existent, and, in fact, the injector process requires more time. Most surgeons prefer to control every step of the procedure, and having someone else load the injector for speed purposes is out of the question.

Ease of use is also very debatable, because maneuvering the optic into the capsular bag in one movement can, in fact, be more risky for the fragile intraocular tissues. However, if one could master this one-step placement without excessive force on delivery or release, the proponents for this type of delivery would increase substantially. The disadvantages of the current systems can be categorized and described as follows:

1. Spontaneous dislocation—This is probably one of the most serious consequences of the unpredictability of these devices. When these lenses are delivered into the capsule with such force, they can begin or extend a preexisting, but unrecognized, tear that leads to displacement into the vitreous.
2. Torn lens delivery—Because the IOL is obscured from full view as it is being advanced through the handpiece and cartridge, there is the potential that a torn lens will be unloaded into the anterior chamber and capsular bag. The lens optic can be torn, which is easily visible. However, in some cases, the superior or inferior foot plate is torn and is not so easily recognized. This is picked up on subsequent exam when the lens is decentered for no readily apparent reason.
   Because silicone is quite difficult to handle when wet, removal of the lens can be a challenge. Cutting the lens for removal is also tricky, because a good grip on the material is difficult to accomplish and maintain.
3. Enclosed sterile delivery—Although this is not clinically documented, there have been some anecdotal comments supporting this benefit of injector technology. A recent study in Germany illustrated no difference in the contents of the anterior chamber (using anterior chamber taps), when comparing an injector with a forceps. Clinical studies and long-term experience will finally settle this issue.
4. Material/injector combination—Perhaps it is the combination of a material with excessive rebound energy and potential for force that keeps so many surgeons away from an injector delivery system. Alcon Laboratories is currently working on a delivery system that, when combined with the viscoelastic (gentle and controlled) properties of AcrySof, may finally make the technology more appealing to the ophthalmic surgeon community. The system is also designed to deliver the lens in an orientation that will not create excessive forces on the capsule but will also require the additional step of trailing haptic placement with a dialing or compression maneuver.
5. Promise of smaller incisions—The current injector systems, although touted as providing the smallest possible incisions, do more damage to an existing incision than the more commonly used forceps. The reason that these systems traumatically enlarge the incision to a greater degree than forceps is that they take up more space in the wound, thereby creating the need for more *give* in the wound itself. Recent studies have shown that delivering the same material, same power lens through the same size incision will result in 16% enlargement for the injector and half that, or 8%, for the forceps.

## Forceps

Forceps is the preferred form of foldable IOL delivery today. The major reason for the preference is that surgeons like to have total control throughout the surgical procedure.

Forceps provides an opportunity to inspect the folded lens prior to delivery into the eye, thereby eliminating the surprise delivery of a broken or torn lens. In the case of AcrySof, this lens is quite easy to grip when wet, so if removal is necessary for any reason, this can be easily accomplished.

Forceps is also in a continual state of evolution, and therefore, it is impossible to provide any listing that stays current for very long. The best approach is to continue to work closely with the company representatives and ask, at every opportunity, if there are any new developments that you should be made aware of.

## POSTOPERATIVE CONSIDERATIONS

There have been numerous anecdotal and clinical observations of postoperative performance characteristics for each of the widely used and currently approved foldable materials.

Perhaps the most significant benefit which is being observed and reported is the reduction in posterior capsule opacification seen with various foldable materials.

In the case of silicone, the plate design lenses have been anecdotally reported as reducing the posterior capsule opacification rate seen with PMMA and multiple piece silicone lenses. However, these reports have never been clinically documented in a well controlled study.

More recently, David Spalton, FRCP, FRCS, FRCOphth, of St. Thomas' Hospital in London, England, has reported on some very innovative work designed to quantify posterior capsule opacification rates with various materials in a well controlled study.

Mr. Spalton's study, which is going to expand to a multi-center trial, concludes that AcrySof lenses produce significantly less posterior capsule opacification than PMMA or silicone lenses, and that this finding has important clinical implications for the prevention of posterior capsule opacification. There are several publications forthcoming on this work by Mr. Spalton.

Mr. Spalton has also undertaken the task of looking at the observed reduction in capsular fibrosis and phimosis seen with AcrySof versus silicone. This work will also be published in the near future.

Additional observations have been reported with respect to overall biocompatibility of the AcrySof material. However, a well-designed clinical study has yet to be completed for this area of significant interest.

The bottom line is that foldables are here to stay, and the market is extremely dynamic. Therefore, it is up to each individual surgeon to select the material and lens delivery system that suits him or her the best and that delivers true clinical benefit to the patient.

# Chapter 38

# FOLDING MANIPULATIONS AND OPTICAL QUALITY OF A SOFT ACRYLIC INTRAOCULAR LENS

*Tetsuro Oshika, MD*
*Yasuhiko Shiokawa, MD*

## INTRODUCTION

Soft acrylic intraocular lenses (IOLs) have been widely accepted as an efficient and safe tool in small incision cataract surgery,[1,2] and its use in the practice has been increasing since appearance on the market.[3,4]

Soft acrylic IOLs unfold much more slowly than other foldable lenses,[1] and thus disappearance of the crease in the optic takes longer than other foldable materials. In addition, cracks of the optic may be formed by prolonged and repeated folding manipulations.[5-7] However, the effect of folding procedures and/or crack formation on the optical quality of this IOL has not been well known.

In this chapter, the authors address the changes in optical quality of the soft acrylic IOL after several simulated folding procedures.

## LENSES

Soft acrylic IOLs (MA60BM, AcrySof, Alcon Surgical) of +18.0 diopters (D) were used in the current study. Lenses were randomly selected from a group of IOLs intended for the clinical use.

Using two IOL folding forceps (E30-635, PMS GmbH), the following manipulations were applied:
1. The lenses were folded for 30 seconds at room temperature (20°C), and were unfolded in a balanced salt solution (BSS) of 20 or 37°C.
2. The lenses were folded for 10, 20, or 60 minutes, and were unfolded at room temperature.
3. The lenses were folded very tightly for 30 seconds or 5 minutes, and were unfolded at room temperature.
4. Linear cracks were created at the central 3 mm zone of the optic surface using a cutter.
5. Strong forceps pressure was applied to the center of the optic, and an impression was formed.

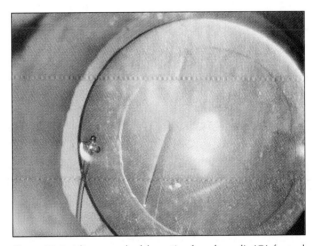

Figure 38-1. A linear crack of the optic of a soft acrylic IOL formed by prolonged and repeated folding manipulation.

## MEASUREMENTS

Following these manipulations, modulation transfer function (MTF) was measured in a model eye at 3 mm aperture size.[8] The model eye was constructed based on Gullstrand's Exact Schematic Eye, which consisted of a front lens corresponding to the cornea, a water chamber where the IOL was immersed, and a rear lens to allow for an air image. Monochromatic light of 546 nm was projected through the model eye and focused on a charge-coupled device (CCD) image sensor. The obtained image was analyzed using a computer.

Resolving power under veiling glare light was also measured. The IOL was placed in a model eye containing a water chamber where the IOL was immersed.[9,10] Veiling glare light source of 300 cd/m$^2$ (30° in size) was placed at 5° to the axis. The contrast visual acuity chart used in the

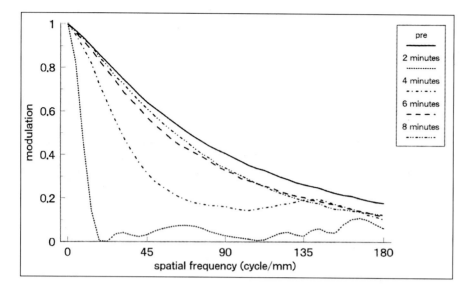

Figure 38-2. Modulation transfer function after a 30 second folding. Lenses were unfolded in 20°C BSS.

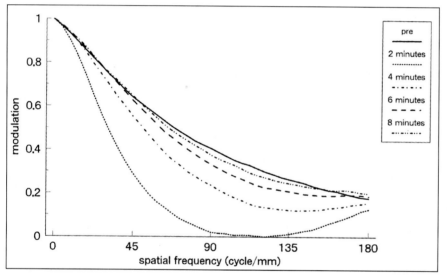

Figure 38-3. Modulation transfer function after a 30 second folding. Lenses were unfolded in 37°C BSS.

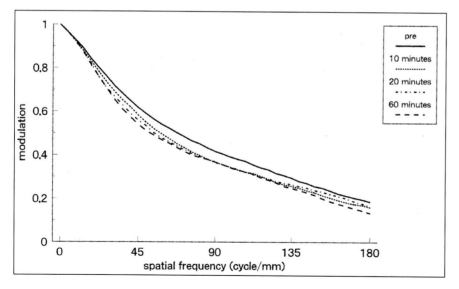

Figure 38-4. Modulation transfer function after prolonged foldings (10, 20, or 60 minutes).

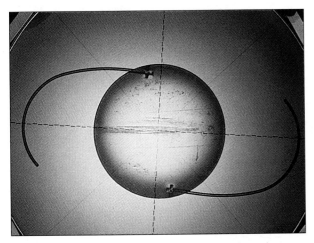

Figure 38-5. Microscopic appearance of lens surface after a 60 minute folding.

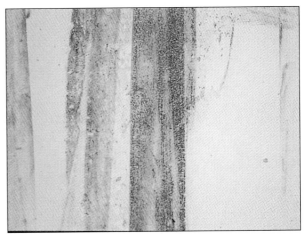

Figure 38-6. Microscopic appearance of lens surface after a 60 minute folding (X 15).

current study theoretically allows the maximum resolving power of 187 cycles/mm (equivalent to 20/10 of Snellen chart visual acuity). A decline of resolving power to 94 cycles/mm (20/20 visual acuity) or lower was judged to be significant.

In each experiment, microscopic examination of the IOL surface was also carried out after measurements of MTF and resolving power.

## FOLDING FOR 30 SECONDS

Immediately after unfolding of the lens in 20°C BSS, marked deterioration of MTF was observed. Changes in the MTF were more remarkable at lower spatial frequencies. Eight minutes after unfolding, MTF almost recovered to the level of untreated IOL. There were no microscopic changes of the optic.

When the lens was unfolded in 37°C BSS, recovery of MTF was quicker than in 20°C BSS, with approximate normalization of MTF at 6 minutes after unfolding. Microscopic examination of the surface revealed no remarkable changes.

## PROLONGED FOLDING

The lenses were folded for 10, 20, or 60 minutes and were unfolded at room temperature. Measurements were taken 30 minutes after unfolding.

MTF was not affected significantly by any procedures. Resolving power under veiling glare was also unaffected by 10 and 20 minute manipulations. However, a 60 minute folding lead to a deterioration in resolving power to 63 cycles/mm (equivalent to 20/30 in Snellen chart visual acuity).

Under microscopic examination, no morphological changes were observed after a 10 minute folding. Damages of the optic material at the region corresponding to the folding forceps were observed, however, following 20 and 60 minute manipulations.

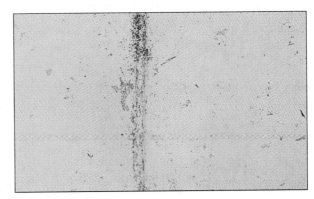

Figure 38-7. Microscopic appearance of lens surface after a 5 minute tight folding (X 10).

## TIGHT FOLDING

The lenses were folded very tightly for 30 seconds or 5 minutes, and were unfolded at room temperature. Measurements were taken 30 minutes after unfolding.

No functional or morphological changes were detected after a 30 second tight folding.

After a 5 minute tight folding, examination revealed several fine cracks on the surface of the optic corresponding to the zone of tensile stress on the convex side as well as the location of forceps. MTF showed slight deterioration at middle and high spatial frequencies. Resolving power was declined slightly to 94 cycles/mm (20/20 visual acuity).

## ARTIFICIAL CRACKS

Linear cracks were created at the central 3 mm zone of the optic surface using a cutter. With cracks less than 10 lines per 3 mm, there were no noticeable changes in MTF. When 10 or more cracks were created, MTF worsened significantly at all spatial frequencies.

Resolving power did not change when cracks were less than 20 per 3 mm. With 20 cracks it dropped to 63 cycles/mm (20/30 visual acuity) and with 40 cracks to 46 cycles/mm (20/40 visual acuity).

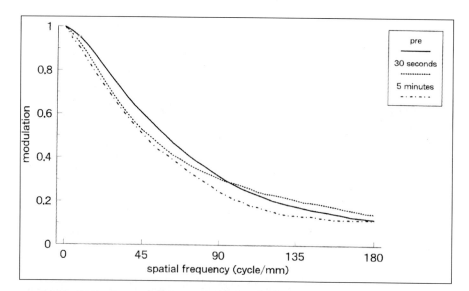

Figure 38-8. Modulation transfer function after a 30 second or 5 minute tight folding.

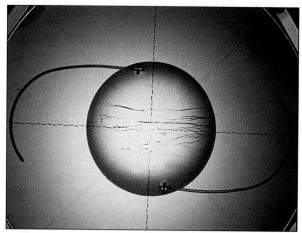

Figure 38-9. Artificial cracks created on the optic of a soft acrylic IOL.

## IMPRESSION OF THE OPTIC

Strong forceps pressure was applied to the center of the optic, and an impression was formed. Immediately after the manipulation, remarkable changes in MTF were observed. At 4 minutes after manipulation, MTF at low spatial frequency recovered. MTF measured at 6 minutes was found to be normal at all frequencies.

There were no changes in resolving power under veiling glare light and microscopic surface quality.

## Discussion

The optical resolution of silicone and hydrogel IOLs after folding simulations was tested previously.[11] It was reported that surface irregularities caused by the grip of forceps could be demonstrated for a maximum period of 30 seconds after manipulation. Only after non-physiological, extremely long manipulation periods did damage of the optic material occur. However, these changes as well as groove-like surface deformities occasionally observed by scanning electron microscopy did not detectably decrease resolution or contrast.

In the current study, we also found that ordinary folding procedures did not adversely affect the optical quality nor the optic material of soft acrylic IOL. Deterioration of the optical quality and damages of the optic material were observed only after extremely non-physiological manipulations, such as prolonged folding for 60 minutes or extremely stressful folding for 5 minutes. Prolonged folding for 20 minutes or less did not affect MTF nor resolution. Tight folding for 30 seconds likewise did not affect the parameters examined in this study.

The effects of artificial cracks and central grooving were also limited. Deterioration of MTF did not occur until the number of cracks reached 10, and resolving power remained unaffected with less than 20 cracks at the central 3 mm zone. Although one or two cracks may be formed in the clinical situation,[5-7] the above mentioned conditions are far beyond the range of clinical settings. A groove created on the lens with forceps lowered MTF up to 4 minutes, but no changes were observed thereafter.

The current tests were carried out according to the methods recommended by the International Standards Organization (ISO) and the American National Standards Institute (ANSI). While these methods are widely used in industry, they have several limitations for evaluating the effects of folding on lenses. For instance, a 3 mm aperture was used to test the lens, but this condition may not apply when major decentration of the IOL occurs. We measured MTF using a line spread technique that may miss astigmatism in the IOL. Monochromatic light was used for the measurement of MTF, but this ignores chromatic aberration. An +18.0 D IOL was used in all studies, but lenses with a higher power and thicker optic may be more susceptible to the folding manipulations. Evaluation of these factors would be the subject of future studies.

## CONCLUSION

Although extremely non-physiological manipulation may affect the optical quality of a soft acrylic IOL, folding procedures within the range of clinical settings are unlikely to affect the optical quality of this lens.

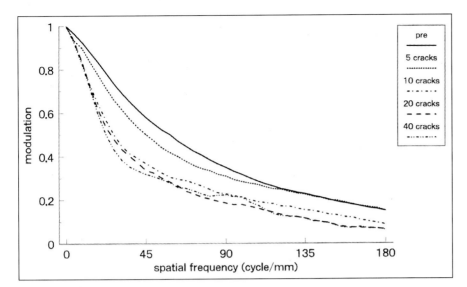

Figure 38-10. Modulation transfer function with artificial cracks created at central 3 mm zone of the optic.

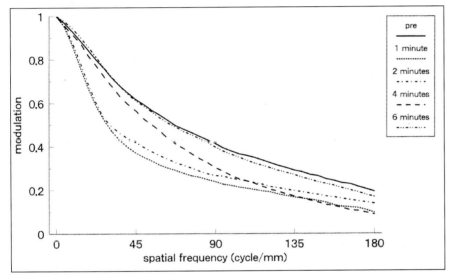

Figure 38-11. Modulation transfer function after an impression was created at the center of the optic.

## REFERENCES

1. Koch DD. Alcon AcrySof acrylic intraocular lens. In: Martin RG, Gills JP, Sanders DR, eds. *Foldable Intraocular Lenses*. Thorofare, NJ: SLACK Inc; 1993:161-177.
2. Oshika T, Suzuki Y, Kizaki H, Yaguchi S. Two year clinical study of soft acrylic intraocular lens. *J Cataract Refract Surg*. 1996;22:104-109.
3. Learning DV. Practice styles and preferences of ASCRS members-1995 survey. *J Cataract Refract Surg*. 1996;22:931-939.
4. Oshika T, Masuda K, Majima Y, et al. Current trends in cataract and refractive surgery in Japan—1995 survey. *Jpn J Ophthalmol*. 1996;40:419-433.
5. Oshika T. Intraoperative complications of foldable IOL. II. Soft acrylic IOL. *Jpn J Clin Ophthalmol*. 1995;49:1614-1615.
6. Carlson KH, Johnson DW. Cracking of acrylic intraocular lenses during capsular bag insertion. *Ophthalmic Surg Lasers*. 1995;26:572-573.
7. Pfister DR. Stress fractures after folding an acrylic intraocular lens. *Am J Ophthalmol*. 1996;121:572-574.
8. Portney V. Optical testing and inspection methodology for modern intraocular lenses. *J Cataract Refract Surg*. 1992;18:607-613.
9. Holladay JT, Ting AC, Koester CJ, et al. Intraocular lens resolution in air and water. *J Cataract Refract Surg*. 1987;13:511-517.
10. Holladay JT, Ting AC, Koester CJ, et al. Silicone intraocular lens resolution in air and in water. *J Cataract Refract Surg*. 1988;14:657-659.
11. Kulnig W, Skorpik C. Optical resolution of foldable intraocular lenses. *J Cataract Refract Surg*. 1990;16:211-216.

# Chapter 39

# TECHNIQUES FOR INSERTING FOLDABLE LENSES

*Vittorio Picardo, MD*

## INTRODUCTION

Foldable lenses have now become the type of implant which is routinely used in cataract surgery with phacoemulsification. The use of this type of intraocular lens (IOL) has allowed surgeons to improve the surgical procedure and reduce considerably the time required for the visual rehabilitation of the patient.

There are many types and models of foldable IOLs available on the market. They have different construction material, shape, and final structure.

As a result, the various manufacturing companies have produced numerous systems of folders and insertion forceps specific for each model.

Regarding these IOLs, it is important that the surgeon be very familiar with the instruments he needs to perform the operation properly with maximum respect for the surrounding tissues.

Foldable IOLs can be inserted both through a sclerocorneal incision or more easily (and now more frequently) through an incision in clear cornea.

For both incisions to the anterior chamber, the size usually shifts between 3.2 and 4 mm depending on the type and shape of the IOL, the instruments, the technique used, and of course the surgeon's experience.

Some studies have shown that at the moment of insertion, with an incision which has been completely sealed by the instruments, the intraocular pressure (IOP) can increase quite considerably. On the other hand, with an incision which is too narrow, the surrounding structures and the walls of the tunnel itself will be subjected to considerable distortion, as reported by Drews. Thus the wider the incision, the easier it will be to insert the lens. However, with a wide incision, undesired astigmatism may result postoperatively.

We should point out that in the past few years, the companies which manufacture surgical instruments have made considerable progress in improving the size ratio between the various holders and folders, and incision size, to such a degree that at present the lower limit of the smallest incision is the thickness of the IOL. Silicone lenses have a low refractive index and are usually consequently considerably thicker than the corresponding PMMA lenses, especially in the high positive power range.

On the other hand, acrylic lenses have a higher refractive index, with a lower overall thickness. Alcon's AcrySof with a 5.5 mm optic plate has a thickness which is less than that of the 6 mm AcrySof.

So it stands to reason that the surgeon will have to add the thickness of the forceps to the thickness of the foldable lens itself.

For implantation techniques using a folder, the dimension of the folder itself will represent the right size for the surgical tunnel.

Common experience has shown that a 3.2 mm tunnel is sufficient for lenses with injectors, while 3.8 mm, 4.0 mm, or 4.1 mm are the most suitable sizes for implanting three-piece lenses of either silicone or acrylic.

In any case, all the techniques for foldable IOLs require the use of a large quantity of a suitable VES with high or extremely high molecular weight, so that the surgeon can completely distend the capsular bag, allowing the lens to unfold without any damage to intraocular structures.

## IMPLANTATION TECHNIQUES

In the past, foldable IOLs were implanted using two instruments, a folder and a holder, used in the opposite manner compared to today's technique. The lens, removed from its container, was supported by a McPherson-type forceps (toothless) or another similar model. It should have thin, cylindrical branches in order to avoid any damage to the optic plate.

| Table 39-1 | |
|---|---|
| **FIRST GENERATION FOLDERS** | |
| Faulkner | Cross-over action |
| McDonald | Cross-over action |
| Livernois-McDonald | Cross-over action |
| Ernest-McDonald | Cross-over action |
| Fine | Straight action |
| Fine Universal I and II | Straight action |
| Shepard-Buratto-Clayman | Straight action |
| Nordan | Straight action |
| Kellan | Straight action |

| Table 39-2 | |
|---|---|
| **SECOND GENERATION FOLDERS** | |
| Barrett's forceps | Storz |
| Mazzocco | Storz |
| AMO Phaco folder | AMO |
| Buratto's universal forceps | Janach |
| Buratto's forceps for silicone IOL | Asico |
| Buratto's forceps for acrylic IOL | Asico |

In this somewhat uncomfortable position, the *folder* rested on the external edges of the optic plate and the surgeon folded the IOL along the main diameter, creating a sort of *sandwich* of the implant. The loading could occur in a longitudinal or transversal direction depending on the final position of the loops, in one case parallel, in the other perpendicular to the lens axis.

During the last 5 to 6 years, the techniques have changed in conjunction with changes in IOL designs and materials so the procedures of implantation vary slightly depending on the type of lens—whether it is a one-piece or three-piece silicone lens, made of acrylic or hydrogel.

## Silicone Lenses

There are two different types of silicone lenses:
- One-piece with a flange-shaped haptic.
- Three-piece with loops of different design and materials (polymethylmethacrylate [PMMA], Prolene).

### *One-Piece IOL*

These lenses have a characteristic *biscuit shape* with a total diameter of 10.5 mm. The optic plate has a diameter of 6.0 mm and is biconvex. The flanges are coplanar so the IOL does not have a side. There is a hole on each flange, different in size depending on the model.

### *Implantation Technique*

The system of implantation with a cartridge and an injector is now used routinely to implant a one-piece silicone IOL. Generally, the disposable cartridge and the injector are both produced by the same manufacturer. These have been modified over the years according to the IOL design.

Preparation of the cartridge and its loading into the injector can be done by an assistant who places the IOL in the system. The launch chamber should be filled abundantly with viscoelastic substance (VES) in order to create a space between the anterior chamber, which is already filled with VES, and the injector which contains the IOL.

Whatever system is used, either the screw-in injector or the syringe-like pressure type, currently produced by Chiron, the IOL must be positioned along its longitudinal axis, closed inside the support system. It takes the shape of a cigar, rolling-up on its largest axis which can be easily introduced into the launch chamber, previously filled with VES. In this manner it will safely move from the injector to the anterior chamber.

For both systems, the surgeon must proceed introducing the tip inside the tunnel, fixing the eyeball laterally to the incision with a fine-toothed forceps (from 0.12 to 0.20 mm), and performing slight rotation movements to the right and left so that the tip will enter the anterior chamber at the center of the capsulorhexis.

The tip should be placed with the edge pointing downward toward the floor of the capsular bag, and from this final position the surgeon will push the injecting system to introduce the distal end of the IOL inside the bag, underneath the distal edge of the capsulorhexis.

The movement will continue very gently under the surgeon's control to expose about 40% of the optic plate inside the anterior chamber. At this stage, the IOL will be close to the *elastic moment*, in which it leaves the injector and enter the capsular bag.

At this stage, a slight downward movement of the tip caused by raising the handle of the injecting system, will allow the final expulsion of the proximal flange, which generally will enter the bag spontaneously.

If this maneuver is not completely successful, the surgeon should slightly press the upper part of the optic-flange with a spatula. The lens will then be correctly positioned. Due to its elasticity, the flange will fold over on itself and avoid the rhexis. Lenses with characteristics of this type are rarely used (shape, overall size, coplanar optic, positioning holes), at least in Europe.

These lenses have enjoyed greater success on the American market because their preparation and implantation is closer to the experience of the American surgeons. They believe that having the lens prepared by the assistant will save time and reduce costs.

The one-piece silicone lenses (with flange) can be implanted without being folded, using a normal forceps through a 6 mm incision. A hook is introduced through a side port incision, and directs the inferior flange inside the capsular bag (two-handed maneuver). In order to position the superior flange, the surgeon must slightly press with the hook on the optic flange junction as described in the previous technique.

Another surgical but uncomfortable technique is always realized with forceps folding the lens in two similar parts along the main axis.

In this case the IOL, supported by a thread-holding forceps along the greatest diameter, will be folded

Table 39-3
**IMPLANTATION FORCEPS**

| | |
|---|---|
| Buratto's universal forceps | Janach |
| Buratto's forceps for silicone IOL | Asico |
| Buratto's forceps for acrylic IOL | Asico |

Table 39-4
**INJECTORS**

| | |
|---|---|
| Staar | Softrans Injector IP (syringe type) |
| Staar | Softrans Injector IT (micrometric) |
| Staar | MicroStaar Injector |
| AMO | Prodigy |
| Chiron | Passport |

between the branches of a McPherson type forceps (toothless) which acts both as a folder and a holder. The technique is not suitable for inexperienced surgeons.

When a one-piece lens is implanted vertically (axis 6-12), it is advisable to rotate it through 90° and place it horizontally. This will allow the tip of the irrigation/aspiration (I/A) system to remove all the VES more easily from the capsular bag and avoid postoperative secondary glaucoma due to capsular block (which can be resolved by anterior peripheral YAG laser capsulotomy).

Regarding toric silicone lenses, once they have been implanted, they should be rotated after VES is totally removed from the bag. This surgical phase must be performed carefully in order to avoid a IOL decentration in the postoperative period.

From the current follow up studies, the possibility of decentration is greatest in the first 2 weeks, even if the lens continues to rotate slightly during the 5 to 6 months following the operation. Sometimes a lens must be recentered.

### Three-Piece Silicone Lens

These IOLs have a traditional shape; they have a biconvex optic with a diameter of 6.0 mm. The overall length of these lenses depends on the material used in the loops but they will tend to be longer if Prolene is used because it is a more elastic substance (generally 12.5 to 13.0 mm).

At this point we should mention the contradictory story regarding the use of Prolene in the loops. Previously, Prolene loops were considered unsuitable for PMMA lenses because of Prolene's premature memory loss and its consequent inability to resist the retraction forces which appear inside the bag postoperatively but was suggested again for use with the foldable silicone lenses.

Several companies are following the new market trends and are producing foldable silicone lenses with extruded PMMA loops (AMO, Pharmacia & Upjohn) or of Polyamide (Staar). The PMMA loops are useful as they are more resistant, have better memory than those of Prolene, and in the long-term follow-up studies these lenses appear much more stable.

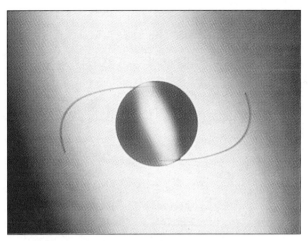

Figure 39-1. Foldable intraocular lens (silicone).

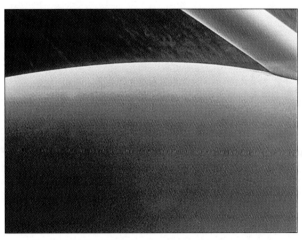

Figure 39-2. Insertion of the loop into the optical zone (electronic microscope image). (Pharmacia & Upjohn 920.)

The loops must be introduced very delicately and carefully to avoid damages so the surgeon must have the right instrument ready—Buratto's forceps for example, Asico AE 42730.

The central thickness of these IOLs is dictated by the low refractive index of the silicone used, and this will have a direct effect on the size of the incision tunnel.

To resolve this problem, the AMO lens has a non-refractive peripheral ring surrounding the optic plate, thus producing a lower overall thickness. For the same reason, Pharmacia & Upjohn has produced a silicone lens with a higher refractive index. This has reduced the thickness of the IOL, especially in the higher positive powers.

Recently multifocal lens technology has been applied to the three-piece silicone lenses (AMO and Pharmacia & Upjohn), but these are still being developed.

### Technique for Implanting the IOL 920 (Pharmacia & Upjohn)

There are two methods for implanting three-piece IOLs: transversal and longitudinal.

Even if IOL with Prolene or PMMA loops are used, two forceps are necessary—one to fold the lens along the

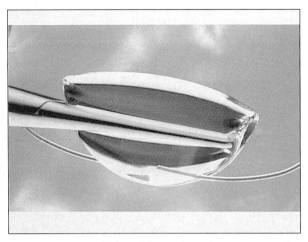

Figure 39-3. Correct folding of the 920 lens (Pharmacia & Upjohn) for longitudinal technique.

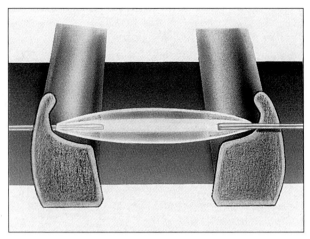

Figure 39-4. The 920 lens (Pharmacia & Upjohn) well positioned in the Buratto folder for transversal implantation.

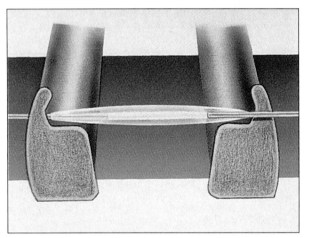

Figure 39-5. Acrylic foldable lens positioned into the Buratto folder; the IOL is thinner than a silicone model, due to the different index of refraction.

diameter and the other to insert the folded lens into the capsular bag (folder, holder). Implantation of this type of IOL is normally performed by an incision and a corneal tunnel (clear cornea; near clear).

The surgeon should remember that this type of lens should never be wet or placed in contact with instruments which are damp or impregnated with balanced salt solution (BSS) or viscoelastic. The resulting hold and thereby surgeon's control of the lens may be poor.

### Longitudinal Technique

First, the 3.0 to 3.2 mm tunnel should be cut with a disposable knife or a diamond blade and the phaco stage completed. Then prior to folding and loading the three-piece silicone lens (for example, Pharmacia & Upjohn 920), the forceps must be cleaned and dried very carefully and the capsular bag must be totally filled with viscoelastic of very high molecular weight. The incision should be widened with a preset blade between 3.6 and 4.1 mm (depending on the diopter of the IOL, ie, its total thickness).

Under low microscope magnification, the surgeon will remove the lens from its container using a dry toothless thread-holding forceps and transfer it to the specific folder of that IOL. The forceps must also be completely clean and dry.

The silicone lenses (Pharmacia & Upjohn 920) can be inserted by Buratto's forceps produced by ASICO AE4253 S or AE 4273.

The folder, held by surgeon in his left hand, will be opened to create the space necessary for the IOL. This forceps has two small walls at the end of each tooth, designed to hold the IOL. They will guide the lens as it folds over itself as soon as the spring mechanism is released, creating a sort of *sandwich*.

The loops positioned parallel to the optic plate, will take on a slightly concave shape which is opened upwards.

In this phase it is important that the lens is really folded in half and that the two halves are symmetrical. By increasing the magnification of the microscope and placing the forceps underneath with the face upward, it will be possible to examine the exact position of the IOL and correct any flaws in the procedure. If necessary, the folding maneuvers can be repeated carefully.

Buratto's forceps produced by Asico because of its crossed arms have two small notches on the walls which are very important for controlling the maneuver.

The lenses folded in this way will be transferred to the implantation forceps, the holder. This forceps, with blunted and slightly curved internal arms, can have either direct or indirect action and the choice depends only on the surgeon's experience.

Both using direct or indirect forceps, the insertion of the IOL can be performed in a Position $C$, with both loops open on the left, or in Position $D$ with both loops open on the right.

Buratto's lens holder produced by Asico has two reference notches halfway along the arm to ensure the surgeon has correctly loaded the IOL.

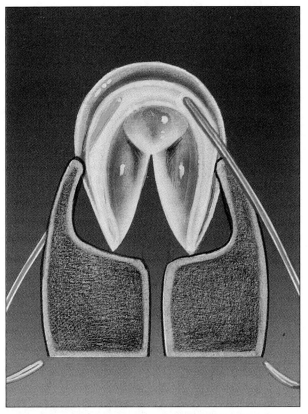

Figure 39-6. Correct folding of a three-piece foldable IOL for transversal technique-the loops are symmetrical.

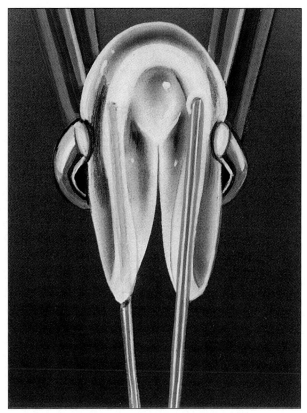

Figure 39-7. Foldable three-piece IOL in the holder forceps, folded for transversal technique: correct position.

## C Position

If the surgeon decides to insert the lens in this position, the holder will be brought toward the tunnel with the right hand slightly rotated to the left. The distal loop will have its *back* to the incision and will therefore be in a favorable position for the implant step.

In this phase some surgeons prefer to catch the free end of the loop inside the folded optic plate to give greater strength to the entire system.

The small device is very useful whenever the surgeon is implanting lenses with Prolene loops due to the elasticity and resistance of this material.

The arms of the holder will be parallel to the edges of the tunnel. The surgeon will open the arms slightly, and guide the introduction of the distal loop and the optical part of the IOL until it enters the anterior chamber well-above the rhexis plane.

At this point the 0.9x /1.0x magnification of the operating microscope should be used in order to have better control of the subsequent phases. The surgeon's wrist will be rotated in a clockwise direction as soon as the distal loop has reached the groove in the bag opposite the tunnel. The surgeon checks that the entire optical plate is at least on the same plane as the rhexis. The proximal loop will be trapped inside the tunnel with the convex part facing the surgeon.

The smooth, gradual rotation of the pulse will set the holder forceps perpendicularly and perfectly in the center of the anterior chamber. The surgeon then begins to release the lens by gently opening the arms of the forceps.

The presence of abundant VES inside the capsular bag and in the anterior chamber will distend the bag, at the same time squeezing the edges of the capsulorhexis which will be very visible. The VES will obstruct the opening of the lens released gradually by the forceps, softening the impact with the intraocular structures and reducing the zonular stress to a minimum.

The proximal loop, which has taken its correct position with the concavity on the right, can be positioned inside the bag either using a toothless forceps, or a positioning hook or a fork which will make the IOL rotate, such that the loop penetrates the anterior chamber first and then penetrates into the bag.

In this phase, the size of the capsulorhexis plays an important role in the stability of the IOL.

The capsulorhexis is the same size as the optic plate, or preferably it should be 0.1 to 0.2 mm smaller to hold the lens better.

If on the other hand the rhexis is wider than the optic plate, the IOL will not be stable in the bag. Slight displacement may occur at a later stage particularly if all the VES is not completely removed from the bag after implantation.

If the diameter of the rhexis is too small, the implantation of the IOL in the bag will be much more damaging and the surgeon will have to examine the situation carefully under strong magnification (10x to 12x). He will have to check that the optic plate is really inside the bag

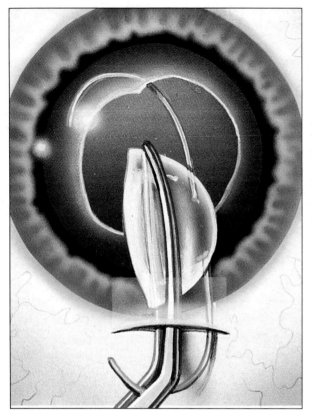 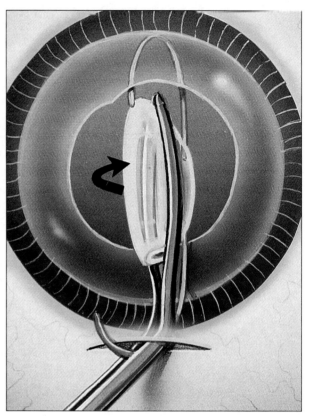

Figure 39-8. Longitudinal technique—The IOL has been inserted in the anterior chamber and the first loop is under the capsulorhexis.

Figure 39-9. The IOL is completely in the anterior chamber; the first loop is in the right position; clockwise rotation of the wrist will be positioned the optic disc in the bag.

and not above it. The rhexis itself must be widened at the end of the operation, as the frequency of anterior capsule opacification is very high in these cases.

The IOL will center automatically because of the special design of the loops.

In the event the surgeon wishes to use a two-handed technique, a button-ended spatula should be held in his left hand, introduced in the anterior chamber through a side port incision. This will be placed gently on the optic plate and pushed gently downward while the holder slowly releases the IOL, implanting it inside the capsular bag.

The implantation of a three-piece IOL can be summarized in three steps:

- Insertion of the distal loop and the IOL first inside the tunnel and then inside the chamber, penetrating with the loop inside the rhexis under the surgeon's constant visual control.
- Rotation of the wrist from left to right to bring the forceps into a vertical position.
- Release of the IOL by opening the arms of the holder.

However, the surgeon must be very attentive:

- During the entrance of the first loop, he or she should check its exact position inside the bag and avoid placing the posterior loop incorrectly above the capsular bag which can damage the zonular fibers.
- In the phase of introduction of the optic plate in the anterior chamber, in order to check whether the distal edge of the folded IOL is positioned below the rhexis plane.
- In the phase of final insertion, to control the correct entrance of the distal loop and avoid it being damaged.

### D Position

This type of implant maneuver is very similar to the C position which has just been described.

The only difference lies in the fact that the lens is brought close to the tunnel entrance with the wrist rotated to the right. The distal loop enters first, and the convex part is to the left, which would appear to be incorrect.

Once the lens has been introduced in the anterior chamber with the same method and care used in the previous C technique, the movement to bring the forceps into a vertical position will be performed in a counterclockwise direction. This will result in the optic plate being centered on the rhexis plane and will also rotate the distal loop through 180°, positioning it correctly, with the convex part to the right.

In this step, it is very important for the surgeon to fill the capsular bag completely with high molecular weight VES (ie, Healon), which will also protect this delicate structure when the loop is being rotated.

The second loop is positioned, using either a one- or two-handed technique. The difference is that with this technique only the internal loop rotates, whereas the external loop is already correctly positioned.

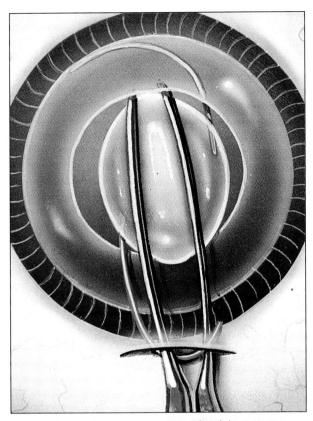

Figure 39-10. The holder is gently opened and the optical disc is released.

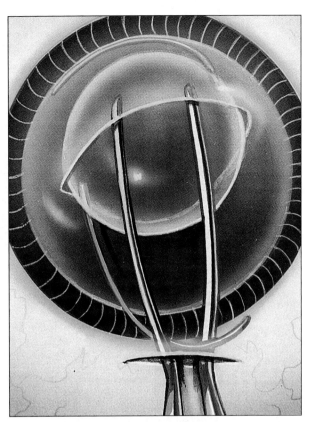

Figure 39-11. The release of the IOL is quite completed. The proximal loop is already outside the capsular bag.

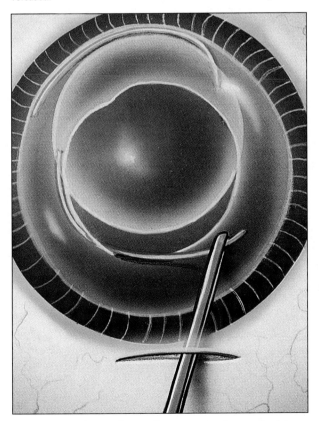

Figure 39-12. The McPherson forceps grasps the proximal loop, starting the maneuver of insertion.

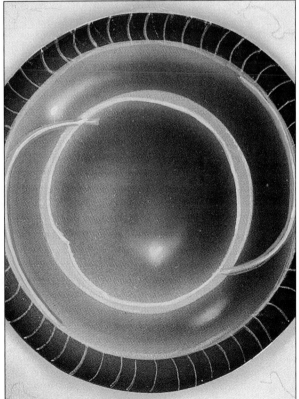

Figure 39-13. IOL implanted in the capsular bag.

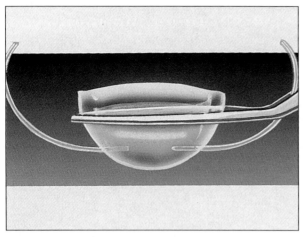

Figure 39-14. Correct position of the lens in the forceps.

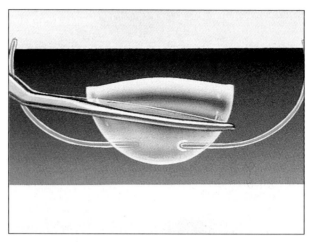

Figure 39-15. Asymmetrical folding of the IOL.

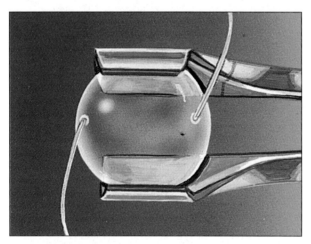

Figure 39-16. The lens has been positioned non-symmetrically for transversal technique; a small under counterclockwise rotation is necessary.

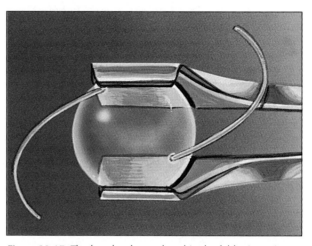

Figure 39-17. The lens has been placed in the folder in an incorrected position; a small clockwise rotation is required for right longitudinal folding.

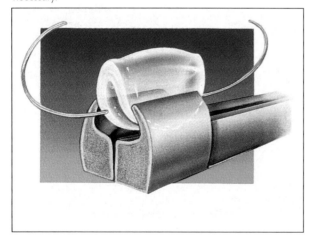

Figure 39-18. Assymetrical folding of the IOL.

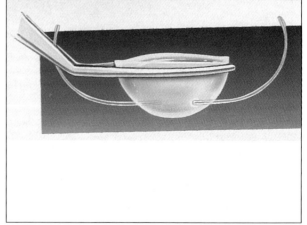

Figure 39-19. Incorrect position of the folder (too high).

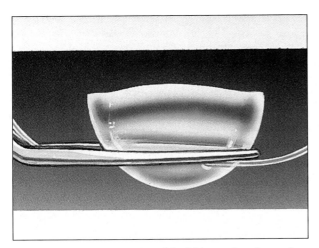

Figure 39-20. Incorrect position of the folder, too low down, close to the loops.

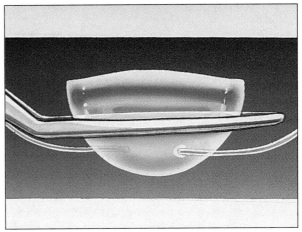

Figure 39-21. Incorrect position of the folder; the edges of the forceps are out of the lens surface.

### Transversal Technique

This transversal implantation technique is a little more traumatic than the longitudinal, but is undoubtedly more effective.

The idea is to introduce the optic plate and the loops into the tunnel in a single movement and then inside the capsular bag by rotating the surgeon's forceps-wrist system through 90°.

The lens should be removed from the container and positioned on the clean, dry folder, with the loops orthogonal to the axis of the folder. The loops look like two small wings on the outside edge of the forceps.

Once the surgeon has checked the perfect adhesion of the optic plate to the holding grooves, and that the loops have the normal clockwise direction, he or she can release the forceps, allowing the arms to close, thus folding the lens in half. It will be D-shaped with the horizontal edge corresponding to the diameter of the IOL, and the convex is formed by the two loops folded over on the same plane, in the same direction, and with the end portions side-by-side or slightly overlapping.

As with the previous technique, the instruments must be clean and dry to guarantee a good, accurate hold of the lens. There are various models of holders, with direct and indirect action, and again, the choice will depend on the surgeon's preference.

In the step between the folder and holder, the lens must be caught just above the holding groove so that it can be held tightly between the arms of the forceps for the subsequent insertion maneuvers.

The IOL and the holder should be as one unit to allow the surgeon to perform the introduction in the tunnel correctly and also to open the IOL correctly without damaging the structures of the bag and the zonula.

A bad or irregular hold may cause the lens to unfold incorrectly in the anterior chamber, with possible damage to the intraocular structures (capsulorhexis, corneal endothelium, iris, angle structures).

The tunnel, sclero-corneal or in clear cornea, is gently opened by a fine-toothed forceps which will raise the upper flap.

The lens will be brought close to the tunnel itself, taking care not to moisten it to avoid losing the holder's grip.

Insertion into the tunnel will always occur parallel to the incision with the loops forming a simple shock-absorbing system. The forceps with the folded IOL approaches the tunnel with the loops toward the lower extreme of the incision and the tip of the forceps very slightly toward the upper limit. Taking advantage of the elasticity of the loops, the surgeon can start introducing the tip of the forceps and the IOL inside the tunnel, changing the direction of the forceps until they are parallel to the axis of the tunnel.

The forceps then proceeds to the center of the anterior chamber which has been well distended with VES, and under high magnification (0.8x to 0.9x), the surgeon rotates his wrist and the forceps-lens system in a clockwise direction.

The forceps will be horizontal, and the loops will extend beyond the rhexis and lie along the visual axis to touch the internal face of the posterior capsule with the curved extremity.

Once the exact position of the entire system has been checked, the surgeon will gradually open the arms of the forceps (direct or indirect), thus opening the lens.

The loops reach the correct final position and the lens will shift down in the capsular bag.

The lens will center itself. The holder brushes the surface of the IOL to check and complete the placement of the implant.

A second instrument is not generally used in the anterior chamber with this implantation technique even though some surgeons suggest that it would be useful to provide better protection of the endocular structure. In this case, the surgeon can introduce a blunt microspatula through a side port incision. It will be placed above the folded IOL and used to help the IOL descend slowly into the bag into the correct position.

Table 39-5

| Manufacturer | Loop shape | Loop material | Diameter of the optic | Overall length |
|---|---|---|---|---|
| Acrylens (Ioptex) | C-mod, i=1.47 opt.r.250 | Prolene | 6.5 mm | 13.65 mm |
| Alcon AcrySof | C-mod, i=1.55 | Extruded PMMA | 6.0 mm, 5.5 mm | 13.0 mm, 12.5 mm |

The final steps of the operation, slight rotation of the IOL and removal of the VES are performed as usual.

### Three-Piece Silicone Lenses (AMO)

The SI30N silicone lenses have an optical zone of just less than 6mm as it is surrounded by a flat neutral edge this makes the lens thinner than other types available. The loops are made of Prolene blue.

This technical feature was also included in the more modern SI40NB lens which has PMMA loops and which has enjoyed considerable commercial success.

Insertion can be performed using the usual team of folder and holder (Asico 4262A and Asico AE 4276) or the more recently introduced Buratto's forceps (Asico AE4253S and AE4273). Using these Asico forceps, the technique and method used to implant the lens is almost exactly the same as the other lenses with a true optic plate of 6 mm.

When the surgeon uses the Asico forceps for the IOL AMO AE4262A, the folder used has direct action with inferior rails. In this case the lens should be placed on a flat surface, ie, the top of its box. The forceps are brought close to the lens with the grooves parallel or perpendicular to the direction of the loops, depending on whether the implantation technique will be longitudinal or transversal.

The surgeon slowly but firmly closes the forceps to fold the lens over on itself, creating a small *sandwich* with loops parallel or perpendicular to the optic plate, depending on which technique the surgeon has chosen.

The reduced thickness of this type of lens undoubtedly makes implanting with a longitudinal or transversal technique through a 3.5 mm incision an easy procedure.

The step from folder to holder occurs in the normal manner. It is important that the closing pressure on the arms is not excessive, given the relatively small thickness of the IOL.

### Other Instruments

Some types of forceps are defined as *universal* because they have a greater range of application due to their unusual shape and technical characteristics. Among them we can mention Buratto's universal forceps with three resting points. These forceps can actively fold the IOL because of the toothed arms (Janach J 21863). In this case, the lens is placed upside-down on the forceps, with the loops open in a counter clockwise direction.

These forceps have another important feature, the two lateral notches which are used to guide the holder. The notches can catch the folded IOL correctly and firmly.

These forceps are ideal for both longitudinal and transversal insertion techniques.

Recently Buratto presented a new interesting folder called a balestra which allows the surgeon to fold both acrylic and silicone lenses, for both the longitudinal and transversal implantation techniques. The instrument is a developed and simplified version of Fine's pyramid.

The folder has two rigid arms, each with the holding groove for the IOL. The two arms overlap slightly and are fixed to the square-shaped external support system.

This instrument is managed in a manner similar to Buratto's folder, but the lightweight and ergonomic shape of this folder make it different compared to other forceps instrument with which the surgeon may be familiar.

## Acrylic Lenses

### Non-Hema Acrylic Lenses

PMMA is used for the optic plate of foldable acrylic lenses. After processing, this material folds easily while maintaining a certain degree of rigidity and consistency which makes these lenses different compared to the foldable silicone lenses.

The acrylic lenses are three-piece with loops of PMMA or Prolene.

They can be implanted through 3.5 mm or 4.0 mm incisions, depending on the size of the optic plate.

They open more slowly and more gradually in the anterior chamber and assume the definitive shape inside the bag just a few seconds after being implanted. This eliminates the longitudinal lines which form during folding.

Acrylic lenses are ideal for implantation in the bag. However, AcrySof MA60BM produced by Alcon with a 6 mm optic plate and overall length of 13 mm can also be implanted in the sulcus.

### The Principal Lenses Available

1. Acrylens (Ioptex) is a lens made with a copolymer of acrylate and methacrylate esters to which a UV absorbing monomer has been added.
   It has i=1.472 and an optical resolution of 250 pairs of lines per mm.
   A plastic instrument for folding the lenses is supplied by the manufacturer; the lens is then held and implanted by a Kelman-McPherson type forceps.
2. AcrySof (Alcon, MA60BM) has i=1.55, C-loops in PMMA, with a 10° angle.
3. Memory Lens by Mentor (ORC).

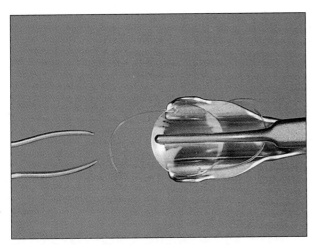 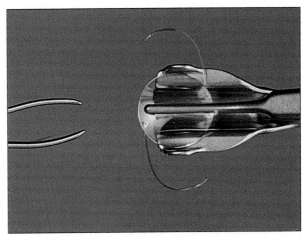

Figure 39-22. The lens has been caught correctly by the insertion forceps.

Figure 39-23. Transversal folding of the same lens with the same instruments.

## Techniques for Implanting the AcrySof Acrylic Lens

PMMA was and continues to be the material of choice for the production of IOLs for cataract surgery, because despite the increasing popularity of phacoemulsification techniques, extracapsular cataract surgery continues to have an important role on the market.

The production of foldable lenses has certainly contributed significantly to the growing interest in phaco techniques, which along with the small incision can be considered to be the future of this type of surgery.

Even though the foldable lenses have been available for more than 12 years, it has never been considered an ideal material for the implants, and surgeons have not been completely convinced regarding their use. Thus, use of foldable lenses was somewhat limited until recently.

When Alcon introduced the AcrySof in 1995, a great deal of interest was generated in foldable lenses and their potential use. This unique acrylic material is foldable and could easily replace PMMA because of its excellent postoperative performance. With all probability, acrylic will also replace silicone as the foldable material of choice.

Recently, David Apple published a very interesting study on a new complication caused by silicone lens implants: the so-called interaction of silicone oil-IOL in silicone. This author has been studying the morphology of pseudophakic eyes for many years. He based his observations on three patients in whom the silicone IOL was completely coated in an emulsion of silicone oil which had been used during a previous vitreoretinal surgery.

The study, reported in *Ophthalmology*, October 1996, was accurate and well-documented. It gave a detailed description of the changes observed in the patients' eyes and in the IOLs themselves, and on laboratory IOLs treated with the same materials (silicone oil) as used in the patients. The IOLs were explanted and the patients recovered postsurgical visual function once again.

The changes, observed in three-piece silicone IOLs with Prolene loops, effected the surface of the optic plate, which appeared to be completely covered by the silicone emulsion seen as bubbles of various sizes on both faces of the implant with obvious alterations of the transparency. Using electron microscopy, the structure of the support loops also appeared to have been changed in the area of extrusion from the optic plate, and all of these findings have a negative effect on the stability and centering of the IOL.

Apple concludes his study by pointing out how the choice of IOL type (foldable, rigid, one-piece, three-piece) is an important step in the patient's visual rehabilitation after cataract surgery. The surgeon not only must decide on the most suitable surgical technique, but also the type of lens to be implanted based on the correct performance of the operation, remembering the preoperative clinical conditions and patient evaluation. This careful management must be done in order to avoid further surgery of the posterior segment via pars plana in patients with a high risk of vitreoretinal pathologies.

The use of vitrectomy techniques, even by an experienced surgeon, nevertheless involves a certain modification of normal ocular anatomy, as well as the use of instruments and different types of endocular buffering systems such as gas, perfluorocarbonate liquid, and silicone oil.

For this group of risk patients, an IOL with a wide optic plate, even with support in the ciliary sulcus, would be the best overall choice.

For these reasons, surgeons should appreciate the research efforts that the manufacturing companies are making regarding materials for safe, long-lasting IOLs. The foldable acrylic IOL appears to be promising addition.

Apart from Alcon, two other companies are working in the field of acrylic—AMO (Ioptex) with Acrylens and Mentor (ORC) with the Memorylens.

Another material which would appear to have potential is Hydrogel. The Storz laboratories have already launched a lens made from this material and other manufacturers including Alcon are continuing research in this area.

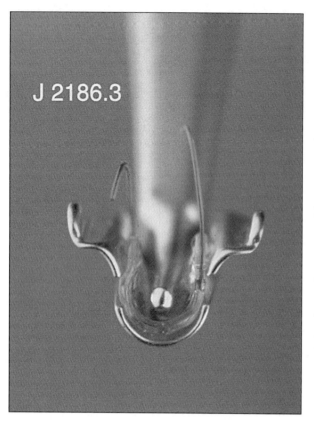

Figure 39-24. Buratto universal folding forceps: frontal view.

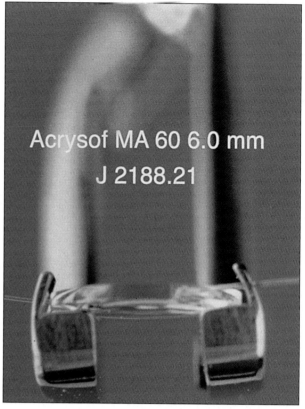

Figure 39-25. Buratto folding forceps for AcrySof 6.00 mm: frontal view.

## Patient Selection

Until acrylic materials were introduced, the use of foldable products (silicone in particular) was limited to no-risk patients and for those patients with a non-compromised, symmetrical capsulorhexis.

High risk patient groups include patients with diabetes, uveitis, or glaucoma. In these patients the foreign body reaction may be considerable and unpredictable. Silicone IOLs were not implanted in these patients due to the risk of inflammatory reactions.

Foldable silicone lenses are not indicated when there is an asymmetrical capsulorhexis or a compromised stability of anterior or posterior capsule. This is due to the difficulty in intraoperative control of the opening of the silicone lens. The lens which is very elastic opening tends to position itself quite abruptly with the possibility of causing damage to the zonular-bag structures.

An abundant amount of VES in the anterior chamber and the bag with excellent exposition of the edge of the capsulorhexis will provide adequate protection of all the support structures for the implant.

The most important characteristic of the acrylic lenses is that they do not have the elastic moment of explosion but rather open slowly, gradually, and in a controlled manner, keeping the demarcation line along the fold line for a short time.

The size of this lens (total diameter 13.5 mm, optic plate 6 mm for the MA60BM) means that the surgeon can either implant it in the posterior chamber or use the technique of planned extracapsular cataract extraction with implantation in the sulcus or in the bag.

Because of the unusual strength of the material, the design which allows implantation both in the sulcus and in the bag, and optimal biological tolerance, the AcrySof lenses have acquired a primary role in the field of foldable lenses.

It is undoubtedly the type of foldable lens that non-skilled surgeons can use when beginning to implant through small incisions.

## Surgical Techniques

The techniques for implanting the acrylic IOLs do not differ greatly from those used for the other models of three-piece foldable IOLs.

## Instruments for the Foldable Lenses

All the lenses available on the market have specific instruments for their insertion and this also applies to Alcon's AcrySof. There are a number of forceps and instruments for use in the phases of folding and insertion.

For these lenses, the general criteria of cleaning, good maintenance, and correct use are to be particularly respected. The surgeon must take responsibility to ensure that he or she has all the correct instruments for the type of lens he or she wishes to implant.

Alcon suggests a variety of folders and holders. Some of the folders are similar to the Stainert forceps, or those

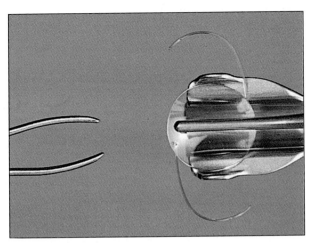

Figure 39-26. Holding of the IOL by the use of Buratto universal forceps.

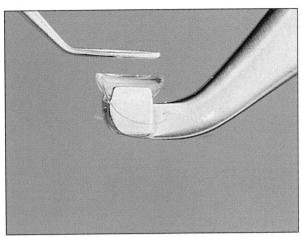

Figure 39-27. Transfer of the acrylic IOL from the holder to the folder.

of Fine, whereas the holders are very similar to the modified McPherson forceps.

It is important for the surgeon to have different forceps for the 6 mm lenses and the 5 mm lenses.

Buratto, in collaboration with Janach and Asico, also produced forceps which were designed specifically for the AcrySof lenses.

So-called universal folders are also available for use with these lenses, as acrylic is a much more manageable material than silicone.

There is one basic difference between the two lenses: the silicone IOL should not be wet at all, whereas the acrylic IOL must be washed well to allow good manipulation during surgery.

Some American authors even suggest dipping the lens in warm water or heating the pack prior to use.

The delicate, easily controlled behavior of the acrylic lenses in conjunction with the easy-to-manage injection systems contribute to the potential success of this technology. Selection of the instruments can play an important role in maintaining the integrity of the incision and its final size.

### Implantation Technique

The implantation technique and the mechanical behavior of the silicone IOL are well-known. Surgeons who have switched from using silicone IOLs in favor of acrylic IOLs have immediately noticed the difference, and especially in the releasing of the latter. The surgeons who began their training with acrylic foldable lenses have been able to perfect the maneuvers, reducing the time required for folding, implantation, and positioning of the lens.

There are no major differences in the implantation techniques for three-piece acrylic IOLs, such as AcrySof, compared to those used for the silicone lenses, at least not in the main steps. The difference lies in the psychological approach the surgeon has towards the two types of material.

The technique of longitudinal insertion (IOL vertical, with the loops external to the optic plate) or the technique of transversal insertion (the optic disc plate and the loops folded into the smaller diameter) with a one-step insertion maneuver can be used.

### Longitudinal Technique

The lens which has already been folded and wet is held in the holder in the surgeon's right hand. The distal loop can remain free or can be folded over on itself, inserting the extremity inside the optic plate. The proximal loop will always be free and coaxial to the entire forceps-lens system.

The upper flap of the tunnel, widened to 4 mm with a suitable blade, will be raised using a fine-toothed forceps. At the same time the holder will bring the IOL, the distal loop in particular, to the entrance of the tunnel.

The IOL is introduced with a sliding movement to reach the distal part of the tunnel inside the eyeball in the anterior chamber, beyond the edges of the rhexis. At this point, the surgeon must twist the tip of the forceps slightly to move the IOL downward to the end of the bag so that the distal loop and the portion corresponding to the optic plate will enter the bag.

The surgeon will then have to twist his or her wrist in a clockwise direction and position the concavity toward the bottom of the capsular bag while the proximal loop will still be partially inside and partially outside the tunnel.

With this D technique, the distal loop is considered fixed and the proximal loop is rotated. If the surgeon wishes to use the C technique, the introduction of the lenses will change. The distal loop will be open toward the right and the proximal loop opened to the left.

However, in both techniques the rotation of the wrist to the vertical position will leave the optic plate correctly on the area of the rhexis and will allow the slow gradual liberation as the forceps gently releases the hold.

Many surgeons, including Buratto, suggest the use of a second instrument, a button-ended spatula, introduced in the anterior chamber through a side port incision. During the first phase of introduction, this instrument will guide the correct positioning of the distal loop inside the bag. Moving backward toward the center of the

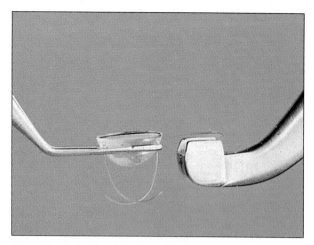

Figure 39-28. The lens is in the holder forceps.

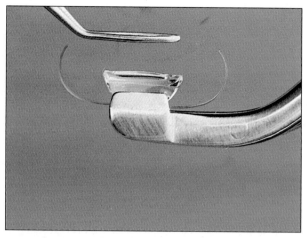

Figure 39-29. Longitudinal folding of the three-piece IOL. Buratto forceps used.

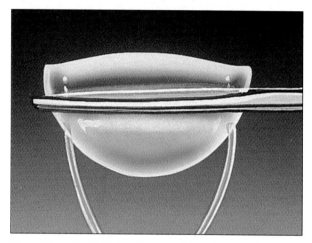

Figure 39-30. IOL folded for transversal insertion technique.

chamber, it will help to guide the distention of the optic disc inside the bag which has been well-filled with high molecular weight VES.

For both techniques, the proximal loop must be positioned inside the bag using a toothless McPherson-type forceps, or with a positioning hook or a push-pull.

Centering of the lens is almost immediate. Nevertheless, it will be useful to rotate the lens slightly to stabilize the position.

At the end of the implantation, the surgeon should ensure that the size ratio between the rhexis and the optic plate is correct. If the rhexis is too small, shrinkage and subsequent opacification may occur. However, data reported in the international literature show that there is a lower frequency of opacification of the anterior and posterior capsules with acrylic lenses compared to silicone lenses.

This feature of the acrylic lenses should not be underestimated because maintenance of good transparency of the bag will allow complete, correct examination of the retina, even long-term after the phacoemulsification operation. In addition, remember that patients subjected to cataract surgery, irrespective of age, are often affected by serious retinal disorders of a dystrophic-degenerative or vascular origin. As they require regular postoperative examinations, it is clear that the transparency of the bag, both the anterior and posterior capsules, becomes very important and of considerable interest.

In addition, no clinical trials have reported the need for a premature YAG laser capsulotomy in pseudophakic eyes with AcrySof lenses.

Buratto, like many other authors, has not observed any of these complications. On the contrary, they all report optimal biological tolerance to the acrylic material and low frequencies of these lenses in producing secondary alterations in the capsular bag.

The Italian Phacoemulsification Association is conducting a multi-center study which is examining the percentage alteration of the capsular bag in size shrinkage and in transparency (secondary cataract). The preliminary findings confirm this positive verdict for the acrylic lenses, particularly when compared to the corresponding three-piece lenses with a silicone optic plate.

It should also be pointed out that due to its size, the AcrySof lens with a 6 mm optic plate can also be implanted in the sulcus. If the IOL is incorrectly positioned with one or both loops outside the bag, it can be left in that position rather than attempting to reposition it—as this could damage the zonules, creating subluxation of the bag.

### Transversal Technique

The transversal technique is an alternative implantation technique. The surgeon folds the lens transversally (or horizontally) so that the loops are superimposed, as shown in the drawing. This type of folding is performed with any folding forceps. The lens is then lifted by the insertion forceps and inserted. In this way, the loops will look like *legs* of the IOL.

The advantage of this technique is that a second instrument is not required to insert or rotate the second loop. Both loops are released in the capsular bag with a single movement, which is neither complicated or risky because the IOL will unfold slowly.

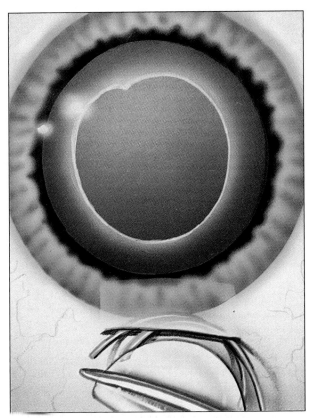 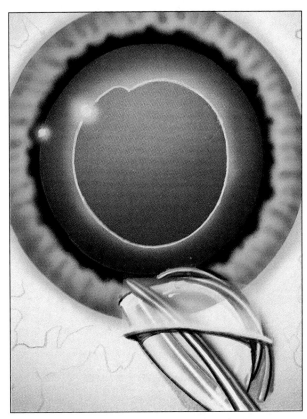

Figure 39-31. Transversal technique—The IOL is positioned in the surgical wound.

Figure 39-32. A gentle rotation of the holder introduced the IOL in the tunnel. Both loops must be preserved from any damage.

The critical step, once the IOL has been folded, is to push the loop symmetrically against the incision edge, thus reducing the volume of the system.

This step will ensure the adhesion of the loop to the edge of the optic zone and will induce a small degree of trauma to the haptics themselves.

The next step is to trap the proximal (or posterior) loop inside the incision edges. The posterior loop is placed at the insertion point (into the optic plate) closer to the surgeon.

For this technique it is very important that the hold by the forceps is very firm and precise to prevent damage to the IOL, in particular the loops, but more importantly, to avoid that the loops open outside the tunnel.

If the posterior loop is not manipulated carefully in this way, there is the potential risk that it will bend and eventually break outside the eye.

The folded IOL is brought close to the incision with the loops placed more peripherally. The loops will be engaged in the tunnel, wherever it has been performed. As soon as the IOL begins to appear from the tunnel, the surgeon will rotate the tip of the forceps in a clockwise direction, introducing it into the tunnel with a movement through 90°. This will be complete when the forceps moves from a position parallel to the tunnel edge to reach a position coaxial to the tunnel itself.

The surgeon proceeds toward the anterior chamber bringing both loops into the tunnel and therefore into the anterior chamber.

He will have to rotate his wrist in a clockwise direction, bringing the IOL-forceps system into a vertical position, and checking that both loops are inside the rhexis and that the end portion of the loops nearly touch the floor of the capsular bag.

Before releasing the lens by opening the forceps arms, the surgeon should ensure that there is no contact with the corneal endothelium.

The use of a second instrument, a button-ended spatula, will be useful in this technique because it will facilitate the gradual sliding of the IOL inside the bag, avoiding any damage to the capsule surface.

The transversal technique is definitely more spectacular than the longitudinal one but the surgeon must be very experienced and be familiar with foldable lenses, VES, and the various instruments.

Implanting foldable lenses should be avoided if the capsulorhexis, the support system, or the posterior capsule have been previously damaged.

Only experience will allow the surgeon to evaluate the possibility of an alternative implant suitable for the individual patient.

### *Hydrogel Lenses (HEMA)*

At the end of the 1970s, Blumenthal began examining new materials with the intention of finding a more biocompatible substance than PMMA—Hydrogel.

Barrett also worked on this project, and in 1983, when Mazzocco was inserting the first silicone IOLs, Barrett designed the Iogel.

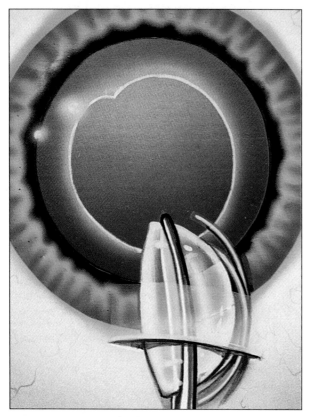

Figure 39-33. Transversal technique—The IOL is completely introduced in the tunnel.

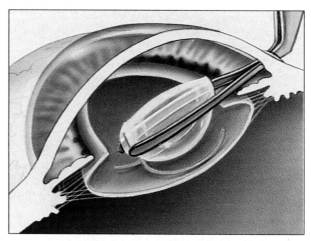

Figure 39-34. The IOL is already maintained by the holder and the wrist has been rotated 90° clockwise.

Hydrogel lenses can be inserted through a small incision, either as a hydrated shape and folded, or dehydrated. In the latter, the lens is rehydrated a few seconds after implantation inside the eye. In the rehydration phase, the surgeon performs a wash-out procedure to remove any debris.

Because of the poor degree of cellular adhesion, the lens can be easily removed, even a long time after implantation.

The lens currently produced is the Hydroview, Storz (P422UV). This lens is defined as a composite one-piece because it has PMMA loops integrated with the optic plate through a special process of polymerization. This gives the lens greater stability. The loops are a modified C-shape, the overall diameter is 13 mm, and the diameter of the optic plate is 6 mm. The water content is 18%, and the refractive index is 1.47. It can be sterilized in hot-damp conditions.

### Implantation Technique

The Hydroview lens is supplied in a container filled with a preservative solution. Because of its structure and the unusual structure of the loops, the lens should be implanted only with the longitudinal technique.

When it is removed from the container, it is loaded into an active folder, eg, Asico AE-4262A.

With the capsular bag filled with VES, the tunnel can be extended to 4 mm with a preset blade.

The moistened lens is then transferred to a normal folder for acrylic lenses, delicately folded with the loops *concavity upward*.

The arms of the forceps will protect the optic plate during the phase of introduction to the tunnel; however, the surgeon must be careful to facilitate the entrance of the distal loop into the capsular bag, below the rhexis, in a position opposite to the tunnel.

The rotation and verticalization of the forceps will implant the IOL as a D if the movement is clockwise and as a C if the movement is counterclockwise.

The second loop and the proximal portion of the optic plate will be introduced with the usual one or two-handed technique.

### Thermoplastic (Memory Lens) (ORC)

These lenses are made from a mixture of HEMA and MMA (cross-linking), with the addition of a UV filter (MOBP).

HEMA gives the lenses special characteristics of hydrophilia (water content 25%) whereas MMA, which is hydrophobic, gives them a relatively high refractive index (1.47) (i PMMA = 1.49).

The resulting material is rigid below 30°C, but above this temperature will begin to soften. The water content will not vary in proportion to the rigid or soft state.

The Prolene loops are thick (6/0, which can be seen under the microscope).

The folding is performed during the manufacturing process. At a temperature of 70°, the IOL is rolled into a cigar shape, measuring 2.35 x 6 mm. It is then cooled and stored at a low temperature (less than 10°C) and supplied to the surgeon.

A new package has recently been developed which has eliminated the need for storage at a low temperature.

### Insertion Technique

This lens, according to the recommendation of the manufacturer, can be implanted through a 3.2 mm incision. However, according to Piovella, it also easily implanted through a 4.1 mm incision. The technique does not require any special instruments, except a McPherson-type forceps.

The moistened lens is removed from the container and loaded onto this toothless forceps; one arm is placed inside the rolled IOL and the other is placed outside.

The thick Prolene loops (6/0) are characteristic of these lenses. They give the haptic support system both rigidity and strength.

To implant these lenses, the surgeon must use quick, precise movements which will transfer the lens from the freshly-opened container to the intraocular cavity in about 20 seconds, the maximum time allowed to keep the IOL from unrolling outside the surgical field.

The longitudinal technique must be used. The surgeon must concentrate his attention on the correct positioning of the distal loop alone, which will be positioned in the well-distended viscoelastic-filled bag in a position diametrically opposite the tunnel.

The second loop will be positioned through a rotation movement using an Osher fork or a push-pull.

Because of the thermoplastic characteristics of the material, the distention of the optic plate will occur within 3 to 4 minutes, whereas fold lines will disappear within 20 to 30 minutes. Therefore, the lens should be removed from the refrigerator immediately before the implantation.

The lens will assume the correct position very quickly with no risk of dislocation as long as the size of the capsulorhexis is in proportion to the optic plate.

## CONCLUSION

If many years ago the transition from extracapsular surgery to the techniques of phacoemulsification represented a giant step forward in improving the quality of cataract surgery, the transition from one-piece rigid lenses to the new modern foldable lenses represents another huge leap.

Foldable lenses are a true innovation because for the phase of implantation of the IOL, the surgeon can use the same tunnel created for the phacoemulsification; this means 3.2 and 4.0 mm self-sealing incisions.

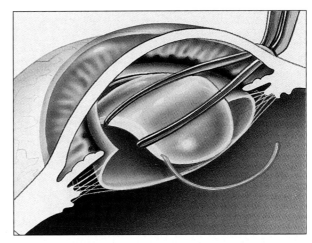

Figure 39-35. The holder releases the lens slowly.

Visual rehabilitation is therefore much more rapid, an advantage for the patient not only from the medical point of view but also in terms of the quality of his or her life.

The future probably holds many more surprises, and there is word of new solutions which are already at an advanced stage of experimentation.

The final objective could be the intracapsular removal of lens material using a phaco laser. the capsular bag could then be filled with a transparent liquid with a refractive index similar to the natural crystalline lens.

This would allow the patient to maintain a certain degree of accommodation, a feature which should not be overlooked in the procedure of complete, perfect visual rehabilitation.

At the moment, foldable bifocal lenses are available so the route has been traced, out but the objective has still not been reached.

So in today's cybernetic world, the problem of the cataract is still a reality.

# Chapter 40

# POSTERIOR ASSISTED LEVITATION

*Charles D. Kelman, MD*

## INTRODUCTION

Posterior Assisted Levitation (PAL) is designed to help surgeons manage many types of troublesome cataract cases. A typical application is with a partially emulsified nucleus, a hard, brunescent lens, in an eye with a shallow anterior chamber, and a miotic pupil. A similar situation occurs when the surgeon is attempting to phacoemulsify a recalcitrant nuclear bowl adherent to the posterior capsule due to inadequate hydrodissection and incomplete nuclear fracture In these cases, continued phacoemulsification in the posterior chamber can result in posterior capsule rupture caused by a tumble of the nucleus or contact with the phaco tip. The surgeons may then be confronted with a lens that has descended into the vitreous. Converting these cases at the appropriate time to a PAL can result in an uncompromised surgical outcome for the patient. A variation of the basic technique can be used in phaco cases where an opening in the posterior capsule occurs early in the case and a large portion of the nucleus remains. PAL has also proven a very effective approach in cases with a subluxated or dislocated lens.

## INDICATIONS

- Small pupil.
- Thin nuclear bowl with significant peripheral lens material behind the iris.
- Confirmed or suspected posterior capsule rupture.
- Zonular dehiscence.
- Conversion to planned extracapsular cataract extraction (ECCE) after partial phacoemulsification.
- Congenital or traumatic subluxated lens.

## TECHNIQUE

### Intact Posterior Capsule

The anterior chamber is filled with viscoelastic utilizing the cataract incision. A 1.5 mm incision is made approximately 3.5 to 4 mm posterior to the surgical limbus. The incision (created with a 15° Sharpoint knife) is angled down and away from the lens to avoid perforation of the posterior capsule.

A Barraquer-type spatula is placed posterior to the lens through the pars plana incision. The spatula is advanced with its distal end angled posteriorly toward the center of the eye. When it is estimated that the distal end of the spatula extends to the far edge of the lens, the spatula is slowly elevated using a slight side-to-side motion to massage one edge of the lens above the iris plane. Once a partial prolapse is achieved, the spatula is removed. A cannula, cystotome, or hook is placed into the anterior chamber through the original cataract incision to complete the prolapse into the anterior chamber.

I typically inject additional viscoelastic on top of the iris on the side of the partially prolapsed lens, to deepen the chamber and allow one edge of the lens to ride further over the iris. With the same cannula, the nucleus can be dialed and elevated into the anterior chamber to complete the prolapse.

With the nucleus in the chamber, anterior chamber phacoemulsification is very easy to perform.

### Open Posterior Capsule

The technique is essentially the same in cases where the posterior capsule has been compromised. However, once prolapse has been completed, a Sheets glide is inserted through the cataract incision posterior to the lens. The glide acts as a pseudoposterior capsule and prevents the nucleus or nuclear fragments from descending during anterior chamber phacoemulsification. Upon completion of phacoemulsification, the glide is removed and an anterior vitrectomy can be performed if necessary. If the opening in the posterior capsule is relatively small and central, a posterior chamber lens can be implanted in the bag. If the opening is small but irregular with the potential of extending into the periphery, convert the rent into a mini posterior capsulorhexis prior to lens implantation. If the opening in the posterior capsule is large but the anterior capsular rim is intact and there is adequate zonular support, I typically implant a posterior chamber lens in the ciliary sulcus. If capsular and zonular support are compromised, I will implant a properly sized flexible anterior chamber lens.

## Conversion to Planned ECCE

When the surgeon wishes to convert to a planned extracapsular technique after partial phacoemulsification, the technique is similar to managing a recalcitrant nuclear bowl or open capsule. Once the nucleus is in the anterior chamber, it is a simple matter to open the incision and express the lens.

## Subluxated or Dislocated Lens

This technique is useful in cases with a congenital or traumatic subluxated lens. In this case, the PAL technique is used to bring the entire lens, capsule intact, into the anterior chamber. Miochol is then instilled to constrict the pupil and trap the lens in the anterior chamber. A spatula introduced through the cataract incision may be used to sever any remaining intact zonules. A viscoelastic can be injected behind the lens to provide further support, followed by insertion of a Sheets glide under the lens. Endocapsular phacoemulsification can be performed in the anterior chamber. The empty capsular bag can be vacuum-bonded to the phaco tip and removed from the eye. I prefer to use a properly sized anterior chamber lens rather than a sutured posterior chamber implant.

# INDEX

anesthesia
    guidelines, 8-11
    limbal incision, 312
    O'Brien's technique, 9
    Packard's technique, 373
    phacoemulsification, 334-336
    phaco Slice and Separate, 390
    topical, 293-302
    Van Lindt's technique, 9-10
    vocal, 296-298
anterior capsulotomy, 49-63
    complications, 216-225
anterior chamber, viscoelastic substance (VES), 264
anterior chamber instruments, complications, 253-258
anterior segment, structure identification, 182
aspiration
    can opener, 176
    cortex material, 176-180, 469-479
        special conditions, 180-182
    description, 171-182
    principles, 172-176

Bissen-Miyajima's technique, 443-445
    anesthesia, 443
    capsulorhexis, 443-444
    epinucleus removal, 444
    hydrodissection, 444
    I/A, 445
    incisions, 443
        closure, 445
    IOL implantation, 445
    nuclei emulsification, 444
    phaco machine, 443
    viscoelastic removal, 445
Buratto's technique, horizontal sutures, 209

can opener technique
    aspiration, 176
    procedures, 49-52
capsular emulsification, rules, 184-185
capsulorhexis, 52-63, 321-332
    advantages, 59, 61
    anatomy, 321-322
    aspiration, 176
    brunescent or black cataracts, 63
    complications, 330-331
    development, 52
    history, 321
    instruments, 53-58, 60

    methods, 325-329
    Packard's technique, 375-377
    phacoemulsification, 337-338
    posterior, 63, 185
    pseudoexfoliation, 62-63
    rhexis difficulties, 61-62
    rules, 54
    techniques, 322-325, 329-330
    viscoelastic substance (VES), 264
capsulotomy, 49-63
    can opener technique, 49-52
    capsulorhexis, 52-63
    Christmas tree, 50
    principles, 58-59
    variations, 49
cataract surgery
    development and techniques, 3-20
    Serafano's technique, 451-454
Chop and Flip, 397-405
    anesthesia, 397
    capsulorhexis, 398
    epinucleus removal, 402-403
    hydrodissection, 398-399
    I/A, 403
    incisions, 397-398
        closure, 405
    IOL implantation, 404-405
    nuclei emulsification, 399-401
    phaco machine, 397
    special cases, 401-402
Christmas tree, description, 50
clear corneal tunnel incision
    equipment and technique, 43
    procedures, 41-44
complications
    anterior capsulotomy, 216-225
    anterior chamber instruments, 253-258
    capsulorhexis, 330-331
    endocapsular techniques, 229-233
    I/A, 250-253
    IOL insertion, 253
    miosis, 258-262
    operation phases, 214-216
    phacoemulsification, 211-262, 225-229
    phaco fracture technique, 346
    posterior assisted levitation (PAL), 511
    posterior capsule cleaning, 253
    posterior capsule rupture, 233-250
    topical anesthesia, 301-302

corneal tunnel incisions, 306-308
    equipment and technique (Buratto), 308
cortex removal, subincisional, 469-479
Crack and Flip technique, 149-157
    Koch's Stop and Chop, 156-157
    Nagahara's Phaco Chop, 150-156
Cut and Suck technique, description, 116-117

Davison's Cut and Suck technique, description, 116-117
Davison's phaco technique, 407-413
    anesthesia, 407
    capsulorhexis, 407-409
    epinucleus removal, 411-412
    hydrodissection, 409-410
    incisions, 407
        closure, 413
    IOL implantation, 412
    phaco machine, 407
    viscoelastic removal, 412
delivery systems, intraocular lenses (IOLs), 481-485
Dillman-Maloney's fractional 2/4, description, 148-149
Dillman's Crack and Flip technique, description, 149-157
direct limbal incision, procedures, 33-34
Divide and Conquer nucleofractis (DCN), 347-353
    crater method, 350-351
    multidirectional method, 349-350
    trench method, 347-349

endocapsular phacoemulsification, 100-103
    hydrodelineation, 65
    hydrodissection, 65
    techniques, 103
endocapsular techniques, complications, 229-233
endothelial pump, theory, 316

Fine's Chip and Flip, description, 117-121
Fine's Crack and Flip technique, description, 149-157
Fine's technique, horizontal sutures, 208
Fishkind's technique, horizontal sutures, 208-209
fluid dynamics, closed hydrodynamic system, 21-23
foldable IOLs, 481-485
    acrylic, 502-503
    delivery systems, 483-484
    hydrogel lenses (HEMA), 507-508
    insertion techniques, 493-509
    manipulations, 489
    material, 487
    silicone, 494-495
    thermoplastic (memory lens) (ORC), 508-509

Gimbel's Divide and Conquer technique
    crater DCN, 143-145
    description, 131-148
    downslope sculpting (DSS), 145-148
    trench DCN, 143-145

Grabow's technique, 415-425
    anesthesia, 415
    capsulorhexis, 418-419
    hydrodissection, 419, 421-422
    I/A, 423
    incisions, 417-418
        closure, 424
    IOL implantation, 422-423
    phacofracture, 419-420
    sphericity, 416-417
    V-groove trifracture, 420-421

Hara's technique, 427-432
    anesthesia, 427
    capsulorhexis, 428-430
    epinucleus removal, 431
    hydrodissection, 430
    I/A, 431
    incisions, 427-428
        closure, 432
    IOL implantation, 432
    nuclei emulsification, 430-431
    phaco machine, 427
    viscoelastic removal, 432
hydrodelamination
    functions and objectives, 70
    procedures, 69
hydrodelineation
    definition, 65, 67
    functions and objectives, 70
    procedures, 69
hydrodemarcation
    functions and objectives, 70
    procedures, 69
hydrodissection
    definition, 65
    functions and objectives, 70
    Packard's technique, 377
    procedures, 67-69
    rules, 65
hydrofracture, description, 69

implantation techniques, foldable IOLs, 493-509
incisions, 303-309
    cataract surgery, 33-48
    clear corneal tunnel, 41-44
    corneal tunnel, 306-307
    definition, 303
    foldable IOL, 481-482
    limbal
        direct, 33-34
        scleral plane, 34
    limbal-corneal tunnel, 304-306
    method comparisons and advantages, 44-48
    operating room arrangements, 307-309

Packard's technique, 374-375
phacoemulsification, 336-337
scleral-corneal tunnel, 34-41
side port, 309
insertion techniques, foldable IOLs, 493-509
intercapsular phacoemulsification
description, 110-116
Michelson and Hara studies, 110
intraocular drugs, 284-288
agents, 287-288
antibiotics, 286-287
anti-inflammatory, 287
miotics, 285-286
mydriatics, 285
intraocular lenses (IOL), 187-203
characteristics, 187
classifications, 187-190
delivery systems, 481-485
foldable, 202-203, 481-485, 487-491, 493-509
implantation, phaco fracture technique, 345-346
insertion
complications, 253
techniques, 192-198, 199-202
material comparisons, 192
phacoemulsification, 339-340
PMMA, 195-199
posterior chamber, 190-195
intraocular solutions, 275-284
antiseptic, 275-276
irrigating, 276-282
limbal incision, 313-314
VES, 282-284
intraoperative primary posterior capsulotomy, 183
intumescent or white cataracts, Modified Phaco Chop, 362-363
irrigation/aspiration
capsulotomy, 176
complications, 250-253
description, 171-182
subincisional cortex removal, 469-479
VES, 267-268
I/A cannula, 183-184, 472
I/A cycle, 171-172, 470

Karate Phaco Chop, 359
Kelman's oculopressor, 11-12
Kelman's technique
description, 71-87
phacoemulsification, 465-468
Koch's Stop and Chop, description, 156-157, 161
Koch's technique, 433-442
anesthesia, 433
capsulorhexis, 433-434
epinucleus removal, 437-438
hydrodissection, 434

I/A, 438-439
incisions, 433
closure, 440
IOL implantation, 439
nuclei emulsification, 434-437
phaco machine, 433
special cases, 437
viscoelastic removal, 439
Kratz cannula, irrigation, 183

limbal-corneal tunnel incisions, 304-306
limbal incision, 311-320
advantages, 314
anesthesia, 312
endothelial pump, 316
history, 311
intraoperative solutions, 313-314
procedures, 312-316
scleral plane, 34
vector analysis and visual results, 314-315, 318-320
Wills feline study, 316
Little's technique, description, 87-93
longitudinal techniques, foldable IOLs, 496-500, 505-506

Maloney's Crack and Flip technique, description, 149-157
Maloney's technique, description, 93-100
Masket's technique, horizontal sutures, 209
miosis, complications, 258-262
Modified Phaco Chop, 361-371
fragmentation techniques, 364-367
hydrodissection, 363-364
instruments, 361-362
Mini Chop technique, 366-367
special cases, 368-371
viscoelastic sandwich, 367
white or intumescent cataracts, 362-363

Nagahara's Phaco Chop, description, 150-156
Nagahara's phaco technique, 355-359
preparation, 355
procedures, 355-359
Neuhann's technique, phacoemulsification, 459-464
nuclear cleavage, description, 117-121
nucleofracture technique
Crack and Flip technique, 149-157
cross or quartering (Shepherd), 126-131
description, 121-170
Dillman-Maloney's fractional 2/4, 148-149
Divide and Conquer (Gimbel), 131-148

O'Brien's technique, blocking facial nerve, 9
ocular pressure, reduction, 11
one-handed phacoemulsification, description, 103-110
operating room
arrangements, incisions, 307-309

eye preparation, 19-20
patient position, 18-19
staff and equipment, 12-17
surgeon position, 17-18
Oshler's technique, phacoemulsification, 447-449

Packard's technique, 373-387
anesthesia, 373
anterior chamber maintenance, 375
capsular cleaning, 384-385
capsulorhexis, 375-377
epinucleus removal, 383
glaucoma and cataract surgery, 382-383
hydrodissection, 377
I/A, 383-384
incisions, 374-375
closure, 387
IOL implantation, 385-387
lens removal, 377-378
nuclei
hard, 381-382
medium-hard, 379-381
soft, 378-379
phaco machine, 373-374
viscoelastic removal, 387
Phaco Chop, 150-156, 158-161, 170
phacoemulsification
anesthesia, 334-336
Bissen-Miyajima's technique, 443-445
capsulorhexis, 337-338
Chop and Flip, 397-405
complications, 211-262
Davison's technique, 407-413
DCN, 347-353
fluid dynamics, 21-23
Grabow's technique, 415-425
Hara's technique, 427-432
history, 3-4
hydrodissection, 338
incision, 336-337
IOL implantation technique, 339-340
Kelman's technique, 465-468
Koch's technique, 433-442
Modified Phaco and Mini Chop, 361-371
Neuhann's technique, 459-464
operating room, 12-20
optimal conditions, 4-8
Oshler's technique, 447-449
Packard's technique, 373-387
phacoemulsifier, 23-31
phaco fracture technique, 341-346
phaco Slice and Separate, 390-396
Philipson's technique, 455-458
physical principles, 21-31
principles, 4-8

technique, 333-340
viscoelastic substance (VES), 264-267
phacoemulsification techniques
Grade 1 nuclei, 166
Grade 2 nuclei, 166
Grade 3 nuclei, 167
Grade 4 nuclei, 167
Grade 5 nuclei, 168
history (1970-1988), 71-100
history (after 1988), 100-170
phacoemulsifier
components, 23-26
operating features, 26-31
phaco fracture technique, 341-346
anesthesia, 342
complications, 346
IOL implantation, 345-346
phaco Slice and Separate, 390-396
anesthesia, 390
capsulorhexis, 390-391
epinucleus removal, 392
hydrodissection, 391
I/A, 392
IOL implantation, 393-396
nuclei emulsification, 391-392
phaco machine, 390
viscoelastic removal, 396
Philipson's phaco technique, 455-458
posterior assisted levitation (PAL)
complications, 511
technique, 511-512
posterior capsule, 183-185
capsulorhexis, 185
intraoperative capsulotomy, 183
vacuum cleaning technique, 184
posterior capsule cleaning, complications, 253
posterior capsule rupture, complications, 233-250

sclero-corneal tunnel incision
characteristics, 38
equipment and techniques, 38
procedures, 34-41
Serafano's technique, cataract surgery, 451-454
Shepherd's technique
description, 103-110
horizontal sutures, 208
Singer's technique, horizontal sutures, 208
sphericity, steps, 416-417
Stop and Chop
Buratto's, 162
illustrations, 163-165
Koch's, 161
Modified, 162
subincisional cortex, removal techniques, 469-479
surgical pharmacology

    intraocular drugs, 284-288
    intraocular solutions, 275-284
sutures, 205-209
    continuous, 206-207
    horizontal techniques, 208-209
    interrupted, 206
    material, 205-206
    objectives, 205

topical anesthesia, 293-302
    advantages, 293-294
    complicated cases, 301-302
    complications, 301-302
    disadvantages, 294-295
    doctor-patient relationship, 296-298
    patient preparation, 298-299
    patient selection, 296
    purpose, 293
    surgical techniques, 299-301
transversal techniques, foldable IOLs, 501-502, 506-507

two-handed endocapsular phacoemulsification
    description, 116-117
    Fine's Chip and Flip, 117-121
    nuclear cleavage, 117-121
    nucleofracture technique, 121-170

Van Lindt's technique, blocking facial nerve, 9-10
viscoelastic substance (VES), 263-271
    anterior chamber, 264
    capsulorhexis, 264
    capsular opening, 268-269
    characteristics, 263
    I/A, 267-268
    phacoemulsification, 264-267
    removal, 209, 269
    using two, 269-271
vocal anesthesia, 296-298

white or intumescent cataracts, Modified Phaco Chop, 362-363
Wills feline study, limbal incision, 316